An Outline of Psychiatry in Clinical Lectures

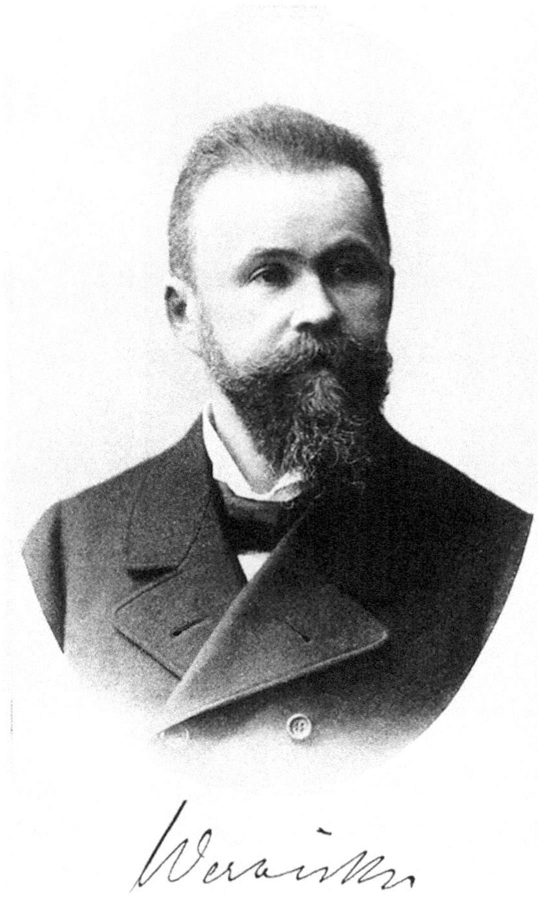

Grundriss der Psychiatrie

in

klinischen Vorlesungen

von

Carl Wernicke

Zweite revidierte Auflage

Mit einem Bildnis des Verfassers

Leipzig
Verlag von Georg Thieme
1906.

Outlines of Psychiatry

in

clinical lectures

by

Carl Wernicke

Second, revised edition

With a photo of the author

Leipzig
Published by Georg Thieme
1906.

Robert Miller • John Dennison
Editors

An Outline of Psychiatry in Clinical Lectures

The Lectures of Carl Wernicke

Translated by John Dennison and Robert Miller

Springer

Editors
Robert Miller, ONZM, B.A., B.Sc., Ph.D.
Freelance Researcher, and Honorary Fellow
Otago University
Department of Psychological Medicine
University of Otago School of Medicine
Wellington, New Zealand

John Dennison, J.P., M.Sc., B.A.
Research Fellow
Department of Anatomy
Otago Medical School
Dunedin, New Zealand

ISBN 978-3-319-34840-7 ISBN 978-3-319-18051-9 (eBook)
DOI 10.1007/978-3-319-18051-9

Springer Cham Heidelberg New York Dordrecht London

Softcover reprint of the hardcover 1st edition 2015

Printed on acid-free paper

Springer International Publishing AG Switzerland is part of Springer Science+Business Media (www.springer.com)

Dedication for This Translation

We want to dedicate this edited translation first to the memory of Valentin Braitenberg, still a source of inspiration. We also dedicate it, a trifle late perhaps, to the many persons whose lives at times of crisis are depicted so graphically in Wernicke's accounts of his patients.

Robert Miller and John Dennison

Foreword

1894 Foreword

It was not originally my intention to let the present introduction to the clinical presentation of mental illnesses stand-alone. While its primary aim is to describe the organ within which such illness is expressed, it also conveys opinions that have developed very gradually, influenced by many years of clinical experience. Therefore its foundation and its integration lie within the facts taught in Pathology.

Through the influence of an advocate of theoretical natural science, I let myself be persuaded to compile a stand-alone volume. His opinion, that the broader scientific community might take a lively interest in it, must be acknowledged as authoritative, compared with my own more reticent opinion. Thus, when this revered man of undoubted competence, and perhaps great foresight, sets his eyes on these apologetic intentions, may he at the same time receive my thanks for his stimulation and guidance over the hours and days of a chance encounter.

Breslau, August 1894 — Carl Wernicke

Foreword

1906 Editor's Foreword

In the middle of preparing this second edition, Carl Wernicke was overtaken by sudden death. His revision had proceeded only to the end of the second section. It was limited to a large number of small alterations and additions, entered in pencil alongside and beneath the text, without the form and content undergoing any other major metamorphosis.

The review copy underwent a collaborative revision by Senior Physician Dr. Knapp, Wernicke's first Adjunct in Halle, and myself, and obviously private notes, not intended for publication, were removed.

During this task I submitted our output to the widow of the deceased.

As for the third, unrevised section, the unchanged copy came from the author himself. That Wernicke had nothing major to alter, and that this section still corresponded with the position of his previous opinions, was testified by some few words, those of the mortally wounded man, worried about the fate of his life's work, uttered on his deathbed: 'Second edition as is'.

Any introductory words about the work are superfluous. It speaks for itself.

H. Liepmann

Preface to This Translation

This translation of Wernicke's *Grundriss der Psychiatrie* grew from the long friendship one of us (R.M.) had with Valentin Braitenberg, born in 1926, and who died in October 2011. Valentin visited Otago, New Zealand, in 1993, and both of us (R.M. and K.J.D.) knew him and recognized in him a person of great generosity, wisdom, and integrity. On his bookshelf in Tübingen were many interesting volumes, some of historic significance. One of them was the 1900 edition of *Grundriss*.

The process of producing this translation was as follows: K.J.D. who is fluent in German produced, lecture-by-lecture, a very literal translation of what Wernicke wrote and sent his versions to R.M., who has basic German, but wide knowledge of many areas of psychiatry and neuroscience. His task was to render these initial versions into fluent modern scientific prose, aware of some of the scientific and clinical nuances which might not emerge in a literal translation. Sometimes, at this stage, words or concepts were unclear, so there were further exchanges of messages between the two of us to resolve uncertainties. In translating and editing Wernicke's text, it has also been necessary to learn a great deal about the life and times when he was writing, and the existing knowledge upon which he drew. In the end, we both contributed to resolving uncertainties about concepts.

As we went through Wernicke's text, a number of editorial comments were inserted, initially as footnotes, to convey such understanding as we could gain, but which might not be obvious to today's reader. These comments varied in length and subject matter from one lecture to another. We soon realized that many themes in the lectures recurred in successive lectures, gradually evolving and being developed. This makes his thinking appear fragmented, if the lectures are read sequentially. This is inevitable, given the context in which any series of clinical lectures has to be delivered, where the lecturer's ideas must be presented in coordination with clinical cases as available (which may arise somewhat opportunistically). The fragmented appearance may also reflect what was certainly a very pressured existence for the author, who probably preferred to spend his time on the ward, talking with patients, and analyzing clinical records, rather than perfecting the write-up of his ideas. We gain this impression from inaccuracies in some of his cited references, inconsistencies in his reasoning, and what seems to be a continuing struggle to find adequate definitions for concepts which accounted best for what he saw in the clinic. As delivered, the lectures probably were not so fragmented for his original audience, for whom, we guess, each lecture would have been followed by discussions which are not recorded. Nevertheless, the 1906 edition of *Grundriss* was a 'work in progress', which sadly never reached completion. It is plausible to suggest that he might have intended to write a comprehensive textbook of psychiatry, to fulfil what was latent in *Grundriss*, just as his thought on the entire field of neurological disorders was presented as his 1881 textbook, *Lehrbuch der Gehirnkrankheiten*. The fact that most of his thoughts on psychiatry are contained in the sometimes difficult pages of *Grundriss*, rather than in a textbook, may have contributed to the neglect of his work, but it is also the reason why we have felt it necessary to write the extended editorial commentary, which follows the translation of Wernicke's 41 lectures.

To give what we hope is a clearer account of Wernicke's thought, we decided that the editorial comments on each lecture should be re-grouped according to their subject matter and coordinated into this substantial editorial essay. This begins with a series of synopses about the subjects dominating each lecture, followed by discussion sections dealing with the numerous matters arising across the lecture series. These topics move from the medical scene in which Wernicke worked, clinical concepts of the day, Wernicke's clinical, didactic, and personal style as far as we could discern it, the scientific concepts he used, his views on underlying philosophical issues, and, most important, a lengthy section on his unique clinical concepts. After that we move to Wernicke's approach to classifying mental disorders and his style of reasoning, including what we identify (from a modern perspective) as flaws in his reasoning. Later parts of the essay give details on his contemporaries whose work is cited, comments to clarify allusions made (mainly by his patients) to matters which would have been familiar in their day, and lastly, to clarify specific issues of terminology. This section came together at the very end of our work, when we compiled a long list of 'problem words' in both German and English and discussed how we could render them in a way which conveyed most accurately Wernicke's intended meaning.

To ensure that anything we write in our editorial commentary can be traced back to their source in Wernicke's text, we identify the lecture in which each point is made (indicated as 'L.' plus a numeral, and our final pagination). In addition, in indexing, we include not only items in Wernicke's 1906 index (translated, and re-alphabetized, with our own pagination in bold typeface) but also, in the same index, items referring to this commentary (non-bold). Wernicke also gave many cross references between lectures in *Grundriss*, as footnotes. We retain these, but include them in the text, with our final pagination. Occasionally, in our commentary, we cite other works, followed by corresponding page numbers (both within parentheses).

To make our version flow well, we often condense superfluities in Wernicke's text. We often replace 'the patient' by a personal pronoun ('his', 'her' etc.). Abstract nouns are frequently replaced by concrete ones or verbal equivalents, and passive by active verbs. There are innumerable re-orderings of ideas within a sentence (inevitably, since sentences are constructed in different ways in the two languages), while retaining the original sense. Sometimes long sentences are split into two or more. When terms are used which are now part of today's technical vocabulary, we use the familiar terms, although, in our commentary, we sometimes discuss concepts, words, and how we choose to render them in English. We are alert to the possibility that concepts do not match words in equivalent ways in German and English. Sometimes, the same word is used in German, for what appear to be two different concepts. These may be related, but differ subtly, and can sometimes be distinguished as different words in English. The German word *Krankheit* is a case in point. Conversely we identify some German words (notably *Ratlosigkeit*, often rendered as 'perplexity') for which no truly equivalent word exists in English. In addition, inevitably, where Wernicke formulates new concepts, with no precedents, and no established terms, he resorts to analogies. In uncharted territory, use of analogy or metaphor is the only way forward, especially in mental abnormality. This necessity is discussed by R. Mojtabai in his 2000 article in History of Psychiatry ('Delusion as Error: The History of a Metaphor'). When translating analogies we prefer abstract to concrete images, as having greater generality. As a priority, we have tried to capture Wernicke's reasoning as accurately as possible, this being more important, we felt, than verbatim translation. Consequently, our translation is sometimes rather free. However, for some words, where we struggle to capture the meaning (perhaps when it is indeed ambiguous), we stick to a more literal translation (perhaps clarified in our commentary). An example is the German noun cluster *Organempfindung*. (Noun clusters in German are not fully captured by adjective-noun pairs in English.) Of course, our attempt to convey Wernicke's meaning depends on how well we understand his work. We have tried hard to grasp the subtlety of his reasoning but, at times, may have missed significant points. At the time of finalizing our translation, our understanding still has some way to go. We apologize therefore for inaccuracies in our rendition.

Wernicke's text uses various forms of emphasis: italicization, quotation marks, and occasionally a third form of emphasis, not familiar in English—the 'spacing out' of letters which make up a word, and with slightly larger typeface—especially when introducing one of his favoured terms. In addition, to make his reasoning as clear as possible, we also often found it useful to add our own emphases, not present in the original. This again is perhaps inevitable, since inflections in German as altered word endings can convey relationships within a sentence, which need to be conveyed in other ways in English. Sometimes we also add emphases to draw attention when the author introduces a new specialist term. Because of this, for all emphases, we have indicated those in Wernicke's original as '[W]', those which were editorial additions as '[Ed]'. All emphases involving 'spacing out' of letters are rendered as italics.

In translating a work over 100 years old, we are aware of changes in sensitivity over terminology. We prefer a flexible style, avoiding stereotyped 'politically correct' terms, but we do try to avoid some terms, such as the generic form, 'the mentally ill'—and we usually prefer 'psychiatric patient' to 'mental patient'. We have nevertheless tried to retain some of the flavour of the time when Wernicke was writing. We see no need to adopt a 'gender neutral' style when using personal pronouns (this being a historical document); and for latinized terms based on Linnaeus' binomial system, we retain the upper case initial character for the first word in the pair. In addition, we have tried to preserve an informal style, of lectures as they might have been delivered, rather than a more scholarly style, as might be found in a journal article.

Wernicke's original text gives references in footnotes to sources upon which he drew, but bibliographic details are often sketchy by modern standards and sometimes inaccurate in detail. In this edition, footnotes are not used. In Wernicke's text, we indicate his citations by number, using the Vancouver system, with a list at the end of each lecture. Since his referencing is often incomplete, we have supplemented the references he gives in footnotes, with relevant publications of contemporary authors he often names without citing their publications. Sources referred to in our Editorial Commentary make up another reference list, appearing at the end of our commentary. Wernicke also used footnotes to make comments, which would break the flow of his argument, or to summarize the eventual outcome for a patient he has just presented. These comments are incorporated into his text (in parentheses, usually at a paragraph end) or in our editorial essay (identified as 'note'), and we omit some of the minor footnotes. Some of his cross references give no page numbers and are hard to identify, and some cross references are clearly to cases presented elsewhere to his students, rather than in earlier lectures of *Grundriss*. Sometimes these appear to be other lecture series (perhaps at a more elementary level), which his students would have attended. There are also many references to published clinical reports (*Krankenvorstellungen aus der psychiatrischen Klinik in Breslau*).

Acknowledgments

We acknowledge, with thanks, insights we have gained on Wernicke and his ideas, either in correspondence or in personal discussion with the following: German Berrios, Eric Chen, Gerhard Heim, Andrzej Kiejna, Mario Lanzcik, Michael Molnar, Andrew Moscovitch, Almut Schüz, Surjo Soekadar. RM thanks Stephen Duncan for help at the proof-reading stage.

Wellington, New Zealand — Robert Miller, ONZM, BA, BSc, PhD PhD (Glasgow)

Dunedin, New Zealand — John Dennison, JP, MSc, BA

Introduction to This Translation

Carl Wernicke: Biographical Sketch

Carl Wernicke was born on 15 May 1848 at Tarnowitz, now south-central Poland (Silesia, at that time part of Prussia). His education included classical languages, since he sometimes uses Latin phrases, and in one instance a Greek one in his text, as if they were common knowledge for educated people. In 1870, he obtained a medical degree from the University of Breslau (Wrocław, to give it its contemporary Polish name), after which he studied for a year with Theodor Meynert (1833–1892) in Vienna. He is well known to English speakers as a pioneer of neurology. When newly trained as a physician, he made major contributions to the emerging concept that specific regions of the cerebral cortex served different psychic functions. He defined an area, now given his name, in the superior temporal gyrus on the left side, in which sensory memories of speech sounds are represented. This was documented by him in 1874, based partly on experiences gained in 1871, as a military surgeon during the Franco-Prussian war. In addition, in the late 1880s, he anticipated findings of Sergei Korsakoff, in defining an amnesic syndrome found mainly in patients with chronic alcoholism, now known as the Wernicke-Kosakoff syndrome (Korsakoff's psychosis or Wernicke's encephalopathy).

After his early success, he held various positions in neuropsychiatry—under Karl Westphal at the Charité Hospital in Berlin (1876–1878); in a private neuropsychiatry clinic he founded in Berlin until 1885; and from then until 1904 in Breslau, first as associate professor, and from 1890, holding the chair in psychiatry at the university there. Patients he met early in his career in Breslau and in the Berlin period are mentioned in his clinical lectures. In later years his relationship with municipal authorities at Breslau became difficult, to the extent that, for some years, he was prevented from using patients for teaching purposes. In 1904 he moved to a chair at Halle. The psychiatric institute there had opened in 1891 explicitly for research and education, was administratively autonomous, and was the first in Prussia to combine psychiatric and neuropathology wards [1].

Sadly, Wernicke died prematurely in 1905, from injuries sustained in a bicycling accident. His lectures on psychiatry were first published in 1894, as *Grundriss der Psychiatrie*, a revision being produced in 1900, and he was revising another edition at the time of his death, published posthumously in 1906.

The original publication ran to only 176 pages, the first 17 lectures of the final version. In a footnote in the very last lecture of the 1906 edition, he writes, commenting on the outcome for a patient, 'I must now put right these lines, written about ten years ago…' The words 'about ten years ago', as in the 1900 edition, imply that drafts of even the last stage of *Grundriss* were being formulated before the partial edition of 1894.

Grundriss is still read in the German-speaking world and indeed is republished from time to time (most recently in 2012). However, English speakers still know little of Wernicke as one who saw neurology and psychiatry as parts of a single discipline (as indeed they were when he was practising), and as a pioneer thinker about mental disorders. Several historians of psychiatry who know Wernicke's work well believe that had Wernicke lived longer and been able to develop his carefully considered, but incomplete ideas closer to the point where their full fruits were evident, psychiatry in the last century would have developed along very different lines, a view also expressed by Karl Leonhard, a successor to Wernicke of a later generation [2]. The idea that mental disorders should be defined in terms of categorical diagnoses, along the lines of diseases in general medicine, was not strong at the time of his first edition, grew stronger in the mid-1890s with the publication of the 1896 edition of Kraepelin's textbook of psychiatry, and was becoming a new orthodoxy by the time of Wernicke's death. He himself was sceptical of contemporary attempts at classification of mental disorders, and, although working within a medical paradigm, appears to struggle with the idea that the 'disease model' borrowed from general medicine dealt adequately with realities of mental disorders, as he saw them daily in his clinical practice.

Wernicke was clearly exceptionally talented in both the detail and exactness of his observations, and his continual attempt to render those observations comprehensible within a wider conceptual framework. However, many basic facts about the nervous system (not least about the basic electrical and chemical signalling by nerve cells) were unknown at the time. Thus, any attempt at theorizing would necessarily often include imaginative leaps based on scanty evidence and vivid analogies. His theories and inferences, while often well ahead of their time, were sometimes far-fetched and lacked empirical support. For this reason his ideas were scorned by some, not least Karl Jaspers from Heidelberg, as *Hirnmythologie* ('neuromythology'). Nonetheless what is presented in *Grundriss* includes such a bounty of ideas, some of which, in our view, are in advance of *today's* psychiatry, that it is important that his work be better known to English speakers. A hundred years ago, an English translation by W.A.McCorn (Superintendent at Elizabeth General Hospital, N.J.) was produced, but is little known. According to a brief obituary of McCorn in 1904 [3], all 41 lectures were translated from the 1900 edition, and many appeared in *Alienist and Neurologist*. However, we have been unable to identify where many of the lectures were published (if indeed they were). In addition, the first eight lectures were translated recently by Gage and Hickok [4]. In producing this complete edited English version of

Wernicke's 1906 edition, we feel immensely privileged to reveal to new readers the observations, ideas, and thought processes of one who was not only a superb clinician but also a profound scientific thinker.

In his day, there was of course already more than a century of careful observation and thought about the realities of mental disorder, yet we discern in Wernicke's writing a freshness of approach, from an acute observer, and careful analyst, encountering many things as if for the first time, with an 'innocent eye' and freshness of mind, unburdened by the weight of a long, unassailable tradition. Thus, he impresses both of us, as an intrepid pioneer, in one of the most challenging areas of inquiry, where few others, before or since, could claim continuity with the broad sweep to the natural sciences. Although his work in psychiatry has been neglected, especially in the English-speaking world, its enduring impact is seen in several terms, now part of psychiatric vocabulary, which started with him, and in a distinct tradition, the Wernicke-Kleist-Leonhard school of psychiatric thought, especially in some European centres. We hope we have done justice to his work, bringing an up-to-date perspective on *Grundriss*, such as McCorn could not have achieved; that we have not imposed on Wernicke's German text too much of our own perspective, which undoubtedly has its biases; and that we have not have not made too many misinterpretations.

Masterton, New Zealand Robert Miller
Dunedin, New Zealand John Dennison

References

1. Engstrom EJ. Clinical psychiatry in imperial Germany. Ithaca: Cornell University Press; 2003.
2. Lanczik M, Keil G. Carl Wernicke's localization theory and its significance for the development of scientific psychiatry. Hist Psychiat. 1991;2(6):171–80.
3. Hughes CH, Hughes MR. Death of Dr McCorn. Alien Neurol. 1904;25:238.
4. Gage N, Hickok G. Multiregional cell assemblies, temporal binding and the representation of conceptual knowledge in cortex: A modern theory by a 'classical' neurologist, Carl Wernicke. Cortex. 2005;41(6):823–32.
5. Mojtabai R. Delusion as error: The history of a metaphor. Hist Psychiatry. 2000;11:3–14.

Contents

Part I

Psycho-physiological Introduction

Lecture 1

1

- Mental illnesses are brain diseases; nevertheless, they differ from them in practice
- Projection system and central fields of projection
- Association organ
- Brain disorders to be defined as diseases of the projection system; mental illnesses as propagated illnesses of the association organ
- Difference between primary and secondary identification in the case of speech

Lecture

Gentlemen!

Our subject here, learning about mental illnesses, is essentially a branch of internal medicine which, because of its practical significance and for other reasons of a more external nature, has required—and has received—special treatment from time immemorial. Sadly, at the same time, it is an area that is backward in its development: It presently stands at the point where the rest of medicine was, about a 100 years ago. You will be aware that at that time an evolved pathology in the modern sense, that is, one supported by pathological disturbances in individual organs of known function, still did not exist, and that, accordingly, people ascribed the status of disease classes to certain frequently-occurring symptoms, albeit in widely varied groupings. Given such an attitude, medical knowledge of diseases did not go far beyond knowledge currently found among the lay public, when it treats coughing, palpitations, fever, jaundice, anaemia, and emaciation as actual illnesses. This is precisely the current attitude towards psychiatry, at least amongst the majority of 'mad doctors'—its proponents. Even for them, some specific symptoms form the very essence of the disease—for example a depressed mood, in the broadest sense, is the essence of melancholy; an elevated mood with excessive movements, that of mania, and so on. People now distinguish many such types of putative disease. However, since in Nature combinations of symptoms are far more diverse and complex, it has been necessary to construct an artificial framework, sometimes more widely, and sometimes more narrowly, accomplished by different observers in very different ways. Despite all efforts to bring the cases of illness artificially into one form fitting within the framework, very many cases remain that cannot be correctly assigned, and in no way fit the framework. Indeed, anyone who can judge without bias, and has the necessary experience, will find that the great majority of cases do not conform to the normal viewpoint. I readily concede that psychiatry has demonstrated substantial progress in more recent times. Work of men like Griesinger, H. Neumann, Kahlbaum, Meynert, Emminghaus, and many others has not been in vain. Yet even these outstanding researchers all still gave in to the

R. Miller, K.J. Dennison (eds.), *An Outline of Psychiatry in Clinical Lectures*,
DOI 10.1007/978-3-319-18051-9_1

temptation of confusing individual symptoms with the essence of the illness; and the low level of average grasp of psychiatry even today can be assessed by the prevailing doctrine of lunacy, the merits of which are realized by a convenient nomenclature. Psychiatry today enjoys more general recognition, and this would have been welcomed as progress by a thinker like Meynert [1] in his time.

Under these circumstances, the teacher of psychiatry is strongly advised that if he wants to apply standards of another discipline, he should stay just with symptoms. However his task is clearly predetermined for him: He should proceed as in the sister disciplines of medicine: Symptoms must be deduced from familiar features of the diseased organ, in order to treat the illness—in our case from features of the brain. Only in this way do we have the prospect of obtaining a classification and overview of symptoms which is both natural (i.e. based on the nature of things) and, at the same time, exhaustive.

The assumption that mental illnesses are brain diseases is probably not contested by any specialist today. If we start from there, we must soon expand, by indicating brain diseases of a particular type, and at a particular site, for they are in no way identical with so-called organic brain diseases with which we are far more familiar. Let us recall the division of brain diseases into focal disease processes and general diseases; mental illnesses will certainly not be subsumed under the former, but possibly under the latter. As is commonly known, two general diseases can be classed amongst organic brain diseases: meningitis and progressive paralysis. Nothing would stop us from proposing mental illnesses as a third category of general disease. However, the question then arises: What are the fundamental characteristics that distinguish this third category of general diseases of the brain from the other two so-called organic diseases?

To approach this question more closely, we must focus for a moment on symptoms of brain diseases. All symptoms of brain diseases are, as we know, either focal or general. The two general diseases of the brain just mentioned amongst organic brain diseases are examples of diseases with mainly general symptoms in their clinical picture. However, they are really characterized by the fact that focal symptoms occur along with general ones. Indeed, one can probably say that these focal symptoms are never totally absent. Mental illnesses in contrast present no such focal symptoms. Accordingly, mental illnesses would represent general diseases of the brain of a particular type that are never accompanied by focal symptoms.

Gentlemen! According to this definition, the significance that focal symptoms provide for our subject matter makes it advisable to examine their essence more closely. We learned from Meynert that voluntary muscles and sensory organs are linked with the cerebral cortex by conducting pathways that extend, in physiological continuity, through the brain, the spinal cord, and the peripheral nervous system. Meynert named the aggregate of these pathways, where the 'law of isolated conduction' [Ed] predominates, the *projection system* [Ed], thus emphasizing the fact of physiological continuity, if not anatomical continuity. More recent investigations have proven this to be valid in every respect—shown clearly and unequivocally. Corresponding with the division of the cerebrum into two hemispheres, the projection system is also divided into two halves, recognized by the connection of motor control and sensibility of each half of the body with the opposite cerebral hemisphere (at least generally speaking). The expression 'projection' [W] is clearly borrowed from optics where, as here, the path of beams is traced precisely through a lens system: Despite all intervening nuclei along these projection pathways, physiological continuity remains, and isolated conduction is preserved throughout. The majority of focal symptoms can easily be traced back to local lesions, or stimulation of conducting links within these projection pathways.

A second series of focal symptoms can be traced back to the fact that the termination or origin of pathways in projection pathways is also localized to different points of the cerebral cortex. The law of isolated conduction prevails in this way until these pathways join with corresponding regions of the cerebral cortex. Such end sites of afferent pathways—we will call them *projection fields* [Ed]—are known to include the optic tract in the occipital lobes; the acoustic tract in the temporal lobes; motor control and sensibility of the leg, arm, and linguofacial region in the so-called upper, middle, and lower thirds of the pre- and post-central gyri; and the motor speech pathway in Broca's gyrus. It goes without saying that, for the type and manner of projection within this region, virtually the same configuration exists as is found in fibres of a peripheral nerve. However, we know that in projection fields of the cortex, regions lying far from one another in the periphery often become united centrally to serve a common function. The most familiar example of this is the projection field of speech in Broca's area. As we shall see later, the principle of function must therefore govern the type and manner of projections in the cerebral cortex, because only a functioning nervous system achieves connections with the cerebral cortex. This is closely linked with a second feature of the projection fields of the cortex: These are also the sites where memory traces of the various functional products of the nervous system are located. Localization of such memory traces thus follows the same principle, so that, at once, the occipital lobe forms the site of the visual memory traces; the temporal lobe that of the acoustic memory traces; the so-called middle third of the central gyri (the arm region) contains memory traces of tactile impressions acquired by the hand. Impairment of such predetermined classes of memory traces also determines focal symptoms of brain diseases.

Focal symptoms appear consistently in the form of disturbed functioning of the projection system—in its pathways, or in the projection fields of the cortex. Therefore, given that focal symptoms of the brain can be collectively traced back to functional disturbances of the projection systems and their destinations in various projection fields of the cortex, then mental illnesses are distinguished from the other two so-called organic general diseases of the brain because in the latter the projection systems and projection fields are *not* [W] affected.

Gentlemen! So far we have only incomplete information about the extent and exact location of projection fields in the cerebral cortex. However, as knowledge increases in this area, we may well find that the entire cerebral cortex is occupied by such projection fields. In searching for a location representing the site of disease, will we not then be led outside the brain and into the transcendental? Not by any means. Beyond the projection fields there is another anatomical substrate of great extent, to which we would quite reasonably attribute the seat of mental illnesses—the system of the association fibres, which serves to connect projection fields one with another. If this applies, then mental disorders are the particular diseases of this association organ.

Furthermore, certain focal illnesses of the brain already force us to assume that there are disturbances in such association pathways; indeed they form a natural bridge to mental illnesses. A case of this kind exists in certain rare examples of the so-called transcortical aphasia.

Gentlemen! From time immemorial, people have hoped that aphasia might be a starting point which leads to an understanding of mental illnesses. That we have not been misled, and that there are, on the contrary, actual cases of aphasia closely connected with known mental illnesses, is shown by the patient who we will now meet.

You see before you a patient [2, 3] who, even now, discernibly bears traces of a severe mental illness that he survived in the years 1885–1889. He stands and moves with a fixed gait, which, however, does not stop him from working as a cabinetmaker, readily providing for himself and his family. Any questions that we direct to him remain unanswered or are answered only by gestures. In fact, he is completely mute, and for 5 years has not been capable of uttering a sound. He understands everything that I say to him, as you can clearly see from his gestures and his performing instructions given to him. However, if I ask other questions or requests of him, he clearly indicates that he does not understand them. He thus shows quite explicitly the extent (within a certain range, yet always the same) to which he understands speech, while he has totally lost the motor ability to speak.

This condition of total motor aphasia and partial sensory aphasia has developed out of a certain mental illness that I will provisionally call *motility psychosis* [Ed]. This has remained as a lasting deficit. In the course of this illness, mutism and verbigeration—two psychotic symptoms that likewise arise in the speech area—had temporarily occurred earlier in the course of his illness.

Now, if we seek a more detailed understanding of this relationship, we must target the various forms of aphasia established by clinical observation. To this end, follow me for an instant into the related area of the so-called organic brain diseases.

Two projection fields of speech are known to us—one motor, and the other sensory. The motor (*m*) is the origin of the motor speech pathway (*mb*), part of the projection system that leads to the nerve nuclei of the extended spinal cord needed for speech. At the same time it is the site of memory traces of movements taking place during the act of speech or of conceiving speech movement. The sensory speech field (*s*) contains the central ending of the sensory speech pathway (*as*) and thus of the auditory nerves; but it is, at the same time, the site of memory traces of speech sounds or, as they have been called since Helmholtz, acoustic traces of words. The clinical picture of motor or sensory aphasia arises according to whether the motor or the sensory projection field is destroyed.

However, if we now stand aside from our patient who, after all, is unique, then generally, mentally ill persons are not aphasic. Normally, in psychiatric patients the sensory speech pathway and the sensory speech field are intact—they can understand everything that people say to them. They are also in full possession of their motor speech ability, insofar as it depends on integrity of the motor speech pathway and the motor projection field. Nevertheless, we do encounter the remarkable phenomenon where responses of mental patients are often nonsensical, and appear to bear only a remote or non-existent relationship with the question posed. How is this to be explained, if we still assume that the corresponding correct answer reflects the usual expression of normal brain function? There is only one explanation—the function of those nerve pathways, which are activated between the two projection fields, must be disturbed. Thus, the mental disorder appears to us as a disease of the association organ. However, I remind you that, in the common account of aphasia which we already use, such association pathways (the sensory speech pathway *as*, and the motor speech pathway *mb*,) are thought to continue beyond the cortical sites (projection fields), *s* and *m*, to a supposed Conceptualization Centre *B*. The transcortical pathways *sB* and *Bm* are nothing but association pathways, and so the site of malfunction must be in their region, betraying itself by the patient's inappropriate answer. Nevertheless, each mental disorder, insofar as it comes to light through a patient's incorrect spoken words, is, for us, an example of transcortical aphasia. The remarkable case of aphasia as a consequence of a mental illness, from which I started, immediately suggests the hypothesis that in some circumstances all the *Bm* pathways and a great part of the *sB* pathways may be interrupted during the course of the illness. Then a genuine aphasia, of the same type as in our patient, can result.

Nomination of a Conceptualization Centre *B* in the aphasia schema has often been misunderstood. However, the impossibility of avoiding it, and why it is necessary, is demonstrated as follows: Sensory aphasia by destruction of the projection field *s*—cortical sensory aphasia, as I call it—is characterized by memory traces of speech sounds having been misplaced by the patient and, as a consequence, words heard are no longer recognized. However, for understanding speech, obviously more is required than just recognition of word sounds: This must be connected with the corresponding meaning. If we distinguish between a word and its conceptualization, then we can only hypothesize that some pathway leads via the cortical centre *s* to other cortical regions that represent the associated concept. In truth, this supposed Conceptualization Centre is distributed amongst cortical sites far removed from one another. Consequently, for understanding speech, we need to distinguish two totally different processes. One, the recognition of word-sound images, is based on known functions of the projection field *s*; we shall call it *primary identification* [W]. The other process, the *sound* of the word by which the concept is identified, is based on functioning of association pathways and that of the supposed Conceptualization Centre. We will designate it as *secondary identification* [W]. If we compare the whole process to the forwarding of a telegram, as others have done, then *s* is the station where the telegram arrives, although the actual recipient is envisaged as *B*. The relationship between *B* and the motor projection field of speech at *m* is exactly the same: Here too *B* is the actual sender, while *m* is the telegraph station that transmits the telegram. In other words: The meaning—the conceptualization of the word—comes first, and this requires transmission along anatomical pathways to the motor projection field *m*, so that the word is spoken.

If we designate the reciprocal connections from *B* to *m* as secondary identification, which we can do by analogy, then we can conclude that expressions uttered by a mentally-ill person, which seem strange to us, are signs of disturbed secondary identification.

Progressive paralysis must be assigned a totally exceptional position among mental illnesses; here, it can even be classed amongst organic brain diseases. However, it is undoubtedly also a mental illness. In the most common cases, where it shows clear-cut focal symptoms, discrete lesions are also demonstrable in which an otherwise-diffuse disease process spreads to the projection system and the projection fields. Occasionally however, there are cases of progressive paralysis where there are no more than hints of such focal symptoms; in these cases, the predominantly transcortical character of the disease is valid.

Gentlemen! Comparison of aphasia with speech symptoms in this mentally ill patient teaches us that disturbance of secondary identification can be a feature common to both mental illnesses and certain cases of aphasia. Concurrence of the two diseases can be explained by changes in the same site in the transcortical or association pathways; but we take note of their difference: Mental illness selectively affects such pathways by themselves, while focal disease processes destroy just discrete portions of these pathways. In exceptional cases, the sum total of individually affected pathways may achieve the same effect as focal processes, and a transcortical aphasia may then proceed out of a mental illness. Our patient demonstrates that such a case can actually occur.

Thus we postulate that, apart from the particular site, there is a particular *type* [W] of illness. As in degenerative neuritis, this type of illness distinguishes individuals to some extent by other concomitant symptoms, and, by analogy with degenerative neuritis, according to the principle of differences in function.

References

1. Meynert T. Klinische Vorlesungen über Psychiatrie auf wissenschaftlichen Grundlagen für Studirende und Aerzte, Juristen und Psychologen. Vienna: Braumüller; 1890.
2. Verhandlungen des Congresses für Innere Medizin; Neunter Congress; 1890 Apr 15–18; Vienna, Austria. Wiesbaden: JF Bergmann; 1890. p. 273.
3. Heilbronner K. Aphasie und Geisteskrankheit. Psychiatr Abh. 1896;1:33.

Lecture 2

2

- To replace the Conceptualization Centre in the speech schema by arbitrary, localized apperceptions
- Registration and objective in the speech schema
- Generalization of the speech schema
- Types of movement: expressive, reactive, and initiative movements
- Disturbance of secondary identification is induced by psychosensory, psychomotor, or intrapsychic means

Lecture

Gentlemen!

So far, restricting our attention to the area of speech, we have contrasted brain disease and mental illness. Speech pathology is one of the best understood topics amongst brain diseases. Likewise, spoken expressions encompass so many of the symptoms of mental illnesses that by themselves they entitle us to view mental patients from this sole perspective. Nevertheless, I hope that in the following more extensive discussion, your understanding will be aided by starting from the simplified conditions of our example.

We must examine further the (arbitrary) fiction of the notional Conceptualization Centre *B*. As our knowledge of aphasia has developed, this preliminary term was clearly essential at an initial stage of our understanding. In the last lecture, I was able to take you back to its true meaning, but only in outline. Let me explain this allusion in more detail.

As already mentioned when discussing the central projection field, we can take it as established that memory traces and ideas are localized, that is, they are linked, according to their content, with different locations in the cerebral cortex. Apart from such localization in the aphasia schema, one can reasonably regard the receiver and sender of those telegrams as being linked to the notional Conceptualization Centre *B*, that is, with all the rest of the cerebral cortex and, as we shall see, its system of association connections. This would artificially separate the two projection fields *s* and *m* from the totality of all other projection fields. Such separation within the cortex is the basis for differentiating the areas for the two projection fields *s* and *m* (whether we stress their subcortical links or their transcortical links beyond the projection fields). In this illustration, the anatomical view was that the aggregate of transcortical pathways *sB* and *mB* formed discrete pathways vulnerable to discrete lesions localized to the neighbourhood of the two projection fields, while beyond there the pathways had to be seen as radiating out to many disparate areas of the cerebral cortex. The discovery of the clinical picture of transcortical motor and sensory aphasia seemingly relied by sheer chance on the fact that these lesions appeared to occupy

R. Miller, K.J. Dennison (eds.), *An Outline of Psychiatry in Clinical Lectures*,
DOI 10.1007/978-3-319-18051-9_2

precisely the postulated site. It is easily grasped that these rare cases were initially attributed to focal diseases of the brain. On the other hand, observation of the patient I already introduced to you proved that such clinical pictures can arise during the course of a typical mental illness, thus forming a natural transition to mental illnesses.

It is essential for our purpose that we go beyond such rare occurrences. However, if we stay with that initial example, and hold fast to the principle of localized representation, then we can conveniently split the centre *B* into two localized representations linked by an association pathway: We shall call them *A* and *Z*. *A*, the *source representation* [W], is linked with the sensory speech field by an association pathway *sA*. *Z*, the *destination representation* [W], is linked with the motor projection field for speech by an identical pathway *Zm*. *AZ* is the association pathway between *A* and *Z*. Altering the schema in such a way corresponds to some extent to processing of an arithmetical problem presented to a patient: Understanding the problem takes place as registration, in *A*; the solution corresponds with the destination representation *Z*; and only when the solution is found does activation of *m* take place. Between task and solution, complex thought processes can proceed, from which it becomes clear that the association pathway *AZ* itself can be regarded as subdivided many times over. We need not assume that the entire process normally follows a set pattern, virtually in preformed pathways, so that the result is predictable. However, we can tentatively assume that it behaves in just this manner in response to any random question; understanding the question is represented in *A*, the meaning of the answer by *Z*, and the intermediate in-series pathway *AZ* makes sense of the case, so that the answer develops from a more or less simple deliberation. If we do not expect a speaker to lead us astray, then we must recognize that in this case, in a normal person, answers will arise in a totally determined manner, to be predicted with approximate accuracy. The regularity hereby observed is based, as we shall see later, on the principle of 'well-worn pathways' [Ed].

This example provides opportunity for expansion, which can become a founding principle for the entire symptomatology of mental illnesses. Instead of projection fields of speech, we have only to insert any other projection field. In place of spoken expression, substitute any randomly expressed movement, and *m* represents the projection field in question, depending on whether the movement takes place in arm, leg, trunk, etc. As is generally known, central projection fields for such movements are contained in the so-called motor zone of the cerebral cortex. Instead of the sensory speech field, the projection field for any arbitrary sensory awareness could take its place. Just the same takes place in vision, for example, as in understanding the speech sounds a person utters. By this means, primary identification occurs in the central projection field of the visual system, in order to comprehend what is seen; but transmission is required to other projection fields (for secondary identification). Without this secondary process, the visual impression is lost to the recipient, remaining unintelligible, just as in the case of transcortical sensory aphasia for the sense of hearing. The same is true for all sensory impressions, as a little thought will confirm.

We quickly see that such a generalization is permitted—indeed recommended—by a more detailed look at our original example. The answer that I expect from the patient need not be spoken—it can be given to me in writing or through silent facial expressions and gestures, or by employing any arbitrary response. Depending on the muscles used for performance, the projection field *m* will have different impact, and correspond with different cortical sites. In other words, my question and my task can be carried out without a word being uttered, whether in writing, or through the spoken word, by expressive hand movements and so on.

I said earlier that our schema, with its modifications, can be used to derive the entire symptomatology of a psychiatric patient. I should have expressed myself more precisely, by referring to symptoms just in so far as they are shown in that patient's movements. However, this limitation is necessary only if we subtract from those movements (admittedly using layman's terms and manner of understanding) speech, facial expressions, demeanour, and all those gestures included in such an expression. Yet even in those cases, everything can be reduced to movement, by which we assess the internal processing of a patient; and for scientific observation, to disregard this fact might be a real error. The more experience you have with psychiatric patients, and come to recognize their symptoms, the more you become convinced that, in the end, there is nothing else to find and observe, than movement, and that the whole pathology of the mentally ill consists of nothing more than peculiarities of their motor behaviour; for obviously, in a given case, a breakdown in movement can be just as characteristic as previously intact movements.

We exclude here only intentional movements of which other people are aware before they reach the consciousness of the patient himself or herself. If these movements amount to speech, we face the same situation although more tangibly and obviously than for other movements. Symptomatology of psychiatric patients therefore has movements as its focus, insofar as they appear to be functions of the organ of consciousness, in other words, the organ of association. Here we encounter the only limitation on the generality of the above sentence: Of course, some movements are independent of consciousness, such as those controlled by the autonomic nervous system, those of the heart, respiration, vessel walls, and viscera; and most reflex movements belong here. As we will see later, these movements can also be affected in mental patients, although they do not form the actual focus of observation. We will further find that, in odd cases, shifts of body temperature and, in almost all cases, of feeding pattern as expressed by body mass are important symptoms. However the exceptions are minor, and should be seen as secondary *sequelae* [Ed], which consistently depend on the patient's movements.

Provisionally then, we can draw an abstraction from the numerous exceptions, and can thus focus more closely on movements as functions of the organ of consciousness. This requires us to classify movements in a pragmatic way. We can conveniently differentiate between 'expressive movements' [Ed], 'reactive movements' [Ed], and 'initiative movements' [Ed]. As we shall see, this classification clearly has the advantage of encompassing the totality of all possible movements, and is thus preferable to Meynert's [1] classification (however far-reaching and fruitful the latter proves to be in other ways) into movements of defence and attack. However, our classification fails in one respect and needs improvement, in that sharp separation of the three different types of movement is often impossible. Inevitably some movements in one area fall also into another area, so that, depending on the observer's point of view, there is dispute over the class to which a particular example of movement belongs. Despite this, we provisionally retain the classification, because it proves useful in the psychiatry clinic.

By the term 'expressive movements' [Ed], we mean, above all, movements through which people's Affect and frame of mind can be recognized. Indeed, speech movements primarily serve this purpose, although not exclusively; and insofar as they serve such a purpose, we should include speech movements in the broadest sense, for example, wails and moans of pain. Most exclamations, as is well known, are words that serve this purpose very well. Laughing and whining are specific expressive movements, as are all facial expressions. Moreover, expression in the face, even when it is *not* [W] in motion, arises from particular muscle actions; likewise posture of the whole body, by the same token, is expressive, just as are words or facial expressions, in revealing a person's state of mind and emotional state. Movements of the entire body serving to express joy, cheerfulness, high spirits, satisfaction, scorn, anger, fear, grief, anguish, despair, hope, hatred, and love are familiar and sufficiently expressive that it would be superfluous to describe them here. Normally the face of an alert man is continually enlivened by an expression; so we recognize *lack* [Ed] of expression as a significant symptom.

'Reactive movements' [Ed] are those arising from actual external stimuli. When a person answers a question, apart from the content of the reply, the answer can always be viewed as a reactive movement. Moreover an answer that is not made up of words but of other gestures—when, for example, the person questioned puts his finger to his lips in a meaningful manner—comes under the definition of a reactive movement. Failure to answer can, in many cases, be taken as a significant symptom. Amongst reactive movements of particular importance in the psychiatric clinic are behaviour of patients: during a physical examination; towards the minor services of the waiting staff; to requests of any kind; to the approach and reception of the doctor; and to the whole unfamiliar situation in rooms of an institution—these merit particular consideration. In addition, expressions of movement that are essential to gratifying bodily needs (even when they can be traced back to internal stimuli) must be regarded as reactive movements. It may, however, be equally valid to include the last-named class of movement amongst initiative movements, and again, many previously mentioned movements can be classed as expressive movements. In any case it can be reiterated that, in psychiatric patients, absence of reactive movements is often just as characteristic and valuable as a symptom, as their aberrant modification.

Amongst 'initiative movements' [Ed] we refer to all movements driven by personal motives, rather than by an external stimulus. This negative definition includes some expressive movements, and some reactive movements. In consequence, for expressive movements, we should always assess the extent to which they belong with initiative or reactive movements. One might ask whether there *are* [W] actual initiative movements, that is, ones which arise without *any* external stimulus, since usually some kind of external trigger can be found for virtually any spontaneous action. However, since such events often are no more than opportune moments connected to prevailing internal motives, identifying them as initiative movements can be justified. In general, initiative movements tend to consist of whole series of individual movements, and can then be referred to as actions. The whole behaviour, demeanour, and 'the doing and the allowing' [W] of an individual in given situations—collectively, all his expressions by means of movement—insofar as they are neither expressive nor reactive movements, belong amongst the initiative movements.

Nervous excitation, which takes place along the pathway *sAZm* can be likened to a reflex process, and we can designate this pathway as a 'psychic reflex arc' [W]. The movement activated from *m* then appears as the result—a discernible consequence—of this activation. Clinical methods in psychiatry consist of studying the end result in order to reveal the process from which it originates.

You will notice at once that it is actually only reactive movements that can be compared with reflex processes in the manner outlined. These may, as in the initial example, be a spoken word or other arbitrary movement; it is always taken as completely spontaneous, yet still the consequence of an external stimulus—one based again on motor processes. However, one can ask: What is the situation for the other types of movement—expressive movements and initiative movements? Obviously, these can be seen from the same perspective; for, quite apart from the question raised about initiative movements, whether they arise totally without external triggers, we can fairly replace external stimuli by memory traces of past stimuli. When an external stimulus is absent, we can regard such memory traces as initial links, with movement as the terminal link in the psychic reflex arc. We can even go so far as to regard movement in progress as evidence of this assumption. Movement without *any* [Ed] kind of cause is inconceivable; yet a visible cause *is* [W] clearly absent. Therefore only a form of 'energy', accumulated somewhere, can induce movement that does actually arise. As we will see later, memory traces *are* [W] such sources of accumulated energy.

From these preliminary remarks we can add to our learning about aberrant disturbance of movement observed in mentally ill people. They are all based on disturbance of secondary identification, as demonstrated above. However, I remind you that we have considered not only the relationship from *s* to *A*, the projection field nearest to registration, but also the activation of *Z* to the motor projection field *m*, operating in the reverse direction. We were justified in this shift because the pathway *Zm* is an association pathway, as is *sA*, and the physical processes taking place through such association pathways should always be the same, regardless of their direction. In like manner we can also include the relationship between *A* and *Z* for secondary identification.

Since all these are nerve pathways, abnormalities of excitability or ability to conduct signals are always the sole basis for disturbance of secondary identification. Three cases cover all possibilities: reduced excitability or conduction ability; increased excitability; and aberrant excitability. We label the pathway *sA* as psychosensory; *Zm* as psychomotor; and *ZA* as intrapsychic. The possible cases can then be summarized as follows:

Psychosensory	Psychomotor	Intrapsychic
Anaesthesia	Akinesia	Loss of function
Hyperaesthesia	Hyperkinesia	Hyperfunction
Paraesthesia	Parakinesia	Parafunction

One could dispute this tabulation on the grounds that these are nothing more than disturbances of movement we encounter in mental patients, as I myself emphasized, and that therefore, the totality of symptoms is exhausted just by three cases—hyperkinesia, akinesia, and parakinesia. This objection is partly true, and requires a thorough explanation. The easiest way to do this is to return to our starting point, the example of speech. When a patient is silent and we would expect him or her to speak, we can interpret this symptom as a circumscribed form of akinesia restricted to speech. If the presenting symptom is an urge to talk, then by the same token this is a circumscribed form of hyperkinesia. If, on the other hand, his or her response is nonsensical speech, we could rightly regard this as a symptom of parakinesia. Here, however, one would need a more detailed account for each of these, because misunderstanding is to be expected. We will always be forced, on practical grounds, to distinguish two totally different aspects of speech: active movement as such, and the content of the spoken words. However, since there may be abnormalities of active movements or, as we can label it, the formal part of speech, then it is more accurate to use the word parakinesia only in this narrower sense. Examples are the symptom of compulsive speech and the monotonous word repetition—the so-called verbigeration. The same reflection that the content portion must be differentiated from the formal part of a movement applies to all expressive movements, and also to reactive and initiative movements. Since patients may gabble a great deal of nonsense using formally correct speech, then the feelings expressed, despite having quite correct form, can still be aberrant; and so can their actions be formally correct but incorrect in content. In these cases therefore, we need not assume any disturbance of psychomotor identification, but are forced to seek disturbance further back in the reflex arc. This corresponds to common idiom, and the habit of completely ignoring a patient's mechanism of sharing his or her internal thoughts, expressing feelings, and so on as self-evident. After this discussion, it becomes comprehensible that, among mentally-ill persons, we frequently see symptoms of disturbed content identification, even though the movement mechanism itself is fully intact.

Reference

1. Meynert Th. Sammlung von popular-wissenschaftlichen Vorträgen über den Bau und die Leistungen des Gehirns. Vienna; Wilhelm Braumüller; 1892.

Lecture 3

3

- Nature of memory images
- Retinal after-images and remembered visual images
- The hypothesis of special sense cells and memory cells is insufficient as an explanation
- Local signs in the retina
- Visual representations

Lecture

Gentlemen!

Before we look more closely at symptoms of mental illnesses we must revisit the aforementioned Conceptualization Centre or, more precisely, those localized memory images. I hope that, on reflection, you conclude that this is not the alleged 'Conceptualization Centre' [Ed] said to have a definite localization, but probably the concepts themselves.

In introducing my first lecture, I presented as a statement of fact, confirmed in pathological cases, that central projection fields are localized to different areas of the cerebral cortex. We must recognize that such fields are also sites of remembered images; and it follows from this that these memory images also have definite locations. However, let us examine these memory images more closely.

First, I want to touch briefly on clinical facts which, in my opinion, totally validate the principle of localized memory images: These are clinical instances of sensory and motor aphasia, and cases of the so-called tactile anaesthesia of the hand. The former are probably well known by now, so I need not go into detail; but the importance of the latter is debated. Two related sets of facts provide support. On the one hand, cases have been seen where circumscribed cortical damage in the middle third of the two central gyri leads to permanent deficit, where the hand fails to recognize objects by touch, although disturbance of sensation itself can barely be detected. On the other hand, there are cases of spinal or peripheral disease where sensitivity, and—I stress—also muscle and position sense, is most severely disrupted, with only minor disturbance of tactile perception. The last-named cases demonstrate to some extent that even a very weak and patchy projection system can still conduct messages to the brain sufficient to support primary identification, provided the central projection fields and therefore the remembered images—tactile images, as we can call them here—are preserved. However, cases of the *first* [Ed] type can be based only on loss of primary identification itself, since disturbance of projection pathways themselves is clearly minimal. The principle that remembered images are localized to corresponding projection fields is established beyond all doubt by such facts, and thus this principle can be fairly applied to all projection fields.

R. Miller, K.J. Dennison (eds.), *An Outline of Psychiatry in Clinical Lectures*,
DOI 10.1007/978-3-319-18051-9_3

If we return to our example of the organ of speech, we find that the process of *recognition* [W]—primary identification (see above)—requires solid ownership of memory images. The question then arises: How should one view such ownership? Evidently this concerns a special characteristic of the nervous system, that it undergoes lasting change in response to temporary stimuli, a property we call *memory* [W]. Such memory is seen, for example, in the fact that Faradic excitability of a nerve can be increased by frequent electrical stimulation [1]. The same stimulation then becomes more effective if it has often been administered previously; and therefore lasting change exists in the nerve as a result of the previous history of transient stimulation. All training is based on the same principle, for any form of learning: 'Practice makes perfect' [Ed]. Pathways that are initially hard to access become more firmly trodden in with each new training experience—you could say that they are 'moulded by experience' [W]. Thus when a memory of this sort reaches a person's awareness via nerve pathways, it occurs specifically in nerve cell bodies. A reflex in the spinal cord mediated via its neuronal cell bodies takes place more easily the more frequently it has previously been elicited; and it has been demonstrated by studies of Ward [2], Jarisch and Schiff [3], and others that this is a special property of the neuronal perikarya. It would be reasonable to relate after-images of the retina mainly to their ganglion cells. Similarly, in the cerebral cortex you would ascribe changes persisting long after instantaneous stimulation, which we call memory images, primarily to neuronal cell bodies.

After this, it appears obvious that possession of such remembered images—*contents of consciousness* [W], we might say—depends directly on the projection system and sense organs by which those images were obtained. The consciousness of a person with poor eyesight, or one with generally deficient senses, is thus quite different from that of a normal person. An individual born blind will certainly have no remembered images of visual sensation. Were his sight to be surgically healed, this would provide a situation we otherwise see only when the pathology of visual agnosia occurs. Just as for an individual born blind, so too for one born deaf, the content of consciousness totally lacks an entire category of memory images originating from the sense of hearing. In partial cortical deficiencies, as observed from time to time in those who are mentally defective from birth and also have sensory deficits such as deafness, there is a similar lack of remembered images due to abnormal development of central projection fields. No less instructive in this connection is a comparison with animal brains. Humans have only a vestigial olfactory bulb, whereas many mammalian species have an olfactory bulb occupying a significant part of their cerebral hemispheres, with a separate ventricle and separate surface gyri. Everyday observation shows just how different is the consciousness of such animals, for example that of a dog from our own. It appears to be full of remembered olfactory images, and the animal, snuffling here and there, revels in all its joyful frame of mind, like the gourmet at table, or the eye of an artist beholding beautiful forms. The content of consciousness shown in this way depends on the state of the projection system and central projection fields, a relationship suggesting the following principle: Consciousness is a function of the central projection fields. If the assumption—that projection fields occupy the entire cortical mantle—is confirmed, then the corollary follows: Consciousness is a function of the cortical mantle.

We can get a better grasp of the notion of a memory image if we use a definite example, such as a remembered image of a visual sensation. For this, comparison with retinal after-images is particularly instructive, since these belong to the same sensory modality. How far is the comparison accurate and justified? As mentioned, we can trace retinal after-images specifically to long-lasting excitation of retinal ganglion cells by a stimulus; and, by special arrangements of such excited cells, an image is formed and referred to a particular position in space. This image is of limited duration. Let us assume that similar cells—call them 'perception cells' [W]—are also to be found in central projection fields of the optic nerve, where projection fibres end.

Could this assumption—that the memory image exists in resonating excitation of such perceptual cells—be sufficient to explain the apparent difference from retinal after-images? Many things contradict this. In my experience at least, the characteristic referral to a preferred position in space is totally different from that of remembered visual images. The latter seem to be spatially referred only insofar as they always occupy a definite position in a particular person. They also appear to be of unlimited duration, a difference that is especially difficult to explain. You would hardly imagine that the same perceptual cell, once recruited, would maintain its long-lasting state of activation, but rather that it could soon be sensitized by a totally different stimulus. You would expect it to be held in the same manner as a retinal image, and, at least, subsequent activation would always wipe out the preceding activation. Let us assume for example that we are dealing with the sensory memory image of a letter or a number. Assume also that retinal images falling on the position of clearest vision, or close to it, will mostly be those leading to development of such remembered images. There, not only is the greatest number of sensory elements to be found, but, in this region, photoreceptors for images are also laid out with particular precision, so that the sharpest images arise there. Correspondingly Nature has arranged it such that, for visual impressions that attract our attention, we locate the point of clearest vision quite involuntarily by appropriate eye movements—a compulsion which, even for adults, makes it difficult for anyone to exert total conscious control over their eye movements. As a consequence of this, many retinal elements that previously represented the image of the letter are soon engaged in forming a new image, e.g. of the number, and correspondingly so also are cells of the central projection field serving perception. Assume (as highly likely) that the point of clearest vision in the retina corresponds to a considerable area in the central projection field. Under these circumstances, the difficulty of explaining the memory of the image by a particular cellular memory therefore remains unchanged. There have been attempts to avoid the difficulty by differentiating between perception-related and recall-related cellular elements, and ascribing the feature of memory only to the latter. Only those elements in the cortical projection area serving perception should correspond to points in the retina. However, it is not just this assumption which raises difficulties. The difference between a perceptual image and a remembered image arises not so much from the diversity of active elements but from the fact that the *patterning* [Ed] of retinal elements or the *form of retinal excitation* [W] in the various examples is different, while mainly the same retinal elements cooperate to create a memory image. It is just the memory of that previous patterning of functioning elements, that is, the *form* [Ed] of activation, which makes up the psychological concept of a memory image. I agree entirely with Sachs [4] and Goldscheider [5] that only by assuming that functional links are acquired between simultaneously excited perceptual elements using existing connections can one explain the specific memory for respective forms of retinal images, defined by patterned stimulation of retinal points. When the same pattern of stimulation returns, and the retinal image, is again detected, one can envisage, as did Ziehen [6], a process whereby the remembered image is reactivated from perceptual elements, because only this combination of cells has been 'tuned in' [Ed], to some extent, to this pattern of activation (somewhat like sound resonators respond only to certain tonal combinations). However, this analogy still requires us to explain this 'predisposition' [W]; and for this we need connection formation between perceptual elements by nerve fibres, that is, the process of association. We shall see later that association of various sensory impressions is always concluded when they take place at the same time; in exactly the same way we can assume here that simultaneously excited perception cells serving sensation become associated with one another; and because renewal of the same sensory impression repeats the same patterning, these perception cells remain associated. A remembered image might then be nothing other than an acquired association of perceptual elements of the central projection field.

You see, gentlemen, that with this concept, we need not assume the existence of any special memory cells. We can reach the same conclusion in a totally different way: Here I stress only that it would not be a convincing account of the discrepancies between sensory activity and memory images if only perceptual elements were involved, and always corresponded with certain points in the retina. The fact that remembered images have no definite projection in space, as do after-images, would remain incomprehensible. Finally, one can take the structure of central projection fields in the cerebral cortex as a counterargument. A simple layer of ganglion cells, all linked to projection fibres, might satisfy the current assumption. However, in the cerebral cortex we find such a large number of nerve cells layered one over another in the visual projection field of the occipital cortex—more than anywhere else—that they far exceed the number of projection fibres. All these thoughts will have to be examined in the future. In the meantime, we should note that we have finally proved a difference between memory images and retinal after-images; namely that the long duration of the former and the transience of the latter can be traced back to an anatomical difference—that *the cerebral cortex has association fibres, while the retina has none* [W].

If the strength of remembered images is to be explained in terms of repetition of patterned stimulation, and this statement is applied to the particular case of visual memory images, we soon encounter difficulties. Retinal images, which are defined by solid objects in the external world, are sometimes big and sometimes small, depending on whether they are near or far; yet their *remembered images* [Ed] are taken as whole units. In fact the relationship of retinal points remains the same, and their respective images can be regarded as perfectly congruent, so that psychological requirements that we place on a memory image are still met. However, there are always a number of retinal points whose patterning must be present on any one remembered image. Even with the simplest assumption that the object is fixed, each memory image would still include countless sub-images which, even though congruent, are of various sizes. The difficulty disappears if we incorporate the brilliant hypothesis of H. Sachs. According to this, so-called 'local signs' [Ed] of retinal points are determined by two measures, namely the meridian on which they lie, and their distance from the midpoint. A specific combination of muscle activity is required for each half of the retinal meridian; through interaction of muscles, rotation of the eyeball brings the macula in register with the light source. This combination of muscle activation remains the same at all points on the same half-meridian, but the intensity of nervous activity varies, and increases with the distance of the retinal point from the *fovea centralis* [W]. On the other hand, for different half-meridians the muscle combination is always different. Differences in image size for fixed objects therefore require no more than shift in intensity of nervous activity; the anatomical factor, the specific combination of different muscle activations, stays the same. In turn, this behavior expresses itself and is transferred to relationships within the cerebral cortex. Visual cells of the central projection field for retinal points of each half-meridian all have similar associative connections with specific points of the central projection field for eye movements. We must think of the latter as broken up into as many different muscle combinations ('eye movement representations' [W]) as there are half-meridians of the retina. Naturally, this must be taken *cum grano salis* [W], since we are dealing with a continually graded series of muscle representations, rather than discrete points. If this concept is taken into account, visual memory images (some of whose properties we already know) are distinguished, in that those visual cells of which they are made up are linked with precisely localized movement representations of the central projection field of eye movements. By repetition of the same visual pattern, associations form not only amongst visual cells themselves, but also amongst matching, similarly localized movement representations. We shall call the widened concept of the visual memory image 'visual *perceptual* [Ed] representation' [W]. We now see that, despite change of image size, the latter components of visual representation remain the same, if they are related to the same object; they therefore characterize remembered images rather than visual sensory images. Similar considerations apply also to retinal images, positioned asymmetrically to the midpoint of the retina, as you will see from reading Sachs' book. (I cannot recommend that book strongly enough, as an introduction to our topic.)

A second, undeniable difficulty is the different vantage points for objects from which clear images are seen. An equilateral triangle or a cross can be recognized whether the triangle is standing on its base or its apex, or whether the cross is standing, lying, or standing at an angle. How could the same memory image be derived? In reply one can say that by far the greatest number of objects in the outside world (and consequently their retinal images) do not present such a difficulty: They provide a firm viewpoint for our eyes. Compared to these, those objects which move and change their position or their retinal images are firstly in the minority, and secondly have mainly a defined, habitual position in relation to our body. In addition, if we count on the ability of our eye to adapt itself in such a way that a familiar image reappears, then the difficulty caused by the changing position of objects will seem only small. However, we cannot deny that in some situations remembered images are insufficient to identify objects in strange locations. We do not recognize inverted letters; several familiar optical illusions are based on the same failing; and how strange appears the image of a person, when viewed through a convex lens, upside down! Even though a few difficulties are raised by these facts, nevertheless the vast number of cell groups needed to accommodate just visual memory images may still seem astonishing. Experience teaches us that a healthy brain can always acquire new memory images; there must therefore still be an abundance of elements for this purpose. However, I draw your attention to a miscalculation that makes us exaggerate the difficulty: As I demonstrate later, we tend to overestimate the number and variability of solid objects in the outside world; and we correspondingly underestimate the frequency of recurrence of the same impressions.

References

1. Mann L. Über Veränderungen der Erregbarkeit durch den faradischen Strom. Deut Arch klin Med. 1893;51:127–40.
2. Ward J. Über die Auslösung von Reflexbewegungen durch eine Summe schwacher Reize. Arch Physiol. 1880;72–91.
3. Jarisch A, Schiff E. Untersuchungen über das Kniephänomen. Med. Jb. Vienna: Wilhelm Braumüller; 1882. p. 261–307.
4. Sachs H. Vorträge über Bau und Tätigkeit des Großhirns und die Lehre von der Aphasie und Seelenblindheit. Breslau: Preuss; 1893.
5. Goldscheider A. Über zentrale Sprach-, Schreib- und Lesestörung. Berl klin Wochenschr 4, 1892
6. Ziehen GTh. Leitfaden der physiologischen Psychologie in 14 Vorlesungen. Jena: Gustav Fischer; 1891.

Lecture 4

4

- The concrete concept: an 'association of memory images' [Ed]
- Awareness of the outside world
- Number of concepts
- Requirement of causality

Lecture

Gentlemen!

Study of remembered visual images taught us that they are acquired associations of perceptual elements of the central projection field, and that, for these, the *form* [Ed] of the stimulus is crucial. You would be justified in transposing this principle to central projection fields of any sensory region. Acquisition of such memory images is generally based on a feature of central projection fields—their perceptual elements, that is, those nerve cells connected directly with projection fibres and also interconnected by association fibres, separate for each projection field. We shall speak in future about olfactory, acoustic, tactile and gustatory memory images without going into further detail about their nature. I need not draw attention to the fact that each sensory area presents its own particular problems [1], and that these simplest mental components, the remembered images, can be more complex in form.

Recognition—or primary identification—is produced by virtue of this property of memory images. If, for sake of simplicity, we restrict ourselves to solid objects, which by themselves make up central aspects of sensory perception, the content of consciousness is made up of the sum of such remembered images of these solid objects. Clearly, within this sum, certain fixed groupings can likewise be differentiated, always corresponding with the features of a particular solid object. One and the same solid object usually contributes to several sensory perceptions, always recurring in the same manner. The simultaneity of these several sensory inputs leads to their remembered images remaining in association. In this manner an acquired association of memory images from different senses corresponds with each solid object, and the association is progressively consolidated the more frequently the same solid object is perceived by our senses. Thus we find an anatomical basis for those psychological dimensions that have traditionally been used to describe 'concepts' [W]. We are now in a position to differentiate the 'strength' [Ed] and 'extent' [Ed] of the concept; however we will distinguish essential and non-essential features of solid objects depending on whether they always adhere to the object or are changeable. Of course, the extent of a concept includes its non-essential characteristics, since these always show a degree of constancy depending on the nature of the object. For any item, we can then easily plot a curve with Extent ('circumference' [Ed] of the item), entered along the x-axis

R. Miller, K.J. Dennison (eds.), *An Outline of Psychiatry in Clinical Lectures*,
DOI 10.1007/978-3-319-18051-9_4

and 'Intensity' [Ed] (or strength) of the concept/ item on the *y*-axis.

We have just seen how secondary identification differs from primary identification, in that when each individual component of a concept is excited, the sum of all the rest, making up the whole concept, can be excited. The anatomical basis for acquiring such related functional groupings of cellular elements is the availability of association fibres between the various projection fields. We shall call these 'trans-cortical association pathways' [Ed], in contrast to intra-cortical intrinsic fibres. The content of consciousness, as we now recognize, therefore includes the *concept* [Ed] of solid objects or, as we will call it, *concrete concepts* [Ed]. We can also identify the sum of such concepts as *consciousness of the outside world* [W], for in these concepts we in fact possess a true picture of the outer world.

As you will notice, also included in consciousness of the outside world is the apparatus for 'simple circuit operations' [Ed]. This process is the same as that which also serves for secondary identification. From audible speech, from the barking of a dog, or from a certain fragrance I can acknowledge the presence of a man, a dog, or a certain flower. Virtually all circuit operations which relate to concrete features are similar, and therefore, as we have seen, are only isolated examples of secondary identification.

The content of consciousness thus consists not only of memory images, but also secondarily of fully-defined *complexes* [Ed] of such images firmly linked to one another through association—concrete concepts. The number of concepts depends on the number of solid objects. Perhaps you are astonished that I have so far presented it as though only a few (and always the same) objects would enter our sensory world. You might ask: Do not things in the outer world come into the realm of our senses in almost infinite number and indescribable multiplicity? Fortunately, a specific answer is possible. The number of words gives us a clue to the number of concepts. The number of concepts that a particular individual possesses is shown by the number of words with which he functions. One of the most comprehensive spirits who ever lived, or will ever live, is, undoubtedly, Shakespeare; accordingly, his vocabulary is also uncommonly comprehensive: extending to 15,000 [2]. How much should we subtract from this, if we want to restrict ourselves to solid objects of the outside world! Not everyone is a Shakespeare, but you will be surprised when we soon pass to the other extreme (amongst civilized nations!): The vocabulary of an English seaman does not exceed a few hundred. The number of concrete items is, in fact, not so great, nor is their diversity so significant, as we can easily appreciate, especially when we realize that the number of nerve cells in the cortex is about a *Milliarde* [W] by Meynert's count. We can now grasp that indeed the same solid object must impinge on our senses quite often, if such a firm connection is to exist of particular remembered images with what we call 'concepts' [W].

Perhaps by now it is obvious that consciousness of the outside world has definite dependence on the outside world, or, we might say, is 'a function' [Ed] of it. Even quantitatively, the above examples show this beyond doubt. However, we should keep in mind, as opposites, not only extremes such as Shakespeare and the sailor, but also the generalized consciousness of urbanites, probably educated, living in complex civilizations, and the man-on-the-land, the fisherman, and the hunter—growing up in secluded isolation with little education. Yet the qualitative variation in awareness of the outside world must also be surprisingly great. Think of the contrast between an inhabitant of the tropics, growing up amidst lush flora and fauna, a world rich in colour, and the polar inhabitant, who experiences only traces of vegetation during a short summer.

It is worth dwelling for a moment on these remarkable facts of association and their essential natures. Most associations that might interest us so far are based on simultaneity of impressions. Admittedly there is no explanation, yet it is undeniable that memory images of simultaneously received sensory impressions remain associated, whether the interaction was brought about by a deeper connection or the loosest random occurrence. However, random occurrences will not be so easily repeated, so their association is not as firm as that for clearly related events.

The association of various remembered images to one another is a second example of the occurrence of the so-called preformed pathways [Ed]; that is, the connection among them is so firm because these pathways have been called upon so often.

Apart from association through simultaneity, we know of another type of association: that by succession. I need only recall that for each attempt to learn something useful, this plays the main role. There is a whole series of associations which, impressed upon us at early age, remain with us for our entire life: I remember the alphabet, multiplication tables, the Lord's Prayer, etc. Through succession alone, this association makes us aware of the regularity of things. Always, when a certain sequence of events recurs without exception, we believe that a law is operating, and are particularly encouraged in this belief when we succeed in arbitrarily evoking the initial event, and then observe the subsequent one. Such an experiment has an irresistible persuasive power over us. However, clearly, this reveals no deeper connection between the two events—it proves merely the presence of that pathway which was claimed earlier in the same processes [3]. Our need to infer causality, in short, is an inborn error or a bias of our brain. Phenomena of the outside world are too far apart to have any kind of connection among themselves; the bond that links them exists only in our brain, and is not used to link the objects themselves, but only the tracks they leave behind in our brain.

We shall see later that simultaneity of sensory perception is not possible, on account of the property designated as the 'one-ness' [W] or perhaps as the 'unity of consciousness' [Ed]. In truth, we always experience only one sensory percept at once; any second, apparently-simultaneous percept happens either earlier or later. Association by simultaneity therefore appears to be but a special case of generic association through succession [1].

Having spoken so much about association, there is no wish to conceal the difficulties in understanding the processes involved. On an earlier occasion [3] I compared it with a wave motion in an enclosed pipe system. Meynert and more recently Ziehen have made similar comparisons. In any case the fact of association can be explained by assuming the existence of pathways connecting the anatomical locations at which memory images for individual senses are localized. Since myriad fibres are detectable as much in the white matter under the cortical mantle as in the cortex itself, whose sole function is to connect various cortical locations, then an anatomical basis for this is also undoubtedly available. When two cortical sites in the same central projection field contribute to the process of primary identification, or when different projection fields contribute to secondary identification, and are simultaneously excited by external stimuli from afferent pathways, the connecting pathway between them is likewise set into sympathetic vibration. Resistance which stood in the way of propagation of the excitation process along such pathways becomes progressively eliminated the more often the process is repeated, and the pathway becomes 'well trodden' [Ed], or as I described earlier, 'well blazed' [Ed]. This does not mean that the pathway is continually needed, but we can claim only its physiological continuity, just as for pathways of the projection system. On the contrary, the fact that it provides a unique layer of nerve cells to the cortex, that of fusiform cells, which by their form and location seem to belong to the association system, indicates in a specific way that such cells too are activated in the association pathways. In general, it indeed contradicts our intuition to accept nerve fibres that cannot prove their origin from any nerve cell. It is simplest therefore to assume that each cell, or association cell, sends out two nerve fibres projecting in opposite directions, which, with their terminal dendrites, enter into association with nerve cells of the projection fields. There is no difficulty in imagining that nerve cells of a central projection field which took part in primary identification are all linked to one another by such association fibres, each in turn provided with an association cell, even though in some situations, depending on the number of perceptual elements involved, calculated according to their combinations, an enormously large number of such association pathways may be required.

But as soon as you go beyond this initial physiological unit, the memory image, and envisage just the next higher level of visual images (see p. 19 above) or even association between visual images and remembered images from another projection field, the difficulty of conceiving the process increases enormously. Recently Goldscheider [4] quite rightly emphasized this fact. However, we still should consider available options. It seems impossible to apply the same scheme that is conceivable in a projection field, namely for each sensory element to be anatomically connected with any other by preformed pathways, nor is it possible for memory images to be connected one with another. Great as the number of fibres at our disposal may seem, it is quite inadequate compared with the almost infinitely large numbers resulting from calculation of combinations in this case. There follows from this the absolute necessity of making some other assumption that simplifies the conditions for association. For reasons already indicated, but above all the last mentioned, one can fairly view the psychological unit of a memory image as corresponding to some kind of anatomical unit. For example, it could be that cells of a certain layer of the cortex receive fibre processes from the association cells mentioned above while at the same time being connected with the perception cells or projection cells. There is absolutely nothing improbable in thinking that excitatory processes (made up of multiple elements) in a particular cortical layer are combined to some extent into a unit with the nerve cells of an adjoining cortical layer. You could also consider that, for our consciousness, remembered images are not perceptions that remain associated, even though acquisition of the association is based on simultaneity of the perceptions. You might consider also how slowly, and with difficulty, firm associations between different sense modalities are acquired, but, once acquired, with what security they are then utilized. Initiation of these pathways may present quite specific difficulties.

References

1. Ziehen GTh. Leitfaden der physiologischen Psychologie in 14 Vorlesungen. Jena: Gustav Fischer; 1891.
2. Meynert Th. Sammlung von popular-wissenschaftlichen Vorträgen über den Bau und die Leistungen des Gehirns. Vienna; Wilhelm Braumüller; 1892. p. 5.
3. Wernicke C. Der aphasische Symptomencomplex, eine psychologische Studie auf anatomischer Basis. Breslau: M. Cohn und Weigert; 1874.
4. Goldscheider A. Über zentrale Sprach-, Schreib- und Lesestörung. Berl klin Wochenschr. 1892:4,5,6,7,8.

Lecture 5

5

- The body is a part of the outside world
- Awareness of physicality is a function of the central projection fields
- Organ sensation and sensory content of sensations
- 'Feeling tone' [Ed] of sensations
- The large intestine represented in bodily awareness

Lecture

Gentlemen!

I can best show you how important to our topic are the intuitions gained so far, by again confronting you with a tangible example: Suppose that someone awakens from deep sleep or morbid unconsciousness. His organ of consciousness is functioning again, enabling him to recognize the outside world and note the normal occurrence of a 'behavioural loop' [Ed]. Consciousness of the outside world had been lost to the sleeper, or rather had not functioned during the time when consciousness was lost. After it returns, how does the person who has lost consciousness behave? We observe that he corrects the uncomfortable position that he had adopted, and feels his body, in order to convince himself of its integrity, and we note that his interest is apparently directed towards his own body. Consciousness of *corporeality* [W] has returned; and we should now examine this process more closely.

Given that sensory impressions and hence information from the outside world reach our brain only by means of the projection system, then most basic considerations teach us that the same is also true of our body parts. Only via nerve pathways which link a particular body part, such as the arm, with the brain, is the brain brought into connection with it; if the pathway is divided, as seen frequently after physical injuries, something quite unrestrained may follow in that body part—it can be pressed, punched, rolled, crushed, or burnt, without the slightest sensation being transmitted to the brain and reaching our consciousness. Incidents of this nature are most commonly observed in the arm, because the brachial plexus lies relatively superficially and therefore is most commonly exposed to external forces.

Since this example applies to all other regions of the body, it is a universal principle that integrity of the nervous system is required to give us perceptions of our own physicality. An unconscious person in whom the brachial plexus is destroyed, upon waking, can no longer identify his arm as his 'property' [W]. Thus consciousness of physicality appears to be a quite general function of the entirety of our sensory nerves, in other words, of the projection system. Meynert's statement, on the significance of a transverse section through this projection system at the level of

R. Miller, K.J. Dennison (eds.), *An Outline of Psychiatry in Clinical Lectures*,
DOI 10.1007/978-3-319-18051-9_5

the cerebral peduncle, also applies to consciousness of physicality: Were that procedure to be carried out, sensation would then arise only from the retina and the olfactory organ. Let us imagine that, instead of such a transection, which cannot actually be carried out, another procedure is carried out which is even less feasible but just as easy to envisage: The skull cap is exposed, and the brain is gently lifted from the floor of the cranium and, with no collateral injuries, raised high above the cranial cavity: Blood vessels, nerves, medulla oblongata, and spinal cord would not have suffered any damage in this stretching process. Then the brain appears to us for the first time, in its true form, as a fully sentient and moving entity, one equipped with a mechanism for registering sensory stimuli, and for executing movements; yet, in relation to the brain it amounts to a part of the outside world, even though it is inseparably connected with the brain. Sensations would, as before, reach consciousness, but with a slight delay caused by the longer pathway; movements would likewise be possible, as before, except that here too delivery of a command would take longer. The brain might then, as in an example already given by Meynert, be compared with a mollusc, bearing both 'sensory tentacles' [Ed]—the sensory nerves—and 'capture tentacles' [Ed]—the motor nerves. The fact that the former tentacles are armed with a complex sensory apparatus, and the latter with a special movement apparatus—the skeletal musculature—does not detract from the analogy. Observations made earlier with regard to sensations will therefore also be useful with respect to our physicality. Also, consciousness of our own corporeality is initially acquired, just as is consciousness of the outside world, by messages from the most widely varied parts of the body reaching their central projection fields in the brain, and leaving there, as residues, memory images.

Some of these projection fields are already known to us in broad terms, localized to specific sites in the cerebral cortex. There is no doubt that cortical regions demonstrated by Munk—which he called arm region, leg region, head region, ear region, and trunk and neck regions—are important central projection fields of those body parts. Human pathology provides irrefutable evidence that such experimental results apply to the human brain, even if we still await precise delineation of corresponding regions in humans. Also, in my view there can no longer be any doubt that each region represents the total sensibility and motility of the designated body part, the arm region, which thus constitutes the central projection field for sensibility and motility or, in other words, the entire nervous system of the arm. Here we face a relationship calling for our full attention: All these body regions are covered by the tactile organ—the skin—and corresponding central projection fields also contain representations of these sensory surfaces. On the other hand, representation of the body will not give us complete 'awareness of corporeality' [W] if central projection fields of the special senses are ignored, since the olfactory mucosa, the retina, the auditory organ, and the lingual and pharyngeal mucosa serving taste, although mediating specific sensory functions, at the same time themselves constitute most important parts of our body. We must therefore put to one side awareness of the physicality of *these* [Ed] sense organs, even if a special projection is not detectable (as for example for the olfactory and taste mucosa via certain trigeminal branches) at their already familiar central projection fields. Therefore, in the cerebral cortex, we are often made conscious of both the outside world and of our own physicality. Here we meet more complex relationships, forcing us again to resort to basic operations of simple sensation.

What we have so far learned for familiar sensation, and which provides material for us to construct our awareness of the external world, can also be described as the sensory content of stimuli. However, we know that any sensation has yet another quality, which we have ignored so far, generally identified as the 'feeling tone' [Ed] of the sensation as opposed to its sensory content. This 'feeling tone' [Ed] of sensation, as I hope to show, is particularly closely related to consciousness of corporeality in that it has a different coloration depending on the site of the applied stimulus, and thus to some extent emits a 'local sign' [Ed] for consciousness—a sign indicating which part of the body has been affected by the sensory stimulus. Stimuli linked to strong feeling tone are closely related to motor responses which appear to serve protective functions for the body. We usually pay no attention to these *organ sensations* [W], which pass us by, our attention being directed to the sensory content of the stimuli. However, slightly stronger stimuli reach our awareness to such an extent that we ignore the sensory content and focus instead on the organ sensation of the affected body part. Already, however, appropriate defensive movements have taken place. A few examples illustrate this: Imagine that your arm is unexpectedly touched in a crush of people; depending on the type of touch, you immediately consider whether the touch came from a person or an object. But if you receive a solid blow, such that the assault is painful, you immediately pull your arm back and try to protect it from further injury. Your attention is directed to the afflicted part of the body. The same response applies to loud noises: Everyone recoils when a shot is fired unexpectedly close to their ear, and nobody remains in the immediate vicinity as an express train rushes past, even though they know that there is no real danger. Here too the 'racket' [Ed] is the essential component eliciting the powerful organ sensation and involuntary rebound. A simpler protective reaction, namely closing the eyes, is seen on exposure to bright light, especially immediately following complete darkness; and in those situations pain can also be felt. When the eye initially focuses on a point source of light, using mechanisms of movement already discussed in the context of visual processing, this also is an example of organ stimulation. All such examples of movement, some simple, some complex, must be considered under Meynert's idea of defensive or offensive movements, and we remember that their origins are innate functional reflexes. I recall Pflüger's famous experiment where a decapitated frog could produce not only protective movements, but even adaptive modification of them, such that, in the attempt to wipe off an area of skin dabbed with acid immediately after its leg on the stimulated side had been amputated, recruited the other leg to assist. Such modifications may be acquired by each individual; they involve at least those regions of grey matter to which only reflex activity can be ascribed; they are doubtless functional as innate reflexes; and they serve protective functions even amongst humans, as in lower animals with predominantly spinal organization. Within this organization the lowest vertebrate can show more than simple reflex movements in that, like the decapitated frog, it has a capacity to make appropriate adaptations. However, where a large cerebral hemisphere is present, as in mammals, and more so in humans, we see similar mechanisms of movement transferred to central projection fields of the cerebral cortex (as shown experimentally by Munk for eye movements). In both cases appropriate modification of the movement is observed, depending on the part of the body affected. This demonstrates that organ stimuli have the immediate aim of protecting the body.

'Local signs' [Ed] in the retina, already discussed in relation to visual perception, now appear in a new light. They originated apparently from organ stimulation of the retina, since we saw that receptive elements, depending on their location in the retina, control movement mechanisms in the cortex in such a manner that the *fovea centralis* [W] always faces the stimulus. They can therefore be considered in Meynert's terminology as defensive or offensive movements. In fact, in the animal kingdom, they must prove equally effective in defence and attack. We have already anticipated when this can be used to explain formation of visual images. However, for this action to proceed, a spatial image of the retina has to be acquired in our own consciousness of corporeality. Thus if receptor cells of the visual projection field assigned to retinal points are to be matched with various points of the oculomotor projection field along the retinal meridian (with the level of oculomotor activity depending on the distance from the centre of the retina), there is an immediate need for a fixed orientation of the location of retinal points, thus achieving a solid image of the retina itself. This arrangement would be achieved through association. The process would be the same as that for acquisition of visual memory images: Through simultaneity or succession of excitation of adjacent retinal points a fixed association arises between corresponding sensory cells on the one hand, and accommodating movements of the eye (between the latter and the points of the motor projection field) on the other. By constant recurrence of the same behaviour under the same conditions, the associations achieve the necessary stability and attain a degree of 'solidity' [Ed]. Evidently consciousness must be initially focused on the retina before the images derived from it can be used spatially.

This spatial sense of the retina—that the retina comes to be viewed as forming part of the body surface—is derived by reasoning similar to that which applies to the tactile organ of the skin, with the associated optical apparatus of the eye merely providing support. Likewise in the skin, a spatial sense can only develop from the fact that consciousness is already informed about the sequence and location of the sensory skin points. Moreover, this information can only be obtained by rehearsal of the associations between sensory elements or perception cells that correspond with points on the skin and mechanisms of movement in the motor projection fields of the thorax, the eyes, and the limbs. However, we must regard the latter as being much more complex than the combinations of movement produced by eye muscles. Just think how relatively easy the movements of the eyeball seem, freely moveable around a centre of rotation within a defined space, compared with the multi-branched tactile organ of the hand. If we focus solely on the simplest tactile movements, such as flexion and extension of the finger, we have known since the time of Duchenne that these cannot take place without reciprocally directed movements of the wrist, which clearly provide fixation for the forearm. The forearm must in turn be fixated in relation to the upper arm, and the latter to the shoulder; however, the latter fixation in turn involves corresponding activation of the thoracic musculature, without which the torso might lose its balance during hand use. Thus, before the hand can be used as a sense organ, it must acquire certain regular relationships between many separate motor mechanisms. This task seems so difficult that we might doubt the possibility of solving it, were it not for the evidence before our eyes.

Gentlemen, I cannot avoid the concerns you might have about my view—it could be a more or less arbitrary construct, and might not stand up to rigorous scrutiny and evidence; but allow me to mention briefly those facts, which I am forced to accept, as essential to the view I have just presented to you so vigorously. One fact is that in cortical diseases, whether in the occipital, or parietal lobe, persisting deficits have been observed: in the former case in the visual fields, in the latter in sensation of skin over the limbs. In my opinion, occurrence of such deficits provides irrefutable proof that adjoining retinal points must project to adjoining cortical elements in the occipital lobe; and adjoining cutaneous areas of the limbs must have similar projections to adjoining cortical elements of the parietal lobe. Occurrence of localized and thus continuous deficits of this type would otherwise be quite inexplicable. The most direct and therefore the most likely assumption is that this projection relates to the most immediate endings of projection fibres—those on the 'perception cells' [Ed] serving perception.

The second fact consists of the secure orientation, which we maintain in relation to the retina and the entire skin surface. I need not present this for the retina. Yet we know this also for the skin of the body: We know it for certain for any chosen part of the body capable of fine spatial discrimination. Any person with closed eyes can immediately indicate a skin area that has been touched. Not only can he describe it, or point it out with his finger, but he can also correctly and without hesitation fix his eyes on the point that has been touched. At locations with a very fine spatial sense, such as the palm of the hand, he can, from the sequence of touching the skin, reconstruct a letter, a number, and even a pattern drawn there. Similar experiments are successful in most people, even for a number of other areas of skin.

Gentlemen, if you have followed me so far, you have gained only the most essential building blocks for building up an awareness of our own physicality, but you will still find it incomplete, in need of some increment to make good the deficit. It still lacks representation from three most important sensory areas, for hearing, taste, and smell. There is no difficulty transferring the point of view that we have acquired to these senses as well. At least this may be clear for the sense of hearing, because there the sensory content of the sensation—think of speech sounds—achieves an importance dominating one's entire mental life. Nevertheless we have already seen an example of circumstances where organ stimulation of this sense is so powerful that it induces a defensive withdrawal response; and not only the intensity, but also the quality of auditory sensations can bring about similar effects. For example, it is common experience that some noises create feelings and movement of shuddering, or are regarded as a pleasant or unpleasant tone. We know that apart from specific spatial sensibility, the organ of hearing is unique, in that the source of an auditory sensation can be specified. However its fine development appears only in abnormal cases, although it does demonstrate that certain local signs indicating the location of an applied stimulus are also present within the auditory sensory surface, quite apart from the organ of Corti, which conveys to us the pitch of a tone.

In taste and smell, organ sensations and sensory content are so closely connected that any separation of the two is quite artificial. As you know, these two exquisite senses for chemical analysis, important for both nourishment and protection of the organism, lie openly exposed.

Also included among organ sensations are sensations emanating from the muscles, joints, and large intestines. The last named show best that organ sensations can have an independent role, and can occur with no sensory experience. Such organ sensations have little impact on our consciousness when we are in a good state of health, although hunger and sense of repletion, the urge to urinate or defaecate, sexual sensations, etc. are familiar to us all. Nevertheless, intestinal illness demonstrates that these senses possess a highly labile sensitivity, and contribute most to our feelings of well-being or malaise. In fact this is the element that you can always identify as the 'feeling tone' [W] of any sensation, i.e. its accompanying feelings of pleasure or pain, with organ sensations from the digestive tract dominating all the others—even those relating to location of sensations.

Localization of these intestinal sensations is always quite vague, even though the sensation is distinct: Think of stomach pains, gallstones, renal colic, discomfiture from an overfull bladder, etc. Thus normal and impaired function of these organs contributes most to our general state; in other words, consciousness of our own physicality clearly depends on the state of our large intestine. We should actually define the aforementioned 'feeling tone' [W] of sensations generally, as afflictions of our consciousness of physicality. We should then assume that consciousness of corporeality also contains special projection fibres from the large intestines, an assumption that gains strong support from some hypochondriacal symptoms in people with mental illnesses. With regard to the location of these projection fields, admittedly, we are at present in ignorance, apart from Meynert's hypothesis that the ganglia of the striatum would participate in this. Seductive as this might seem, obvious considerations, both anatomical and morphological, leave the idea still floating in mid-air, and allow no practical applications.

The entirety of memory images of all organ sensations forms the content of our consciousness of corporeality, just as memory images of sensations constitute consciousness of the outside world. We can now attempt to define psychologically the viewpoint we have acquired, realizing that the former refers to *location* [Ed] of stimuli, and the latter to the their *form* [Ed] or the mutual organization of their stimulated elements.

We can also now define, in a few words, the essential difference between a sensory percept itself and its memory image: Sensory percepts are always accompanied by organ sensations and are therefore projected to certain spatial locations; memory images, on the other hand, are not. Apparently it is the 'perception cells' [W] immediately connected to retinal and to cutaneous points, which convey organ sensations.

I have already indicated that all projection fields, which encompass consciousness of bodily sensitivity, must be considered as intimately connected with each other by association pathways. Since the messages that the body itself transmits to consciousness are always the same, under the same conditions, this results in a permanent link from bodily sensations to memory images, because the former can never be thought of as memory images of the outside world. Various parts of bodily physicality are quite immutable in their relationship with one another; in contrast, external entities are more variable. We can more or less cut ourselves off from the external world; by contrast, sensations provided by our body are always with us. During sleep, the effects of the outside world seem to pass us by, virtually without trace; however the body surfaces, on which we lie, continue to send their signals to our consciousness. Whatever posture we adopt when awake, we cannot escape the continual pressure and our perception of it on some part of our skin.

Such awareness of bodily physicality accompanies a person throughout their waking state, and is seen unmistakably in their behaviour. If a person's attention is attracted to an object in the outside world so strongly that, at times, he is deeply entranced on hearing a melody, the body still maintains its upright position, continues to walk, avoids obstacles, adapts unevenness in the terrain, makes widely varied defensive movements, etc.

It is now clear that, from any organ sensation, the entire complex of memory images of the body's organs is brought to consciousness. Thus, if we adhere to the analogy based on 'consciousness of the outside world' [W], then what is built up here is, so to speak, simply one large concept, that of corporeality. This refers at least to those defensive movements with which we are familiar through powerful organ sensations, since virtually the entire body musculature can take part. In the formation of concepts of specific body regions, defined as firmly as befits concepts of the outside world, these seem not to encroach on consciousness of corporeality, or only incompletely so. Since sensory perception is not possible without evoking relevant organ sensations, consciousness of corporeality *in toto* [W] is also evoked by any sensory perception. Consciousness of corporeality therefore also arises from every act of sensory perception.

Organ sensations certainly then have two sources: In addition to stimuli from the outside world, they are also evoked by internal stimuli. Think of warmth or coldness of the skin due to vasomotor processes; perverse taste sensations during catarrh of the oral mucous membrane; subjective tinnitus—so-called noises in the ear; light flashes that are unrelated to the retina during total darkness, etc. None of these organ sensations relate to the outside world. The reciprocal relationship that exists here is that although sensory perception is inconceivable without corresponding organ sensations, the latter occur only when stimuli lack connection to the outside world. *Perception has organ sensation as a precursor* [W]; but, decisively, organ sensation has no corresponding links to perception. This also suggests that the idea of central projection fields that I already developed—namely, that consciousness of corporeality is represented by perception cells—implies also that the first station in the cortex must be no more than an intermediate port of call, to be passed before a sensory stimulus conveys consciousness of the outside world. The laminar layout of nerve cells of the cerebral cortex favours this assumption, according to which the cortical layer (or layers) immediately adjacent to white matter would represent consciousness of corporeality.

At certain times a person's body—already well developed—can still undergo noticeable change—the time of entering sexual maturity, or puberty; the climacteric; pregnancy; puerperium; and senile involution. In our opinion it is no longer strange that these are times of special vulnerability for development of various diseases of consciousness.

The relative immutability of our consciousness of corporeality explains why our body appears as constant in size, compared with other contents of consciousness—as one unit, as opposed to the impressions of the outside world, which are subject to changes. Through experience, our consciousness learns that corporeality is indivisible; the outside world however can be more or less broken into its component parts. Thus our body comes to form a 'primary ego' [W] (Meynert), under which we comprehended our consciousness of corporeality.

Lecture 6

6

- Concept of spontaneous movement
- Distinction from reflex movement
- Position sense and position representation
- Sensations of nervous activation of muscle, and their memory images
- Sense of motion and movement imagery both derive from organ sensations
- Also, tactile sensations and touch representations from the hand's tactile organ are derived from organ sensations

Lecture

Gentlemen!

You may already have noticed that so far I have completely ignored a group of phenomena that have close connection with our awareness of physicality, namely our entire apparatus for movement. I have avoided this until now, because it is quite complicated. How can we understand that any comparative mollusc learns to master its muscular system so completely—as is indeed the case—if we avoid consideration of its innate abilities? We now examine this point more closely.

It is known that humans like all vertebrates still bear the clearest traces of their lineage from the invertebrates, in that the spinal cord preserves a segmentation, designated by the numbered vertebrae. We must also remember to take this metameric structure into account along with that 'motion machine' [Ed] which supports the brain. This operates by reflex mechanisms of the spinal cord, which, right from the start, bring sensory and motor apparatus of the same transverse level into mutual relationship. This is probably why a gentle prick applied to the plantar surface of the toes immediately elicits a plantar flexion reflex. This metamerism not only determines the structure of the spinal cord, but also, as shown in Pflüger's 'irradiation of reflexes' [Ed], recruits larger muscle areas, according to the stimulus strength, even almost all muscle groups, involving connections which are presumably built into the grey matter of the spinal cord. These reflexes have no immediate link to awareness; they are innate, taking place even in the absence of consciousness, as in deep sleep or coma. However, later, when awake, we become aware of them. That mollusc, by comparison, receives information from reflex movements based on innate characteristics of its body. Without immediately prejudging more detailed statements, we can call these messages 'sensations of movement' [W], and their residual memory images 'representations of movement' [W] or motor memory images. Now, let us try to understand those 'sensations of movement' [W] in greater detail.

In reflex movement, a whole series of different sensations arise. First, let us denote the joint which is moved, by *g*. Joint sensation depends on the excursion of a given joint movement, and is associated with a certain skin sensation *h*,

R. Miller, K.J. Dennison (eds.), *An Outline of Psychiatry in Clinical Lectures*,
DOI 10.1007/978-3-319-18051-9_6

because, on the flexor side of the joint, skin surfaces are shortened to a specific extent, and approach one another; on the extensor side, on the other hand, surfaces are stretched and move apart. Thus there is a constant relationship between g and h, which applies if the joint reaches the same position passively. However, muscles are also demonstrably involved, since during flexion they are relaxed on the flexor side, and elongated and stretched on the extensor side, the opposite occurring during extension. Observations from pathology demonstrate that these muscle sensations m are independent of—and can sometimes occur in the absence of—skin and joint sensations. The highly specific ratio of these three sensations to one another, that is, $g{:}h{:}m$, we call 'position sense' [W], l, so that $l = g{:}h{:}m$.

We can call memory images formed from this 'position representations' [W] L. The same position sense must arise when the joint is moved passively, and is in no way linked exclusively to reflex action.

A subject's position representations can be examined clinically, because a person passively adopts some arbitrary position for his joints. A healthy person is then in a position to either imitate these positions, or to make some alteration; at least we recognize that he has full control over the position of his limbs. This investigation is particularly relevant for easily moveable joints of fingers and toes. Successful testing of position sense depends on total exclusion of the subject's own activity, that is, elimination of his own motor impulses. This, of course, is not equally possible for all individuals, because it presupposes the person to have a degree of control over his movements.

Muscle sensation has previously, and incorrectly, been given a dominant role in position sense, and therefore presence of position representations as a unique sense has been called the 'muscle sense' [W]. We prefer not to use this word, since it can lead to further misunderstanding.

Suppose now that position sense l is generated by reflex action; this creates the sensation of movement b; but another feature must be added to what has gone before: It may be nothing more than sensation linked with nerve cell activity z, which can be taken as the origin of nervous activation of muscle at the moment of the reflex. Muscle contractions which occur at this moment trigger certain muscular sensations m_1; and these stand in constant relationship with activity in nerve cells z, thus $m_1{:}z$. We can then designate the message which reaches consciousness, as the sense of nervous activation i, and then $i = z{:}m_1$. The movement sensation b, taken as a whole, then contains both components of the reflex movement—the sense of nervous activation—and the position sense—and these, as is readily apparent, stand in constant relation to each other: $b = i{:}l$.

Muscle sensation m_1 can also be tested directly, by electrical stimulation of the muscle. In this case, the most that can be determined is the current strength that can be perceived, and whether changes in this measure are perceptible. The resulting joint movement requires a separate position sense, perceived like any other in normal awareness. However, a regular connection between muscle sensation and position sense does not exist in this experiment, because isolated contraction of one muscle never occurs normally, the experimental conditions thus being a novelty for conscious awareness.

Sensations of movement which reach consciousness in this way, and which, through their content, always recur in like manner, develop into movement representations, as robust features of consciousness, which we can denote as B. Although they give rise to memory images limited to reflex movements, definite patterns of muscle activation are nonetheless represented, since reflex movements are undoubtedly coordinated, in the sense described by Duchenne. According to Duchenne's classification of muscle coordination, as impulsive, collateral, or antagonistic, reflex movements are impulsive and collateral. Reflex movements are not lacking in usefulness, and can be considered more clearly as protective reactions, which defend against a stimulus, or remove part of the body from the vicinity of a stimulus. These two occasions can be regarded as the most important preconditions leading to spontaneous movements. A person recalls that during reflex movement a message reaches consciousness not only from the movement itself, but also from the sensation *e*, which elicited the reflex. The memory image *E* of this stimulus, whether it be tactile or directly painful, will consequently remain associated with the movement representation *B*. We will then only speak of spontaneous movement, when the memory image *E* evokes the movement representation *B* through the association pathway *EB* in such a manner that the movement actually takes place. A necessary assumption is that a centrifugal pathway *p* stretches from *B* to the nerve cells which went into action previously during the reflex response. This pathway has, in fact, been demonstrated: It is the pyramidal tract.

Two examples will illustrate in more detail the essential difference between reflex and spontaneous movement. A needle applied to the sole of the foot is followed by reflex flexion of the lower limb at all three joints, thereby removing the foot from the sharp point. In spontaneous movement we only see [Ed] the needle; the memory image *E* of the tactile sensation *e* thereby is brought into consciousness and, via the association pathway *EB*, elicits the movement that had previously taken place by reflex. The pathway *Bz*, which is still required, is the pyramidal tract. It behaves in the same way if the eyes were to be closed as the needle approaches: Initially visual perception occurs; this is associated with the memory image *E*, as is the latter with movement representation *B*. We can now define spontaneous movements in general as responses to external stimuli mediated by memory images. In reality most spontaneous movements throughout life are constructed from all kinds of external stimuli, although we cannot exclude the possibility that external stimuli are totally absent; thus spontaneously emerging memory images are the start for association processes which end ultimately in movement.

The first spontaneous movements a child makes are apparently under control of organ sensations. Suckling movements, which are reflexes in the newborn, later become spontaneous movements brought about by bodily feelings of hunger. Later still, the sight of the nipple is sufficient to elicit suckling movements. A child's sensitivity to bright light, in eliciting eyelid closure, is another indication of dominance of bodily sensation. Amongst spontaneous movements, those which are overwhelmingly dominant in the first years of life are *defensive movements* [W], as more or less faithful imitations of reflex movements, again based on bodily sensations. There are also very complex combinations of movement persisting throughout adult life, such as the combined response to a shock, including jumping backwards and leaping sideways, controlled mainly by bodily sensations, as we already know from earlier examples; and if you accept a hereditary influence on development of language—which is hard to deny—you should trace the drive to imitate audible sounds back to bodily sensations from the auditory nerve. In other words, you must assume that excitation of the auditory nerve at a given moment is connected with a pleasant feeling, and that a child's discovery that they themselves can produce sounds can be used to create such pleasant sensations by its own vocal gestures. Bodily feelings in the visual sense are still detectable in adults when they acknowledge pleasurable sensations hinting at titillation in the play of colours, where various saturated colours follow one another in rapid succession. We can hardly doubt that, in the auditory sense, pleasure provided by producing a particular tone has a similar basis.

This simplest scheme for spontaneous movement, as just described, can soon be applied to the active acquisition of tactile representations. As in reflex action, a movement follows a stimulus, for instance when visual perception of a needle leads to eye closure mediated via association pathways; so, undoubtedly, visual perception of an object may trigger tactile movements—'attack movements' [W] in Meynert's sense. Given that our entire skin surface functions as a passive tactile organ conveying obscure tactile perceptions in the absence of any bodily movement, we still possess specific moveable tactile organs, actual *feelers* [Ed] for discriminative sensation in the limbs, and also, in the first stages of life, the mouth. A child examines by touch every object that he sees, with hand or mouth. For the retina, as described above, each memory image was the residue of a particular spatial arrangement of excited retinal elements, and this principle must also apply to memory images from the passive tactile organ. For the retina, there was a definite point of clearest vision which we can then use as the site for acquiring memory images. For the skin, there are also places of greatest sensitivity, such as an infant's mouth and the skin of hands and fingers. We may still suppose that such a limited skin area by itself can give rise to memory images; but they can also be acquired from any skin surface. With certain limitations this is of course also true of the retina, since objects perceived outside the fovea can be recognized accurately, and one can postulate that, for the retina, memory images acquired in this manner will gradually become associated with images obtained in central vision. A similar association between memory images applies to the various skin surfaces, once it is grasped that they originate from the same objects; and one can consider them to arise in central projection surfaces of a passive tactile organ. Nevertheless one cannot deny that finer representations of touch are acquired through the *movable* [Ed] tactile organs—the hands and fingers. Let us take a closer look at how this happens.

If a solid item such as a penknife is touched, assuming this to be done with only one hand, and we let palmar surfaces of the fingers, with many changes of position, play over it to convince us of the consistency, smoothness or roughness, surface temperature, and overall form and dimensions of the object. We then consider all these sensations together, as a single unit, which recurs only on subsequent occasions when a penknife is felt—but for no other solid object. If we call this unit the 'tactile sensation' [Ed] of an object t, then it is made up of a series of skin sensations $e_1+e_2+e_3$ ..., and a series of motor sensations $b_1+b_2+b_3$ ... standing in simple—yet also complex—relationship with the former. Simple, in the sense that any major muscle contraction reinforces the pressure sensation from the object; complex in so far as a series of successive movements is required, under conditions of constant pressure, to sense the object's shape. Just how complex the integral $t=e+b$ must be comes from the fact that each component of the series b_1+e_2 is itself already a composite integral, as I just discussed: Remember that $b=i{:}l$, implying a particular relationship between position sense and feelings of nervous activation; and now comes an added association with passive tactile sensations of the series e_1+e_2 .... We can call this complex integral t, the tactile sensation of an object. We then denote as T, a memory image, tactile representation, or probably a tactile image. In practice, we test for tactile representation by requiring a person to recognize specific objects merely by touch, using their hands, with eyes closed. A normal person solves this problem with ease, for every object he knows.

Gentlemen, by more detailed examination of this topic it should have become clear to you how important are the unique body movements in our sensory perceptions. Memory images from the sense of touch which, when we started our enquiry, could be traced back to a type of passive projection process (like other sensory perceptions) now appear to be assembled simultaneously from memory images of spontaneous movements. However, these motor memory images must correspond to consciousness of our own corporeality—our body form—so here we enter an area where awareness of the outside world and that of our own physicality lose their fundamental separation, refuting the proposition that only changes in our own physicality give us knowledge of objects in the outer world, and reverting to the most obvious: The similarity between the outside world and our own physicality, in their sensory connections, shows that all spontaneous movements give us mastery over the outside world ('attacking movements' [W], according to Meynert). Each skill or adroitness amongst our known movements, from walking and speech movements to the most complex movement sequences of a creative artist, must be learned laboriously. All these occur only under continual guidance from the sense of touch: They are made possible only by our possessing a large repertoire of most complex tactile representations. If we undertake to test such varieties of movement representation, we tend to concentrate on the simplest evidence of manual dexterity.

For example, a patient is given the task of unbuttoning his clothes and then buttoning them up again with eyes closed, or sharpening a pencil, winding a clock, writing numbers or letters in the air, or writing in the normal way. With few exceptions, handling one or more objects is always required, and, in order to carry out the required movements, tactile representations must be available.

Since in the tactile representations just discussed movements are linked to skin sensations, there is a quite complex muscular apparatus, whose movements are under control of impressions from the retina. If the form of an object is to be perceived precisely, then, with familiarity and by appropriate eye movements, the point of clearest vision is scanned across the contours of the object, a process entirely analogous to scanning by that tactile organ, the finger, and to be described just as for scanning by the *macula lutea* [W]. The intricate eye movements required to leave behind motor memory images form a series of associations, very similar to those discussed above, obtained by scanning with the hand. When these are merged with passively acquired memory images of principal sensations *E*, then together they represent the complete tactile concept of an object. The motor memory images—so to speak—of scanning eye movements, are a new component which, when associated with those with which we are already familiar, constitute a single unit which we may justifiably call a 'visual representation' [W]. For eye movements it is unfortunately not possible to analyze position sense and position representations separately. Nevertheless their importance in spatial orientation can hardly be overestimated—they are a further striking example of how organ sensations can be surveyed to build a coherent picture of the outer world in our consciousness. In conclusion I draw to your attention a similar relationship between tactile exploration and auditory perceptions: A child's vocal gestures are tentative movements unrelated to skin or retinal sensations, but which are related to and guided by auditory sensations.

In so far as we have been able to survey the contents of consciousness, up to now we have seen definite localization of function made possible through the fact of projection. As visual memory images are explicitly localized in the central projection field of the optic nerve, and acoustic ones in the central projection field of the acoustic nerve, we cannot doubt that the tactile representations of solid objects are localized in like manner. Simple figures, such as numbers, a cross, a circle, and a triangle, can be recognized by touch, when drawn on the skin surface with the subject's eyes closed. Therefore central projections of the passive tactile organ—the skin—develop a *space* [Ed], like the retina, wherein reciprocal arrangement of skin points aroused by a stimulus influences the resulting memory images.

As stated above, these cutaneous memory images become tactile representations through their association with movement representations of the tactile elements.

The same tactile images thus reach various projection fields, but are connected with one another not only by secure associations, but also, above all, by visual representations held in common. Tactile representations of solid objects should be localized exclusively to the arm region, although, of course, in different hemispheres for right and left arm because such tactile representations are acquired, in adults at least, exclusively through hand movements.

It is also to be understood that we have no innate orientation of the position of retinal points, these needing to be acquired. Orientation 'above' [Ed] and 'below' [Ed] or 'left' [Ed] and 'right' [Ed] refers exclusively to one unique body, meaning no more than the acquisition of strong associations between perception cells, associated with points on the retina, and the 'concept' [W] (see above) of our own corporeality. This brings two kinds of movement sensation into consideration: firstly those originating as deliberate gaze movements upwards, downwards, and to right and left. These could be called mass eye movements. Second are those serving to adjust the eyeball to the light stimulus or rotating it—to be distinguished as adjustment movements. The fact that such eye movements can occur reflexly at any time during life is a necessary physiological postulate. The most likely movements are adjustments that, using appropriate preformed connections of primary visual centres with eye muscle nuclei, are triggered by a light stimulus. Sensations of nervous activation ($i=z{:}m_1$, see above) arising in this way have particularly fine sensitivity for eye muscles in this situation, given that you might not want to assume a special position sense in the eyeball (via the ciliary nerves?). Their memory images are movement representations for eye musculature. According to the manner of their acquisition, they become associated with perceptual elements in the projection field of the retina in such a way that, from each such element a particular form and particular degree (extent of excursion) of associated muscle combinations can be evoked.

Trigger points found by Munk in the canine occipital lobe, from which adjustment movements can be elicited, evidently correspond to such muscle combinations. In the dog they correspond in location with cortical projections of the retina and its centrifugal fibres, *Bz* (see above), and run conjointly with projection fibres of the retina in the sagittal cortical bundle of the occipital lobe. Thus far, they adopt a special position, and differ from fibres of the pyramidal tract.

Lecture 7

7

- Consciousness of personhood, or individuality
- Is its localization accessible?
- The mystery of self-awareness

Lecture

Gentlemen!

With the overview that I have given you of two great areas of awareness—of the environment and of our own corporeality, we have by no means exhausted the content of consciousness; those areas are just the first foundations of awareness we share with animals, albeit with quantitative differences. Higher mental development of humans must start from these fundamentals, but extends far beyond them: It sets sail—so to speak—from the point where these basics have already been acquired. The normal unfolding of mental development results in the formation of a 'personality' [Ed], or an individuality. An unconscious individual, who we choose as a subject for our study, must regain consciousness of his own personhood before we can consider him to be fully reconstituted: That is, he must remember not only that he has the same body as before his accident, but has remained the same in terms of his whole mental status. A prerequisite for 'consciousness of personhood' [W], which we should now consider in detail, is the possibility of development of an 'ego' [Ed]. The main condition for this is the possible existence of an unchanging sense of corporeality, in contrast to the ever-changing environment, as we have already seen. As soon as a child begins to operate with the word 'I' [W], constraints are felt from these facts. If mental development were cut short before this time, the outcome would be an imbecile who would speak of his body in the third person. Awareness of personhood therefore includes everything that you tend to understand linguistically as intellectual 'property' [Ed] and intellectual *acquis* [Ed]—everything introduced to the child through teaching, education, and child-rearing, so that the individual infant can be transformed into a person.

The first distinguishing hallmark of each human is undoubtedly the social environment in which he grows up. Living examples have always been the most effective means of education, the more so when they combine with the obvious implicit authority of parents towards their child. Family life of parents is indubitably imprinted as the ultimate stamp on the child, his intellectual personality, and his future character. Consciousness of personhood thus includes all those properties arising as instinctive regularities in the social environment in which each individual grew up and lived. These properties include notably all those so-called character traits, which develop in specific ways in each family environment, according to whether it was a more brutal or a more refined 'temper of life'

R. Miller, K.J. Dennison (eds.), *An Outline of Psychiatry in Clinical Lectures*,
DOI 10.1007/978-3-319-18051-9_7

[Ed], and on which depend the predominance of more egotistical or more altruistic objectives of a person's future actions. Such characteristics can also develop quite strongly, even where the most powerful, even half-instinctive method of child-raising, the spoken word, cannot be used, as witnessed for example in deaf mutes.

Possession of language itself must in some sense be associated with awareness of personal identity, insofar as it reflects the style of the environment in which each individual has lived. The variety of language used by different nations has a special place within 'intellectual property' [Ed] differing from that used almost everywhere else, despite similar consciousness of the outside world and of the body's physicality. Within one and the same population there may be differences in dialect, which remain with an individual throughout his life and betray where he has lived. An individual's entire style of speech, which differs quite markedly according to the manner of his upbringing, and his level of intellectual development, adds to the evidence of personalized consciousness. Through language, the entire mental acquisition of an adult, and not only of each individual but of countless generations whose intellectual heritage he has encountered through language, is transferred to the child's brain. This is done with a certain logical order and structure, somewhat comparable to skill on a musical instrument, yet not complex enough to be considered as virtuoso performance. Orderly, logical thought and all finer intellectual operations undoubtedly have their main roots in the comprehensive yet traditional art of language. It is therefore also distinctive of the complete mindset of each individual—the language handed down from parents, whether poor and rough for a person of lowly status, or rich and more refined from highly educated parents. The altered manner of speech found in those with mental illnesses indicates a change in their intellectual personality.

If we disregard the child-rearing medium of speech, then everything that an individual otherwise learns is from instruction and what is handed down—the sum of all knowledge—which he adsorbs as part of his personality. When we speak of a person's memory we understand mainly the sum of his acquired knowledge; at least we usually examine memory by inquiring about such acquired knowledge, and a person's ability to recall it, compared to what is accessible for most normal people. The sum of such skills or knowledge varies widely, not only quantitatively but also qualitatively, depending on each individual's developmental processes. I need not explain the quantitative differences in more detail. Qualitatively it is so great because knowledge gained in early stages of education consists mainly of a series of associations devoid of any deeper connections—historical facts, memorized sayings and songs, the Ten Commandments, and even multiplication tables. As long as more new knowledge is acquired, it is assimilated into the existing repository of information, and is further refreshed and reinforced in memory. However this is not all of equivalent value since a child's brain is distinguished by its ability to retain what has been learned, and the knowledge needed and most commonly made use of early in life. Reading and writing usually belong to temporary acquisition of knowledge, although the acquired associations of letters with speech—associations that are often interrupted remarkably by focal lesions of the brain—are laid down very firmly.

To personalized consciousness belongs the sum of experiences peculiar to each individual. The individual we see before us always represents this sum total—be it knowledge, or experiences—a sum having a definite value only at a specific point in time, but which undergoes new growth every hour and every day. The current state of the brain is always this final summation of all previous states. Hence, after a person has recovered from a mental illness, it is required that we ensure that he has achieved insight into the abnormality of the state he has experienced, for the sum must necessarily be inaccurate if it contains false elements.

In like manner, personalized consciousness encompasses the range of each person's interests, be they self-centred, showing interest in other people, family, etc., his occupation, or clinging to daily work routines. In particular, interest in family, friends, and other people while laying aside personal concerns often occupy centre stage in the contents of an individual's consciousness—think of the intimate relationships between mother and child, between husband and wife in sexual love, etc. Willingness to go to one's death for others, or for an idea, a principle, or a predetermined ambition to die on the one hand, and the over-weaning, selfish world of interests of most people on the other demonstrate extreme opposites and infinite variety of intellectual personality types, all still falling within the normal range. Further varieties are added by illnesses. All this explains how difficult it is to describe mental status—be it that of a normal person, or of a mentally ill person; it also explains the slow progress of clinical psychiatry.

Personalized consciousness obviously depends on awareness of corporeality and of the environment. A man with keen senses and a healthy body must also develop differently in his intellectual personality, compared with one endowed with dulled senses and a feeble body. Character traits such as courage or cowardice, openness or concealment, vigorous action or doleful shyness—these can often be traced back to those same fundamentals in consciousness of corporeality and of the environment. Adaptability to the outside world, which Herbert Spencer identifies as a normal mental condition, itself varies according to such preconditions. One can express such a mutual relationship in this sentence: Personalized consciousness is a function of awareness of the environment and of corporeality. However, if you include impressions that come from the social *milieu* [W] within a person's awareness of the environment—which is justifiable—this sentence is still quite illuminating. It is then self-evident that such personalities develop in civilized conditions, while on the other hand antisocial personalities arise in criminal families. You will clearly not take a mental illness as an explanation of criminal tendencies, but can speak of such only when a person's intellect has developed in defiance of the external world, as in cases of the so-called moral insanity [W]. In any case, personalized consciousness is far more complex than consciousness of the environment and of corporeality, because it is based on those processes of association, which, from the outset, have certain intrinsic individual differences.

The position that each individual believes he occupies in a human society depends on his awareness of his own personality. If he is ill, we may see relevant symptoms of grandiosity, belittlement, persecution, etc. Later we will have much to say about such disease phenomena.

What spatial sense can we make of a personalized consciousness? Or have we already reached the limits of spatial representation, and confront the incomprehensible?

It seems that consciousness of corporeality is most accessible to cerebral localization because it is most closely connected with the normal arrangement of the projection system. Awareness of the environment likewise allows us to partition according to relevant projection fields, in which its components, the sensory memory images, are presumably stored. In our consciousness of being a person, localization according to such norms of the projection system is out of the question. Does it therefore remain totally inaccessible to the principle of localization?

Clinical experience teaches us that this is not so, because some mental illnesses draw attention exclusively to a person's awareness of their own personhood, others almost exclusively to their awareness of the environment, or of their own corporeality, while yet others reveal some other combination, of disorder of personal identity with a person's sense of bodily physicality or of his environment. Thus, the disease process appears to distribute itself in various locations. Mental illness which develops progressively and perniciously *κατ' εζοχηv* (to a prominent degree), such as progressive paralysis, attacks in turn an individual's awareness of their own personhood, of their environment, and of their own corporeality, and seems to begin quite often with atrophy of fibres in the outermost purely grey cortical layer. Still other clinical experiences present, and even suggest further localization for awareness of personhood. It so happens that in the wake of serious illnesses, including brain diseases, large fragments may disappear from an individual's awareness of their own personhood.

It may turn out that all ideas acquired recently—a period ranging from a few months or years, and sometimes up to half a lifetime—have been lost. Dr. Freund has published such cases from my own clinic [1], under the heading 'general weakness of memory' [Ed]. Patients in question have a fairly good memory—about as accurate as you would normally expect—for all events that took place before a certain period of time, for instance before the age of 30 years; all those happening later have vanished from their memory: Often this includes their most important personal events, such as marriage, birth of their children, loss of assets, and the like, but also well-known public events of the time, skills acquired during this time, etc. In a word, the loss encompasses the entire chain of events that has become linked to awareness of personal identity after a certain point in time. Consequently, one such patient, who is an elderly woman, still behaves like a young, blossoming girl, thereby becoming prey to a mocking contrast with reality. To a lesser degree, similar loss of memory is encountered almost normally in advanced old age where, commonly, old memories can be preserved in every detail, while memory for daily events of recent days, weeks, or months may be totally lost. The fact that experiences from a certain period in time can be lost as a result of gross physical illness allows a precise interpretation that the site of these complex memories is predetermined in the cerebral cortex from the time of their being laid down. From this, we can conclude, approximately, but most directly, that a kind of layered deposition of memories takes place in the brain, similar to sedimentary formations of the youngest strata of the earth. You might be tempted to assign the outer cortical layer facing away from the projection fibres to awareness of personhood, this being the youngest structure. Without letting the crudity of this notion to make us recoil in alarm, other considerations stand in the way of interpreting such experiences in terms of layer-wise localization. Occasionally we see circumscribed loss of recently acquired memories after focal lesions of the brain. Cases are known, and well documented, where a stroke occurs in people who are strongly multilingual, and this skill is lost, except for their mother tongue. Quite recently such a case was published by Charcot. Unfortunately, the distinction between skill in speaking and in understanding language has not been sufficiently analyzed, so that localization of the lost function in a strict sense is not possible. However, from reported facts, this much can be concluded with certainty: that the loss is quite analogous to any other focal symptom arising in a part of the brain. Now, suppose that a purely motor deficit was the issue here, one that, according to all our previous knowledge, would be attributed to Broca's convolution: Then, from our above assumption, quite specific layers of this convolution would be totally destroyed as a result of the stroke, while layers immediately above or beneath, and serving skills in the mother tongue, would be left completely unharmed. This seems highly unlikely. By contrast, the following idea has, in its favour, a whole series of other known facts. Cells and fibres of the cerebral cortex are extremely delicate structures, tending always to remain in an embryonic state until they begin to function. Only through functioning do they obtain a certain resilience, which increases in proportion to their functioning. This hypothesis is completely analogous to that which Cohnheim attributed to muscles—that they grow and increase only during their functioning. Now suppose that in the vicinity of focal brain damage, there is a centre, like that of Broca's convolution, where besides cells and fibres that have been functioning for a long time and therefore have a certain resilience, there are those placed at risk by slight injury. It therefore seems quite plausible that a side effect of acute focal damage spreads to surrounding tissue, and destroys one element while leaving others intact. The same explanation also applies to cases of general weakness of memory. As with the circumscribed location just described, it must be assumed that a harmful effect spreads throughout the cerebral cortex, where only resilient elements can survive, and it is then little wonder that the level of this resilience is a function of time; in other words, only those memories laid down most recently would disappear.

Personalized consciousness includes a specific highest level faculty of the brain, which has always been considered the mystery of mysteries, the phenomenon of *self-consciousness* [Ed]. In this aspect it appears that the same organ, the brain, in which you probably place your trust, is able to perceive, and at the same time, that it is also perceived. However, it seems impossible that one and the same being, or thing, which *makes* [W] a perception, could itself, at the same time, *be* [Ed] the object of perception. We can already see from this comparison the lack of clarity about matters at issue here that prevails amongst philosophers, who still feel the need to warn us against overestimating the importance of anatomical and physiological views on the subject. We should remember that personalized consciousness is a sum, whose value is a function of time; in other words, the perceiving individual, at the moment of perception, is a certain mental personality, differentiated from the personality of the previous moment, by a significant value; so it can be no surprise that this latter value is capable of perceiving previous values from recent times in that sum, as well as objects of sensory perception. In other words, the intellectual personality does not perceive *itself* [W], but only that personality that existed a few moments, hours, days, or years before. It is mere self-deception to believe oneself to have remained exactly the same.

Reference

1. Freund CS. Klinische Beiträge zur Kenntniss der generellen Gedächtnissschwäche. Arch Psychiatr. 1889;20:441–57.

Lecture 8

8

- The activity of consciousness dependent on the content of consciousness
- 'Preformed' [Ed] organization of the connections of thought
- Narrowness of consciousness
- Level of consciousness
- Attention and will
- Ability to be attentive
- Affect
- Normal value of apperceptions

Lecture

Gentlemen!

Let us take a backward glance at our journey so far. The organ of consciousness has been revealed as populated by a collection of potential energies, remembered images in their various groupings, from the simplest up to those of complex dimension, for which the name 'memories' [Ed] seems appropriate. For such contents of consciousness a natural division into three areas emerged—environment, corporeality, and personhood—an organization that, as we shall see later, is also required in practice for any observant physician. You will notice, however, that in such 'quiescent consciousness' [Ed], as it were, you face an inanimate machine. It is now our task to examine in greater detail the *activity* [Ed] taking place in the organ so constructed. However, we must acknowledge that this organ is composed exclusively of nerve fibres and nerve cell bodies, and that therefore we can demand no more from it than the sequence of certain excitatory processes, and, during its disease states, a morbid change in such processes. Moreover, in what we have considered so far, we needed no other precondition, because the contents of consciousness—the sum of all acquired perceptions—had no meaning for us other than that of permanent molecular alteration in purpose-built fibre and cell masses, resulting from excitatory processes that had taken place. We referred to the ability of nerve elements to undergo lasting changes elicited by stimuli that had occurred as their 'memory' [W], a phenomenon with analogies in the natural world of inanimate matter, since iron can be magnetized. Thus we deal here with excitatory processes in a complex organ, whose activity depends on excitation that it underwent in previous times. We should therefore examine, first of all, the nature of such dependence.

When a question from a particular field of knowledge is addressed to a person who is unfamiliar with that field he may find the very question incomprehensible. A fundamental principle applies here, which should surprise no one, about newly acquired perceptions: Understanding the question can be gained only on condition of preexisting acquired perceptions. If we refer to processes currently playing out in consciousness as 'mental activity' [W] and activity triggered by

R. Miller, K.J. Dennison (eds.), *An Outline of Psychiatry in Clinical Lectures*,
DOI 10.1007/978-3-319-18051-9_8

the question as 'registration' [W], and the result of mental activity included in the answer as 'execution' [W], then, in the present case, mental activity remains incomplete because the individual cannot produce activity corresponding to 'registration' [W]. If we bear in mind that mental activity is, as a rule, connected to an external stimulus, that is, any sensation, then sensory perception in general depends on such stimulation. Sensory perception that has never occurred previously and therefore cannot produce the usual consequent mental activity remains not only misunderstood, but also very imprecisely perceived: This fact convinces anyone who concentrates on the sounds of a foreign language. Thus if perception itself is to be precise, it requires certain preexisting 'mental acquisitions' [W]. Quite similar to these simple examples of mental activity is behaviour involving more complex thought processes, where registration is often merely casual sensory perception, which escapes our attention. Moreover, such complex thought processes usually take place along prescribed paths from which emerge relatively rare ideas that are truly new. Overall, mental activity shows itself to depend on a long history of acquiring ideas, and arranging them in special ways; that is, it usually means simply repetition of the same excitatory processes in the same order as have repeatedly taken place in the past.

What is the basis for the 'order' [W] prevailing in these perceptions, which is expressed in routine mental activity? As you may recall, we gave the name 'association' [W] to the network of perceptions; order prevailing in perceptions therefore allows us to unlock our cache of associations, which are roughly the same for all individuals. Our question can therefore be rephrased in the following way: In what way are such universally valid associations formed? In part, I build here on what was said earlier, and is already familiar to you. In speaking of consciousness of the outside world, I pointed out that the natural order and succession of things represented in our brain are, to some extent, a reflection, of what is present in the outside world. It is therefore legitimate to link phenomena found there, to those also found in our consciousness. Amongst those properties of things that we learn to be relatively constant and changeless are their relationship with other things, be they inanimate or animate, and, in particular, with our own person. The fact that water becomes ice when cooled, and becomes water vapour when heated, is an experience that we take as valid because of its constant occurrence. In our brain this is reflected by association between the perceptions of water, ice, and water vapour, and hot and cold, happening in a completely regular way. The cold sensation of the skin can then, by association, awaken the perception of water freezing. The association is somewhat more complicated when observation of a thermometer leads us to the same conclusion. Here, visual perception linked to the registration is learned, as well as its association with the other perceptions. Just as the simplest natural phenomena impose themselves in regular order so to speak, so it is for more complicated associations of perceptions that we learn from examples in our environment. Our innate drive to imitate is analogous to the compulsion with which natural phenomena impose themselves on our brains. From earliest years we are used to behaving always in the same way as others. For example a person learns, in the crudest sense, from the example of others, that you dig up crops, cook them, eat them, and thus satisfy hunger. Even this simple example suffices—the person plants crops *now* [Ed], with planting of crops itself as an objective, to satisfy hunger *later* [Ed]. This highly complex action is ultimately driven, after interpolation of a whole series of associations, by initial feelings of hunger. In the simplest condition, every activity is driven by similar examples from the environment. The environment in which the person grows up, or where he lives, therefore extends back to fill his consciousness with a whole series of perceptions in a very specific arrangement, and the more monotonous the flow of his life the more strongly and immutably is this arrangement of perceptions fixed, undisturbed by details of more complex living conditions. Collective consciousness requires that you should behave like everybody else, and may often still be effective when mental activity is totally dislocated as a result of mental illness; so the otherwise inaccessible—and always reluctant—mental patient adopts the examples of fellow patients. The entire institutional treatment of mentally-ill people is based on this principle. On the other hand, we can see how deeply this herd consciousness is ingrained in us too, when we participate in a group gathering, or any kind of mass demonstration, intending to remain passive, yet being dragged into the same feelings that inspire the crowd. Teaching by example is also effective in deaf mutes who have had no other instruction. If he has no other deficits, such a person may often be a useful member of society within a narrow walk of life.

However, the main way to acquire a particular order to one's perceptions is through articulated speech. Through this medium all finer and more precise relationships are made with ease, not only among concepts of solid and fixed objects, but also between these and events or activities—the latter in chronological order—and, by subtle nuances, the status of the personality in question is recognized. For more complex associations, abstract concepts [W] become familiar to us mainly through language, and shorthand labels are found, so that we learn to use a whole series of perceptions; and just by using such abbreviations for various states of mind, everyone learns empirically about such things as love, hate, fear, anxiety, hope, sorrow, etc. In such terms we have at our disposal a whole series of experiences in summary form, comparable to our conceptualization of solid concrete objects. The syntax of language, and its logical structure, gradually leads and guides the run of our thoughts. At least it may distinguish the educated from the uneducated, in that the former can follow every logical nuance of expression.

What I have just said requires further explanation, since you might easily think that I wanted, above all, to elevate the role of speech in relation to mental activity. Far from it, I merely point out that an essential condition for understanding language is not only our possessing the same language as that being spoken, but also the same 'apperceptions' [Ed] as those of the speaker. We therefore assume a degree of commonality between intellectual personalities, whereas so far we have emphasized individual differences; and it cannot be denied that the traditional heritage that we are given through sentence structure and terms for abstract concepts in language is chiefly responsible for this. Despite all differences in social milieu, and the epoch in which we live, all individuals in full possession of their senses have firmly laid down in their store of apperceptions combinations of identical thoughts. In this regard therefore, we must guard against overestimating the diversity of individuals. This is definitely an advantage for psychiatry, making clinical observation possible. Here, the question mentioned in passing was whether mental activity has to take place using words, and how far it depends on words. Renowned scholars have argued for such dependence, and cited certain abstract concepts as evidence that ordered thought cannot proceed without the abbreviations contained in language. However, these very abstract concepts are little more than a means of communication, and it seems inconceivable to me that anyone familiar with modern ideas of aphasia could entertain the notion that a person with total aphasia has lost all his concepts of faith, love, hope, fear, anxiety, hatred, grief, sorrow, and the like, or of the nation state, society, religion, time, and space. The behaviour of such patients does not imply this in any way. Each word may still be closely linked with a whole series of perceptions; yet we qualify this by pointing out that the associations are not just with the word, but include association of each of these series of perceptions among themselves, even though the latter may have been acquired only via the word itself. Language is only the means of training the disciplinarian, by means of which perceptions are arranged, once and for all, in rank and file.

What we referred to above as mental activity probably coincides with processes that Fechner called 'psychophysical motion' [W]. Fechner compared such psychophysical motion to the passage of a wave of excitation, which we considered to run between registration and execution. Thus we seem to be shifting our viewpoint on the course of excitatory processes from a specific nerve pathway to an entire system of interdependent fibres and nerve cell bodies, interrelated in a manner dependent on various, already acquired associations. We would make the same mistake if we were to compare the movement of a wheel with that of a whole, complex machine; yet in both cases, the processes of motion are at least similar. Let us imagine, by way of illustration, that we plot this excitation on rectangular coordinates: We are interested in the shape of the resulting curve, and we think of spatially extended awareness of corporeality as the abscissa. On this, the curve must extend as a flat plateau across its full extent, since awareness of corporeality accompanies us throughout our waking state, albeit in only a moderate degree of arousal. We can then add the use of speech, by which, when we are conscious, we imply not only the content of consciousness but also its activity, or the level of arousal of the movement going on within it; therefore in this sense we must differentiate various *levels* [Ed] of consciousness. The level of consciousness is plotted on the ordinate by the height of the curve, while the 'extent' [Ed] of consciousness corresponds with distance along the abscissa. We gain quite a low level of consciousness from our physicality; but, since external stimuli continually play on our bodies when we are awake, it follows that 'the body' [W] can be taken as such a solid unit that it is always being activated in its entirety. A steep wave of activation can rise anywhere from this uniform plateau, indicating the position of the currently highest peak of excitation. It is characteristic of the human brain that only one such peak can occur at any one time. That peak indicates the highest level of awareness—the most intense excitation—and, from experience, only a single peak at any given time. It was therefore totally appropriate that we envisaged the wave of excitation in psychophysical movement as migratory, and it is the peak—that second elevated component—which shifts its place, while the initial plateau retains its overall extent.

The experience that only a single peak is ever present on each curve is identified by the phrase 'unit or intensity of consciousness' [W]. A person cannot think of two things at the same time, nor carry out two actions, nor even perceive two things. An astronomer who records the time at the stroke of a pendulum when a star passes over the cross hairs of his telescope sees either the star first, and then hears the pendulum, or he hears only the pendulum and then sees the star; and between the two moments, a measurable time interval has elapsed; this differs for different observers, but remains a personal constant, to be taken into account in astronomical formulae, when results of different observers are compared. In this example, the peak must be thought to migrate between central projections for visual and auditory perceptions. The fact of unity of consciousness or intensity of consciousness leads us to assume that the volume of the curve, when it can be calculated, remains constant; in other words, there is always only a certain store of [Ed] 'life force' available in the brain for psychophysical movement. Fechner illustrated this statement as follows: A miller, who is used to sleeping through the clatter of his mill, awakens fully alert when the mill stops. It must be assumed that the sleeper's auditory perception of the mill's equipment sets up sustained psychophysical motion in the auditory projection field, which then, suddenly, disappears, whereupon psychophysical motion at some other brain site undergoes such an increase that the raised level of consciousness awakens the sleeper. Numerous similar examples can be cited. A further conclusion can be drawn from these that the volume of the curve remains constant even in sleep, but the shape of the curve differs from that in the waking state, in that the aforementioned peak is not so pronounced. On the other hand, Fechner expressed his view that sleep and wakefulness differ in the location of their psychophysical motion, which is correct if one concedes that the shape of the curve influences its location.

If the peak designates the site of most intense thought activity, then you can imagine that the most closely associated concepts would be contained in ascending and descending limbs of the curve, which are in continuity for the sequence of thoughts between initial perception and goal.

We use various terms for the migration of peak of activity—we speak of 'attention' [Ed] when referring to the act of perception or thought, and of 'will' [Ed] when we prepare for activity or a process of association. Let us take a specific example—contemplating a work of art. Prolonged attention is then focused on visual perception, and so the peak must lie in the central projection field of the visual system. Guided by this peak of activity, all associated apperceptions are successively brought into consciousness; indeed this is the purpose of our scrutiny. Attention directed to an object thus corresponds to mental activity in which, without our intervening at all, a large number of pre-existing associations rise 'above the threshold of consciousness' [W]. As we experience this over and over again, we come to believe that we can arbitrarily focus our attention, a self-deception analogous to that of self-awareness. The more intensely a viewer directs his attention towards the picture, the more does awareness of the environment and of corporeality and the rest of his personality retreat. Absorbed in contemplation he may forget who and where he is; yet consciousness of corporeality is nevertheless shown by the fact that he involuntarily shifts his position, dodging about or making defensive movements, etc., according to the situation. The dominant peak of activity may even exclude from awareness parts of our own body, when visual sensations are of great intensity; any further associations then become inaccessible. However, should pain or unpleasant sensation occur in any part of our body, when attention is directed to a selected portion of the outside world, attention is immediately deflected and redirected to our own physicality. Very intense pain, such as violent toothache, immediately signals to our subconscious to redirect attention to our senses. The artwork that gave rise to our sensory perception is still there; associative processes come together just as before, but they prove inexcitable, because the peak is tuned into consciousness of our own corporeality, and to special regions of it. Thus a severe pain prevents one from thinking, despite the arguments against this always given by followers of Stoic philosophy. The pain may be tolerable, yet one's attention certainly cannot be arbitrarily redirected to any other object. Apart from the strength of a stimulus which may be encountered by any body part, great importance to momentary discomfort can be conferred more or less arbitrarily by its associations: The slightest hoarseness catches the attention of a singer, and the slightest damage to the foot becomes the focus for a trekker. For all senses, the so-called threshold for sensation depends on our general attentiveness. The fact that it has a certain measure differing little between people, suggests that attention—in other words the height of the peak on the ordinate—is approximately the same in all normal people. The threshold level can have a spatial extent seen when we assess visual fields; concentric narrowing of the visual field, as applies to the clinical picture of retinal anaesthesia, indicates nothing more than a reduction of awareness. In neuroses following head injuries, railway accidents, and the like, reductions in awareness play a major role, and do so no less among mentally ill people.

Gentlemen! You can see from this that in determining the threshold value for sensations we have a method to measure awareness, that is the ordinate height of the excitatory process, specific to each faculty of awareness we study. Even in neurology this fact should be taken into account, and methods set up so that patients direct their attention, as we examine them, towards corresponding targets. You will remember that I presented to you in an earlier lecture a female patient in whom it was entirely my choice whether I demonstrated either total cutaneous anaesthesia for touch or normal tactile sensitivity, depending on the nature of the methods we used for investigation. Let us bear in mind that a reduction in such threshold values may, under certain circumstances, imply a reduced level of consciousness.

A prerequisite for acquisition of new remembered images and for sensations is the very possibility of normal awareness. In future we shall refer to this aspect of the 'organ of consciousness' [Ed] as 'memory' [Ed], including also the normal use of language. To avoid misunderstanding, in future I will speak of memory only in the sense of the long-acquired store of concepts, whereas under 'retentiveness' [Ed] we can understand the 'ability to lay something down in memory' [W]. We can test the latter ability by giving a patient the task of recalling a multi-digit number, an Affect or Mood. Here too unfamiliar word, etc. If it is lost or half-remembered, then this may sometimes be due to a lapse of attention. However, you will soon become familiar with cases where memory is markedly impaired, despite good attentiveness. In memory we can therefore see a way to test independently the activity of the 'organ of consciousness' [Ed] and the neural elements in question, and only conditionally of attentiveness.

Between memory and the *capacity for recollection* [W], we encounter a similar relationship as that between attention and memory. The test of memory just mentioned showed us that a *memory deficit* [W] can sometimes be detected. In the above test this consisted just of a patient forgetting a task he had been set. From my last lecture however, you saw that such memory deficits can cover long periods of time so that all experiences, insights, and knowledge acquired in memory, obtained along with those same impressions, appear to have vanished. In particular we encounter the same phenomenon amongst mentally ill people, or, after a mental illness has run its course, for the entire period of illness, or for certain phases of their illness. If we tested the memory of these patients, and memory was seen to be lost or diminished, then the deficit would have seemed to be a comprehensible consequence of the reduced encoding, at the time when the memories should have been acquired. In addition, the conclusion that a memory deficit is always based on loss extending over a given period is not correct. Without doubt there are mental deficits arising from other causes. I remind you of the remarkable cases of the so-called retroactive amnesia in which head trauma, an epileptic seizure, or a stroke led to total loss of recall, not only for the subsequent period but also for experiences immediately prior to the attack, that is, at a time of full mental clarity and health. Also, cases of general weakness of memory mentioned in the last lecture allow us to recognize such retroactive effects of the illness that caused the impairment. In such cases memory acquired subsequent to the onset of illness is shown to be permanently and markedly diminished.

Graded levels of consciousness, right down to loss of consciousness, are usually taken to differentiate states of the sensorium, subdivided by terms such as dizziness, somnolence, and coma. However, this does not match our language for small reductions in activity of consciousness, which we can call 'drowsiness' [Ed], whose detection is possible only by special, focused investigation. Among psychiatric patients, only exceptionally do we encounter marked drowsiness, although, by contrast, we frequently find reduction in attentiveness or retention in memory.

Gentlemen! We now come to a set of phenomena which until now I have intentionally avoided, but which very often have effects of slowing down the course of mental activity, which are decisive and disruptive, in equal measure. These are the moods or 'Affects' [W]. People find it difficult to define 'frame of mind' [Ed], and the same goes for pain; both are facts of inner experience, which we assume to be present in all people, because their utterances and behaviour suggest it. We know that pain has a contrast: the feeling of pleasure. We know also that the conditions in which pain can arise can be stated in a general way, and that such pain-causing excitation may exceed any useful performance of nervous pathways—such as conduction of sensations—and it may damage the nerves. We also know that pain then arises when isolated conduction is interrupted and the grey matter of the spinal cord is brought into consideration. Pain is an Affect of such grey matter, without which, it seems not to exist. In all this, no definition of pain is given; however given that pain is a functional property that can be ascribed even to the least developed nervous system, not just in vertebrates, organisms seem to be endowed with a type of alarm signal, enabling them to avoid harmful effects that would cause structural damage to the nervous system. The converse, namely nervous arousal that is beneficial to an individual, seems to apply to simple pleasures such as tickling and erotic excitement. The same importance which attends feelings of pleasure and pain in the spinal cord also seems to confer Affect to the 'organ of consciousness' [Ed]. Whatever is conducive to consciousness of personhood—the ego—evokes a pleasant state of mind; whatever is harmful to it evokes an unpleasant state of mind. According to the degree of this state of mind we speak of Affect or mood. Here too, we see a protective or defensive device that the brain may have acquired during its development. Normally, all more complex processes of association—'mental processes' [W] as we called them—are accompanied by a moderate degree of Affect, a kind of pleasant 'sense of self' [Ed] (see Lecture 7), which Griesinger aptly named the 'Psychic Tonus' [W]. This nonchalant, slightly elevated mood of healthy people does not affect either mental activity or other Affects when it remains within moderate limits. We distinguish this uniform, smooth flow of mental activity as a state of equanimity. During all stronger, or stormy Affects, be they exuberant joy, or sorrow, anger, and rage, such equanimity is lost: The flow of our mental images can no longer follow through in their inherent predetermined order, but are dominated, without any check by certain overriding circuits of mental activity, which might otherwise be counterbalanced by opposing apperceptions. Also, a form of unrestrained mental activity may occur, such that hints of diametrically opposite perceptions emerge in passing, without the line of thought being pursued; we call this 'bewilderment' [Ed].

Gentlemen! Allow me again to connect this to a fact that I just hinted at, that mental activity itself is usually associated with a slight degree of Affect. After the somewhat teleological definition of Affects—as you may have found it—which I have given, it will not surprise you that the content of apperceptions in mental activity also exerts its influence on accompanying Affect. Suppose that a train of thought, whose content is advantageous to an individual, is often repeated—a condition brought about deliberately, for instance for educational purposes and character-building—then we meet in the intellectual property of such an individual a group of apperceptions associated with strong motivations. Other groups of apperception in the same individual are acquired in such a way that a strongly aversive Affect is consistently linked with them. Apart from that, excitability of certain groups of apperceptions, and the ease with which they can be re-enacted, will also depend on how often they have been used. Both conditions are especially clear for lines of thought which become individual motives for action. In this sense, we come to realize that, with apperceptions with normal links to personal values, there may be a well-defined gradation of arousal relationships, which vary over a certain range in different individuals, but require in each individual a preformed range. Content of consciousness in each person thereby gains richness and individual colour. The diversity of personalities is mainly due to the different value of each person's apperceptions, from which come their actions in different circumstances. In the normal case, we expect that *overvalued apperceptions*, [W] which might lead to action, cannot be accessed easily, due to opposing apperceptions, and their requiring a loss of constraint before action occurs. The concept of honour, modesty, cleanliness, and the like are guiding principles for actions of civilized people. It is required that normal values of apperceptions should prevail within conscious activity. Among mental patients we often encounter deviations from such normal values of apperception.

Part II

The Paranoid States

Lecture 9

9

- Overview of clinical results
- Mental disturbance
- Mental illness
- Paranoid states
- Unrecovered mental patients
- Patient demonstrations

Lecture

Gentlemen!

Before we approach clinical examination of mental patients, we shall try to get an overview of the tasks we face. Taken altogether, we call the subject of our study 'mental disturbance' [Ed]—a term quite familiar to lay people, and well suited to include all mental conditions deviating from the norm. Among such conditions it is useful first to select the simplest ones for study, i.e. those that we might hope to understand with no prior specialist knowledge, but just on the basis of general notions, such as were discussed in earlier lectures. The simplest are those with persisting alterations in the content of consciousness after recovery from mental illness. These in turn are divided into two major groups depending on whether they are qualitative—falsifications of consciousness, or quantitative—deficit states of consciousness. We encounter far more complex symptoms in 'real' [Ed] mental illnesses; the more so, the more acute and stormy their course. The contrast is between stable conditions and diseases actually in the process of developing; and to understand the former intrinsically presents fewer difficulties. This is just the same distinction as discussed earlier between the content of consciousness and conscious activity: Dealing with alterations to the content of consciousness in the course of normal or near-normal conscious activity is a simpler task. On the other hand, when actual mental illnesses unfold, we are spectators of conscious activity whose actual course is abnormal. Conscious activity shifts as a function of time, and its output is the specific content of consciousness; thus we can define acute mental illnesses as the process of altering the content of consciousness, which we see taking place in a defined time period. Such changes are often linked with Affects and changing moods, just as they are under conditions of healthy mental life. Acute mental illnesses are therefore almost universally accompanied by vivid Affects, and we note that these complicate understanding and treatment of acute mental illnesses. The shorter the duration of the acute mental illness, the more stormy the accompanying Affects tend to be; and in the event of the outcome not being an actual return to health, the greater are the resulting alterations in content of consciousness, be they qualitative or quantitative.

We thus have to assume that equivalent normal mental activity can take place within consciousness, despite the richness of content being

R. Miller, K.J. Dennison (eds.), *An Outline of Psychiatry in Clinical Lectures*,
DOI 10.1007/978-3-319-18051-9_9

of infinite variety. You can hardly doubt this, since, as mentioned earlier (see p. 22), amongst people who function with only a small number of concepts can be found individuals whose intelligence matches that of people with extensive learning.

Gentlemen! Our immediate task might therefore be to get to know cases of mental disturbance which, after recovering from actual illness, carry its residue in the form of altered or defective content of consciousness. Activity of consciousness has returned to normal, and the strong Affects, which accompanied the emerging changes in content, have disappeared. Patients therefore do not lack Affects, and their Affects are not generally abnormal. Thus, the latter, even when related to altered content of consciousness, are not specific signs of illness, and can be understood using the same criteria as for healthy people. We come across quite similar behaviour in many patients with very chronic mental illnesses. These reveal a very slow and gradually-occurring change in the content of consciousness, a process also occurring when the organ of consciousness is healthy, but which here is due to internal morbid changes in the organ. In fact, content of consciousness of mentally healthy individuals undergoes steady increase right into old age. This applies particularly to consciousness of personal identity, since such awareness assimilates the entirety of individual experience. If the same is accomplished by similarly slow disease processes, we observe a very gradual change of personality, without this requiring the normal changes to have occurred in external conditions. Extreme Affects, from which the healthy are not spared either, are here not in themselves abnormal, but are often built upon an abnormal shift in personality. If we seek an analogy with brain disorders, the gradual change in the content of consciousness may be likened to the gradual accumulation of focal symptoms in the case of a slowly growing tumour substituting for (and not just displacing) brain tissue. As in such cases, symptoms of mental illness in extremely chronic cases thenceforth also bear the hallmark of an incurable disease. In our case, this is due to complete amalgamation with the healthy content of consciousness, and in the tumour due to purely local effects of destruction. It is almost superfluous to point out that, in exactly the same way, content-related alterations after recovery from acute stages of mental illness—with exceptions yet to be mentioned—represent incurable conditions. Thus our clinical material will consist primarily of incurable, so-called old cases [W], and also of some patients with ongoing conditions who, in outward appearance and in expressions of their conscious activity, are very similar to cases that recover. Most long-term inmates of large mental institutions are such patients, usually without differentiating the two categories based on their very different modes of origin. If we eliminate conditions of deficit from this material, we can summarize the still very large number of remaining cases under the heading 'paranoid states' [W] because they share the common feature—an aberrant alteration of content of consciousness, in other words, a falsification of consciousness. The content of the falsified consciousness may be either residual, if it is retained after recovery from a mental illness, or may be an expression of a chronic, progressively developing mental illness.

The full range of 'residual falsifications of consciousness' [W] will, of course, be relevant for further classification. We have already seen that we can speak of three different aspects of consciousness—personhood, the external environment, and the physicality of a person's own body; for a brief description of symptoms related to each of these areas, I propose the names: autopsychic, allopsychic, and somatopsychic. 'Residual autopsychic falsification of consciousness' [W] includes, for example, the many cases who are discharged from institutions, following recovery from mental illness, as only 'improved' [Ed], yet unable to be classed as 'recovered' [Ed], because they have not achieved full insight into their mental illness (see p. 39). Misconceptions, mostly false judgments made by these individuals, usually relate to the manner of their treatment and the necessity for their staying in the institution, to which they owe their relative recovery; and since they are reinforced in their opinion by similar false judgments about other patients during their stay in the institution, and believe that they have witnesses amongst the latter, it is understandable that they complain about, and discredit, the institutions more or less vigorously and constantly, according to their individual temperaments. I remind you of the high school teacher with a doctorate, discharged only as 'improved' [Ed], who subsequently resumed his teaching activities, and the wine merchant treated here years ago who even now conducts a flourishing business: They have both gone to highest authorities with their complaints over injustices suffered at the hands of the clinic. A portion of these attacks, which in recent years have also been expressed in the press against our treatment of lunatics, can be traced back to such sources.

Gentlemen! As you see, the point just touched on is of great practical importance. Not only the position of the 'alienists' [Ed] but also that of the medical profession in general, and the public in need of their help, have an interest in ensuring that the explanation of this is expanded in the widest circles possible. I will therefore go into even greater detail on this than I did when commenting on consciousness of personhood in my seventh lecture. Lack of insight into illness is, in effect, the same as an increase in the sum of a person's memories by a body of data not corresponding to reality, as we might gain from the experiences of a dream. If we were to string these often highly adventurous dream experiences onto our store of memories, what incalculable consequences for our actions or our judgment of people might it lead to! Yet this is precisely what happens in totally incorrect assessments of experiences subsequently preserved in memories of mentally ill people. I must quickly note that lack of insight into an illness may be manifest to varying degrees. In acute mental illnesses it is not uncommon that the peak of the illness declines shortly after its beginning, and the patients indeed gain insight into the more severe phenomena occurring at this most acute stage, but not for subsequent occasions. It is in the nature of things that special credence be attributed to accounts of such apparently insightful patients, which is indeed justified with respect to their admission, but not to their remaining in the institution. Should insight be acquired about an acute stage in a subsequent episode, then the conclusion seems justified to the patient, as to all lay people, that merely the enforced admission to the institution, and the impressions gained there, would have caused the illness. Furthermore, lack of insight into illness is not always an incurable condition: Quite often, memory of supposed experiences of illness and its associated effects fade away progressively with the passage of time, especially when there is no lack of regulated activity in the patient's normal experiences. These same patients, who have previously complained bitterly, then tend to revisit their institutional experiences only reluctantly; they appear to have partly or completely forgotten them, and any aversion to doctors or staff of the institution no longer has any practical consequences. You will remember that we frequently used this fact to enable patients, who could not gain full insight into their illness despite a long hospital stay, to return to civilian life and take up an occupation appropriate to their abilities.

Gentlemen! A second major category of patients unfortunately is not destined to return to civilian life, even though their mental illness has run a similar course, and quite favourably. These differ however from the first group in that, apart from complete lack of insight into their illness, they exhibit fixed delusions to be classed as 'explanatory delusional ideas' [Ed], which we will study later. As I already suggested, if such patients regard their stay in an institution as an injustice inflicted on them, this can only be seen as a logical consequence of their lack of insight into their illness. A further inevitable step leads to the idea of persecution that the purpose of a period in an institution was to remove the patient from a profession, or even to harm him civilly; or to eliminate him temporarily or permanently; or even to make him insane by enforced mixing with other mentally-ill people. Usually then, there are people who are perceived as persecutors and enemies, even though they are identified as some sort of 'higher power' [Ed]. More detailed development of this delusional system may differ widely, depending on a patient's consciousness of their own personality (or individuality), just as the vigour of their action may be based on motivation obtained in this way. If the source of persecution is sought among large organizations, such as the Church, the Freemasons, or state authorities, then those organizations may be excused, on the grounds that they are acting under compulsion; however, the initial suspicion, and later the certainty about the source of persecution, is often directed at individual persons, depending on individual experiences, as in regular cases where one spouse suspects the other—the real purpose of detention in an institution then being to enable an adulterous relationship. In such cases, the doctor is almost always saddled with the blame, and is the first participant in the conspiracy to be identified. In many cases the first explanatory delusion of persecution has a sequel in ones of subsequent explanatory delusions of *consecutive grandiose delusions* [W], followed by requisite cooperation of the authorities, leading to the view that such an unseemly process had probably been brought only against a major personality, and that the power of the state had been rendered subservient to the persecutor. None of these patients can be given their freedom, because they make no secret of their violent tendencies and danger to the community. The root of their delusional system, namely their detention, cannot be eliminated and therefore their system of delusions is constantly supported and reaffirmed. However, within the institution, over time, and especially as they become accustomed to useful activity, their Affects can be moderated, and a tolerably peaceful existence brought about.

Gentlemen! As a representative of a third category of old institutional inmates, I present to you the 61-year-old patient, gardener Rother, who I have known for the last 24 years, since 1871, as a past case of acute mental illness, and about whom further information is unfortunately unavailable. Since that time he has led an active life in the institution, and apart from temporary, short-duration episodes of excitation occurring years apart, connected mainly with external disturbances in his professional activity, he has shown calm, attentive behaviour and a normal physical condition. He goes in and out freely, and has keys to the garden and his work area. As you see, his appearance is quite appropriate to the situation. He is polite and accommodating without being obsequious; he evidently puts his trust in the doctors in the institution; he is satisfied with his stay in the institution and its activities and, indeed, expresses his wish to be discharged, but he can easily be dissuaded by the opposing view that he has a carefree existence here. His plans after possible discharge, to reestablish his position, seem quite reasonable. His answers come promptly and their content is appropriate to his level of education. Also his sphere of interests appears to be no more restricted than to be expected from his now 24 years of life secluded from society. He reads the most important political information and daily news in the newspaper. Attention and retention in memory are demonstrably normal. Therefore we appear to be dealing with a sane person, one of the unfortunate victims of negligence and recklessness by alienists, so often illegally detained in institutions, if you believe reports appearing daily in the press, written by well-meaning but untrained and therefore (at least probably) imprudent philanthropists. I have no doubt that a commission of lay people armed with the right to discharge patients at their own discretion—the familiar reformatory idea of those philanthropists—would declare the patient healthy, especially since, towards strangers, he is extremely careful and cautious. However, once he puts his trust in us, in the chatting stage, he regales us unreservedly with his experiences. At first we are struck by the fact that he knows nothing about having overcome a mental illness; for his part he might have come into hospital only because of an acute febrile illness, and he actually considers it wrong—a mistake—that he has been held for so long, even though he admits that the doctors had always been kind to him. Then he tells of a conflict with one of his gardener's boys shortly before his admission to the institution. During the struggle he had been thrown down the stairs by this man, and had broken his neck.

I ask: 'Who?'
'Well, me'.
Question: 'But aren't you alive and sitting here?'
'Well, yes, but the other one is probably still there'.

Question: 'What other one?'
'Well, Rother'.
Question: 'So, once you have been dead; is this possible?'
'Of, course, everyone has a double'.

The patient then recounts how he had experienced other quite different things that no one would believe: He had once been a bull and, as such, had been tortured in a quite inhumane manner and then been slaughtered. He describes how they had drawn a ring through his nose and dragged him along. He had also been crucified once, together with two robbers.

Question: 'Like Jesus Christ?'
'Yes, exactly like that'.
Question: 'Then you are probably Jesus Christ?'
'Yes, I am Jesus Christ'.

The patient goes on to explain that he had also been Gottfried von Bouillon, describing the steel armour he wore, and had also been a *brummer* [W] (meaning a blowfly), and flew around like one.

We stumble here across most fantastic ideas, in the realms of consciousness of bodily physicality and personhood, but this patient also carries around with him equally perverse ideas about the outside world. From the stately garden where he had just recently busied himself, a staircase was alleged to lead down into vast underground spaces. There you might encounter all kinds of fabulous monsters, great snakes, dragons, and wild beasts. The underground space extends right under Breslau, and beyond there into the unknown. The sun shines above, and, around it you can see the earth rotating, a respectable ball in itself.

Question: 'Does it not then fall down, or is it supported?'
'It rests on a big pointed stone'.

In his journeys the patient has travelled far. He is on foot, and in 3 days has gone from Europe to America on a causeway that was about as wide as an ordinary road. From time to time he came across a guesthouse where he could spend the night. To right and left he saw the blue sea and the most beautiful ships. Then once he walked around the Black Sea, in a few hours. People were busy drying it up.

Gentlemen! For the moment, let us leave the question unresolved as to how the patient arrived at this enormous number of misconceptions; you will concede in any case that we are dealing with falsification of content of consciousness on a grand scale. All three areas are affected equally, but in such a way that the most contradictory ideas coexist without interfering with one another, and that things that are quite impossible are not considered to be contrary to everyday experiences of reality. It is, in a sense, a crumbling of consciousness into fragments that you see before you, a state of 'decay of individuality' [W], that totally eliminates any systematization. Therefore we cannot talk of any actual *system* of delusions in this patient. The absence of delusions of persecution and grandiosity coming into existence as a result of logical thought activity will seem only natural; but the surprising lack of judgment that he shows through his morbid content of consciousness makes only a minimal impact in the rest of his life. In his profession, he presents even as though he is fully mentally competent. However, he judges his fellow patients for the most part as fraudsters, in that he recognizes only the disturbed and excited among them as mentally ill. The fact that such a patient cannot live in a society, cannot care for himself nor 'stand on his own two feet' [Ed] needs no proof; he is dependent on hospital care forever.

Gentlemen! The patient before you can be taken, in a sense, as the paradigm for all cases of extensive, residual falsification of consciousness. The extent of the disturbance itself prevents the development of a delusional system. However, the relatively complete recovery from the disease *process* enables him to develop approximately normal mental activity within the boundaries of his professional interest, and thus an active life.

Lecture 10

10

- Patient demonstrations (continued)

Lecture

Gentlemen!

The patient I present to you today is a typical example of slowly emerging 'allopsychic falsification of consciousness' [W]. She is a 45-year-old agent's widow, Frau Reisewitz, whose illness developed gradually over the last 5 years, from barely noticeable beginnings, and is expected to develop further. She has already surprised you as she enters, by her measured and somewhat dignified bearing, and her facial expression is similarly rather solemn. She says, when asked, that she had lived in Dalldorf, from where she was brought here, and that her surroundings there must have been brought with her here to Breslau. She does not recognize the building where she is as a hospital; these are 'sacred places' [W], a 'house of God' [W], all bearing the stamp of religious solemnity. The purpose of her stay is probably to prepare for a future important position; she is still very unworthy, and great honour falls on her by her being included here. Possibly she owes it to a high priest, to whom she turned in her misfortune. The fact that she has been through a great deal of misfortune and suffering is well known; her name is known throughout Breslau. Apart from the interpretation she conveys of elevated self-assurance, she is persistently submissive by nature; she rises at each salutation and bows, doing this to every fellow patient, even to a very feeble-minded female paralytic patient. She often apologizes that she has not behaved in a seemly manner, and begs that her words not be taken as too sharp. She regards her fellow patients as men of the cloth, usually high-ranking clerics who are here in part for repentance. The doctor too belongs to the clergy, although he may previously have been a physician. She declares a 13-year-old girl to be the Duchess Arco, chief wardress to His Majesty Kaiser Friedrich, and others as guards for certain princes. All of these people had been around her in Dalldorf but would have made changes in their appearance since then. She alone remains unchanged.

Gentlemen! The information we have just obtained suggests a so-called systematic delusion based mainly on recurring religious themes, and an autopsychic falsification has developed, leading the patient, having now survived the examination period, to play the role of a priest or prophetess. Particularly striking to us however is her reinterpretation of people and the whole surrounding to fit this religious delusion. Given the apparent prudence and the peaceful behaviour of the patient, we cannot assume that her senses have deceived her, such that she could not observe objects and events in the outside world correctly; yet everything is identified in a reconfigured manner to match certain prevailing notions, and, as is

R. Miller, K.J. Dennison (eds.), *An Outline of Psychiatry in Clinical Lectures*,
DOI 10.1007/978-3-319-18051-9_10

often the case, within just such a religious framework. And so she presents us with a striking example of disturbed secondary identification resulting from delusional content of consciousness altered by mental illness. I intend to return later to the amnesia very characteristic of such cases. With regard to her current mental status, it was noted only that she was not entirely free from sensory deceptions. Very few auditory hallucinations seem to occur, whereas olfactory hallucinations and subjective skin sensations are fairly common. The former are interpreted as audible blessings, perhaps the voice of God; in the latter two sensory domains, the 'vaporization' [W] of chloroform and the 'electrical treatment' [W] are usually accepted patiently as tests, and leave behind bodily weakness; but sometimes they provoke outbursts of anger and energetic ranting. A prolonged conversation is perceived as stressful; but nevertheless you can obtain accurate information about personal details of the patient right up to the time of onset of her illness; memory deficits do not exist; attention and memory are approximately normal.

You will observe the contrast between this case with such pronounced allopsychic falsification of consciousness and another patient, in whom consciousness of the outside world is in no way involved over the entire course of the illness right up to the present time, while the main alterations are in awareness of physicality, and, in due course, also of personhood. We can take it as an example of residual, mainly 'somatopsychic falsification of consciousness' [W]. This is a 46-year-old female cook, Tscheike, who had been treated for 4 months in our clinic 5 years ago, and was then transferred to the asylum in the city of Berlin. She was discharged from there as relatively improved, but after multiple attempts to resume her employment finally came back to our clinic. The period of her first stay could be regarded rather as the most acute stage of a mental disturbance, which up until then had been gradually increasing over a 2-year period and had been accompanied by all kinds of serious disturbances of general health. Currently, she is entirely free of such complaints and presents a healthy appearance; her bodily functions are controlled; she maintains a roughly constant body weight; and her behaviour at today's clinical presentation shows nothing remarkable. Her answers are prompt and meaningful. She is fully orientated with respect to her surroundings, her current situation and her former illness, and also about all her personal circumstances; namely, she has good memory for certain details of her illness. The sum total of her knowledge is consistent with her stage and level of education; despite a degree of malaise, her mood is elevated rather than depressed. On the ward, however, she does not always behave appropriately and comes only from time to time to her occupation in the sewing room, usually preferring to become involved in all kinds of things that do not concern her, giving advice, and harassing her fellow patients through jokes and childish behaviour. For example she pulls the bedclothes off them, or throws water in their face to surprise them, steals from them, or perhaps steals food she is not entitled to from the kitchen. She is in the habit of disrupting clinical rounds by interjecting. She disobeys doctor's orders, and if she is sent to bed for disciplinary reasons is unabashed to wander naked in the corridor. So you see, gentlemen, that the patient's behaviour is in no way normal, but, on the contrary, requires so much patience and forbearance on the part of her surroundings that she can exist only within the special confines of an institution. You will see later that many patients are in the same situation: After recovery from actual mental illness, they prove themselves incapable of living anywhere else than in an institution, on account of their social incompatibility, and their demanding and mainly egotistical behaviour requiring constant supervision. On closer investigation our patient shows that she is also full of a vast number of misconceptions. At the time of her illness she suffered from bronchitis. She was so full of mucus at the time that she felt that a prehistoric man, a bloodthirsty man, or a lancelet—she uses these three terms synonymously—had entered her body. The prehistoric man disturbed her greatly—he had been housed in her body as if a living child was therein. He was originally created in the diaphragm; he has a transparent pink body consisting of phlegm—as might be seen in an aquarium—an angel's head, and a pointed tail. He lies within her in such a way that the head is in her brain, the body along her spine, and the tail above her anus. He often wanted to get out, forcefully, which she noticed from stitches on top of her skull and below at her anus. He lived on what she ate, but mainly on what she drank, which was why she had to drink so much. Since that time she had doubled everything—double nerves, double heart beat, and even a double brain. From that time on she also had gained a very young face like that of a 15-year-old girl with the head of an angel, and her pockmarked skin had become smooth. (The patient actually has numerous pockmarks on her face.) At the time of her illness the right half of her brain had broken out on one occasion: She had suffered from severe headaches and nausea; the vomit looked like brewer's yeast; she felt that the right half of her brain had suffered damage. The diseased half of the brain later replaced itself. Through the illness she had also received doubled thought—'on the one hand the epitome of everything that had been my work, on the other hand politics and science'. In fact, she seems to differentiate between her earlier mental status, which corresponded well to her areas of interest as a cook, and her mental activity since the onset of her illness. She believes that she has 'genius in everything', and has apparently read a number of books, which aroused her interest but with no comprehension. She mentions the book by Häckel, 'Urmensch oder Lanzettfisch' [W], but believes that Häckel means something like binding, or belonging together. According to her, a person has 27 senses: profundity, combativeness, hygiene, sense of language, word meaning, sense of colour, and artistic sense; the others she just could not recollect. She writes treatises on political conditions, of which I shall read you only the beginning of one: 'The lowest class of people is used to save the life of the higher. As a consequence, the poor individuals receive an acute or the opposite of it. This stomach ache is related to chlorosis' etc. She emphasizes that she understands something of medicine, can treat fractures, apply bandages, cure diphtheria, etc.; and it is this that leads her to interfere during ward rounds. Gentlemen! We will talk later about the processes by which such falsifications of consciousness—partly somatopsychic, partly autopsychic—actually arise. I want to emphasize just one point here: That we have observed in these patients the time at which somatopsychic delusional ideas actually originate, and can thus provide evidence of their origin from abnormal physical sensations. If such fantastic ideas could arise from one's own body, we need to remind ourselves of the peculiar situation in which these patients find themselves: Patients experience morbid feelings which are hitherto quite unknown, totally devoid of any analogy with normal bodily sensations, for which patients lack any vocabulary to describe their experiences. Parables, similes, or analogies are then forced up to conscious levels in distinctive ways for each patient, and are then used as a means of description. During the acute, Affect-laden stage we hear patients complaining all too often how indescribable, unspeakable, and unique are the feelings which afflict them. The bodily localization of these feelings—which may be more or less definite—then provides the main evidence leading to the development of a delusion, by way of explanation, whose building blocks are then adaptations of each individual's scientific knowledge. Our patient was probably influenced by Häckel's undigested writings when she conceived her delusional system. A further delusional explanation is based on the autopsychic notion that, due to the illness, she has come into possession of a new way of thinking, extending to politics and science. In this, she expresses her own perception that her mental activity has changed direction, due to alterations in the content of her consciousness, a point to which I shall soon return. The nonsensical, apparently feeble-minded aspect of her thought processes, here associated with elevated mood—a contrast with the way her thoughts had formed previously—can thus be fully explained.

Gentlemen! You will recall an even purer picture of residual somatopsychic falsification of consciousness from last semester. I presented to you a 65-year-old woman about whose past we could find no detail. According to her own account she had been through a serious illness

18 years previously, that left her entire body, especially her outer body, permanently disfigured. She complained about her horrible ugly face, her plump ungainly limbs, her altered skin shade, her imbecilic facial expression, and the like, while in reality she was a graceful, finely built, and relatively intelligent, introverted, elderly lady. She had no abnormalities of sensation, nor did her general condition reveal any disturbances. Nevertheless, more extensive examination showed other severe changes, noted as deficits, which encroached principally on the allopsychic and autopsychic domains. In addition, close scrutiny showed that her memory had decreased significantly, from which we reach the conclusion of a residual falsification of consciousness, complicating mental disorder of the elderly. The initially striking purity of the case was thus proved mistaken.

Far purer was the clinical picture in the other example I presented at the same time of a residual somatopsychic falsification of consciousness. You will recall, this was the case of a young man of 20 years age, Biega, who as a result of his illness claimed to have experienced a deformity such that he had become a hunchback; his upper ribs had become sunken, while the lower ribs had expanded angularly, and his shoulders had slipped down considerably. Objectively, nothing could be seen of all these changes, and they no longer caused the patient any discomfort; but probably he was recalling the time when the change had set in, with pain and indescribable sensations—a period that lasted for years. While this had opened up conversation with the patient, it demonstrated that he had no deficits of any kind; and by very careful testing it could be shown that attention and memory were normal. Nevertheless, the whole demeanour and external appearance of this patient gave the impression of profound mental disturbance—his broken posture, his meagre responses, his 'out-of-tune' [W] face, cool extremities, and morbid complexion surprised us right from the start. We also learned that he was quite reclusive in his behaviour on the ward, hiding away from other patients, eating inadequately, and severely neglecting his appearance. The suspicion we therefore had, that he was still suffering physical sensations, was confirmed when we examined him; for it revealed that the patient still felt an obstruction and constriction of the bowel immediately proximal to the anus, and complained about extreme discomfort and all sorts of abnormal sensations during defaecation, albeit conveyed with a sense of hopelessness and requested medical treatment for his actual suffering.

Gentlemen! The 57-year-old master mason's widow, Frau Schmidt, who I present to you next, makes a perfectly healthy impression in physical terms; she does not complain of any disturbances in her general condition, and calmly and reasonably gives the following information about her discomforts. The occasion for her forcible transfer here would have been the harassment to which she was subjected at home, and to which she had responded with threats against their families and other residents; she had mainly been sprayed and hosed, and shot at from all sides. But let her speak for herself. 'I felt as though I had been injected with a syringe in fine jets on my skin, usually affecting my head. It happened when I stood at a window that I heard a signal, and then received a spray, often in my eyes as well, so that I could not see. At first there was bone damage as well—they were red and inflamed, and I also heard shots fired, injuring my arm, chest and other parts of my body. Something had been painted on the skin of my feet, the heel especially, so that I could not walk for 8 days. Sometimes, when I went to bed I got sharp splashes, which stung me. Anyway, the walls were hollow and passages had been dug out. I was sprayed from there. I do not know who could be persecuting me in such a manner. I think it is a punishment but I do not know who has the right to punish me so'.

She then tells how the medical check-up that would have preceded her transfer did not go properly. Somebody had put a woman in the clothes of her well-known physician, Dr H. However; she recognized from his beautiful teeth that it was not a man but a woman. Here in the institution the enactments ceased, for the most part. Yet we learned from the case notes that the patient had complained of being harassed around her genitalia during the night and of having seen a shadow. In the ward she has complained of other physical abuse. At home someone had forcibly broken her teeth and glued her lips together with a greasy substance and closed them tightly. At times she complained of burning facial pains, which she explained by somebody having poured a caustic substance over her face. Regarding the development of the illness, we learned from the patient's son-in-law that she had felt herself persecuted in this way for 5 years, and a few years ago had became unsociable and distrustful, and did not go out anymore. Occasionally she had complained of voices emanating from a wall, without going into any greater detail. Out of mistrust she finally dismissed her housemaid and did the housework herself. She failed to recognize one of her grandchildren, and claimed that the child had been planted on them. Finally, she had threatened to smash every window pane in the house.

The patient was apparently suffering a slowly developing paranoia, the basis for which could be found mainly in a series of morbid sensations and tactile hallucinations. She notices changes in her body but, in contrast to the previous patient, attributes these to outside influences; and thus she reaches allopsychic—in addition to somatopsychic—falsification of consciousness. We will encounter a similar paranoia in the following case, but with a very different origin:

The 50-year-old, flourishing, well-nourished gunsmith's widow, Frau Reising, complained that she had been cunningly lured from her home by a policeman and brought here. This involuntary transfer to the asylum was obviously an act of revenge by Frau W., who was known to the district police chief, with whom she associated. This would have enabled her to involve the police in her plans. She had known this Frau W., a busy midwife, for 6 years. Since she, the patient, was childless, and had noted that Frau W. treated her daughter badly—'the kid got in the mother's way' she interpolated—she had taken the child to raise herself. Two years later the child was taken away again, for no reason. In the meantime she had learnt that Frau W. led an immoral lifestyle, and was a malign and quarrelsome person. She had noticed soon after taking over the child that she must have been slandered in some taverns; amongst other things she had been accused of sexual intercourse with Frau W.'s husband; at every opportunity she had been insulted and harassed; on the street she had been told to her face that she was a whore, etc. Emphatically, only Frau W. could have been to blame; this could all be attributed to her. In the end, after 'years of malicious persecution and deliberate enticement of the child', she had filed a lawsuit, but did not know what had become of it. Finally, to have some peace, she had moved to the little town of K., but had noticed that she was also abused by people there. Apparently Frau W. had written to this place, and stirred up people there. She then returned to Breslau and found it worse than ever. She heard the words whore, mad bitch, and the like even from small school children and, undoubtedly, the midwife Frau W. was to blame. Three weeks ago the latter made a complaint about her to police headquarters, upon which as she correctly describes she had been visited by a police medical specialist. She, the patient, however understood the process quite differently: She believed that the police chief was engaged in an illicit affair with Frau W., and had agreed with her to bring her [the patient], a person with completely normal mental health, into the asylum.

You can see, gentlemen, that this woman regards her delusional system with a semblance of probability. She speaks correctly in accord with her level of education, and gives a smart and energetic impression. She has been hospitalized for 3 months. Initially she was most insistent that she be discharged, became easily excited when this was refused, and frequently gave utterances indicating a continuation of her auditory hallucinations. Gradually, she became affable and friendly, and auditory hallucinations appeared to have subsided. Moreover, she knows nothing of 'voices' [W], but apparently projects her hallucinations onto people round about.

She explains her detention in the asylum by the doctors having to act according to the instructions from the police. In addition, apart from occasional stomach pains, we have heard of no physical complaints. Her body weight decreased by about seven pounds over the first 2 months, and has increased somewhat since then.

Gentlemen! The patient, Frau Reising, is a typical example of a commonly encountered form of chronic progressive falsification of consciousness. Auditory hallucinations of morbid and threatening content appear to form its basis, so that we can formulate it provisionally as a particular form of allopsychic falsification of consciousness. Later, we shall come to deeper understanding of the case.

Lecture 11

- Interrelationship of lapsed so-called old cases to chronic psychoses
- Explanatory delusional ideas of autopsychic, allopsychic, and somatopsychic origin
- Autochthonous ideas and hallucinations

Lecture

Gentlemen!

Before we make acquaintance with new patients, we should dwell for a moment on patients we have already seen, while they are still fresh in our minds. Firstly, let us face the question of nomenclature. According to current labels, all those patients would be examples of 'chronic insanity' [Ed] or 'paranoia' [Ed]. However, if we wanted to *comprehend* [W] it in this way—that paranoia was a well-characterized clinical form of illness—then the floodgates of greatest confusion of concepts would be opened, for the cases show very great differences from one another. We can avoid this misunderstanding if we talk of *paranoid states* [W], which include all those chronic mental disorders where we encounter falsification of content of consciousness, while conscious activity remains well preserved. In so doing, we believe that we cater for the view, often expressed by earlier authors, that we should include under paranoia an overriding disturbance of intellectual activity. Under this very broad definition, we might accept that, amongst cases I have shown, there are conspicuous differences not only in terms of presenting findings but also of their histories and origins. The diversity of presenting medical conditions could easily be characterized in greater detail if we were to use the terms autopsychosis, allopsychosis, somatopsychosis, and their various combinations. For any material falsification of consciousness covering all three areas of consciousness, the term would then be 'total psychosis' [Ed]; but when it was just a portion of this totality which had been attacked, the name in question would be some appropriate combination of these terms. According to this classification, the first patient presented, the gardener Rother, would be classed as an example of a total chronic psychosis; Frau Reisewitz, a chronic auto-allopsychotic; the patient Tscheike, a chronic auto-somatopsychotic; the Biega case, a pure somatopsychotic; Frau Schmidt, a combined chronic allo-somatopsychotic; and Frau Reising, a chronic allopsychotic. By addition of 'residual' [W] you could emphasize the importance of that group of patients in whom the disease process had apparently run its course, with the patients returning to health, without their having gained any insight into their illness.

The necessity of the latter distinction can, however, lead us to introduce other, somewhat simplified terms into the field. It might, perhaps, be advisable to reserve the term 'chronic mental

R. Miller, K.J. Dennison (eds.), *An Outline of Psychiatry in Clinical Lectures*,
DOI 10.1007/978-3-319-18051-9_11

disorder' [Ed] just for residual cases, and apply the term 'psychosis' [Ed], with appropriate combination of words, only to those cases of mental disturbance actively in progress. If we were to prefer this nomenclature, then all cases which, relatively speaking, have recovered (but without insight into their illness), and the two patients Rother and Tscheike, would be included in the area of chronic residual mental disorder. All cases I presented—and others mentioned in passing—belong in the area of actual chronic psychoses. All psychotics who do not progress to full recovery but reach a standstill fall in the group of chronic mental disorder, under this classification.

Gentlemen! If such a distinction (as we acknowledged is no more than a clinical requirement) still has to be made, you will ask whether it would not have been better to separate past cases and chronic psychoses from the beginning. Now, it will still be fresh in your memory from my introductory remarks that we can recognize falsification of consciousness occurring in both categories of mental disturbance, and, as you gradually get to know all inmates of our clinic, you will find many patients amongst whom it is quite impossible to decide immediately which of the two categories they belong to, since information on their past is missing. But even when it *is* possible to obtain detailed information, it is often so far back in the past that inaccuracies and distortions are inevitable; and therefore, just as for the obvious inadequacies of lay observations, one can no longer reliably distinguish these two groups of illness. Combining all such 'old cases' [W] into a single large group, that of 'paranoid states' [Ed], therefore meets a practical need.

However, if we dig deeper, we come to understand an indisputable connection between the two. Allow me to suggest what is for me the critical aspect, even if I cannot now treat it with the breadth it deserves from a theoretical point of view:

The content of our consciousness was presented to you in introductory lectures as something acquired, indeed acquired through functioning of the organ of consciousness itself. Each new acquisition corresponded to a specific pattern of associative elements functioning in concert. We came to recognize that the strength of these functional links varied, depending on how often they were used. However, since this strength was intrinsic to the most complex, highest level of associative links, we were led to conclude, quite generally, that there existed a balanced and regular organization in the flow of mental activity in any normally developed person. So, let us assume that in the reverberations of the same combination of associative elements, the same mental processes always take place. We would then not be too bold were we to conclude that, in this sense, the set of 'specific energies' [Ed] of sensory elements may be transferred to the entire organ of association. The way in which such associative links are triggered into action is thus somewhat irrelevant: Under some circumstances it can be an aberrant internal stimulus which starts off various psychic processes, depending on its localization. For purposes of this analysis, all changes in content of consciousness can then be likened to focal symptoms, and will behave just as do more familiar focal symptoms of brain diseases; but these naturally will have different clinical 'weighting' [Ed] depending on whether they correspond with the stimulus state or the paralysis state.

Let us take examples from neurology: A major cerebral haemorrhage of the well-known marginal artery of the lentiform nucleus or an embolism of the f. S. artery generates during the period of acute illness not only hemiplegia, but also a series of severe accompanying symptoms, to be seen as secondary effects of local brain injury. Residual hemiplegia remains as a permanent outcome, while side effects of the focal damage disappear. However, exactly the same finding of hemiplegia may come about when a slowly-growing tumour or chronic brain-softening causes tissue destruction only very locally; at first (usually) there is a slowly developing monoplegia affecting for example the leg; then a brachial monoplegia may arise, then one involving the facio-lingual area, so that, finally, hemiplegia emerges. Corresponding with such slow progression, there may be total absence of severe general symptoms. However, the site of brain destruction is the same in both cases, so it is fair to compare a residual focus with a chronically developing one. In exactly the same way we can fairly equate residual alteration in content—as a localized process—with changes in content when psychoses progress slowly.

Gentlemen! The comparison we have made with brain diseases has proved so instructive that we should apply the analogy to another major—and unavoidable—question. When can a mental illness be considered to have run its course, apart from cases of it actually having been 'cured' [Ed]? When can it be regarded as still present, or increasing in intensity? For residual hemiplegia, we have no doubts about this matter. For mental illnesses on the other hand there is often great difficulty in deciding this; and I have already pointed out (p. 55) that in cases we might otherwise deem to have run their course, new psychotic symptoms have emerged, associated with explanatory delusions, and, in practice these can be of the greatest importance. I must note here that such explanatory delusions only rarely stay limited to the initial delusional ideas (usually of persecution, see above) but often develop further in the most consistent manner, forever giving rise to new delusions. Precisely this process, the so-called systematization [Ed], has always been seen as indicating that a patient is incurable—albeit erroneously, as we shall see later. Should we now believe that such progression of delusions runs in parallel with progression of the disease process itself? As I already indicated, we should not assume this automatically; rather, we should recognize that, once established, without any new adverse processes needing to be in play within the brain, an alteration of content of consciousness can have most disastrous consequences for the entirety of subsequent mental life of the individual, possibly even in direct conflict with it, because normal flow of mental activity and strict logic has been preserved in the individual. We must soon duly consider this effect of once-established change in content of consciousness—the emergence of explanatory delusions.

Gentlemen! It would be going too far and take up too much of this clinical lecture were I to discuss here 'delusions of explanation' [W] more broadly. Suffice it to say that we can trace back explanatory delusional ideas to every single one of the acute symptoms that we will encounter later. Here, only certain types of explanatory delusions are evident. We follow the guideline that they should lead in part to understanding cases as presented, and in part to recognition of pathological principles, as necessary and essential hypotheses in the psychiatric clinic.

The area of *somatopsychic explanatory delusions* [W] is almost indescribable in its variety. We met an example in the case of the patient Tscheike. Her conceptions arose at a time when supposed changes in the body would have been directly experienced; but seldom do they remain as harmless as in this naïve admirer of Häckel. More commonly, changes which the body has supposedly suffered are regarded as arising from external influences, and then become channels for the patient's resentment and hatred against people or institutions—and I remind you here of the patient, Frau Schmidt. Another patient of the same type, who I presented to you recently, expressed his indignation in a more drastic way, in that he believed that this type of treatment had degraded him virtually to a pig; he repeatedly called himself a pig, yet leaving no doubt that he did not mean actual change in his body but only linking it figuratively with the aforementioned meaning. The real change in his body—his main complaint—was that his head had been divided by the impact of hammer blows; his face had slipped down; the cranial vault had been pushed upwards; and thus his entire head had become broader. The entire alteration had taken place quite rapidly, over one night. Somebody had imposed these changes on him; how this had been done, he left to the doctors, because he was a layman. You will probably still remember the clarity with which this intelligent patient, a 27-year-old merchant who had been mentally ill for 3 years, developed his explanatory delusions in relation to their motive. This shifted between three different assumptions. To him, the most likely one was that someone wanted to drive him mad and so eliminate him. When I then asked whether he was therefore insane, he responded, you will remember, by declaring that this was highly likely. The other explanation to which he was inclined was that the physical abuses were intended to test him and prepare him for a higher calling. In particular, the disfigurement of his head might serve to give him the outward appearance of a high-ranking personage, the Duke of Sagan. He added indignantly, 'However, I will not assume the name, because then I might actually be a pig in my innermost heart'. A third possibility floated before the patient: The purpose of such manipulations was to entertain other people and have fun. 'The whole thing is perhaps a human game, or a fashion game, or pure theatre'. By presenting these three possibilities he undoubtedly counted on the assumption that a whole conspiracy had been set against him. Gentlemen! I have no doubt that in a few semesters I can present to you the same patient, in possession of the same, well-preserved formal logic and dialectics, and that he no longer ranges across various possibilities but offers a firmly founded, uniform delusional system. Whether this corresponds to one of the latter dubious possibilities or is rather a new, far more complex delusional structure cannot yet be determined. The second of these assumptions seems more likely, because, at present, we see the patient constantly revising, under the influence of new psychotic experiences. We do not always get the opportunity to see the very process of systematization itself, as we can in this patient, due to his level of education, his well-maintained logic and prudence, and willingness to share it with us. Usually we have to deal with explanatory delusions only as ready-made facts, leaving no doubt about their meaning. I merely make you aware of one of the most common somatopsychic explanatory delusional ideas because it is of great practical importance. There is a predilection for people in the immediate environment (e.g. family members), or the institution's administration to be blamed for the physical agony. A patient of this nature, with such a round-about description of the change in content of his consciousness, is seen by many doctors as a hypochondriac, that is, suffering from neurosis rather than psychosis. This patient laid the blame on his wife, who in the end had to invoke a separation, to protect herself from his verbal and physical ill treatment. In another patient, indisputable general malaise was blamed on the institutional administration—and all his thoughts and endeavours were then consequently directed towards shifting to a different institution, since he felt far too ill to do without institutional care.

For *autopsychic explanatory delusions* [W] we have already found an example in the patient, Tscheike. She claimed, since her illness, to be able to think 'in double' by her embracing a newly acquired ability, enabling her to argue about learned, political matters and the like, in addition to her kitchen duties.

One of the most important sets of explanatory delusions of autopsychic origin is built around what we shall call 'autochthonous ideas'. [W] Patients notice the emergence of thoughts which they consider to be alien to themselves, not perceived as normal, that is, probably not created by the usual processes of association. Interpretation of this symptom presents no problem, since it is exactly what we would expect from aberrant stimuli acting at a particular location in the organ of association. We assume that such an aberrant stimulus is stronger than normal excitatory processes involved in the act of association; that consequently, such a stimulus occupies a peak of the psychophysical wave of excitation; and that it disturbs otherwise normal and ordered thought processes. In any event, attention is forcibly directed towards such autochthonous ideas, and others are perceived as annoying intruders. In this connection such ideas bear close resemblance to equally annoying, so-called obsessional ideas, but differ in that the latter are never perceived as foreign and alien to the personality, and consequently do not attain the disastrous importance for the entirety of mental life as do autochthonous thoughts. Apart from that, disturbances of association, brought about by autochthonous ideas, in many patients—especially those with more finely organized personality—are equally distressing, often even so more than physical feelings and pain; they are almost always a fruitful source of autopsychic explanatory delusions. Hence, amongst mentally-ill people, only as an exception do you find an 'objective' [Ed] observer who experiences just the 'foreignness' [Ed] of emerging thoughts without attaching to them any far-fetched interpretation. Almost always, these thoughts are said to be 'made' [W], 'looked for' [W], 'inserted' [W], and probably also that they 'took it to be' [W]; how and in what manner this occurs depends entirely on each patient's individuality, and his not-unrelated store of innate ideas. Pious thoughts come from God; evil thoughts are instilled by the Devil; more enlightened individuals rely on physical tools, for whose handling they usually put their trust in doctors. So it also was with the merchant, whose somatopsychic explanatory delusions have just occupied us; he complained about 'strange thoughts' [W] afflicting his mind, especially those that disturbed his sleep and which, at the onset of his illness, incapacitated him in his professional role. He was also able to indicate the direction whence his thoughts 'pursued' [W] him; probably this was due to simultaneous abnormal physical sensations: They came from above, from the ceiling. At the most critical time, he actually revealed, insofar as he presumed to explain his thoughts as being based on suggestion and hypnotism, that he had not noticed the act of his being hypnotized, and it would have taken place against his will. You will probably still remember how hard it was for me to get the patient to divulge information about these thoughts—only after prolonged pleading on my part did he deign to impart them. There was no need to give the reason for his refusal, his thoughts already being known to me. We will come across this phenomenon of 'thought becoming sound' [1] [W] from other sources. One of the most common explanatory delusional ideas for the symptom of autochthonous thoughts is that patients see doctors as authors of their thoughts, and therefore assume these to be known already by them. The response heard so often from quiet sufferers, 'You already know that' or 'You know that much better yourself', usually conveys this meaning.

Gentlemen! You see from this example just how much the era we live in can influence the specific content in all appearances of explanatory delusions. We currently have no fewer than three chronic patients in the clinic, whose explanatory delusion is built up from received ideas about hypnotism and suggestion. In the Middle Ages, religious beliefs, belief in miracles and superstitions ruled their minds, and corresponding contents of explanatory delusions in everyday parlance, for which you can find most telling examples, were extorted confessions of unfortunate victims of numerous witch trials.

We find similar dependence of specific content of the delusions on prevailing ideas of the period, these being specially prominent in *allopsychic delusions of explanation* [W]. The most common bases for delusional 'explanations' [Ed] are sensory deceptions, under which heading we include both hallucinations and illusions. In our sense, sensory deceptions are defined as psychosensory hyperaesthesias and paraesthesias; further detail is reserved for a later lecture. The effect is always that content of consciousness is increased by various false components in the allopsychic area. They are usually construed by patients as 'foreign' [W] phenomena, which provoke the explanation; however, for reasons that we will come to recognize later, their reality is usually not doubted. The explanation is usually achieved by adopting some 'physical medium' [Ed], for which any enemy and persecutor—in rare cases friends and patrons as well—can serve. The nature of the medium varies for each individual, and the system based on it corresponds exactly to each patient's level of education. To explain auditory hallucinations, uneducated people usually refer to a device similar to a simple speaking tube: Either holes are bored through the wall, or the walls are hollow, or there are underground passages, and so on. For a while, the telegraph played the same role, for all those for whom it conveyed only sound, and now it is almost universally replaced by the telephone. For those with some education in physics, absence of visible wires creates no difficulty since experiments on the heart have established that electricity can be propagated without fixed conductors. False perceptions in the visual sense are attributed to more or less complicated optical instruments; simpler mirror devices and projectors are popular here. Tactile hallucinations lead to the idea of being sprayed or sprinkled, usually of course with harmful substances, and, if there are tingling sensations, most people know this to be due to electricity. The sensation of pricking, of being attacked and touched on various parts of the body, etc. are projected externally by patients. Deceptions in smell and taste may vary, depending on the knowledge, the school of thought of each individual, and the supposed effect; but these are mostly interpreted as harmful or toxic. The so-called *physical persecution complex* [W], of which you saw an example in patient Schmidt, is based, as you can see, on just such attempts at explanation; we will therefore not evaluate it as a clinical form of illness, or at least only in the same sense as any other type of explanatory delusion. To assign persecution complexes formed in this way to the correct place in the science of disease requires totally different criteria. This is clear from the single fact that in rare cases the same hallucinations can also be interpreted in a favourable sense, as a source of advice, a supervising agency, a treatment for the body to toughen or harden ones' self against injurious influences, etc. This cannot be based solely on individual differences in coloration of the hallucinations, since we will gradually find that this content is not itself a random selection but varies according to how the illness presents itself, and can therefore be regularly codified.

Reference

1. Cramer A. Die Halluzinationen im Muskelsinn bei Geisteskranken und ihre klinische Bedeutung, ein Beitrag zur Kenntnis der Paranoia. Freiburg: Mohr;1889.

Lecture 12

12

- Sejunction hypothesis
- An attempt to explain pathological symptoms of stimulation
- Delusional explanatory ideas resulting from motility symptoms and from intrinsically normal functions

Lecture

Gentlemen!

In the previous discussion of allopsychic delusions of explanation we could not avoid the fact that a large proportion of chronic psychotic states, whether they be temporary or permanent, are accompanied by sensory deceptions, admittedly—in the former case—just insofar as they coincide with episodes of acute illness. In addition, sensory deceptions can persist, even in cases of residual chronic mental disturbance, sometimes permanently, sometimes temporarily, or only on certain occasions. This appears to contradict all our preconceptions that conscious activity has returned to normal in residual paranoid states, since it is notable that, for sensory deceptions, there is a clear disturbance of conscious activity. If it has not returned to normal, then we ask ourselves whether any definite signs of a more florid, evolving disease process remain, when chronic mental disorder is accompanied by sensory deceptions. Gentlemen! The very fact that this question is raised proves to you the difficulty that often confronts us in deciding between residual mental disorder and chronic psychoses.

We would do well to avoid answering, until I have introduced a hypothesis about language, which, on its own, in my view, can guide us to deeper understanding of the essence of all mental illnesses. Here I remind you of our first patient, the gardener Rother who, incidentally, also suffers from sensory deceptions, albeit rarely and then only temporarily. How is it possible, we wonder, that in the same head such a vast quantity of misconceptions and misjudgments can exist side by side, in such contrast both among themselves and with reality, with well-preserved formal logic, apparent prudence, and totally accurate appreciation of the reality of his situation? Well, gentlemen, compared with the indisputable facts seen after the origin of his current condition, the answer is undeniable: It was the acute mental illness that created the gap in the solid structure of his associations. We will give this process of detachment an appropriate name and call it 'sejunction' [W]; we cannot fail to see it as a deficit, a break in continuity, which must correspond with failure of certain lines of association. The fact that, in the brain, different ideas and idea complexes are not merely juxtaposed, but are normally combined into larger groups, and finally into unity of the ego, can, in the final analysis, be due only to associative processes. The very fact that this patient is unaware of

R. Miller, K.J. Dennison (eds.), *An Outline of Psychiatry in Clinical Lectures*,
DOI 10.1007/978-3-319-18051-9_12

contradictions between his various misconceptions suggests that the combination of all higher associations into a single unit, the ego, has ceased. This individual consists simultaneously, as it were, of a number of different personalities: We could boldly call his condition a 'disintegration of individuality' [W]. It is perhaps just coincidence that this is so little evident in his outer appearance, because of the small demands made on his whole personality by his occupation. A gardener's monotonous work is similar in this respect to that of an agricultural labourer, many factory workers, and even busy people whose work is single-mindedly manual, conforming to definite patterns. If it were a profession requiring development of a highly complex personality, such as a judge, a doctor, or an industrialist, disintegration of the personality would be revealed all the time in such occupations.

Gentlemen! We will see later that most signs of disturbed secondary identification, which make up symptoms of acute mental illness, can be explained by assuming the same sejunction process. Changes in content of consciousness, remaining as consequences of errors in identification, can therefore be traced back to sejunction.

Nevertheless, we also know that, other than healing, or persistence of changed content, there is a third way in which acute mental illness can develop: to varying degrees of dementia or feeble-mindedness. We can also derive dementia from the sejunction process, as we shall see later, because according to this, we define it just as a failure—or reduction—in associative activity.

With acute mental illnesses, you can often observe a shorter or longer stage, where, after a period of acute illness, a state somewhat similar in form may be present, albeit with changes in content, or with reduction in processes of active association, before a definitive return to full health. This stage of acute mental illness, whether paranoid or demented, is therefore still accessible to restitution.

All such considerations compel us to see in the sejunction process the real nature of acute mental illness. As the Rother example teaches us, prior episodes of sejunction can be readily seen in many old cases. In other cases, unmistakable progressive changes in content suggest the same chronic progression, albeit less obvious. Whether the disease eventually merges into a state of deficit, namely dementia, depends on the extent of the sejunction.

Gentlemen! We thus see that the sejunction hypothesis provides us with a key to understanding the most important phenomena of such conditions, which we can equate with deficit symptoms of brain diseases, equally for chronic as well as for acute mental disorders. However, a number of other symptoms appear to have no explanation in such terms, by which I mean ones we have regarded as 'irritant' symptoms, such as hallucinations. The better researched pathology of organic brain diseases gives us no explanation here, because the origins of even the most common symptoms of irritation—localized spasms and contractions—are still totally unknown to us. We learn only a little here from brain diseases: that these irritant symptoms are almost invariably linked to neurological deficits, and only from the latter do the former gain their clinical status. In some way, therefore, we should assume a causal relationship between deficit symptoms and irritation symptoms. But in our case, gentlemen, it is different, insofar as some irritant symptoms, such as hallucinations, are the most important symptoms of mental illness, apparently often occurring on their own. Should we not try to find some relationship to deficit symptoms, as an example of sejunction? This requirement is virtually forced on us by our clinical experiences, because we know of some mental illnesses which offer almost exclusively—throughout their entire course—only such irritant symptoms, and yet result in the same fateful outcomes, either falsification of content or dementia. As irritant symptoms are extinguished, deficits, whose full extent was hitherto unsuspected, then become apparent. With all due caution, you can at least say that the process of sejunction is accompanied by irritant symptoms, and may be obscured by them. It is entirely within the current framework of our ideas of disease processes that destroy nerves that they simultaneously act on nerves as a stimulus: The current theory of stimulation is indeed based on this. The same view probably prevails for ganglion cells. The time course of processes leading to death of nerves would then be a critical determinant of the occurrence of irritant effects. But perhaps also a purely mechanical concept of irritation, both plausible and comprehensible, is possible: As you will recall, we have taken mental activity to be a form of movement, which progresses in a closed chain of association *sAZm* in our schema. Memory images were, for us, sites of stored energy, always being refreshed from the ascending pathways, which access projection fields. This energy is being continually drained away, we may suppose, as charge on the projection field *m* declines, in readiness for their being called into action. Such continuous balancing up of energy can be inferred from the so-called unconscious mental activity, and from the circumstance that you always wake up from sleep with thoughts running through your head. According to general principles of mechanics, you would expect that disruption of such a flow of energy by sejunction would result in a build-up of energy, and thus localized enhancement of excitatory processes. Were this 'nerve stream' [W] to be readily comparable with fluid movement, you could then speak of a reflected wave in the nerve stream; but even without this, you might expect in ganglion cells—the main sites of stored-up energy—that voltage would increase, when run-off is impaired, but with continuation of influx, and this can easily overcharge the psychophysical movement to reach a wave peak (p. 46). In this sense it is probably not too bold to speak of 'accumulated nervous energy' [Ed]. Then the location of the sejunction process would be a critical determinant of any resulting irritant symptoms. Occurrence of hallucinations would suggest that sejunction on pathways *sA* would occur in a relatively confined range of pathways, or at least in one of the sensory projection fields, for example in an area of their output representations *A*.

In the case of autochthonous ideas, of course they appear at first sight to be a 'pure stimulus' [Ed]; but comparison with compulsive ideas shows this assumption to be insufficient to explain the phenomenon. In fact, patients differentiate quite well between their own thoughts, which in the case of compulsive ideas compel them against their will, and 'alien' [Ed] thoughts, in the case of autochthonous ideas, for which they initially have no explanation. We might also be tempted to seek a distinguishing feature related to sejunction, so that at one time—for compulsive thoughts—we might be dealing with an excitatory process whose continuity is preserved, and at another time—for autochthonous ideas—with an excitatory process where it is loosened.

This consideration throws light on the internal relationship between hallucinations and autochthonous ideas. Both are based on sejunction processes; both appear to the patient as alien invasions, and are usually projected externally. We will have to look for the real difference between them in the different locations where sejunction occurs: for hallucinations in the pathway *sA* and for autochthonous ideas in the pathway *AZ* of the mental reflex arc.

We can now understand that these two activation symptoms are also closely related clinically, and that transitions are found between the two. I can demonstrate this to you, for example, in the case of the 24-year-old mechanic who had interpreted his autochthonous ideas near the beginning of his illness as promptings from the Holy Spirit. However, a few weeks earlier, he heard the voice of the Holy Spirit speaking to him. Also, in the patient Böhm, according to his own precise account, at one stage his autochthonous thoughts led to his hearing 'voices' [W]. Furthermore, the finding that patients themselves do not know exactly whether they hear voices or only experience related thoughts corresponds to a transitional state between autochthonous thoughts and hallucinations. Such uncertainty on the part of patients about their own perceptions is commonly reported.

A second implication of our study deals with the status of hallucinations in the whole science of disease. If our hypothesis is correct, hallucinations may occur even without any actual abnormal process being in place, merely by accumulation of nervous current at the point of sejunction. From this site of discontinuity, one may expect the perceived magnitude of the stimulus to be amplified beyond the norm, and consequently, for excitation of sensory regions of the brain in *s* to occur, even without an external stimulus, especially if the same process has occurred often, and therefore become habitual. I remind you of what I said in my introduction about memory, and 'exercising' [Ed] of the nervous system. There, I finally went so far as to give you reasons to assume that under some circumstances hallucinations cannot claim to be intrinsic to any active disease process but are to be regarded as pure *sequelae* [Ed] of disease processes that have run their course. A clinical case that will occupy us later appears in a very interesting light, after this discussion. It is not uncommon that healing of acute mental illnesses is delayed through an intermediate stage, which, unfortunately, is often of very long duration, and where—apart from the delusions, of which more later—no psychotic symptoms other than hallucinations make their appearance. I call this condition 'residual hallucinosis' and have presented one or more examples of this every semester for many years. You may guess how we should interpret these findings: The acute disease processes are over, but highly localized sejunction is perhaps still not completely balanced, or pathological habituation has so relieved retrograde movement that even normal stimulus intensities drain away into sensory projection fields. In such patients all stronger Affects tend to induce hallucinations—as is entirely consistent with our understanding of the symptom. It seems to be just in such cases that a slightly feverish co-morbid illness can bring about speedy recovery. An example of this is a gentleman with whom I am still in contact, who, after a severe acute hypochondriacal psychiatric illness, suffered lively hallucinations for some years, and he was considered incurable. Following influenza, he became quite healthy within a few days.

After this digression into theory, let us return to the purely practical topic of symptomatology, by turning to a further large group of explanatory delusions:

The particular type of explanatory delusions which emerge from elementary disturbances of motor behaviour [1] fall in a position intermediate between somatopsychic and autopsychic: For the former, insofar as people's motility is expressed only through visible bodily changes, and for the latter, because movement makes an increasing contribution to the entire personality, as levels of schooling increase. At least one can say that so-called actions [Ed] (but also most simpler movements which are under conscious control) can be taken as functions of 'consciousness of personhood' [Ed]. We need not deal with florid hyperkinetic states here, because they occur exclusively in acute psychoses, or in the rare—but not acute—exacerbations in chronic psychoses. In contrast, parakinetic and akinetic states are not rare in chronic psychoses, and then, their more coherent occurrence (limited to certain muscle groups) corresponds to slow summation of focal symptoms. Here we deal with the subject provisionally, just insofar as it is essential to understand related explanatory delusions. Independent development of akinetic and parakinetic mobility symptoms, separate from normal mechanisms of association, is one of the most instructive examples of the sejunction process. A key to the resulting explanatory delusions is provided by the impact of autochthonous thoughts and hallucinations, namely their being perceived as subjective processes foreign to the personality. I remember an elderly female psychiatric patient whose incessant activity was to arrange a circle a few feet in diameter, and then to rotate about its axis. The explanatory delusion related to this was that she was the world, and had to rotate. Such a fantastic delusion, not driven by any Affects, is of course encountered preferentially among long-term patients for whom there are already various alterations of contents of consciousness. But is it any less adventurous when a completely fresh patient claims that he must be in the immediate vicinity of a machine, admittedly hidden from him, that turns him continually around in circles? Of course in such cases magnetic and electrical forces are commonly to blame as the effective agents. More rarely, but more conclusively, parakinetic symptoms are described by patients, without their being connected to any explanatory delusion. Thus, during one clinical presentation, a female patient began to sing, and you may still remember how clearly she spoke about the fact that she did this against her will, and did not feel like doing it. This was the same patient in whom I was able to demonstrate another interesting phenomenon: She typically showed a defective pattern of breathing, which I call 'phrenic nerve insufficiency' [Ed], that is, during inspiration her epigastrium was drawn upward and the normal enlargement of the lower chest circumference was prevented. When singing however, she suddenly presented a normal respiratory pattern. I believe that I have demonstrated conclusively that the explanation of this phenomenon is possible only based on the sejunction hypothesis. A similar case distinguished by the absence of any explanatory delusion is that of a woman I am currently treating. From time to time she must both laugh and cry, without the corresponding Affects; she complained especially about her 'silly laugh' [W], which might lead her to be regarded as feeble-minded. In this case we are dealing with waning of a subacute psychosis, distinguished by mutual separation of successive psychotic symptoms, progressing even to retrospective associated delusions (see later). These examples, though incidental to our actual topic, may find a place here, to show you the symptom itself, in all its purity. Very often it is expressive gestures which occur in this manner, some simple, like angry facial expressions, threatening with the fist, outbursts of moaning, wringing of hands, and the like, but often also complex attitudes and series of movements, such as a praying posture, different types of fencing positions, dance movements, and the like. Such complex series of movements, such as exercising, or describing circular motion (as above), fall more into the category of initiative movements. As soon as such movements become permanently established, corresponding explanatory delusions seem to arise without fail. Sometimes the content of delusions depends more on the fact of the movements themselves, and sometimes more on their form. A physical persecution complex can draw on such parakinetic states—in brief, on a belief in supernatural powers, be they good or evil, of an obsession, and not infrequently of the idea of being transformed into an animal: outbursts of inarticulate sounds giving rise to the latter idea, along with biting movements, facial distortions, and using limbs in an animal-like manner, for example, walking about on all fours. Where such parakinetic states occur only briefly during chronic psychosis, explanatory delusions likewise tend to be short-lived; at most it may happen that memory of such explanatory delusions resurfaces, a patient believing that he had earlier undergone some kind of animal metamorphosis.

It is not infrequent that a limited set of movements, usually reactive in nature, become fixed and habitual for a patient, so that they persist for the rest of his life. More or less clownish, strange facial expressions and gestures of older mental patients are often based on such acquired habits. For instance, I know an elderly female patient who, at every interview, used the index figure of her right hand to turn the upper eyelid on that side upwards, probably a parakinesia, originating in abnormal sensations—and therefore 'psychosensory' [Ed]—which then became habitual. Another male patient you saw recently in the department tends, during conversation, to place his hand on the crown of his head, and another you will recall has the habit when speaking of putting his hand over his mouth. In all such cases the movement is now quite unconscious, or at least motiveless, and if the patient's attention is drawn to it, he can give no reason for it. The 'crazy' [W] veneer of many old psychiatric patients, so striking to lay people, is based on such peculiarities. Various explanatory delusions can be related to these.

Akinetic and hyperkinetic states are similar with regard to the range of phenomena. States of general immobility occur only very exceptionally in chronic psychoses, seeming to be reserved for acute and subacute ones. If they do occur, they seem to have psychosensory sources, as in well-known examples from the literature, of the man who avoided any movement, because he believed an infernal machine dwelt within his body that could explode if he moved, and similarly, the woman who claimed to be made of glass, and feared that any movements would shatter her. But perhaps in such famous cases we are also dealing with residual, more acute motility psychoses. On the other hand, you often see motility becoming impaired only partially during chronic psychoses. Such partial akinesias, such as the inability to swallow, are also predominantly psychosensory in origin, and could lead to the symptom of food refusal, which can then proceed entirely chronically. The accompanying sensation is usually described as closure of the throat, and independent explanatory delusions, somatopsychic in nature, may be connected with this. Next to food abstention, dumbness or mutism is the most frequent form of circumscribed akinesia, and here too, in some cases, it is psychosensory in origin. One learns from such patients, sometimes in writing, that their tongues seem to be totally missing and are swollen, paralyzed, curled up, or completely stiff; however, the sensation probably extends beyond the tongue, for in such cases accompanying lip movements are often also absent. At other times the symptom is of a pronounced psychomotor type, since such sensations as those just described are expressly denied. Mutism and food refusal are often combined. These very localized akinesias with psychomotor links often present themselves as forbidding 'voices' [W]; the fact that such hallucinations have no meaning other than that of verbalized intentions becomes clear from instructive examples in which the direct physical cause of the movements in question is attributed to the voices. Accompanying explanatory delusions that only certain people—whose voice is recognized—can 'take away' [Ed] speech, or prevent food intake, thus are easily understandable.

Although general states of immobility, as already indicated, do not really belong here as a source of manifold explanatory delusions, they still deserve early consideration, because they occur preferentially during acute episodes in chronic psychoses. Patients' subsequent interpretation of such states commonly employs the belief that they have already died and returned to life. Recovery of mobility is usually seen to be an act of resurrection, specially connected with all those explanatory delusions of a religious nature suggested by comparison with the suffering and death of Christ. Patients therefore consider themselves to be the returning Messiah. If this idea does not occur, a relationship with the prophets easily arises, and they are tasked with redeeming the world on the basis of alleged supernatural experiences similar to the passion of Christ. In other cases fantastic interpretation of akinetic states is still strongly coloured by memory of visions and dreamlike hallucinations that took place during the acute episodes, and then have a preference for ecstatic, religious content. There is no need to emphasize that the state of consciousness during times of the akinetic states cannot be observed directly, but must be inferred only later from the statements or behaviour of patients; yet so far, we can be certain that these are very different circumstances, under which akinetic symptoms can have a completely separate status.

In other cases you hear of patients who, once they have awoken from a motionless state, have experienced a variety of morbid sensations: pain of unbearable intensity, the feeling of cardiac arrest, failing breath, stasis of blood in every vein, etc. These, then, would be cases of psychosensory-based akinesia. Sometimes patients portray their feelings as continuing death throes. Hypochondriacal feelings are often accompanied by corresponding skin sensations and visual hallucinations, such as the feeling of dying from blood loss, and the visual hallucination of pools of blood in their beds. Such combined hallucinations are, as we see later, not uncommon in all situations of reduced sensation. It can be seen what an abundant source for explanatory delusions is provided at times of such suffering. Here too, there are comparisons with the suffering of Christ, or any similar martyr; most often this is linked to the grand delusion of redemption or the 'calling' of prophets.

Gentlemen! It is not always actual psychotic symptoms that give rise to explanatory delusions; it may also be normal processes of the organism, or some kind of functional disturbance, which of themselves would be of little importance. But here the relationship is shifted, so that explanatory delusions have no independent significance, occurring only in relation to other pre-existing delusions, and serving to expand these. Of such quite normal processes, sleep is the first to be mentioned. Deep sleep occurring at the moment of newly emerging changes of content is often perceived by patients as their having been 'stunned' [Ed.] to play a part in some manipulation. The feeling of pregnancy seen as 'validation' [Ed.] can be interpreted in this way; and the opposite idea, that sexual intercourse had never taken place at all, can thus be eliminated. Yet allopsychic alterations in the content of consciousness can also lead to delusional interpretations of sleep: Patients have been stunned, and, while in this state, have been brought into a strange environment. The situation is similar when dream experiences, albeit recognized as such, are held up as divine enlightenment. Of existing—but delusionally interpreted—functional disturbances, discomforts of menstruation and pregnancy deserve mention; and next there is ongoing heart-burn and digestive disorders, also found in hypochondriacal mental illnesses, often as actual pre-existing constipation. You see, gentlemen, that a pre-existing tendency to delusional interpretation is also fed by abundant normal or near-normal material for processing and evaluation, and that here too, occurrence of explanatory delusional ideas provides a means to satisfy consciousness with a number of ideas.

Reference

1. Kahlbaum KL. Klinische Abhandlungen über psychische Krankheiten. Vol. 1: Die Katatonie. Berlin: A. Hirschwald; 1874.

Lecture 13

13

- Sensory deception of speech sounds or phonemes
- Delusions of relatedness and reference: of autopsychic, allopsychic, and somatopsychic origin

Lecture

Gentlemen!

Given the major role—which we can hardly exaggerate—that sensory deceptions play in the symptomatology of mental illnesses, seen also to some extent when they have run their course, we should start by using part of the theory of sensory deception, which is indispensable for understanding these symptoms, and for their clinical assessment. Let us stay with the sejunction hypothesis, which I developed earlier, without arguing whether this is the only possible way in which sensory deceptions can arise. Indeed, we will later come across sensory deceptions that probably originate in the stimulation process in projection fields of sensory centres; and it must then be clear that their *causa efficiens* [W] and the target of the stimulus must be sought in projection fields themselves, regardless of whether these fields are directly affected by an aberrant stimulus, or are affected only indirectly as a result of a sejunction process and the hypothetical backflow of nervous current from complex associative structures. We can say one thing already: The sejunction hypothesis is probably valid for the vast majority of hallucinations, especially those of paranoid states, which are our main concern here.

Certain basic features of hallucinations emerge directly from our hypothesis. These include, first, the 'incorrigibility' [Ed] of hallucinations: The reality of a sensory deception is maintained against the testimony of all other senses, and most fantastic attempts are made to explain it, leaving no room for doubt, or the possibility of their sense being deceptive. As you already know, comparison with the other senses is the only possible means of correction; but once attention has been captured by morbid activation, which rides the 'crest of the wave' [Ed] of psychophysical motion, then constraints imposed on consciousness make instantaneous correction impossible. Formation of associations with any normal ideas, which such an image excites, thereby raising to prominence contradictory images, is made difficult or quite impossible by sejunction.

Exactly the same arguments explain the familiar incontestable nature of those hallucinations that either command or prohibit behaviour. Again, countervailing signals become inaccessible by the very fact of sejunction, so that the nerve current, confined to a narrow pre-formed channel, discharges with its elemental force upon motor projection fields. However I have to add that the compelling nature of such hallucinations

R. Miller, K.J. Dennison (eds.), *An Outline of Psychiatry in Clinical Lectures*,
DOI 10.1007/978-3-319-18051-9_13

is usually overestimated, and you often find patients who can resist unreasonable demands, and who even complain about them. Thus, for example, a patient may have a hallucinatory urge to hit his doctor, which may not reach fruition, when faced with that same patient's attachment to the doctor; but even this fact may be explained, by the different degrees of the sejunction process, as is readily apparent.

A second striking fact is the predominance of auditory verbal hallucinations, usually identified by patients themselves, as a 'voice' [W], which, by virtue of their special clinical status, deserve a special name—a 'phoneme' [W]. Occurrence of other auditory hallucinations is no more frequent than in other sensory domains. However, the fact that hallucinations of many patients are exclusively speech sounds, and that, for all hallucinations—with few exceptions—hallucinated speech sounds predominate, must be taken as one of the most fundamental characteristics of sensory deceptions, to be traced back in the final analysis entirely to the manner of their formation [1]. Let us remember that we developed our concept of secondary identification using the specific example of the sensory projection field of language. The sound of a word is not sufficient for us to understand it, without, first of all, memory images, which make up the corresponding concept being activated, so that secondary identification can take place, and the sense of the spoken word can be grasped. Although we can generalize this, we cannot fail to recognize that it is just the sensory speech centre which has such close links with the simplest patterns of association: These are the terms for solid objects, if you do go as far as to equate a sound image with its concept. For a mechanical conception of processes taking place during a hallucination, you must now realize that in no other sensory area does a more intimate connection of a concrete concept exist than in the sensory speech centre. Experiments show that the name of a specific object—which, we can assume has five different sensory qualities—can immediately be found when just one of them is activated, excluding all the others. Let us assume that similarly deep-rooted associations exist between s, the auditory speech centre, and each of the five sensory projection fields: Then we will realize that during central excitation of the concept resulting from the 'damming up' [Ed] of nervous energy, excitation spreads to the sensory speech field, multiplied fivefold, and in this way will achieve the abnormal level of activation needed to generate a hallucination. Equally favourable conditions are not to be found in any other sensory projection field.

When introducing psychophysiology I commented that you should assume that there are individual variations in this relationship: Sometimes a more conceptual side prevails, sometimes more 'thinking in words' [Ed], that is, in speech sounds. Before I made that suggestion, I had felt it necessary to warn you that in some quarters it is claimed that thinking takes place only through speech sounds. However, if we accept that individual variation in thought mechanisms does exist, then we have found a key to understand an important clinical fact, which is probably quite universal: For a single form of illness (such as an acute 'anxiety psychosis' [Ed]), which entails an essential mental content, one individual might portray the content itself, while another produces phonemes representing the same content. In this example, in one case only ideas full of anxiety or 'anxiety ideas' [W] as I call them, in the other, frightening and threatening phonemes, that is the same ideas, but put into words. We can assess such experiences not only among acutely ill psychotic patients, but in exactly the same way amongst those psychoses arising slowly, and progressing chronically. To some extent, pent-up nervous energy amongst individuals predisposed to hearing 'voices' [W] (and who, by the way, are in the overwhelming majority) [Ed] can find greater excitability of the sensory speech field and its converging incident pathways.

In some chronic mental patients you can observe a particular form of hallucinated speech sounds, in that they believe that they hear quite complex dialogues. Patients often tend to show a preference for such hallucinations; they obviously find them to be the best entertainment and the most preoccupying. Probably these are always the individuals whose mental activity has habitually taken place mainly through resonating images of words.

Gentlemen! I have repeatedly pointed out that the content of hallucinations is usually not random but depends on other more or less familiar conditions. This is especially true, you might expect, for phonemes. Indeed, I have already mentioned anxiety ideas, commands, and prohibitions, which often take on the guise of 'voices' [W]; later we will encounter the grandiose ideas of manic patients and the self-accusatory ideas of melancholia, each taking the form of isolated voices. The situation is similar for explanatory delusions of paranoid states. These often occur as voices and lead us to understand that voice content is predominantly threatening and abusive, corresponding to ideas of persecution, ideas that often make up the content of the delusions. Equally we encounter phonemes in the content of grandiosity when the urge to explain leads to progressive elaboration of the grandiosity. Here we encounter a phenomenon similar to that we came to recognize earlier, as a source of explanatory delusions, but with quite a different significance, in that it brings together a verbal delusional explanation, and the supporting impact of 'sensory perception' [Ed]. A delusional view of the outside world thus finds new avenues to exert its influence. When, as often happens, the same elementary system of phonemes is not recognized as something alien, it is even more disastrous, the explanation then being taken as a provocation, referred to not as 'voices' [W] but projected onto the people in the vicinity. This more severe level of phonemic symptoms is a particular way in which 'delusions of relatedness' [Ed] are made manifest, to which I come very soon.

Although this is not the place to address the theory of hallucinations in an exhaustive manner, I must point out in advance that we must consider the overarching processes of stimulation whereby elements of sensory projection fields, which we previously identified as perception cells (p. 30), contribute to awareness of our own physicality. Despite only cells representing a definite location on the sensory surface of the body being stimulated, we can still explain the main characteristics of hallucinations, which we will study later. The difference from actual sensory perception is then limited, in that the origin of the stimulus in one case lies in the periphery, while for hallucinations it lies in central, transcortical, sites, although the target location is the same in both situations. We already saw in an introductory lecture, that all stronger sensory stimuli arriving from the periphery are provided simultaneously with 'feeling tone' [Ed], to be regarded almost as a sign of 'corporeal Affect' [Ed] (p. 27). We have recognized defensive movements following sensory stimulation linked with strong feeling tone as a protective mechanism of the body, indicating in part a remote ancestry. Here, it is of great interest that something quite similar occurs also in chronic psychoses, except that the emphasis of the feeling tone is due not to the strength of a sensory stimulus—which is in fact the most ordinary and, in content, most familiar of sensory perceptions. Rather, because of the mental illness, that emphasis becomes an element of normal sensory perception in itself. The feeling tone given to commonplace sensations per se [W] leads to falsification of secondary identification, in that, amongst all possible interpretations, the one relating just to the single person is preferred—Neisser's morbid self-reference—and in this way leads to development of 'delusions of reference' [Ed]. The so-called delusion of reference [W], like paranoia, is only a collective name for a wide variety of delusions, which, however, are somehow linked to the act of perception and occur along with it; it consists of falsification of perceptions themselves. Examples may serve to illustrate this symptom. Anyone walking down the street will find the bustle of other people unremarkable and mainly quite random. However, a mentally-ill person, suffering from a delusion of reference, may make the observation that, because of his presence, people stand still, step to one side, or make some kind of gesture. When they spit, they are spitting in front of him; when they speak, they are talking about him; when they wait, they are waiting for him. Oncoming people want to confront him; those behind are following him; random looks and facial expressions of other people are directed at him. Sensory perception is undoubtedly accurate, the illness process being only in their being referred to himself, this being inseparably linked to perception itself, in other words only to the fact of sensory stimuli being provided with strong emphases of feeling tone.

With regard to elucidation of this symptom, we follow the path that led us to understand hallucinations. The symptom has an apparent internal relationship with hallucinations, one perhaps to be described such that delusions of reference arise from abnormal accrual of stimuli operating at the same site as hallucinations, yet not reaching levels needed to trigger hallucinations. Therefore, the symptom is valid only in connection with real sensory perceptions. We can easily accept the heightened activation, derived once more from the sejunctive process, occurring at the same site, but lower in intensity than in the case of hallucinations. Experiences in the clinic provide the most telling evidence for such a view: In very chronic psychoses of increasing intensity, the initial stage commonly consists of such a 'delusion of reference' [Ed] to be followed by a hallucinatory stage, mostly again of phonemes; and it is quite characteristic that the content of the phonemes consists overwhelmingly of delusions of reference. However, delusions of reference tend not to stop immediately, once phonemes of the same content become established; they usually continue at the same strength. Therefore, it follows from this that, as abnormal excesses of activation continue, phonemes, which tend to appear only intermittently in such cases, require a special amplification of activation before they come to a standstill. Similar conclusions apply to residual hallucinosis (p. 74), which goes hand in hand with delusions of reference. Here too content of auditory hallucinations is derived mainly from delusions of reference, and, in the aftermath of phonemes, the delusions of reference can still remain on their own, for a time.

Circumstances leading to referential delusions are by no means limited to mental illnesses. Indeed, quite typical examples of this can be found in healthy mental life. A high-school graduate appearing for the first time in tails and white gloves may easily feel all eyes fixed on him; and, likewise, the young man entering the ballroom for the first time accordingly acts in a very awkward manner. A picture of such a delusion of reference is masterfully drawn by Fyodor Dostoevsky, when his hero Raskolnikov, conscious of having committed murder, finds nothing but indifferent expressions and meetings, but will eventually betray himself, just in relation to this fact. Should anyone experience a feeling of deliberate rudeness when a greeting is omitted, etc., then this also is an echo of a referential delusion.

Examples just mentioned of 'physiological' [Ed] delusions of reference—or if you want to avoid the word 'delusion' [Ed] in this context, 'referential ideas' [Ed]—present themselves to us as primary causes: a self-perceived change in personality; and we can distinguish this as an 'autopsychic' [Ed] origin for the delusion of reference. It is an Affective state based on an autopsychic sense of 'disarray' [Ed], seemingly quite intrinsic to the context—a perception of something foreign, not-belonging, not-yet-assimilated, or 'digested' [Ed] (forgive the word)—in a word, the new experience encounters difficulty forming associations. In a brutal habitual criminal, the state of mind of a Raskolnikov would be impossible. As in these examples taken from normal situations, so too do autopsychic delusion of reference of mentally ill people assert themselves as very specific ideas or domains of thought. There is, therefore, a 'circumscribed referential delusion' [W] developing autopsychically. In some quite common cases of chronic mental illness, such circumscribed delusion of reference—apart from certain 'overvalued ideas' [Ed] (see later!)—two single psychotic symptoms become manifest, relevant to emergence of mental illness, which may be followed later by a lengthy chain of explanatory and analogous secondary symptoms. I return to these later. We encounter a more common autopsychic delusion of reference when patients believe that events they encounter in the environment, or spoken sounds they hear, are connected to their own thoughts. Instead of real sensations, visual hallucinations or phonemes may underlie this delusion; and so patients prefer these experiences to be followed by explanatory delusions, namely that their thoughts are heard out loud without their having been enunciated. Patients reach this view with particular ease when the phonemes represent answers to thoughts that pose questions or which refer just to a patient's imaginary responses. According to information provided by good observers of mentally ill people, there is no doubt that this is often the origin of the phenomenon of 'thoughts out loud' [W] (p. 80).

By analogy with autopsychic delusions of reference, we can speak here of an *allopsychic delusion of relatedness* [W] (perhaps an expression of allopsychic 'disarray'? [Ed]) when there is a clear change in a patient's awareness of the outside world. We will need to return often to such cases amongst the acute psychoses. At other times falsification of allopsychic consciousness cannot be shown directly; however, the symptom is so distinct that there is no doubt as to its allopsychic origin. Examples mentioned above (p. 82) fall into this class.

Finally, we can conveniently distinguish a 'somatopsychic delusion of relatedness' [W] even when, in itself, commonplace sensations become linked to subjectively perceived morbid sensations or other changes in a patient's own body. Corresponding examples can be subsumed partly under the heading of *somatopsychic delusions of relatedness* [W], but differ to some extent from these when special emphasis put on commonplace perceptions appears necessary to understand the conclusions which are reached. A typical example came to my attention when I was asked for a second opinion about a diagnosis. I will describe this here briefly to illustrate such a symptom for you. A young man in his formative years came before the court because he had carried out a murderous attack on his father while the latter lay sleeping in bed. He readily admitted that he was extremely embittered against his father, and had the intention of 'setting him straight' [Ed], without murdering him. The source of his embitterment lay in observations he described as follows. It was not uncommon, while they were sitting at the table, for a quarrel to break out between them, in which other family members would take part, sometimes on his behalf and sometimes on the side of his father. It often happened that the father pounded the table, which drove him into the most powerful sexual arousal. Also while he was engaged in farm-labouring out in the field, his father would appear every now and again, and arouse him sexually. The very sight of his father was apparently associated with a morbid feeling tone that in this case was linked to morbid physical sensations about which he was uncomfortable. Such examples would probably have been called reflex hallucinations by Kahlbaum [2]; the best known examples are when soup is being ladelled out and distributed, and a mentally ill person alleges that he too would be ladelled out; or when a fire was being lit that he too might be burnt, etc. However, to me, the name does not appear appropriate, because morbid physical sensations, although having some analogy to sensory hallucinations, should be differentiated from them in practice. (The same can be argued for Cramer's so-called hallucinations of muscle sense.) Somatopsychic delusions of relatedness are indeed particularly common amongst acute psychoses, but they also play a major role amongst chronic psychoses. Sometimes this state merges gradually into chronic somatic psychosis; sometimes it appears late in the course of chronic progressive psychosis to which somatopsychic symptoms are added; and sometimes, within an otherwise stable state, patients may even experience acute exacerbation in which morbid physical sensations occur concurrently. So-called *hypochondriacal persecutory delusions* [W], which may soon be joined by grandiosity, come from such somatopsychic delusions of relatedness. In every mental hospital there is a series of such patients who, through occasional outbursts of angry exchanges, demonstrably motivated by delusions of reference, disturb the peace.

References

1. Cramer A. Die Halluzinationen im Muskelsinn bei Geisteskranken und ihre klinische Bedeutung, ein Beitrag zur Kenntnis der Paranoia. Freiburg: Mohr; 1889.
2. Kahlbaum KL. Die Sinnesdelirien: Ein Beitrag zur klinischen Erweiterung der psychiatrischen Symptomatologie und zur physiologischen Psychologie. Allg Z Psychiat. 1866;23:1–86.

Lecture 14

14

- Retrospective delusional explanation
- Falsehoods of memory

Lecture

Gentlemen!

The sejunction hypothesis clearly shows us how to reach a mechanistic understanding of psychotic symptoms. As with brain diseases, it turns out that when we penetrate the nature of mental illness more deeply, then functional *deficits* [Ed] give us a valuable clue to aid our understanding. However, more complex circumstances underlie aberrant processes of *activation* [Ed], and in some way must be seen to depend on symptoms of deficit. In this regard we can never ignore lessons from brain pathology. In the light of our hypothesis, the patient with whom I started our first clinical demonstration becomes more comprehensible to us, and appears to be more consistent with this abnormal process in the organ of consciousness, made up solely of neural elements.

We set out initially to study alterations in the content of consciousness. We identified acute and chronic mental illnesses according to the processes by which they arose, and acknowledged their mutual relationship in terms of our knowledge of brain pathology. We may think that, by now, we know what is the main process that brings about substantive changes of consciousness: It is sejunction, or the uncoupling of associations. We can now define as mental illness, the occasions when, due to disease of nervous tissue, such dislocations of association take place. In such a way breakdown of nervous structure—a change occurring at a definite location—leads to signs of deficit, with no possibility of recovery by regeneration (as indeed is common in the peripheral nervous system), or its replacement by establishing new associations. However, we should also consider curable acute mental illnesses, as examples of just such regeneration or replacement. It seems that dissolution of associations in some circumstances is equivalent to destruction of certain psychological units. Later we will be able to assess a loss of concepts, that is, a reduction of the number in use, as a deficit state occurring in the wake of mental illnesses.

First however, we have more to learn about the sejunction hypothesis and how to use it to understand other clinical phenomena that we observe every day among so-called old cases. This primarily involves correction of the contents of consciousness in the aftermath of mental disturbance—or *retrospective explanatory delusions* [Ed]. We see this process taking place, always in the same manner, during recovery, or at the beginning of a chronic mental illness, or finally in acute mental illnesses that have reached a chronic stage. The modified contents of consciousness must be reconciled, according to our prevailing

R. Miller, K.J. Dennison (eds.), *An Outline of Psychiatry in Clinical Lectures*,
DOI 10.1007/978-3-319-18051-9_14

notions of causality, with old, as-yet unchanged domains. The more that discernment can be regained or has been retained during chronic psychoses, the more mental activity takes place according to strict standards of logic, and the more imperative it is to restore some semblance of order in structures brought into disarray by illness. Normally, in a complex brain mechanism, there should not exist the remotest corner that is in discord with all other parts, and which does not function under their influence. An example will best illustrate this process. You will remember the patient, a Doctor of Philosophy, whose explanatory delusion was built on teachings about suggestion and hypnotism. This patient had already survived an episode of mental illness 8 years earlier, but had recovered from it to the extent that, for many years, he had full insight into the symptoms of his acute illness. When I met him recently during a new episode, to my great surprise I found a remarkable development that his insight into his illness was lost, so the patient now asserted that the basic symptoms of his first illness, namely phonemes, had not been the result of an illness, but of the effects of hypnosis induced by some adversary. However, he had accurate recall of the fact that for many years he had regarded his auditory hallucinations as signs of an illness; but now he noted quite correctly that such a conceivable insight into his illness could be explained as effects of suggestion. You will see from this example the ease with which judgments, which, for many years, he regarded as having 'made his own' [Ed], as hard-won products of complex thought processes, could be overturned by a supposedly new insight, itself aberrant. Nevertheless, if, as I do not doubt, we should regard this process not as aberrant in itself but only as a reaction of a normally functioning brain mechanism when challenged by a material change, you will not be surprised that often, a patient's limited knowledge of the physical basis of most mental illnesses is overwhelmed by the testimony of their senses as they experience hallucinations, such that assumptions about supernatural effects, subterranean tunnels, hollow walls, and the like, used to explain alien, subjective perceptions, lose the outlandish and grotesque character they might have in the judgment of those same persons when they are in good health. Often, previous knowledge might have stood in the way of resolving a problem, for instance when belief in the principle of conservation of energy constrains acceptance of 'perpetual motion' [Ed]. Here, however, such knowledge is modified in such a way that the obstacle no longer applies, and can then explain many of the craziest inventions and discoveries.

In particular, specific earlier experiences may form the subject of such reinterpretations. Guided by newly acquired and supposedly better insight, demonstrations of love appear as hypocrisy or cunning calculation; hostile actions as good deeds; insignificant incidents as highly significant events; and a random event as a deliberate action by some patron or adversary.

The process of subsequent correction achieves special importance as soon as it extends beyond knowledge, judgment, and more complex end processes, to include memory of earlier perceptions, and in this way leads to subsequent falsification of secondary identification. We want to designate such retrospective correction of earlier memories as *retrospective delusions of relatedness* [W]. They involve events analogous to those in normal mental life. Every one of you will know of times when, only retrospectively did you remember having encountered an acquaintance to whom, because you were preoccupied at the time, you had paid no attention. This late recollection can just as well be accurate as inaccurate in its content, and normally a person takes this into account. Amongst mentally ill people there are also often those, perhaps identified subsequently, except that their most superficial features usually suffice to identify them. In such patients with established grandiose delusions, such reinterpretations are often based on memories of their youth. The patient remembers for example that once, as a boy, he had been spoken to by an officer, who, as he subsequently recalls, was Kaiser Wilhelm, or Kaiser Frederick, or some other highly-ranked, popular personage. In school at the same time he was asked by his teacher who were his father and grandfather. This question was about that same high-ranking personage, and should indicate where he had to look for his father or grandfather. Should the objection be raised that this could also have been an inconsequential question, such patients rebut this by pointing to a meaningful glance or a telling gesture by the teacher in his statement—clear proof that the perception itself has been falsified in memory. Amongst such patients, you can listen for hours to stories of childhood memories described mainly just as they had been experienced. Overall however, their perceptions show every nuance of referential delusions, which an outstanding psychiatrist has described succinctly with the words '*tua res agitur*' [W].

Retrospective delusions of reference can easily lead to completely false notions among uneducated and uncritical people, not used to separating their subjective impressions from objectively perceived material; and it is often difficult under these circumstances to single out the facts as they had actually happened. Nonetheless, clinically, it is necessary to make a clear distinction between retrospective delusions of relatedness and another elementary symptom, which is inclined to be preferred in similar patients: so-called *falsifications of memory* [W] [1]. This symptom involves either of two equally significant changes, one positive, and the other negative. The *positive* [Ed] form of falsification of memory [1], also called *confabulation* [Ed], consists of appearance of memories and experiences that are certainly not real. The content of such confabulation is usually so coloured as to signify prevailing mania. Thus, for example, in previously mentioned cases of established grandiose delusions (p. 87) the content provides much of the evidence for the patient's claim to his having high-status parentage, or a relationship to such; in cases of systematized persecutory delusions (often directed at a person) confabulation may contain most fantastic, alleged persecution. In other cases the symptom again reflects incoherence in content of consciousness (decay of individuality, see above) as in the case of Rother, and very often also in the fantastic and audacious stories of the paralytic. An internal link to memory disturbances, which one may already suspect *a priori* [W], can also be detected clinically, since the symptoms belong with three groups of disorders, whose components are seldom absent and all feature memory deficits starting in a timely fashion: hebephrenia, presbyophrenia, and progressive paralysis.

No less remarkable is the *negative* [W] form of falsification of memory, in which circumscribed gaps in otherwise well-preserved memory might occur, with no sign that any clouding of the sensorium or loss of retentiveness could have intervened at the time of the experience in question. For correct understanding and description of this symptom, high value must be placed on the latter precondition. No one would be surprised if a patient with initial symptoms of abdominal typhus or meningitis has totally lost memory for hours and days, for example the distance travelled under these conditions on a journey from Rome to Berlin. Nor should we wonder about the total loss of memory during epileptic twilight states, alleged experiences of *Delirium tremens*, or any other delirium from severe intoxication, hysteria, or, lastly, during normal dreaming. So, for any such experiences occurring during a mental illness in which simultaneous memory loss can be shown, complete amnesia seems quite understandable. The behaviour is quite different for the symptom of negative falsification of memory. In that case, individual actions and events that occur when mental clarity seems to be perfectly normal are wiped from memory, while events occurring nearby in time are still recalled exactly. However, two circumstances, never lacking as features of this symptom, should serve to suggest its explanation: The incident in question, and the action taken, always seem to fall at times of particularly high Affect. In addition, they are related to a specific 'overvalued idea' [Ed], such that either they both appear as an emanation of the latter and are thus motivated by it, or have their significance in its rebuttal and refutation. I have found the most typical examples of this to have occurred in so-called querulous delusions and related conditions of chronic partial psychoses. To put the previous points by way of an example, I cite the case of a master craftsman, living here—incapacitated but still busy—who, in public and on a public street, insulted a policeman with that insulting phrase familiar from *Götz von Berlichingen* and the accompanying gesture, and afterwards denied under oath that he did this. This man was under the influence of an overvalued idea that, for some time, had compelled all his actions; he regarded officials as his personal enemies and watchdogs; shortly before, he had suffered mortification connected with this idea, and no doubt at the time of the offence was acting under the influence of strong Affect. However, given both the precise knowledge of the person and the whole state of affairs, it was inconceivable that this decent-minded, religiously-inclined man could consciously commit perjury, although he had actually given false testimony under oath. With respect to aetiology, only a strong family predisposition to mental illness was established in this middle-aged man.

Gentlemen! While the process of correction could itself be regarded as normal, those last three symptoms, linked to subsequent corrections of the content of consciousness, are an abnormal excess of such corrective action. All three phenomena clearly belong together, and their mutual relationship can be expressed by subsuming the first as a 'qualitative falsification of memory' [Ed], and the other two as 'quantitative falsifications of memory' [Ed]. Instead of the terms 'positive' [Ed] and 'negative' [Ed], it might be more appropriate to call them 'additive' [Ed] and 'subtractive' [Ed] so that we would now have a uniform nomenclature to differentiate three forms of falsification of memory: one qualitative, one additive, and one subtractive.

If we now want to attempt an interpretation, it would be best to treat all four phenomena in context. Turning first to the subsequent correction, you will soon notice how closely the phenomenon is related to explanatory delusions, which you have known for a long time. However, the subsequent correction possibly corresponds to a more refined psychological need, while explanatory delusions are driven by a coarser motive. Explanatory delusions take advantage of consciousness, usually quickly, through unconscious processes, and thus with much elemental power; subsequent corrections, on the other hand, take place slowly, as real, conscious thought processes leading to a conclusion after long brooding, when the patient has clarified various things that previously seemed incomprehensible. The patient Böhm who you will remember was just beginning such a process of clarification, and said that he could not, at the time, decide which of the various assumptions was the correct one.

However, it stands to reason that the very slowness and thoroughness of such retrospective correction must lead to irreparable falsification of intellectual acquisitions. Even the waning of elementary symptoms, such as phonemes arising from explanatory delusions, leads to falsification of mental ownership, which, once acquired, cannot be amended. Explanatory delusions and subsequent corrections are the two foundations of any so-called systematization; it is therefore no surprise that you find the theorem still applied everywhere, and that systematization signifies 'incurability' [Ed]. However, as a generality, the theorem is incorrect, and certainly does not hold true for most systematizations in acute mental illnesses based on explanatory delusions in the sense just described. On the contrary, as we see later, there is one mental illness—one of the most curable—where systematization almost always occurs: acute hallucinosis, or strictly 'acute hallucinatory allopsychosis' [Ed] (p. 103).

In contrast, the theorem should apply with no restrictions to chronic psychoses. Yet even here, how much more favourable are the conditions for retrospective correction, albeit in an aberrant sense! In the acute illnesses we dealt with, there are weeks or months during which abnormal components increase, usually to such an extent that one displaces the others, all flowing into consciousness. Afterwards, elementary symptoms go quiet, and what remains of them is no longer strong enough to overwhelm earlier acquisitions, but is subject to the combined power of restored normal functioning of the identification process and of earlier acquired ideas. In chronic cases on the other hand, new acquisitions carry too much of the stamp of normality for the old repository to be treated in any way different from normal new acquisitions.

Gentlemen! As we have just seen, the excitatory processes, which are the root of elementary symptoms of chronic psychoses, can all be interpreted as consequences of sejunction; we must therefore also consider the associated explanatory delusions and retrospective correction in paranoid states as inevitable, if indirect, consequences of the sejunctive process. The phenomenon of retrospective delusions of relatedness, on the other hand, allows us to recognize a direct connection with sejunction. We saw that we must trace delusions of relatedness back even as far as an excitatory process asserting itself in secondary identification. Once we accept this view, nothing stands in the way of the further assumption that the same level of activation generated in the act of perception by external excitation of a projection field also increases excitability for memory images in association pathways, and can thereby misrepresent the relationship of that image to the person himself or herself. However, the required increase in level of activation can, as we have seen, arise from nervous energy accumulated as a result of the sejunction.

The positive or additive form of memory falsification requires a preceding break-up of associations. This needs no extensive discussion. The strength and reliability of our memories are due mainly to strict correlation in timing between them; and, as an image that you may envisage, along the time axis, memories are strung so close together that alien elements find no place between them. This temporal association must therefore be broken if the pseudo-experiences of confabulation are to be taken as true. Of course only the *possibility* [Ed] of occurrence of a symptom is explained by this; therefore, the *actual* [Ed] mechanism of formation remains obscure. But it is precisely the manner of occurrence of the symptom and its origin that requires discussion.

The most obvious assumption, that we are dealing with memories of pseudo-experiences of acute mental illness, obviously does not apply to all those confabulations occurring without any previous acute stage of illness, which is what we envisaged, while virtually excluding other situations from our concept of confabulation. Somewhere those situations must define every detail of the vividly described events that were never experienced. Assumptions which come to mind and seem to any knowledgeable person to exhaust all other possibilities are that they represent arbitrary productions, deliberate misrepresentations, or lies in the usual sense of the word. These confabulations are definitely not lies, because mentally-ill persons are totally convinced of their truth. Since the content of this confabulation often also has a fantastic character similar to dream experiences I think it is quite possible that they are actual memories of dreams.

One might argue for this possibility as follows: Even a mentally-healthy person may have the experience that, on awakening from a dream, for a short time he believes in the reality of the dream events. However, this happens only when the content of the dream does not contradict precedents from reality too severely, and also if it can be related easily to experiences from the recent past. The latter condition would be fulfilled, for example, if memory of an experience from the previous night were lost, or could be recalled only imprecisely due to mild intoxication. A mentally ill person can completely lack these two constraints: Temporal continuity of memory becomes a weaker chain, so that insertion of alien intervening links is more easily permitted, nor are precedents from reality as unassailable to him as they are to a sane person. Obviously, it is again the fact of sejunction that removes normal barriers to the storage of dream experiences in the memory banks; but perhaps something else may still be needed to bring about confabulation, such as abnormal vividness of dream experiences. However it would lead us too far off course, if we were to address in more detail the associated conditions, which in themselves are not inaccessible.

For the negative or subtractive form of memory falsification a familiar analogue is seen amongst post-hypnotic phenomena. Familiar commands can be given to a hypnotized person, which he or she later carries out while awake, while failing to remember the command. For our purposes, execution of the command is irrelevant, being no more than a check on whether consciousness had been affected at all at the moment of the command. What is significant for us is the complete amnesia for the palpable reality of the command, and also that the action is certainly not to be regarded as a real act of will. We must trace back any suggested effect to the fact that alien components have been implanted in the organ of consciousness without their recruiting associative links with remaining contents of consciousness. This is a circumstance, incidentally, that brings the compelling influence of such transplanted components of an alien consciousness to be grasped in a gross, mechanical way in terms of movement. In any case, we must also refer to the absence of associative links to account for gaps in memory, the symptom we are concerned with, to explain the fact that the previous history of events cannot actually be recalled. However the close relationship between the content of these memory lapses and the overvalued idea points to the fact that the associative link is not entirely missing, but is heavily biased towards and limited to the overvalued idea, without which insight the apparently conscious act could not be explained. So this probably represents a narrowing of consciousness, as is known otherwise only in states of high Affect. Since actions occurring during periods of memory lapse often appear to be due just to Affects, we can also see here an opportune moment for future forgetfulness. However we cannot exploit this moment, because it remains unexplained why only certain types of mental patient show this symptom.

Reference

1. Kraepelin E. Über Erinnerungsfälschungen. Arch Psychiatr Nervenkr. 1886;17:830–43.

Lecture 15

15

- Retrospect of earlier account of elementary symptoms
- Overvalued ideas

Lecture

Gentlemen!

An overview of elementary symptoms occurring during paranoid states allows us to make the following distinctions: First, we found several changes in content of consciousness, namely delusions and delusional judgments, expressed within an unbroken train of conscious activity, in so far as they were in a logical form, preserving attentiveness and memory, and in their moment-by-moment adaptability to any given situation. However, the intactness of these faculties in no way prevents the remaining content of consciousness appearing to have disintegrated, to a degree, into fragments a fact to which we gave the name 'sejunction' [Ed], in other words, the detachment of individual components one from another. Such components initially form tight-knit structures, as complete experiences, but their sejunction is shown by the fact that memories that flatly contradict each other can coexist. The sejunction hypothesis then led us to a closer understanding of certain symptoms of activation, first, of manifestations of disturbed conscious activity itself, then of autochthonous ideas and obsessions [1], and then of hallucinations and delusions of relatedness and reference. Explanatory delusions, which took up much of our discussion, could then be likened to normal expressions of conscious activity, in contrast to the aforementioned primary psychotic symptoms. We then came to recognize subsequent corrections of the content of consciousness as conditions essential for the so-called systematization, itself related closely to explanatory delusions. We also found amongst these corrections a process, which we viewed as normal conscious activity reacting against 'false intruders' [Ed]; and we also saw psychotic symptoms in various types of memory falsification, seemingly quite aberrant in themselves, yet appearing to stand in regular relationship with existing disturbances of the content of consciousness, such that their occurrence depended on the extent of changed content. Amongst such psychotic symptoms we distinguished at least three different points of origin, all emerging in part as a reaction of intact conscious activity to alterations of content of consciousness. These included explanatory delusions and subsequent corrections, either of which occurred as a direct consequence of sejunction; the latter included contradictory contents of consciousness in many old cases, and additive and subtractive ways in which memory can be falsified. Lastly, there were excitatory processes arising out of the sejunctive processes: these included hallucinations, delusion of relatedness,

R. Miller, K.J. Dennison (eds.), *An Outline of Psychiatry in Clinical Lectures*,
DOI 10.1007/978-3-319-18051-9_15

and retrospective delusion of relatedness, and finally autochthonous ideas.

The last mentioned group included *overvalued ideas* [W] already mentioned repeatedly; these have an obvious relationship to obsessions and autochthonous thoughts, the questions then being how they differ from such symptoms, and whether any sharp boundaries can be found. Overvalued ideas are sharply distinguished from the autochthonous ideas in that they are evaluated within a patient's consciousness, and thus, by no means are to be viewed as alien intruders: Indeed patients see in them expressions of their very being, and quite rightly take a leading role in their elaboration—a struggle for their very own personality. Nevertheless they are often perceived as painful, and patients may complain that they cannot think of anything else. However, they still remain quite distinct from obsessions because they are seen to be normal, to be accounted for fully by their mode of origin, while obsessions are recognized as untrustworthy, and often as manifestly nonsensical.

Clinically, one can easily distinguish this symptom from the two other closely related ones; yet the mechanism of their formation remains unexplained. In this regard, note that, in general, we can define overvalued ideas as any kind of memory, but especially of Affective experiences, or a whole series of related experiences of this kind. So, for example, the following incidents led to the emergence of overvalued ideas: the discovery, by a man who had taken over the administration of an inheritance and, as an heir, was then involved in its distribution, and that he had significantly disadvantaged himself; news of the suicide of a personal friend; the death of a husband; an older girl's delusion that a gentleman had paid her attention; a wife's remark that her husband, despite her objections, sniffed a lot; the sight of cleansing of a person infected with lice; and, finally, one of the most common cases, judicial condemnation, or judgment by superior authorities perceived as an injustice. The Affects revealed can be very diverse in character, and can soon manifest themselves as anger or insult, sadness or disgust, or as sexual arousal. In any case we can infer from this list that almost any cherished event can lead to emergence of an overvalued idea; that it does not depend at all on the type of emotion; and that there must be overvalued ideas that are in themselves completely normal; yet the way that an individual is treated can determine whether they acquire an aberrant character. People who commit suicide after loss of a fortune, after being sentenced to dishonourable punishment, or after death of a loved person, are certainly acting under the influence of an overvalued idea; and we should regard their conduct as abnormal, even though not due to mental illness. Therefore, in every single case, we should establish whether an aberrant, overvalued idea is present, or whether it falls within the bounds of normality. Your decision on this will probably depend on whether the motive triggered by the relevant memory, and which leads to its acquiring a dominant role, is sufficient grounds, or not. However, this criterion is sometimes left completely undecided, as in examples of malcontents: Some such patients *have* [Ed] actually been unjustly judged in the first place, and have every reason to feel indignant about this. A reliable criterion is that in cases of aberrant overvaluation of ideas, the symptom does not remain in isolation: A number of other psychotic symptoms soon appear, especially delusions of reference characteristic of such cases, yet quite circumscribed (p. 82).

The following is a typical example of an aberrant overvalued idea: A 61-year-old person of independent means, who was recently presented to you, gives, as reason for his being admitted, the 'hounding' to which he had been exposed outside the institution. Inside the institution he is completely free of such annoyances, and feels so well that he is already in his fourth year here, and intends to stay. Several attempts to discharge him have failed because, repeatedly, the same harassments have led to police intervention and internment. Originally it was a certain gentleman, known to him only by name, who lived in his neighbourhood and who he therefore often encountered on the street. He came to believe that this gentleman stopped and waited for him, standing as though counting windows of a house. He therefore crossed to the other side of the street but noticed next time how the same gentleman, at the same spot, was talking to an acquaintance, no doubt about *him* [Ed], of which fact he was convinced, without being able to hear what was said. He therefore went close to the two men and said, 'Do you perhaps want something from me?' He then went home and observed that the men followed him and remained standing in front of his house. Having reached his home he then went to the window and waved his stick, calling out to them 'Come right up! I'll give you what for!' A similar encounter on another occasion led to the two men actually following him to his home, who then found out his name, and laid complaints with the police. That event led to the patient's initial admission. I took him into the clinic soon after, and established that the patient's delusion of reference was directed solely against one of these two, a master carpenter; and I then asked him: 'How did this gentleman come to harass you?' The answer was quite typical. He could think only as follows: The gentleman in question was the brother of a close friend, who 6 years ago had been, like himself, a regular guest of a particular wine merchant. The patient himself had been interested in this businessman's daughter for years, and had even proposed to her, but had then broken off the engagement, because he had been told that her father was in financial difficulties. As the master carpenter had spoken to the other gentleman about him, he had probably said, 'There goes the scoundrel who left the girl in the lurch'. Detailed investigation and observation of the patient failed to find any kind of psychotic symptoms, other than his continuing to insist on the accuracy of these allegations. Therefore he was discharged, at his own request, after a few weeks, but was soon readmitted; and this was repeated a second time. Since then he no longer tries any more. The harassment that the patient was exposed to when outside the institution occurred far more frequently on the two further occasions than before; also, other people were involved, as well as the police. However everything always came back to the one master carpenter who, meanwhile, had served up the old story to other people, and notified the police of his observations of mental illness. Nowhere in the institution has anyone observed even a hint of a delusion or any other sign of mental illness in this patient.

We see here, in a typical case of *circumscribed autopsychosis* [W], how the overvalued idea linked initially to a very circumscribed delusion of reference, expanded subsequently, yet never comes to light within the institution, where the patient meets only with strangers. The basis of the overvaluation of the idea is therefore the same as for delusions of reference: namely the inner conflict between the not entirely honourable course of action, which he described, and the otherwise righteous character of the patient. We can probably assume that, at the time of the first mentioned incident, the patient was busy internalizing his previous experience, which felt like his own failing. A passing glance, the expectant attitude of the man who might know his affairs, led to an abiding association with the currently dominant distortion—albeit not in content but in the falsified evaluation of thought content, a falsified secondary identification very similar to that based on the delusion of the young murderer, mentioned earlier (see p. 83). As you will remember, it happens in just the same way even for physiological delusions of reference, as described so well for Raskolnikov. It is probably no coincidence that Dostoevsky's central character (from *Crime and Punishment*) has already been described as a man of almost unhealthy nervousness, and softest, most compassionate heart: Under such circumstances alone, memory of the murder he had committed must have remained, so to speak, as utterly unique in his consciousness. As in all cases of autopsychic delusions of reference we meet the difficulty of assimilating these to pre-existing contents of consciousness, that is, by associative processes, this being the basis for his overvaluing the idea.

Judging by features of the present case, we might propose that such experiences would favour emergence of an overvalued idea, which, in its content, would be particularly difficult to bring into congruence with existing content. Since such experiences are no stranger in the mental lives of even the most healthy of us, some special conditions must prevail before such overemphasis takes on an aberrant character.

Normally there is contradictory evidence, which gradually corrects any overvaluation. For aberrant overvaluation however, these counterarguments, demonstrably, are no longer available, and, at the same time, clinical signs of delusions of reference also appear, all in accord with the activation hypothesis, which I connected earlier to the sejunction process.

If we want to pursue these clinical features further, it turns out that the 'damage' [Ed] proceeding from the present symptom is well known, to be sought in the high levels of Affect accompanying particular experiences. Since this frequent antecedent cannot be discovered for other psychotic symptoms, this one serves also to characterize aberrant overvaluation of ideas.

As in the case just described, a fairly stable and enduring disease picture can be seen in a series of similar cases, and, on account of its strong inclination, bears the traditional name of *obsession* [W]; yet in most cases, delusional explanatory statements are added on, and these can continue to grow in strength. Subsequent corrections to the content of consciousness and the various ways in which memories can be falsified thereby join in, giving rise to a close-knit delusional structure, whose complex content does not match its relatively simple, and often minor, point of origin, and serves to conceal or disguise the latter. In old cases of this kind, one can easily determine such a delusional structure, but often one cannot go beyond *assumptions* [Ed] about the underlying overvalued idea, and the experience to which it is linked. For all such cases we can understand why patients can no longer reach a full recovery, as is the case for all other cases with more extensive systematization. However, when the extent of the disease is limited just to the first psychotic elements, it is possible for health to be restored through the gradual appearance of more powerful countervailing arguments. Two cases of this type, where recovery has taken place, are related to the typical scenario of a so-called malcontent's delusion. The clinical presentation of such cases has proved useful to me several times, as is the process of 'internalisation' [Ed] itself, that is, a conscious ability to recognize mental illness, and to constantly accept paternal guidance: These are powerful and salutary corrective experiences. Healing itself always happens very gradually, the principle being that, by avoiding occasions when Affect is renewed, the Affect itself disappears, and necessary correctives gradually gain acceptance and prove to be effective.

It would take too long, were I to introduce all individual cases of overvalued ideas here; even then, I might not exhaust the topic, since there must naturally be almost limitless variations, topic by topic, on this otherwise well-characterized theme of chronic autopsychosis. For practical reasons I allow myself just the suggestion that, when anyone has the possibility of acquiring an accident-related annual payment, it can easily lead to overvaluation of ideas. Finally, I do not want to shy away from the idea that almost every other psychotic symptom, as well as being an overvalued idea, can be the initial stage of an acute or subacute psychosis which progresses, including progressive paralysis, and this it is seldom absent as a feature of melancholia.

To conclude this discussion, I want to describe an instructive case, as far as systemization goes. A single woman in her 40s, a science teacher at a secondary school for girls, who is very keen and capable, possibly a little too intense in her profession, believed that she noticed that one of her male unmarried colleagues, with whom she had enjoyed friendly relations over many years, had serious intentions towards her. The idea came to her that during lessons in his class he often stood at the window, from which it was possible to glance into her classroom; that in his free time he often stood on a landing which she had to pass with her pupils on their way to her classroom; and that he greeted her very sincerely. She soon found this perception to be confirmed by all sorts of random encounters, which aroused strong Affect; she spent days and nights in inner turmoil about how she should respond to this, and especially how she should behave as inconspicuously as possible, so that pupils and colleagues would never notice. When she believed that she could no longer stay in control of her actions, she tried to avoid such encounters, and even went so far as to deliberately refrain from replying to his greetings. Around this time she also noticed that her students seemed to be aware of what was going on; remarks were dropped that referred to it; perhaps there were isolated phonemes, for she heard, 'How distressed he looks'. Female colleagues who had previously kept apart from her now visited her more frequently, and spoke quite often about the young man; good female friends, on the other hand, withdrew from her and appeared to disapprove of her 'relationship' [W]. Even the Director intervened, by speaking with the male teacher in the breaks, and keeping him in a completely different location, further from her than he would otherwise have done. After some time the male teacher in question left the school to continue training overseas. At a farewell visit he was utterly confused, with altered complexion, and, in particular, a long glance told her that he knew very well what was going on inside her, and also returned her affection. After he had left, she noticed that, in exchanges with her female colleagues, they were sometimes derisive and gleeful, and at other times also sympathetic and considerate; in any case her relationship was generally known, and any mention of the teacher in question contained allusions to it. The Director must have mentioned the subject at a staff meeting; she could tell this from the expressions of all those present, when once she attended a staff meeting. All these events took place over 2 years. No direct messages came to her from the teacher, and she began to doubt whether he was a man of honour. Although she had to acknowledge that her behaviour would have repelled him, she believed that, as a righteous man, he should have explained himself. Quite satisfied by having sacrificed her own interests through her behaviour, in favour of school discipline, she even made a violent scene with the Director, whose indelicate interference she had not forgotten, and she was put on leave, with advice to go to a mental hospital for 6 months. The head of the institution she visited diagnosed grandiose delusions and delusions of persecution, and declared her incurably insane. When I saw the patient for the first time about 3 years after the onset of her illness, she was a guest of a friend's family, and made herself useful by giving lessons to the children. Since she did not strike me as odd, either in her behaviour or her expressions, the news that she had been declared terminally insane by the director of an institution of course astonished me; she was therefore persuaded to accept my counsel. I found her an educated, sensitive lady, who was quite clear that she should have had the right to arrange her relationships with that young man as she saw fit; however her sense of duty to the school left her with no choice, 'She had the right to sacrifice herself to her duty'. She was in no doubt that the young man would have intended to propose to her. Yet she had to admit that not a single word had ever come from him which, similarly, could not be interpreted in an indifferent sense either. That he never did declare himself, which she had thought was a little unfair on his part, was due mainly to the intrigues and indelicate interference of the director and the entire teaching staff. She gave no credence to my assurance that all her perceptions of events could be explained by an abnormal preconceived opinion which was deceiving her; yet she had allowed herself voluntarily to be admitted to a hospital, where she remained I should say for a few weeks only. Now, 2 years later, I learned that the patient has resumed her teaching activities at a private school, has proved herself perfectly efficient there, but has now completely broken with all her former friends, and holds them partly to blame for the fact that she has been cheated out of her happiness. Explanatory delusions and falsifications of memory will have become building blocks of a now-completed system.

Gentlemen! I cannot help but add a brief comment here. Had it been a rather more ruthless personality, instead of a tender-minded and educated lady, she would certainly have asserted her claim on the teacher more vigorously, and become a typical example of the 'persecuted pursuers' [Ed], so often mentioned in recent times [2]. I am convinced that the majority of such cases can be traced back to some aberrant overvalued idea, save that the very base of the system often remains hidden in the self-conscious prejudices of observers [3]. Even the head of the institute whose above-quoted dictum aroused the not entirely unjustified indignation of the lady has focused just on the surface of the matter, apparently with no idea of the true nature of the illness.

In this lady there was no psychopathic basis from which the overvalued idea would have grown. However, you will not go far wrong if you take note of the 'critical' [W] age she had reached, combined with an excess of mental energy, and resulting in improper lifestyle, as sufficient reason for occurrence of a sexually-coloured, overvalued idea.

References

1. Friedmann M. Über den Wahn, eine klinisch-physiologische Unterstellung, nebst einer Darstellung der normalen Intelligenzvorgänge. Wiesbaden: JF Bergmann; 1894.
2. Magnan V. Psychiatrische Vorlesungen. Vol. 1. Ueber das 'Delire chronique à evolution systematique' (Paranoia chronica mit systematischer Entwickelung oder Paranoia completa). Leipzig: Georg Thieme; 1891.
3. Hitzig E. Über den Querulantenwahnsinn, seine nosologische Stellung und seine forensische Bedeutung. Leipzig: FCW Vogel; 1895.

Lecture 16

16

- When has a mental illness run its course?

Lecture

Gentlemen!

The question—if and when a psychosis that has not reverted to full health is to be regarded as having run its course—is, from everything we currently know, one of the most difficult we can pose; and yet it is at once of both theoretical and practical significance. From a theoretical point of view, its importance is clear from the idea that in autopsies of deceased cases we can see only *remnants* [Ed] of the disease process in the organ of association [1], but no longer the changes themselves, in the organ. In practical terms, cases where active illness is fully extinguished implicitly intermingle their healed deficits with ones that remain in other areas of pathology. Nothing would stand in the way of a patient being discharged from a mental hospital as soon as the change in content of consciousness, taken by itself, becomes harmless, as is often the case for an alleged inventor and founder of new world views. Evidence by which we can answer this question must of course be found exclusively in the area of symptomatology. Our task then is to examine psychotic symptoms we have met so far, with a view to determining whether, and to what extent, they are expressions of a more active disease process.

This question is of paramount importance because of the overwhelming significance of symptoms, especially explanatory delusions, in almost all paranoid states. In fact, this often shows up as an endless succession, in that one symptom can always emerge out of another; and so the process of delusion formation takes place over and over again. By contrast, in other cases the same substantive changes persist, to be joined by delusional explanations only in outline. An obvious difference here is certainly defined by the different ways in which patients react; the question then is only whether this has a basis in actual pathology. I have already mentioned that a vigorous reaction to change in content of consciousness, once that has happened, is to be seen as *normal* [Ed] mental activity; accordingly, explanatory delusions which subsequently correct the content of consciousness cannot be based on pathological processes. After all, such subsequent correction is conditional upon substantive change of consciousness remaining to command each patient's interest.

The simplest example on offer here is that of a delusional idea of a psychiatric patient lacking insight about his illness, who at the time of that illness had been illegally detained and robbed of his freedom. We can assume that such a patient, on resuming a regular job and returning to a normal way of life, would find so many other normal interests that, only if his main interest remained focused on the alleged injustice, would

R. Miller, K.J. Dennison (eds.), *An Outline of Psychiatry in Clinical Lectures*,
DOI 10.1007/978-3-319-18051-9_16

he reveal any particularly unfortunate traits. But let us assume instead that a lawyer, full of legal concepts, suffered the same fate; then his main interest would focus on the injustice he had suffered; and accretion of new delusional explanations would probably become obvious. He might file a complaint claiming compensation. Since 'what befalls one befalls another' [W]—there would be no more closely linked notion than that others too might have suffered the same injustice. If his complaints are then rejected, he might come to believe that not only he himself but also his fellow sufferers are deemed guilty; and so he continues to pursue his rights. Constant rejection shakes his faith in Justice; he comes to suspect that judges were bribed, possibly by the same faction that had seen fit to put him away in the mental hospital; or that the law was bent, to cover up the institution's alleged crimes. Even his earlier personal experience becomes generalized. He now considers every lawsuit from the same point of view, and therefore constantly arrives at new false judgments. Let us make the quite plausible assumption that his wife had arranged his admission to hospital. Even in the institution, he has harboured the suspicion that she has taken up with another man; yet he has fought—and temporarily overcome—this belief. Now however, when outside the institution, the suspicion re-emerges: He begins to observe all of his wife's comings and goings from this point of view; he pays attention to things he had never noticed before; he highlights remarks of an incriminating nature, and so on. If, following from normal expression of Affects, abnormal jealousy were to arise, delusional jealousy with all its conflicts may end up in the patient's being readmitted. In all these trials and tribulations the patient now assesses his relationship to other people and to legal institutions incorrectly, according to his biased viewpoint, focusing on whether they support him or his opponents. Thus, we see a whole chain of false judgments being formed; expanding delusions, with each subsequent link as the logical consequence of the preceding one; and, for malcontents, each station along the entire pathway as a possible starting point for their insults and violence. In fact, such non-recovered mental patients are unpredictable in their actions.

We now want to examine conditions under which, despite the fact that he survived a mental illness, such a disastrous outcome could have arisen. The fact that special individual factors play a major part was already pointed out. I have already emphasized the importance of suitable employment, as this may draw out the patient's interest—usually in a quite normal way. Of greater importance however is the social milieu in which the patient finds himself, and his acceptance there. If he has to deal with foolish people who offer support for his misconceptions about the past, and reinforce his beliefs, he will delve just as injudiciously into newspaper reports about his fellow victims; he will again be excited by these and can hardly escape from delusions, which continue every day and week that passes after his discharge, unless he puts his allegations to the test, thinking this to be in his best interests, thus helping the inherently false focus of his attention to fade away. Thus an Affect-laden frame of mind must be seen as the most common precondition for explanatory delusions. Gradually, and in favourable cases, patients themselves notice that return of awareness of their illness period is unhelpful; and I could show you several such patients who are 'right back into' [W] their life, and who are independent enough to earn their own bread; yet they are very reluctant to talk about their periods of illness, even setting up major barriers to clinical probing. In practice, it follows from this that one cannot be too careful when planning discharge of mental patients who are only 'improved' [Ed]; yet the issue cannot be side-stepped, as it is a means of strengthening each patient's normal interests as they make their way forwards independently, thereby granting them further possibilities of subsequent rehabilitation. Unfortunately, however, it is often inevitable that patients return to a life with no structure of regular activity, nor any ordered social engagement, conditions that are harmful both through the lack of normal interests and also even by pre-disposing them to emergence of depressed Affects. Their main interest may then remain focused on experiences of injustice; an Affect-laden state of mind sets in, and further delusion formation is inevitable. Thus we see that individual circumstances can decide the outcome—another argument supporting our view that the formation of explanatory delusions cannot be based on an ongoing disease process. Further evidence for this lies in the fact that certain acute illnesses are characterized by clear *absence* [Ed] of explanatory delusions, this going hand in hand with pronounced deficit symptoms, that is, an apparent dearth of mental activity. Delusion formation cannot occur in such cases, precisely because normal processes for contextual change by the association mechanism are lacking.

The situation for most other symptoms that you already know is quite different from such explanatory delusions. The first things that come to mind here, as the principal means of systematization, are symptoms of additive and subtractive falsification of memory, and retrospective delusions of reference. As shown above, their readjustments seem to occur only when the solid structure of associations has been loosened by sejunction processes. However, since those same symptoms may be absent in the presence of this condition, without this being explained by any actual deficit state, we must assume that these symptoms, so essential for development of a delusional system, must have another basis. The most obvious assumption is that it is not sejunction which has already happened that is essential, but that which is still in progress, as an ongoing disease process. At least, this assumption is most likely for the three other symptoms: autochthonous ideas, hallucinations, and delusions of relatedness, albeit with some restrictions.

I remind you that in the case of residual hallucinosis we came to know a stage of illness, which along with the accompanying delusions had been viewed mainly as a sequel to the sejunction process, after the latter had died down. This formulation may be conveniently modified, so that it corresponds to the stage of 'dying away' [Ed] of 'subsidence' [Ed] of the sejunctive processes; a stage therefore in which the most acute sejunction processes have already faded, along with all other severe symptoms of acute psychosis, so that just the aforementioned elementary symptoms emerge in their purest form. The assumption was made above that habituation of excitation occurs through backflow of 'nerve current' [Ed]; and thus aforementioned symptoms could become habitual, while the pathological process itself had reached a standstill. This assumption would seem to apply only to cases in which phonemes and delusions of relatedness had already existed for a long period, especially during acute phases of the illness; and for such cases one must concede the possibility that these symptoms persist to some extent as a purely functional disorder. Apart from that, it will always be justified to take the above-mentioned symptoms as signatures of a still active disease process, even if it is in decline.

A second exception is the occurrence of a circumscribed delusion of reference, as we came to recognize it on p. 92. Amongst very stable findings seen in these patients in every other respect, and with emergence of delusions of reference always limited to very specific situations or the sight of certain people, here too we can see delusions of reference as relatively fixed, now quite habitual, and thus to be viewed as the *outcome* [Ed] of a functional change. At the same time this urges us to consider that these delusions are nothing new as regards their content, and therefore represent no further development of the delusion.

If we apply the same criterion to the now-habitual phonemes and the delusions of relatedness in each previously mentioned case, we might expect, by their characteristic content, that they too can be seen as *expressions* [Ed] of current delusional ideas, without their leading to any further development, or incorporation of new delusions. In fact, there are related cases of illness in which, despite persisting hallucinations and delusions of relatedness, actual systematization never occurs.

In general, from a patient's displays of Affect, one has an indication of whether the hallucinations and delusions of relatedness move just along familiar paths, or contain new items. Fading Affect is therefore often a sign of favourable outcome, in that it indicates fading of hallucinations and delusions of relatedness, and their gradual cessation. Apart from that, internal links between Affects and occurrence of those symptoms of active psychosis cannot be underestimated, since those Affects, given their origin, must be considered normal, but clearly are often occasional precursors of sporadic occurrence of phonemes and delusions of relatedness in otherwise stable states. We have already met an example of this in a rare case where isolated phonemes occurred among malcontents. This is also the reason why patients in whom the sejunctive processes were only moderately pervasive must often continue, even after their relative restoration of health, to rely on life in the institution. Any attempt to return to the hard struggles of life outside leads to relapse, with acute psychotic symptoms; and only a well-equipped institution offers such patients constant thoughtfulness and benevolent treatment, as well as the freedom from material wants, which for them is a precondition for permanent mental equilibrium.

Gentlemen! As a generalization, one could state that a fine measure of how secure the constitution of a person's brain might be is to be found in the brain's ability to withstand Affects of especially distressing kind. Therefore you sometimes see apparently strong men, who have never experienced mental illness, steering clear—with anxious dread—of those occasions when powerful Affects are unavoidable in their mental processing of annoying events. In contrast, I know of nothing more conclusive for the partial nature of the disorder and healthy performance of the brain (in contrast to the alleged 'degeneracy' [W]) than the elation and joy with which many malcontents join their fight, and who, despite all disappointments and adversities, continue to fight to the utmost for their rights.

Gentlemen! As a main criterion for the disease process being really over, we must consider a critical test: whether the return to civilian life meets with success. This test should therefore be carried out, if at all possible; and the task of the institution, to create conditions of an active and free life in an artificial way, should be reserved only for those invalids who cannot exist otherwise. A second criterion is just as important, but sometimes fails in individual cases. It consists of the 'general condition' [Ed] of a patient. The crudest measure of this is for a patient to have a constant, relatively high body weight. Disturbed sleep and appetite are already excluding factors. We face as a fact, which for laymen is quite surprising, that the brain has a large influence on diet. This confronts us particularly in acute psychoses. However, this is also revealed in chronic psychoses, and particularly in paranoid states where each more severe exacerbation and every state of intense Affect are associated with a decrease in body weight, often in striking contrast to apparently unaltered balance between intake and output, to be explained only by specific trophic influences. This offers a rewarding task for metabolic experiment that, doubtless, will lead to an interesting and instructive result.

Reference

1. Weigert C. Beiträge zur Kenntnis der menschlichen Neuroglia. Frankfurt: Moritz Sierterweg; 1895. Aus d. Abhandl. d. Senkenberg. naturforsch. Ges. 1895; 63–209.

Lecture 17

17

- Course of chronic psychoses
- Aetiological classification
- Griesinger's primordial deliria

Lecture

Gentlemen!

With the summary knowledge of paranoid states that you have acquired so far, I realize that so far you have become acquainted only with certain dominating symptoms; but many others that occur concurrently can also be found only as acute psychoses. However, you will now be able to discover the main features of the vast majority of paranoid states—and so satisfy the requirement which must be fulfilled, with examples, in each psychiatric report, namely that psychotic symptoms which constitute the mental disorder in each specific case must be recorded in precise detail—a requirement that sadly is seldom met in reports of even so-called authorities. I cannot emphasize strongly enough that you have the right to declare a person mentally ill only when you can produce evidence of this by establishing definite psychotic symptoms; only then will you be spared the embarrassment of your opinion being exposed to justified attacks by lay people. The 'general impression' [W] sometimes relied on even by better known representatives of our profession, when they fail to elicit definite psychotic symptoms, is no better than everyday parlance and must elicit the deepest suspicion, when used as the basis of diagnosis of a paranoid state. It deserves to be rejected most strongly when, in such cases, the claim is made that we are dealing with a well-known and relatively simple disease state, given the accurate name of *paranoia chronica simplex*. Then, it is easy to arouse the impression of intentional deception, for both judges and lay people, thereby harming the reputation of the entire alienist profession. If you want to avoid such mistakes, please note that the most obvious self-aggrandizement is far from any grandiose delusion; mistrust and hatred of a few—or many—people is not a persecutory delusion; and paranoid states are mental disorders which are always relatively easy to grasp, detected by very specific psychotic symptoms.

In some of our most widely read textbooks you will see sub-classification of paranoia into *paranoia chronica simplex* and *hallucinatoria*. You can infer from my comments how much or rather how little such distinctions are justified. There is no merit at all in independent terminology for hallucinations, at least for phonemes, which almost always predominate.

Perhaps it requires a certain apology, when, with motives such as I have just outlined, I choose the term 'paranoid states' [W] to cover all chronic mental disorders in which material alterations of consciousness are dominant. One might object by demanding that I at least make

R. Miller, K.J. Dennison (eds.), *An Outline of Psychiatry in Clinical Lectures*,
DOI 10.1007/978-3-319-18051-9_17

an attempt to delineate clearly the supposedly well-known *paranoia chronica simplex* [W]. I deliberately avoid such an attempt because, in my opinion, there is no well-known illness of this type, unless you want the name to monopolise that very small number of individual cases that happen to match one another. I come back to those cases shortly (p. 102).

With regard to the broader range of paranoid states, our lack of our knowledge is particularly noticeable when we try to subdivide them according to their respective course and later development. In this regard, we are familiar with only some limiting cases. I shall briefly recapitulate these here, according to data that I have often touched on. Among residual mental disorders are some we have come to recognize as stable states, usually characterized by low incidence of symptoms, and integrity of other functions. Then, there are other cases, about which we know little, which are characterized by very gradual, creeping development, and an equally slow, steadily progressing course, never amounting to actual acute attacks or severe exacerbations. For both types of illness, as for all major changes, we can construct a disease curve corresponding to the expansion of the disease state. In the first situation the corresponding curve remains parallel with the x-axis; in the second—it rises uniformly and slowly away from the x-axis.

A few remarks are directed to those latter cases with an extremely chronic course. They correspond to the rather more common type, of slowly emerging persecutory delusions, which, after some time, may evolve into grandiose ones. The period of slow, imperceptible development in such cases, which often makes it difficult to determine the precise starting date, is characterized by occurrence of delusions of relatedness, and, shortly afterward, by isolated phonemes with the same content. An overvalued idea may take hold as the first and foremost symptom, and determine the substance of delusions of reference. Gradually the phonemes get out of hand, and other sensory hallucinations and abnormal sensations may even join in. Persecutory ideas are then systematized in two ways. One is via delusions of explanation, which refer to the hallucinations themselves: the so-called physical persecution complex [Ed], with hallucinations related in turn to the agent behind the persecution, and his motives. Grandiosity preferentially links up with a series of explanatory delusions, because of the logical necessity of explaining how such a large following—an array of so many people—should develop. If discernment and formal thought processes are well preserved, this finally leads to formation of technical terms of a more or less adventurous nature, often appearing at first as phonemes, providing patients with newly formed words. Such patients express themselves in a changed manner, which is very characteristic. By means of their intact sense of logic, their entire world view is gradually transformed and, depending on the sick person's state of mind, philosophical systems may be advocated with quite outlandish structures. Formally correct logic and unmistakable intellectual productivity remain right to the end. In the philosophical literature of the last decade, you may have been struck by a multi-volume work written by an apparently mentally ill scholar, which would have left you shaking your head. The final outcome of the full disease process is a material change in all three domains of awareness, because the patient sooner or later becomes aware of physical changes in his body. Thus, if you want to choose a name for such cases, then in the later stages you are dealing with 'chronic total psychosis' [Ed]. The initial symptoms are likewise beyond any question, the entire first period of the illness manifest predominantly in the allopsychic area. Delusions of relatedness are detectable by themselves for a long time, entirely of an allopsychic character as just described. Hallucinations with explanatory delusions bring about gradual, but inexorable, reinterpretation of the outside world; and for initial years of illness, the designation of 'chronic worsening allopsychosis' [Ed]—also 'chronic hallucinosis' [Ed]—is justified. The qualifier 'worsening' [Ed] indicates that the psychosis gradually becomes total, since, from the time of onset of grandiose delusions, it also encompasses the autopsychic domain. That it never comes to more severe symptoms in the area of motility also seems characteristic of such cases. While relatively common (pp. 63, 64), only a small absolute number belong to the class of 'purely chronically progressing' [Ed] cases. These correspond most closely to the commonly alleged *paranoia chronica* [W]. The two female patients, Schmidt and Reising, are examples of this—the latter, right from the outset, in conjunction with an overvalued idea.

A third trajectory for paranoid states has become known to me over the course of time through several cases. It develops in a special manner, representing continuation of a bout of acute psychosis, after surviving several such bouts in previous years with total recovery. Up to the present, I have seen such a disease process after acute hallucinosis, or acute hallucinatory allopsychosis (see later), usually in alcoholics. Progression of the chronic condition, which always takes the form of a physical delusion of persecution, here seems to be more rapid and deleterious than for the aforementioned chronic forms.

I can mention a fourth form of paranoid state only in anticipation here. Amongst acute psychoses, about which we will learn later, is the state of depressive melancholia, an acute general illness characterized by intermingling of Affect and general akinesia of intrapsychic origin. Such a melancholic state can, for a long time, imply existence of pure melancholia, until clues are provided from a patient's altered behaviour that intrapsychic dysfunction is subsiding, but at the same time, delusions of relatedness and corresponding phonemes appear. Usually it is any outbreak of indignation that prompts a patient to speak out, and with one stroke, to reveal an entirely different picture. The paranoid state, which is now revealed, is usually made up of persecutory and grandiose delusions in equal measure. Outbursts of wild ranting and a tendency to violence accompany it in nearly characteristic ways, leading quite soon to falsification of the entire contents of consciousness, to the point of material confusion. Patients seem to be able to remain in this stage of major confusion for a long time, although with decreasing energy in their actions, but without actual dementia. I am not yet clear of the final outcome. To avoid misunderstanding, I notice that the substantial confusion is by no means due exclusively to this course of events, but occurs with any extensive falsification of consciousness. Patients ultimately function using a series of idiosyncratic terms, making them unintelligible to other individuals, and they may even be understood falsely by others. Such confusion is then only apparent confusion, not noticed at all by another individual with just the same falsifications of consciousness.

Undoubtedly, in years to come, there will be success in determining a well-characterized set of trajectories amongst paranoid states, apart from the four just presented here; but for the time being I content myself with these hints, and confine myself to indicating the task that awaits us here. It will consist of establishing the regularity with which individual psychotic symptoms and significant changes follow one another, for it cannot be accidental how the symptoms are grouped together, any more than it is mere coincidence that in the entire domain of other nervous diseases it often comes down to particular, well-characterized groups of symptoms. In the latter case, the reason for this is no secret: It lies in the particular arrangement of the nerve pathways in certain parts of the brain. If I remind you that we could likewise regard those major changes in consciousness as, in a certain sense, focal points, then we can apply the same principle here too, enabling us also to think of particular groups of symptoms as the expressions of definite anatomical arrangements in association pathways. For the time being, as I have said, we are right at the beginning of our knowledge of such groupings, and I would caution you to interpret the manners of progression outlined above only as groupings of the most common cases. In reality, they are only a fraction of the many variants of unknown type included amongst the many paranoid states.

Gentlemen! It may perhaps seem surprising to you that I neglect classification by the principle of aetiology when trying to organize the many forms of paranoid states. If I were actually to carry that out, I would certainly be taking a false path. However, in what I specifically described, for a psychosis that begins in bursts and then progresses towards physical persecution mania, you will find an aetiology of alcoholism. The question of aetiology is the second task that needs to be addressed, one of equal importance. Thus, just as it would be wrong to deal with palsy due to lead poisoning before you are familiar with its most common form, namely bilateral radial nerve paresis, so it would also be incorrect methodology if you wanted to start classifying psychoses on the sole basis of aetiology. I can easily show how one-sided is this approach by the fact that acute hallucinosis of a drinker also occurs in non-drinkers. Let us assert that the psychoses are brain diseases, and that we can assume that one and the same site always produces the same symptoms. Here then is an area accessible to research. For some causes however, we cannot expect that the effects will always point to the same sites, just as if a brain haemorrhage always has to be in the same site in the brain. The aetiological factor must therefore be only secondary in this area of research. I know full well that under some circumstances the site that is attacked is also determined by the aetiology, particularly the paresis already mentioned; but disease of the posterior columns, produced by alcoholism and syphilis, and, finally, the best known type of progressive paralysis are also examples of this. Later too, in acute hallucinosis of alcoholism, and in presbyophrenia we will learn about psychoses where the same is true. In general however, I cannot emphasize strongly enough that the forthcoming principle of classification must be that of anatomical arrangement, giving a natural grouping and sequence of material changes.

Gentlemen! I must content myself for the time being, with explaining my point of view on these important issues, reserving the right to come back later, with more detail, since acute psychoses necessarily require a definite opinion on these issues. However, I cannot side-step mention of a specific point here: Chronic psychoses are, to a large extent, no more than outcomes of acute psychoses. Given that, it seemed to me advisable, concerning certain phenomena mentioned in the literature, not simply to remain silent on these undercurrents. Works of an eminent French psychiatrist, Magnan, have drawn us, even here in Germany, in his direction, in the back-and-forth swirl of public opinion. You could easily gain the impression that a new, opportune expression had been found for several universally known clinical facts, and that there were actually only two major disease groups to be distinguished amongst chronic mental disorders: mental disorders of degeneration on the one hand, and mental illness which is probably well defined clinically, but not by aetiology, and which the French author calls *Délire chronique à évolution systématique* [W] but which the German translator calls *paranoia completa* [W]. As you can see, basically I have to reject such a classification because of what it leads to: a supposedly clinical, well-known form of chronic mental illness—the supposedly well-defined chronic paranoia—separate from all other mental illnesses, and the so-called degeneration, acknowledging the latter to have only one aetiology. You encounter here, in my opinion, just the same exaggeration, which has so far led to failure of all attempts at classification of the psychoses. The class of 'complete chronic paranoia' [Ed] is, in my opinion, far too broad, containing a wide diversity of different chronic psychoses, which are yet to be differentiated. Only in this way could that author get to the contrasting idea of 'degeneration' [W] accounting for the entire field of psychoses. As for these latter cases, I do not doubt that even this aetiological point of view, as well as many others, will prove fruitful; in Magnan's work however, it is grossly overestimated; and I believe that I should point out to you, as a core of the notion, just one fact: In 'degeneration' [W], psychotic symptoms appear preferentially, either in isolation like overvalued ideas or just at such low intensity that it remains in doubt whether the individual in question is to be regarded as already mentally ill. Evidence for the fact that such borderline cases are particularly common among the 'degenerates' [W] can hardly be found anywhere except in Magnan's studies. There again it is based on exaggeration, where the author appears to regard cases of illness—that I described as circumscribed autopsychoses or overvalued ideas—as occurring only among degenerates. This is not the case at all, unless you want to acknowledge occurrence of psychosis itself as evidence of existing degeneration.

Gentlemen! Allow me to end this discussion with a remark intended to prevent possible misunderstandings. I am well aware that I have fulfilled the task that I originally set myself—that of constructing for you a lifelike portrayal of paranoid states—in only a very inadequate way. You will find later that I have not even touched on several important symptoms, and, on the other hand, have already mentioned some things that actually belong in the field of *acute* [Ed] mental illnesses. But the difficulty here lies in the subject matter. It is actually impossible to give a vivid portrayal of even a single area, such as I have selected here, without expanding to the entire area to put it into perspective. This impossibility has, however, come to my attention even more in acute mental illnesses, so that after many years of work I had to decide to reverse my strategy, and to start working from the ground upwards, placing acute mental illnesses, which are still the main source of paranoid conditions, as the precursor of the latter. It is just the same with individual symptoms: Each newly-emerging symptom of mental disorder may have an acute character. Most chronic mental illnesses can even be characterized by their acute episodes, with new symptoms, which may occur at any period along their course. I have intentionally avoided describing these states wherever possible, because they belong with the acute psychoses; but this was not wholly successful for separating such episodes from newly-emerging individual symptoms, because even there, just as everywhere else in nature, imperceptible transitions take place.

Gentlemen! The history of psychiatry is probably an area that is extremely interesting to experts, but for you, who still require instruction in the rudiments, it must take a back seat compared to the greater needs of the moment. Nevertheless, I should not omit one topic here, whose place in the history of our science we cannot deny. This concerns what Griesinger called primordial delirium. In in-patient clinics you will have heard so much about this great clinician that you will not be surprised that his textbook of psychiatry is still one of the most widely read books, and produced downright amazement in its day. Yet in this book Griesinger takes a position not shared by well-known older authors, in that he denies that primary material changes can occur without preceding melancholy mood; and only in 1867 [1] did his view shift to a more accurate one with his proposal of a 'primordial delirium' [W], this coming after a preceding lecture by Snell [2] entitled 'Monomania as the primary form of mental disturbance' [W]. Given the dominant status going along with Griesinger's strong personality, you can imagine that the teaching of primordial deliria now proclaimed by him shifted everybody's perceptions, and was welcomed as a great step forward for our science. I know this myself, from the beginning of my career in psychiatry in 1871; and I still clearly remember that this point was always a focal point of discussions, whenever psychiatric topics arose. However, one of the unintended effects of the book, and of Griesinger's teaching, was that primordial deliria rarely happened, and the interest of all young psychiatrists was focused mainly on diseases of nerves and brain. In this regard it will seem strange to you that amongst psychotic symptoms, which are regarded as the foundations of paranoid states, I have not yet mentioned 'primordial deliria' [W]. Let me now explain this; but first, please let me pass on a remark about Snell's position, in that he indisputably had priority over Griesinger. Why then was the famous concept of primordial deliria linked not to Snell's name but to Griesinger's? The answer is simply that, although the same phenomenon was recognized by both researchers, the versatile, thoroughly-trained clinician, complete master of the clinical method, felt the need to trace it back to certain elementary psychotic symptoms which he had just named 'primordial deliria' [Ed]. Both authors started from the same clinical experience, that in a certain type of mental illness, which Griesinger called 'primary craziness' [W], and Snell called 'monomania' [W] without prior melancholy (in the sense of older authors); primary ideas of persecution apparently arise at a time of elevated, self-confident mood. But while Snell was satisfied with sketching the general course taken by these cases, with intelligence remaining intact, yet with frequent additions of subsequent grandiose ideas, Griesinger sought to penetrate more deeply into relevant pathways, to find, in primordial misconceptions, and specifically, in false judgments, the source of those ideas of persecution, and possibly also of grandiose ideas. To clarify what I mean, I give detail of such judgments: The idea emerged in one patient, by way of example (a case of anxiety psychosis) that his parents, his wife, and his children were dead, and he was readily convinced of this. To another came the thought that he should be executed, and to a third that he was a millionaire, or of princely descent. Thus, there are 'emerging ideas' [W] that are held to be true, a phenomenon that may remind you of obsessions and autochthonous ideas.

So I find that I can understand only Griesinger, and thereby catch a glimpse of his real stature. Let us see how he himself spoke, in his lecture at the opening of the psychiatric clinic on 4 May 1867 [1]: 'In ganglion cells of cortical grey matter, according to our current assumptions, processes that *trigger* [Ed] the imagination come first' [W]. Abnormal transmission is then the result of *tabes dorsalis* [Ed], a disease of dorsal columns; and 'then abnormal action of those cortical cells immediately triggers images, words and ideas of all kinds, which no longer correspond with reality' [W]. Here we see Griesinger putting forward a proposition that is close to our own. However, it is not lost on him that such nonsensical judgments should be constructed from pre-existing material within the thought processes. To explain why, he indicates two sets of phenomena. *First* [Ed]: Disturbance of ganglion cells can be purely functional, they being excited from other distant sites. He calls this phenomenon 'associated signs' [Ed], in which the first activation may, for example, be produced by sensation in the bowels. We can simply accept this view, and you will remember that I repeatedly indicated such a development of specific manifestations using the term 'anxiety phenomena' [W]. In acute psychoses their location can be traced back to this in a comprehensive manner.

The *second* [Ed] set of clinical phenomena, in which he contrived an analogy with primary occurrence of certain erroneous judgments in the insane, is the occurrence of obsessions in neurasthenic patients; the overwhelming incidence of 'animal delirium' [Ed] in *delirium potatorum* [W]; and finally the subjective sensation of a particular colour, red, in certain pathological brain states (e.g. epilepsy). Here a connection with legitimate false judgments of mentally ill people is produced only by taking obsessions into account. So, the great mystery remains for Griesinger: how such regularity of content can arise—the occurrence of ideas of grandiosity and persecution, in which 'perhaps among ten patients, only five throughout the whole duration of the disease, form the main content of the delirium' [W]. Now we have known since Meynert that it is the properties of the primary Ego of the child, and of primitive people, that are reflected in this regularity, and I need only refer you to his essay *Über den Wahn* [W] [3] to allow you to get your orientation on this. In the natural state, people interpret as actions any events that touch their well-being or might harm them; and on this basis, ideas of persecution or grandiosity develop as two basic ways in which an individual might react, as does anybody, to impressions from the outside world.

We now must ask: Is there really such a primary mode of origin for delusions of persecution and grandiosity, in Griesinger's sense? I can give an affirmative answer only in a very limited sense: To my knowledge, the supposed primary delusion of persecution of chronic psychoses generally develops from either delusions of relatedness, as described above, or explanatory delusions; and, in my opinion, other modes of origin for paranoid states can be excluded, if you do not want to include paranoia of feeble-mindedness as well. The same goes for grandiose delusions [4]; but I submit that besides the consecutive grandiose delusion, which develops in a logical succession from persecutory delusion, and furthermore besides the grandiose delusion of the feeble minded about which we shall speak later, there are two other sources of the so-called grandiose delusions, which can easily be overlooked, and can then mimic the appearance of a grandiose delusion in its primary sense. One is the substantive somatopsychic change mentioned once or twice earlier, a hypochondriacal feeling of happiness, with a feeling of anxiety located in the chest region, and probably varying along with this. Usually this is correlated with the process of respiration, and is described as very light, easy breathing. Such was the case for example in an earlier mentioned patient (p. 73), Schulz, who believed himself to be filled with the Holy Spirit, preached inspired sermons to people, and travelled to a nearby region to have himself consecrated by the court chaplain. Grandiosity in this case is merely a case of what I call 'ideas of happiness' [W] and forms the complement of occasionally mentioned 'ideas of anxiety' [W]. The second source is again delusions of reference, often connected to certain overvalued ideas, or at other times to the hypochondriacal happiness described above. Autochthonous ideas emerge in such cases, with falsifications of memory, and retrospective delusions of reference, which dress themselves up as facts, to fulfill a scheme, and are made manifest in the elevated mood and enhanced clinical facts.

I would like expressly to state only one exception, so as not to distort the clinical facts. There seems to occur, although very seldom, in young people developing a chronic mental illness what Sander [5] calls 'original craziness' [W], in which the primordial deliria, in Griesinger's sense, form the original source of grandiose ideas. Yet pure cases of this kind are seen only quite exceptionally. Closer examination of these cases almost always allows grandiosity to be traced back to one of the other previously named elementary psychotic symptoms. Apart from this, the majority of such cases of so-called original craziness [Ed] belong to borderline feeble-mindedness, which may remain undetected for a long time, since the so-called original craziness usually occurs as a hebephrenic psychosis; and only in some extreme—yet undoubted—cases, can it be distinguished from them. In my experience, in the majority of such cases, not one of the above-mentioned, actual psychotic elements is detectable, on account of their long-term feeble-mindedness identifying them as hebephrenia.

Gentlemen! I cannot end this historical digression without mentioning a significant literary event, in which somebody spoke eloquently about Griesinger's primordial deliria, but unfortunately found defenders shooting wide of the mark. Friedmann, in his book *Über den Wahn* [6] [W], investigated the essential nature of delusions—let us say the substantive falsifications of consciousness—in paranoid states as such, according to the false judgments, corresponding to the type of primordial deliria. Closely related obsessions are regarded by him as a fundamental symptom of 'paranoia' [W] which he also accepted, but understood in a very broad sense. We shall see later that his assumption about acute mental illnesses is true in many cases, but we must reject his attempted generalization. In chronic cases it is contradicted by experience, and we are not mistaken if we attribute the one-sidedness of this astute researcher to his lack of a large sample.

References

1. Griesinger W. Vortragsur Eröffnung der psychiatrischen Klinik zu Berlin am 2 Mai 1867. Arch Psychiatr Nervenkr. 1868;7:143–58.
2. Snell L. Über Monomanie als primäre Form der Seelenstörung. Allg Z Psychiat. 1865;22:368–81.
3. Meynert Th. Ueber den Wahn. In: Sammlung von populär-wissenschaftlichen Vorträgen über den Bau und die Leistungen des Gehirns. Vienna: Wilhelm Braumüller; 1892. p. 83.
4. Snell L. Die Ueberschätzungsideen der Paranoia. Allg Z Psychiat. 1890;46:447–60.
5. Sander W. Übereinespezielle Form der primären Verrücktheit. Arch Psychiatr. 1868;1:387–419.
6. Friedmann M. Über den Wahn, eine klinisch-physiologische Unterstellung, nebst einer Darstellung der normalen Intelligenzvorgänge. JF Bergmann: Wiesbaden; 1894.

Part III

Acute Psychoses and Defect States

Lecture 18

18

- Definition of acute, as opposed to chronic, psychoses
- Presentation of an almost recovered case of acute psychosis
- Features and special coloration of ideas of explanatory delusions
- A few new sources of delusional elaboration:
  - By analogy
  - By failure of attention
  - And by aberrant restructuring of associations

Lecture

Gentlemen!

Acute psychoses are characterized primarily by their manner of creation: We should consider as *acute* [Ed], using the word 'acute' [Ed] as it is used in other organic diseases, all of those mental disorders which develop within hours, days, or over several weeks to produce a significant level of symptoms. Further development of the illness is then subject to whether and for how long the patient remains in the acute stage, whether there is recovery, or whether the disorder progresses to a chronic condition. In the latter situation, acute psychosis merges into an acute initial stage of a chronic psychosis. With the same logic, acute stages of chronic psychoses presenting at times other than the initial period must be regarded as acute psychoses.

However, were we to focus solely on the time course to determine whether a psychosis was acute or chronic, it would have little bearing on the complexities of real situations and the terms used to describe them. Instead, it is the characteristics of the clinical presentation, its 'acute nature' [W], which immediately denotes it as being the result of rapid development. Even with a long duration of illness, or where the onset is not rapid, these characteristics are sufficient that they provide independent criteria for recognizing an acute psychosis. This shows the special position that must always be given to diseases of the nervous system: Long-standing sciatica or other neuralgia, or an old *Tabes* [W] can go hand in hand with severely racking pain; and the overwhelmingly chronic suffering due to brain tumours brings with it regular periods of the most acute neurological symptoms, such as combinations of headaches, dizziness, vomiting, and general convulsions. Thus, acute reactions of the nervous system reveal themselves quite generally as depending on the timing of stimuli, which has little apparent connection to the basic progression of a disease process, namely change in anatomical tissue. In our efforts to characterize acute psychoses in more detail, we must consequently rely, essentially, on other more detailed criteria. May I remind you, gentlemen, of remarks (p. 54, Lecture 9) I made on the mutual interactions between content of consciousness and conscious activity and, in consequence, on the resulting

R. Miller, K.J. Dennison (eds.), *An Outline of Psychiatry in Clinical Lectures*,
DOI 10.1007/978-3-319-18051-9_18

effects that abnormal alterations in *content* [Ed] of consciousness produce on the main object of our study, as we dealt with chronic psychoses. We must now add, in so far as this is familiar to us, permanent or irreversible changes in content of consciousness. However, we will have no problems with the further conclusion that abnormal changes of conscious *activity* [Ed] help define the form for acute psychoses.

Gentlemen! If you now recall the schema (p. 13) I gave you at that time, for deriving psychotic symptoms, you will soon find that it also represents a schema of the abnormal changes in conscious activity, changes which we identified wholly as disorders of secondary identification. To show how symptoms of mental illness are derived from this schema, and to put their occurrence and importance in various mental illnesses in their proper perspective, would be a separate and independent teaching exercise; yet any such attempt might take us too far from our real task, which is to become familiar with specific cases of illness. I shall therefore restrict myself just to the most important problems of identification from a theoretical point of view: I shall discuss these separately, in some detail, as ones which are quite essential for understanding the general pathology of mental illnesses. These are mainly symptoms falling in the domain of hallucinations, or which have internal links with such symptoms. Otherwise, I must restrict myself whenever I present an illness to shedding light on the meaning of the new symptoms you will encounter, in relation to our schema.

Gentlemen! Simple reflections will show you that, for symptoms derived from our schema, the symptomatology of acute mental illnesses is a field with no boundaries. Earlier we had come to realize that the activity of consciousness generates the content of consciousness, so that altered activity of consciousness must also result in changes in the content of consciousness; and we could thus define acute mental illnesses as the changes in content of consciousness taking place within a certain time frame (p. 54). However, now we can assume a priori [W] that such changes in content of consciousness during acute mental illnesses will be less fixed or shorter in duration than those in chronic illnesses. Nevertheless, the clinical significance of substantive disturbances of consciousness during acute mental illnesses is so significant and crucial for establishing the characteristics of illness that any teaching on illness which neglected this point of view in a one-sided manner would turn out to be insufficient to encompass the clinical facts. While in chronic psychoses or paranoid states we could limit ourselves mainly to changes in *content* [Ed] of consciousness, you should understand how much more complicated are our tasks in describing acute psychoses, where changes in activity of consciousness are just as important as the changes in its content.

In addition, secondary processes, which we saw added to various elementary symptoms in the chronic psychoses are, to a great extent, also present in acute psychoses. They may even be enhanced—for instance the principle of explanatory delusions; and, just as explanatory delusions do not in themselves represent abnormal activity, so in acute mental illnesses we will get to know *new sources of delusion formation* [W], which likewise are aspects of normal mental life. Experiences that we will gain in this respect, forming, in one sense, an addition to the theory of paranoid states, are also quite appropriately included here. A patient who is now due for discharge, and who has been free from psychotic symptoms for 3 months, offers us a good opportunity. He is a 27-year-old, academically-qualified mechanical engineer K. who is considered to have recovered from this, his second episode of a severe mental illness, complicated by his lack of insight into a few symptoms of his illness persisting from the time of its acute onset. He has a complete memory for the entire period, approximately 1½ years of illness, and his intelligence and training in scientific observation make him quite rare, as a reporter about certain symptoms.

I skip over the fact that this patient can give us a detailed account of the voices and autochthonous ideas at the time of his illness. We learn from this only that these familiar elementary symptoms of paranoid states often also occur in acute mental illnesses. Much more important for our purposes are the explanatory delusions which the patient connects to these experiences. He was, in fact, always fully aware that the voices, which he could see as having no objective basis, could not be explained by any physical means, and so there remained for him only the evidence of his senses, and—much as he struggled against it initially—the assumption of supernatural effects of 'spirits' [W]. He then attributed the strange thoughts as coming from these spirits; and the fact that they never led to a physical delusion of persecution but rather to the assumption of supernatural effects can, to some extent, be ascribed to this person's scientific training. We see also from this example that *delusions of explanation in acute mental illnesses* [W] play no lesser role than they do in chronic states. Of course, as a prerequisite, there must be, to a certain degree, a retained ability to think—that is, there must be requirements of logic and the logical ability to provide explanations for these strange phenomena. In general, this condition corresponds, to some extent, to his discernment, as was mostly present in our patient. In addition, the content of explanatory delusions depends on individual characteristics of each patient. How much this is the case, you will see from a second case. Among thoughts that had been instilled in him, our patient announced that he had already been in the world several times, as Wotan, and as Ahlbrecht the bear. He therefore believed in transmigration of souls. When I asked him how he had imagined it, and if it was an act of resurrection, the patient expressed his view that the personality of every person should be viewed as a specific arrangement of material components, and he thought it possible that precisely the same order of molecules could be repeated at various times, and could produce the same person. Much as the patient himself now laughs at this assumption, you must admit that only a scientifically-minded person could formulate such an explanatory delusion.

When the conclusions a patient reaches amount to more complex explanatory delusions, a degree of discernment may be an indispensable prerequisite, as is likewise the case in his assessment of autochthonous thoughts. Assume that a false judgment, such as that just mentioned—of having lived twice previously, at different epochs—had been formed in this way. If such emergent thoughts are to be recognized as alien, a minimum level of judgment must nevertheless still remain. We should therefore not be surprised if acutely ill mental patients who lack such discernment find themselves in a state of more or less total bewilderment, and then express rather outlandish ideas without offering any critical opinion, or attempt an explanation. In this sense I recognize the occurrence of what Griesinger called primordial delirium in people who are acutely mentally ill, as mentioned earlier (p. 107), referring to Friedmann's book on delusions. Although, in his more recent work on origin of delusions, this author has persistently maintained his point of view—an excessively far-reaching one in my opinion [1], based on comparative ethnology—it nevertheless contradicts clinical experience, exactly in relation to the exception just presented. Incidentally, you can immediately see that development of obsessions or rather the correct judgment which protects patients from developing those ideas which might result from aberrant stimulation is generally conditional on a patient having a certain level of discernment and judgment. In future, we should remember that gradations of this sort can be obscured by new thoughts, which emerge suddenly among the acutely mentally ill, to be replaced by primordial delirium in Griesinger's sense. This is no cause for surprise, because the stormy Affects that interfere with orderly thinking often occur naturally in acute mental illnesses.

This patient also describes to us a form of delusion that we have not met before, and which he refers to as a 'vision' [Ed]. He believed that during his illness he experienced whole scenes and situations that sometimes played out in other historical periods. He described to us, for example, that he had seen his father in a French Marshal's uniform, standing by the scaffold, the threatening crowd below, and the hangman next to him; he heard the howling of the crowd and the hangman calling out, 'You have to go up' [W]. When I questioned him, he stated that he believed that he had been transported to the time of the

French Revolution, and had no doubt about the reality of the events, which he now regards as a vision. We will study this type of hallucination in greater detail later, under the heading of 'dreamlike hallucinations' [Ed]. Here we are interested in the conclusions that the patient drew from this. He believed, in fact, that he had been transported to other lands and time periods, and explained this by wizardry. However, when I objected that he should not have believed the experience to be real, because his father had not even lived during the time of the French Revolution, he weakened in a quite remarkable manner. He stated that he had believed at the time that his father, and other people as well, such as the head warder, had previously lived during different time periods. Apparently we have encountered here a conclusion made by analogy, as the source of the delusion, and the patient himself confirms that he reached this conclusion, because he was firmly convinced of his own former existence. You will recall the patient (Rother, p. 56) who claimed to have a *Doppelgänger* [W], and who generalized this by saying that everyone has a double. You see, gentlemen, how the mentally ill apply Goethe's line—'What befalls one, befalls the other' [W]—in practice, a rich source for forming of delusions, with incalculable scope. However, a prerequisite for such *delusions by analogy* [W] is a facility for relatively well-ordered thinking.

Gentlemen! We shall see later that hallucinations that combine several sensory modalities, of which you have just seen an example, are linked preferentially to dreamlike states. Also, in the present case, careful observation revealed that the patient often seemed quite absent minded, and unaware of events in his surroundings. He is now able to explain to us in a satisfactory and very instructive way some strange utterances he made at that time. On one occasion he expressed his astonishment that the head warder had disappeared through one door of the hospital and simultaneously entered through another door. On another, food suddenly stood before him without any delay, a process that reminded him of the fairy tale 'the wishing table' [W]. Both events seemed supernatural and magical to him at the time. Now the patient gives us the explanation that he made errors of observation due to lapses in attention. He was often so preoccupied with auditory and visual hallucinations that he paid insufficient attention to events around him. Mostly he even had his eyes shut, a statement I can verify. Here, in a most instructive way, we are confronted by a new source of *delusion formation* [W], following a familiar principle of attempted explanation—the *diversion of attention by internal events* [W]—and we see how, in this manner, very minor and ordinary events take on an obscure and eerie appearance to patients, but with delusional explanations differing according to individual characteristics, in this case leading to an assumption about magic. We can guess just how uncanny and disorientating such experiences will prove to be in all cases, whether or not explanatory delusions are added, according to each patient's powers of reasoning.

If we continue examining our patient, we soon come upon a new source of delusions, again an unfamiliar one for us. At one point during his illness the patient had addressed the ward physician in familiar terms, and later made the remarkable statement that he regarded him, to some extent, as his son, also indicating that one of his fingers signified the physician in person. We learned later that each of his fingers represented a particular person: one as his father, one his mother, one as Napoleon, while it remained in doubt who is represented by one finger. The patient spoke occasionally of the lawful role of *pater familias* [W] in Roman law, evidently in accord with the sense of this delusion. He could shed light on this for us as follows: The idea that one of his fingers represented the person of the physician arose because every time the physician came into view, even in dream images, and when he heard his voice, a peculiar sensation arose in this finger. The other fingers behaved similarly. The patient was unable to describe the sensation in more detail, although he indicated that it had not been painful. We see here a new kind of concept formation fulfilling itself, the result of an abnormal process, namely the occurrence of certain localized morbid sensations, simultaneously with—be they real, or aberrant—perceptions with a certain content. We shall designate this process as *aberrant new formation of associations* [W], and will encounter it very often in acute mental patients, even if it is rare to get such clear evidence for it. Incidentally, when I asked the pointed question on whether his finger was to be identified with the doctor, the patient firmly denied this: He had meant no more than that the latter stood in a certain legitimate relationship towards him.

Gentlemen! The example from which we have just learned will certainly call to mind things you already know. You may recall the young man (p. 83) who at each sight of his father became sexually aroused. I presented this to you as an example of a somatopsychic delusion of relatedness; however we cannot doubt that here too it was based on a process of aberrant elaboration of new associations. In our patient still other examples showed up in this connection, with somatopsychic delusions of relatedness forming via processes of aberrant association. Thus, on one occasion during his illness he requested that nobody should touch his bed lest blood be pulled out of his heart; he had a phase when he would not let himself be touched, because it would cause him discomfort; he once declared that his head would burst if one of the warders uttered a certain word. We can also perceive all these as examples of somatopsychic delusions of relatedness. It is also readily apparent that such aberrant associations can exert a decisive influence on the behaviour patients show towards certain people, and on their actions in general. Some whimsical, strange actions that are quite incomprehensible during healthy thinking, but are also dangerous at times, and certainly unpredictable, can be the result of such aberrant elaboration of new associations.

Gentlemen! A favourable coincidence provides us with the opportunity to show a case of distraction through internalized processes, just as patient K. described it, as a first-hand account. This is a very similar, complicated case, just as patient K., and, by chance, also a young person with some technical expertise. Initially we could not get a word out of him. He looked quite absent minded in the auditorium, and seemed to ignore my questions. All of a sudden he turned towards me, addressed me by name, showed himself well orientated about the situation he was in, and at my request correctly named Pythagoras' theorem. He refused to prove it, when I asked this—saying it was too hard for him. Suddenly, and quite abruptly, he interrupted in a lively tone: 'You don't know Saxony and England' [W]. But then he became lost in contemplation once more. He indicated that he was very preoccupied with alleged mishandling by the warders, who were also present, and talked about this extensively, always returning to the subject. Here in Breslau there was something odd. External voices had already appointed him as Mayor of Breslau. The voices came out of the air, and from many sides. They were heavenly voices; but he concluded that he could not see anything. In addition, thoughts were piercing him: He was both a Christian and a Jew, and had had a previous existence; and he refuted my doubt by pointing to the third article of Faith that relates to the resurrection from the dead. Suddenly, and quite abruptly, he again said animatedly: 'The run of life' [W].

You can see that he understood my questions and willingly engaged with them, and yet it is striking that he sometimes looked distracted, and initially answered my questions with the counter-question: 'How?' [W]. Clearly, to sustain his attention to external stimulation required ongoing effort, and otherwise he seemed to sink into a type of dreamworld, with vivid hallucinations. Nevertheless, in between such times, he was fully attentive and showed himself able to reproduce a four-digit number correctly after a delay of 10 min. He promptly gave the date of his first most acute illness, 5 years previously; he was also aware of a later relapse; and he considered it quite possible that he was now sick again. On inquiry we learned that he was not suffering headaches but experienced very unpleasant sensations in his head, which he described as dull and dragging—they were a result of mistreatment by the warders. He added this information as we delved more deeply, along with more about mistreatment by relatives, who had been committed at the same time. Suddenly, with another glance at the warder, who by chance had risen from his seat: 'I am not guilty' [W]. He claimed that he had observed that the latter had spoken to him. As I bade him farewell, I tried to explain the purpose of the clinical presentation. He left us with the reply: 'But you also judge those who inflict something on me. Every officer has his honour; I am no common man' [W].

We see in this patient changes between very different states of consciousness: sometimes distracted by internal processes, making him almost inaccessible, and most reminiscent of the physiological state of the so-called bewilderment; at other times well attuned to the demands of the moment, and, despite repeated changes of his mental states, with a well-preserved memory. The state of distraction is reminiscent of delirium, and appears to be associated with a dream-like clouding of consciousness. We can conceive of no sharper contrast than the attentive, razor-sharp consciousness, which follows immediately afterwards. We can discern amongst the internal stimuli mixed together in the centre of his radiant mind abnormal sensations, autochthonous ideas, and simple, disorientating phonemes. Disorientation occurs predominantly in the autopsychic area, followed by the allopsychic area. It is quite possible that later, this patient, supposing that he recovers from this, his second relapse, will report on magical occurrences during the time of his illness, and will even be in a position to explain them quite accurately as diversion of his attention, as did patient K.

Delusion formation through analogy; by diversion of attention from proceedings in the outside world; and by abnormal newly formed associations—are often also encountered in chronic psychoses. In contrast to other changes with which we are already familiar, whose substantive changes are much easier to comprehend, these appear to be of secondary importance. However it is different in acute cases where, in consequence of multiple alternate disruptions of content, first one and then the other dominate, and, through their influence on the patient's actions, gain attention. In this regard the report of our patient is instructive, and should not be neglected. Yet, understanding of acute mental illnesses demonstrates itself to be far more difficult than comprehension of chronic cases.

Reference

1. Friedmann M. Weiteres zur Entstehung der Wahnideen und über die Grundlage des Urteils. Monatsschr Psychiatr Neurol. 1897;2(1):10–22. 120–33, 353–76.

Lecture 19

19

- The science of hallucinations
- Hallucinations in various senses
- Combined and dreamlike hallucinations
- Historical section
- Theory of hallucinations

Lecture

Gentlemen!

Learning about hallucinations, which we merely touched on in previous discussions, is probably the most important topic in the general pathology of mental illness; and we therefore have to know about their basic features before we can proceed to studying examples of the various clinical pictures seen in acute psychoses. Since the time of Esquirol [1], sensory perceptions have been differentiated into two major groups: hallucinations and illusions. Hallucinations are sensory perceptions that occur without excitation of the relevant sense by any external object or external stimulus; illusions are false perceptions—misconceptions in perception of objects that are actually present. For the purposes of our schema, hallucinations belong to the group of psychosensory hyperaesthesias (p. 13); that is, they represent a pseudo-identification produced by aberrant stimuli; illusions are attributable to psychosensory paraesthesias; that is, they represent a falsification at the level of secondary identification.

We must consider how far primary identification is involved, when we come to discuss the theory of sensory perceptions.

The main experiences of hallucinations are to be found in the sense of hearing; so let us start with these, especially since they can claim, by far, the greatest clinical significance. Here again I limit myself to essential points in clinical experience.

Auditory hallucinations take two different forms, namely voices (or *phonemes* [W]) (p. 80), and auditory perceptions of a different kind. The latter, also called *acousmata* [W], can show up in the widest variety of ways, so that, for example, sick people hear slamming, banging, clattering, knocking, thunder, drums, shooting or chirping, hissing, boiling, howling, barking, neighing, or roaring. Such noises are seen particularly in very acute disease states, often accompanied by severe morbid changes in the general condition of a patient. If there is a dry tongue and oral cavity, the mucous membrane of the Eustachian tube and inner ear may also be affected, so one cannot exclude the possibility that hallucinations classed subjectively as tinnitus are of peripheral origin; and this is particularly true for simple, elementary sounds. You would have heard of the group of hallucinations arising from peripheral irritation of the inner ear, singled out by Kahlbaum [2], the *Phenazismen* [W], to be classed as disorders of primary identification. This type of acousma is apparently very close to

R. Miller, K.J. Dennison (eds.), *An Outline of Psychiatry in Clinical Lectures*,
DOI 10.1007/978-3-319-18051-9_19

an illusion, since the fact that it originates peripherally does not prevent its being interpreted and used by a patient in a fantastic way. This manner of origin draws on occasional experiences of every healthy person of a subjective tinnitus, and also on inner ear peripheral irritation. It is also known that pure tones can arise in this way. Acousmata such as distinct melodies, an orchestral piece, or other auditory impressions of more complex nature, such as groaning, moaning, whimpering, or screaming children—these cannot be explained in such a way, and must have some other origin.

The 'voices' [Ed]—or phonemes—also occur in two different forms, namely when they are expressly identified as 'voices' [Ed], which a patient himself perceives as something special and different from ordinary experience, or when they are attributed to another person who is actually present, or to a person nearby. The first case is a clear instance where a patient himself creates his own form of expression to describe it as a symptom. If you ask such patients to say whether they hear voices, they usually affirm it without hesitation, conveying also that they fully understand the question. Other patients also will come out with the description of 'voices' [Ed], without any external prompting with this term. This clearly indicates that auditory hallucinations made up of words seem to be inseparably linked to a very specific vocal quality. Patients can usually specify with certainty whether the voices come from known or unknown persons; in the former case they can name them, and distinguish men's, women's, and children's voices. The terms 'angelic voice' [Ed] and 'voice of God' [Ed] occasionally issue from an unusual, alien tone of voice. The voices seem sometimes far away, and sometimes nearby; often they come from close-up, so that it seems to the patient as if someone were whispering, speaking, or screaming into their ear. Usually the direction from which voices appear to come can be precisely specified; and patients often develop, in this regard, quite striking ability to localize, found only in cases of illness. The source of the voices is indicated not only by the direction, but even by the very precise location and distance from the ear. It also happens quite often that the voices seem to change their location independently of each other. The patient thereby acquires some form of personification of a voice: He complains that the voices fly or buzz around him; he looks for them under his pillow and hunts for them as if they were an annoying insect. Our engineer K. heard them, among other places, in his food bowl. At other times, it is not so much the abnormally fine localization, but the vivid perception that the voices are accompanying the patient, for example when he changes his location, or on a walk, and this leads him to conclude that the voices can also change location.

In the case of unilateral hallucinations, which occur quite often, the direction from which the voices come changes with the patient's own position, a manifestation that under favourable circumstances can lead to our investigating the subjective nature of the symptom. In such cases we usually succeed in detecting either a high level of deafness or reduced acuity in one ear. Hallucination in these cases may be encountered sometimes on the side of the healthy ear, and sometimes on that of the damaged ear. Perhaps there is some regularity in this respect, which is apparent if we pay attention in a medical examination to the localization of ear impairment. Our patient K., who is hard of hearing in his right ear as a result of old middle-ear catarrh, reported a voice that had been so loud and so close to the ear that the ear began to bleed and in fact he once found a small bleed in the external auditory meatus.

Those voices that are interpreted as originating from persons present, and which are projected onto these persons may perhaps owe this property to the aforementioned abnormally precise localization of phonemes. This type of voice, through which patients reach a misconception about surrounding people, therefore deserves to be called *disorientating phonemes* [W]. Such experiences are of particular importance for their practical consequences, since they often lead patients to direct their anger, wrath, and hatred towards certain people, and may provoke them to dangerous actions. Patient K. explained his attack on the head warder in this way. Thus, disorientating phonemes represent the worst manifestation of voices; and in fact it is often noted that the first-described form of voices develops into the second, while at the same time the patient's whole condition worsens. The same observation can be made in reverse order.

Hallucinations can force themselves upon a patient's attention, even if erroneous sensory perception is not understood. So, by way of example, indefinite noises precede distinct phonemes; and quite often the phonemes fade out in such a way that patients no longer speak clearly but hear only a whisper. In both cases, patients give a clear indication that they need to listen to the sound, even though they do not understand its meaning. Even with the new patient K. it was the same. Like many others, he felt a compulsion to listen, as a physical torment, to an intrusive act of abuse.

A second feature of hallucinations is their incorrigibility. It has been known for a long time that, even using the strongest reasons, and the witness of all other senses, one can never prevail in convincing mentally-sick people of the subjectivity of their hallucinations. The main supporting argument that patients use is heard quite often, when they say 'I have seen it with my own eyes or heard it with my own ears' [W]. They necessarily trust the testimony of their own senses when the focus is on actual sensations; but this is always also the case for hallucinations, and we hear it from our own patients. The fact that consciousness can be narrowed—which you will recall from my eighth lecture—gets in the way of every corrective strategy at the moment of hallucination; only after disappearance of the hallucination can correction become effective, always when it is already too late. Even the most intelligent patients faced with a choice whether or not to trust the testimony of their senses would rather resort to outlandish attempts at explanation than concede that their hallucinations are essentially subjective. Phonemes are not generated continuously, but mainly leave breaks in between, during which, with proper instruction, some doubts about the objectivity of the voices can gain ground. Sometimes voices occur only in spasms. At the height of such bouts the accompanying symptom of anxiety occurs quite regularly, but often throughout the whole duration of the attack. Unceasing, overwhelming hallucinations, occurring without any break, are observed only in the most severe cases of mental illness, with simultaneous disorientation. Apart from that, you usually find it possible, with some medical encouragement, to distract a patient during the act of examination, and the hallucinations may even subside or cease altogether during this time. In general, solitude, silence, and especially seclusion from busy sensations have a favourable effect on occurrence of hallucinations; yet every now and then, cases are seen in which the very same conditions can bring about the disappearance of hallucinations while, on the contrary, stimulating them (*functional hallucinations*, Kahlbaum) [W].

Under *reflex hallucinations* [W] Kahlbaum includes those produced either by actual perception or by another hallucination, whether these are brought about by the same or a different sensory modality. For example, one of Kahlbaum's patients heard, every time, on first catching sight of strangers, the nickname 'Uncle August' [W]. A patient under my observation, in early stages of *delirium tremens* [W], heard with great fear, from the ticking of a clock, and from the swirling sound of a water outflow, the words 'Mangy dog' [W] and 'Go hang yourself' [W]. When a patient who had behaved very badly for a long time became highly motivated, because I usually made an insulting comment at the end of a conversation with him, this also probably indicates a reflex hallucination. Some patients, at the sight of the meal set before them, hear every time quite contradictory instructions—'eat' [Ed] and 'don't eat' [Ed]—and this is probably also based on reflex hallucinations. In their inner disarray only a resolute command by a physician can tip the balance and motivate them to eat.

Following auditory *hallucinations* [W], we should next consider those of *smell and taste* [W], mainly because of their major clinical significance. Most often these take the form of patients believing that they are tasting and smelling poison, the word poison apparently being used by patients to refer to the widest variety of strangely occurring substances. There is no lack of detailed descriptions of these substances: chloroform, phosphorus, and sulphur are smelled; nauseating things like dog or human flesh mixed with manure, mud, or urine might be tasted. Olfactory hallucinations alone are often of very long duration and continuous, especially that of putrefaction, or some other disgusting odour, interpreted as a disease process in the body. Taste hallucinations usually tend to occur only at the time of food intake. They are, by nature, often inseparable from tactile hallucinations of the tongue, which also usually relate to alien admixtures to the food. The above examples show the content of hallucinations usually to be unpleasant, and threatening. Accordingly, the importance of this symptom is that patients partly or totally refuse food as a result of their perceptions. Taste and olfactory hallucinations are among the most important and most common precipitants of food refusal. In general hallucinations of taste and smell tend to indicate a particularly bad prognosis. However, in acute and especially the most acute forms of mental illness, smell and taste hallucinations do not allow a specific conclusion on the prognosis.

A familiar exception to the general principle that content of hallucinations is mainly unpleasant is to be found in later states of general paralysis. Such patients tend to indulge in scents, and you often see them spending hours or days chewing, tasting, and making tongue-clicking mouth movements with all the signs of satisfaction, and often without any previous intake of food. Likewise, in certain ecstatic states of hysterical mental patients, and in the wake of some acute intoxications, such reveling in pleasant hallucinations can occur.

In all cases of acute mental illness, as a consequence of powerful Affects and associated restlessness, dryness of the mouth and nose may set in, which must provide fertile soil for the development of illusions. Such sensory illusions appear to be even less easily separated and distinguished from actual hallucinations in the realm of taste and smell than for other senses.

Hallucinations of the sense of vision [W] have a general peculiarity that they do not bear the stamp of tangible reality, but appear as solid images seemingly lacking the depth dimension. Very often patients themselves refer to them as 'images' [Ed], and at other times as phenomena, shadows, or even as ghosts, a term implying some form of explanatory delusion. Common expressions such as 'It shows me something' [W] suggest that hallucinations in the visual sense are distinct in their appearing to be deceptions of reality. An exception to this most common experience may occur when the sensorium is clouded; when drowsiness, or stupor, or an ecstatic condition is present; or when half-asleep. So it is quite common for these same patients who see only 'images' [W] during the day to report visions of a physically tangible type during the night. Likewise, states of extreme Affect make physically tangible visions more likely. A hazy state of consciousness can be the basis for visions of an alcoholic delirium, which sometimes even have the hallmark of reality, just as other acute intoxications provide fruitful soil for this. We will examine the content of such visions later. Just as for phonemes, we will find that it depends to some degree on a patient's Affective state.

Intelligent and discerning patients who can talk about their visions describe them as capturing their full attention. For example, a female patient sees a man appearing at a certain place in the room, at night. She must look at him, she cannot take her eyes off him, and her gaze follows him as he slowly approaches the bed and bends over her; all this is accompanied by feelings of anxiety, gradually rising to unbearable intensity. Likewise, amongst delirious visions, such feelings of anxiety not uncommonly surround the entire delirium with an aura of fear. The content of the visions matches this: the devil comes to fetch her; hell opens up; an abyss opens at her feet; walls move; the ceiling threatens to collapse; and the like. In situations of melancholia we encounter occasional hallucinations that are a true reflection of the prevailing feeling of misfortune: deceased relatives, corpses, a coffin, and an entire funeral.

In so far as we hear clear descriptions of these visions, they are projected to precise parts of a room. You will remember the patient with numerous and varied visions who described accurately to us that an image was about 1½ feet in front of him, the whole thing being no bigger than the palm of a hand; nevertheless, he saw an entire landscape—the bank of a river—and recognized quite clearly the form of a former friend who was swimming. When patients speak of shadows, this sometimes provides us with the detail that their visions are transparent; in this way, a male patient described among others the vision of a deceased loved one.

Visual hallucinations are far less common than phonemes; and their clinical importance is in no way comparable with the latter. Since they do not usually bear the full stamp of reality by themselves, they are far less effective in producing feelings of disorientation or disarray than are phonemes. Nevertheless, they are a common source of explanatory delusions, coloured in different ways, according to each individual's personality. As you will recall, our Engineer K. fluctuated between assumptions of magic and that the spirits which he also heard wanted to conduct various procedures on him on purpose, for the spectators, even the dream images that he described.

Hallucinations of touch [W] or, perhaps more accurately, of cutaneous sensation are best known in *Delirium tremens* [W]. Patients experience the sensation of creatures crawling on their bodies, whether they be vermin, reptiles such as snakes, lizards, toads, and so on; and they show themselves incessantly trying to sweep them off by appropriate movements. Possibly, such cutaneous hallucinations can occur in other acute mental illnesses as well. More often, however, they take another distinct form, in which patients feel that they have been sprinkled or sprayed with powdered substances or fluid in droplet form, naturally of a harmful nature. This hallucination is also extremely common amongst chronic patients, usually those classed as hypochondriacal paranoia. An abnormal flushing of the skin may underlie this, so that delirious, raving patients feel that they have to strip off their clothes. The tingling sensation described precisely by many mental patients, interpreted as if they have been electrified, and also morbid sensations of heat and cold are likewise probably attributable to hallucinations of cutaneous sensation, while bites, blows, thumps, and other inflicted pains represent hallucinations of common sensation.

Hallucinations often are not limited to a single sensory modality, but embrace several modalities. The most common combination, already mentioned, is a combined hallucination of smell and taste. The result of such a combination is, of course, that abnormal sensory perception in one domain is taken as confirmation of hallucinations in others. The prerequisite for this is a degree of 'kinship' [Ed] of hallucinations so that combining sensations belonging to two different sensory domains occurs in the same way as happens in reality, in perceiving specific objects. It is precisely this process that appears to be the rule for *combined hallucinations* [W]. Simple combinations—such as that of taste and smell just mentioned—occur most often in those sensory modalities characterized by lively organ sensations, such as—besides those mentioned—those of touch and the so-called hallucinations of common sensation [Ed], which we will deal with in more detail later. More striking manifestations are those combining so-called higher senses, and which are therefore characterized by predominance of sensory content. Thus by congruent interaction of hallucinations in the senses of taste, sight, and touch, the most complete deceptions of reality are created. A patient believes that he has been transposed into a certain situation and environment, for example to his home in the bosom of his family, or into a churchyard in the middle of a burial service. He sees the people in action, hears them speaking, and hears all kinds of associated noises such as the rattle of carriages, funeral music, and the like; in short, an entire event is reproduced, rather like in the theatre, the patient even being able to interact. Once the hallucination is over, the patient sometimes explains that 'it had come to him' [Ed], or that it had been as if he found himself in that particular environment—statements that allow a patient insight into the abnormality of the event. Combined sensory hallucinations of a delirious patient are quite similar: He might see himself as a coachman sitting on the box, with the horses and road before him, and required to take evasive action when he hears the horses neighing and people screaming, while in reality he is in a hospital room lying in bed. Such combined hallucinations are rarely seen among mentally ill people, except in *delirium tremens* [W]; they are however peculiar to fevers in severe physical illnesses such as typhus, in the specific brain disease of meningitis, and in certain acute states of recovery, and characterize them all. In all such cases, a precondition seems to be a mild to moderate degree of drowsiness along with diminution of the sensorium. Since they also appear to have greatest similarity to sensory delusions of dreams, we can appropriately refer to them as *dreamlike hallucinations* [W]. Epileptics and hystero-epilectics can experience such dreamlike hallucinations for hours or for days; in pathological intoxication, they occasionally present as though under the influence of ether, chloroform, belladonna, or similar poisons. In people severely predisposed to nervous diseases, they can occur sporadically, without our ever being able to infer a mental illness.

Kahlbaum already pointed out that such dreamlike hallucinations commonly escape medical detection, and can be revealed only retrospectively from conversation with patients. We are not then entitled to conclude the genuine presence of hallucinations, except in cases outlined above; our focus should rather be on the already familiar stages of progressive falsification of memory. Another combination of hallucinations not belonging to dreamlike states deserves mention here because of its frequency. It consists of hallucinations in other sensory domains, or in the domain of hearing being interpreted and confirmed along with the 'voices' [W], and eventually put into words. For example, nothing is more common than for patients with taste and smell hallucinations occasionally to hallucinate the words 'poison' [W], 'human flesh' [W], and the like, or that patients with abnormal physical sensations use particular names for them, which they use all the time, made manifest as further auditory hallucinations.

Gentlemen! Our understanding of hallucinations as symptoms of acute psychoses is of such importance that I cannot omit introducing theoretical considerations, by way of some comments on history. The oldest theory of hallucinations, which prevailed for a long time, developed under the influence of the great physiologist Johannes Müller [3], and is derived in the simplest way from physiological processes of sensory perception. It started from the fact that we can normally make a clear distinction between memory images (fantasy images) and real sensory perception. For physiological investigations however, the difference is based on the fact that, with sensory perception, there is always excitation of a sense organ or of sensory nerves. So, to explain the same perceptions—which cannot be avoided, bearing in mind the nature of hallucinations—and with excitation of memory images (fantasy images) as an exception, then such perceptions can only become a hallucination if aberrant excitation takes place simultaneously in the periphery, that is, in sensory nerves; and then such excitation forms the most essential prerequisite for a hallucination. Following from this viewpoint, people have developed a theory along the line that hallucinations are diseases of sense organs or sensory nerves which lead to such excitation; yet only very rarely have such changes been detected in sense organs or nerves, and some apparently confirmatory findings have aroused valid concern about the correctness of the theory. Thus in visual hallucinations the optic nerves were found to be completely degenerated, and transformed into a mass of connective tissue, even in cases where long existence of this change had been proven before the onset of hallucinations. The same happens in other cases of blindness due to destruction of both eyeballs. In such cases, it seemed to be a very forced conclusion that after years of inactivity of the optic nerves, the assumption should be made that they became operational once more with the onset of a mental illness, or that from the very sites of disease from which nothing at all had been previously noticed, you might expect activation to arise. The outcome of this difficulty was that the required stimulation process was moved from sensory nerves themselves at their central end and indeed according to one source (Schroeder van der Kolk) [4] to the so-called nucleus [Ed], and according to another to the thalamus. It was considered anatomically proven (by Luys) [5] that the thalamus represented a central station for all sensory nerves. This assumption, first established by Hagen [6], now has the most followers. Its latest and most effective proponent, in slightly modified form, is Meynert [7]. His views can be summarized roughly as follows: If a mentally ill person has a hallucination and, despite normal functioning of other senses still available to him, has no insight into the abnormality and subjective quality of this deception, then this shows a certain weakness of intelligence or hemisphere performance. However, the hemispheres are not only supporters of intelligence, but have a second major function consisting of inhibition and suppression of automatic and reflex effects of stimuli within the subcortical ganglia. A reduction of hemispheric performance means abolition of this inhibition, and therefore has an effect on subcortical ganglia, such that stimulation processes taking place there are amplified to the level of stimuli otherwise transmitted from the outside world. Thus hallucinations are explained by a state of 'irritable weakness' [Ed], whereby the stimulus and the weakness have their locations in two different regions. This hypothesis has the flaw that it is based on several other hypotheses: such as the assumption that abnormal stimulation occurs in subcortical ganglia, which must surely be present if it is to be amplified to an aberrant level, and further that hemispheric performance is reduced in hallucinating patients. We will see later that this assumption is quite superfluous. However, if you want to accept it, it would still all lie within Meynert's train of thought first to think about the fact of mutual inhibition of hemisphere performance, and to seek a location of both these opposing states within the hemispheres themselves, so that we might envisage some degree of functional weakness as being distributed in remaining parts of the hemisphere, while the amplification of function, on the other hand, is distributed in central projection fields of the sensory modality in question. In this case, nothing forces us to make the further assumption of a change in stimulation in the subcortical ganglia.

Gentlemen! If I am forced here to argue against one of Meynert's hypotheses, then I should guard myself against possible misunderstanding: I am far from making the mistake that the hypothesis of this deep-thinking master finds support merely in his very special view of the intervention of the vascular system in the cerebral mechanism, and that I have singled out only one member from a chain of hypotheses whose force lies in its solid structure. But merely from the descriptions emerging in our clinical studies we are forced to renounce the hypotheses as not strictly necessary for our understanding. Moreover in fairness I should mention two of Meynert's predecessors, following his train of thought. In his work, already mentioned, Kahlbaum (on the basis of anatomical views of Schroeder van der Kolk) suspected that the site of the stimulation process in some types of hallucinations was in subcortical centres and indeed in the nuclei of origin of the nerves. Finally we must mention a purely psychological viewpoint, of H. Neumann. Neumann explains hallucinations as being due to the elimination of those normal activities of the brain, which he called a 'critic' [Ed]. He treats hallucinations as diseases of this critic. That this consideration, which dispenses with any experiments on localized function, coincides perfectly with Meynert's assumption that hemisphere activity (which would do just as well as the 'critic' [Ed]) is reduced is readily apparent. Neumann's approach, at least, is noteworthy for its great impartiality.

These brief remarks on the history of hallucinations may suffice to show how, in pursuance of Johannes Müller's original assumption, previous authors have been forced to wander further centrally, and to relocate the aberrant stimulus from the sense organ and sensory nerves, first to sensory nerve nuclei, and then to the next higher station—the subcortical ganglia. Involvement of the central projection fields therefore remains indispensable, since supposed stimuli from subcortical ganglia could not possibly engage in associative activity presupposed to account for the ordered character of the real perception.

Our position on this question is given simply by considerations that I developed for you in my introductory lectures (pp. 15–50, particularly pp. 27 and 30). The difference between a memory image and a visual image becomes blurred in hallucinations, by an abnormal process. We found this difference earlier, when the first termination of the projection system in the central fields of the cortex, which we named 'perception cells' [W], was co-stimulated in the act of perception. We became acquainted with these cells as carriers of the organ sensation and components of consciousness of our own physicality. We can therefore also identify the essence of a hallucination by saying that the aberrant stimulus extends via the memory image to these carriers of the organ sensation; and a memory image becomes a visual image, and next becomes a hallucination, as soon as it makes contact with the associated organ sensation—by excitation of those perception cells. Thus it is a disorder of consciousness of corporeality, which constitutes the main feature of hallucinations. The essential features of hallucinations analyzed above thus become explicable to us. Above all, as an example, we can explain the compulsive demands on attention. Each intense organ sensation exerts such compulsion, as I already demonstrated to you in various examples (p. 27), and you will also recall that this compulsion is, at the same time, a protective measure for the very essence of corporeality—Meynert's 'primary ego' [Ed]. We can also now understand that the Affect of fear itself shows such an intimate connection, often depending directly on hallucinations. Such an Affect, you will recall, always occurs when corporeality, the 'primary Ego' [W], is threatened.

Thus we also gain an understanding of the remarkable observations of abnormally precise localization of hallucinations. Organ sensation as a constituent of overall consciousness of corporeality always refers to a specific location on the cutaneous sensory layer, or of the retina, or of the epithelial layer lining other sense organs. Thus, in the retina, the entire specific projection is mapped upon space, a property which, as we saw, is entirely fitting for vision. It has been pointed out previously that adjustment movements of the eyes must be derived from the organ sensations of the retina. Such preformed adjusting movements can also be seen in relation to the organ of hearing in all animals with moveable ears; and the vestiges of aural mobility, which humans still possess, are proof that humans could also once make such adjustment movements. It has indeed been reported by primitive peoples that their greater acuity in the sense of hearing enables them to locate the source of sounds or noises in a surprisingly accurate manner. Civilized humans have lost this ability. However we see it reappear in cases of illness and, as seems quite understandable to us, linked to abnormally strong organ sensations that, in part, are directly felt as painful, capturing attention to such an extent that the patient is forced to listen to a hallucinatory hiss even though he cannot understand a word of it. As we shall see later, such abnormal localization seen for phonemes also occurs internally in the body, in a leg or 'a boot' [Ed], as one patient expressed it. From time to time we will also find the Affect of fear located in this strange way. In this, we will see examples of abnormal association in the domain of consciousness of corporeality, and we will no longer find them so strange.

References

1. Esquirol E. Des maladies mentales considérées sous les rapports médical, hygiéniqueet médico-légal, vol. 1 and 2. Paris: Chez J-B Baillière; 1838.
2. Kahlbaum KL. Die Gruppirung der psychischen Krankheiten und die Eintheilung der Seelenstörungen. Danzig: AW Kafemann; 1863.
3. Müller J. Ueber die phantastischen Gesichtserscheinungen. Eine physiologische Untersuchung. Coblenz: Jacob Hölscher; 1826.
4. Schröder van der Kolk JLC. Bau und Functionen der medulla spinalis und oblongata und nächste Ursache und rationelle Behandlung der Epilepsie. Braunschweig: F Vieweg und Sohn; 1859. p. 105.
5. Luys JB. Recherches sur le système cérébro-spinal, sa structure, ses fonctions et ses maladies. Paris: Baillière; 1865.
6. Hagen FW. Die Sinnestäuschungen in Bezug auf Psychologie. Heilk Rechtspflege. Leipzig: Otto Wigand; 1837.
7. Meynert Th. Ueber Fortschritte im Verständniss der krankhaften psychischen Gehirnzustände. Wiener med Blätter 9. 1878.

Lecture 20

20

- The science of hallucinations, continued
- Cohesiveness of preformed associative organizations
- Involvement of the projection fields in hallucinations
- Special localization of memory images
- Paraphasic speech compulsion of paralyzed patients
- Compulsive repetition of phonemes
- Different intensity of memory images
- Hypermetamorphosis
- Hyperaesthesia
- Modification of the schemata for disturbance of identification

Lecture

Gentlemen!

The view just developed raises a problem deserving our attention. How is it possible, we might ask, that a pathological epigenetic activation, whose localization is in one sense subject to chance, replicates the very activation pattern of a particular visual memory image, or an artificial grouping of unique impressions such as the acoustic memory image of a word or a melody? Should we not rather expect that a process, whose aberrant action depends on its affecting a chance location, would likewise result in totally-random stimulation of perception cells in the relevant central projection field, with no relationship at all to those functional units for remembered images and the corresponding *concrete concepts* [Ed]? We encounter this difficulty more sharply, in the case of unique hallucinations in a single modality, or in the case of dreamlike—or indeed any type of—combined hallucinations. However, we should take notice of the peculiarity in such dreamlike hallucinations that the excitatory process causing the hallucination takes place in a similar manner in the different projection fields, that is, with just such an organization of stimuli as reflects an accurate picture of reality. In fact, to explain this strange coincidence we cannot dispense with a hypothesis that I proposed earlier (p. 66) that clinical experiences force us to transfer the theory of specific energy of sensory elements to the entire organ of association, and to assume that resonance of the same combination of associative elements always leads to the same mental process taking place. We previously applied this only insofar as we needed it to explain the emergence of certain thoughts, as just such a resonance of a very specific combination of associative elements. We now have to go a step further to consider the emergence of dreamlike hallucinations as resonance of such functional units by *any* [Ed] type of activation. In other words, in whatever way excitation of elements making up functional units and pathways occurs—and however, by repeated function, they always act—the effect is invariably the production

R. Miller, K.J. Dennison (eds.), *An Outline of Psychiatry in Clinical Lectures*,
DOI 10.1007/978-3-319-18051-9_20

of a definite content, specific to them. So the congruence of the parts of combined hallucinations gives us an exact example of the firmness with which those functional connections [1] are established, which represent the outside world. In particular, the hypothesis just proposed should apply to propagation and spread of activation from *any* [Ed] site, onto the intact central projection fields, although diseases of the projection fields are themselves capable rather of generating *abnormally altered* [Ed] hallucinations. In this way we can understand A. Pick's [2] remarkable observation in an individual who had earlier suffered sensory aphasia. Here auditory hallucinations had a pronounced paraphasic character, consisting of distorted words, sentences with malapropisms, and the like. The same author [3] reported on a patient with a hemianopic deficit of homonymous quadrants of both visual fields. The visual hallucinations of this patient had the peculiarity that they were concerned with gaps corresponding to the quadrant in question, so that, for example, a head appeared with the corresponding, sector-shaped cut-out. In progressive paralysis in particular, which always leads to a localized pathology in projection fields, distorted or completely meaningless words are often hallucinated, but elementary sounds can also occur, which are likely to owe their origin to the random activation *in situ* [W], in a projection field which is itself disturbed. In the visual area, most diverse visual phenomena—visions of lightning, and fireballs—may be experienced. The vast majority of hallucinations, however, are certainly attributable to spreading effects of stimulation, since we learn from neuropathology that the majority of symptoms of activation are based on a propagated activation, often from quite distant parts of the brain.

Gentlemen! From views just developed, we cannot construe hallucinations as localized processes, assuming their location to be confined to projection fields of corresponding modality. Indeed we are forced to overlook any initial stimulus in the location corresponding to memory images, and thereby to assume further activation of associated sensing elements—'perception cells' [W] as we named them earlier—arranged according to the norms of that projection system. Clearly, this view can only be seen as supporting an assumption that memory images are transferred to spatially separate sites in the cortex, rather than to the site of perception itself. The latter assumption has already gained significant support from a study by H. Sachs [4] in my clinic. As you will recall, in my Introduction, I portrayed the *form* [Ed] of the stimulus—a reciprocal relationship of stimulated perception cells—as the essence of memory images; and Sachs has proven, or at least made very likely, that memory of this relationship in the visual sense is to be conceived not as distributed amongst specific elements of what he called the 'light field' [W]—the cortical endings of *tractus opticus*—but in the *oculomotor projection field* [Ed]. We must think of vision as coming about in such a way that certain memories of oculomotor images are immediately aroused as a result of the sejunction process, and only from there are associated perceptual elements of the so-called light field [Ed] aroused. This second action is known to be beyond our voluntary control, so we must conclude that only activation of abnormal strength can overcome those resistances preventing the enforced reversal in the direction of conduction. We conclude that such resistances are very important, from the fact that most visions are manifest as shadowy and less bright, while the other fact, that they appear only as two dimensional, and as 'images' [Ed], indicates that propagation of activation from one oculomotor field to the corresponding one in the opposite hemisphere usually does not occur—possibly because no preformed pathway for this exists. We cannot expect activation caused by aberrant processes to be symmetrical at identical sites in both hemispheres; or we regard this possibility to be exceptional, found only under special conditions. For perception of depth, insofar as it is mediated through the eyes, interaction of the oculomotor projection fields of both hemispheres appears always to be necessary. You see, gentlemen, that by assuming a more or less arbitrarily localized pathological point of activation, the simplest explanation is provided for certain fundamental characteristics of visual hallucinations. Of course we cannot exclude the other possibility that pathological activation achieves exceptional salience in the 'light field' [Ed] itself; thus we do encounter so-called elementary [Ed] hallucinations, the most diverse kind of light experiences, whose form is irrelevant. If someone sees lightning flashes, a fiery cloud, a flaming sword, or a sea of fire before him, or if he rejects milk because he regards it as blood, or sees a pool of blood in his bed: These will be forms of primary activation of the light field—due of course to the sejunction process.

The fact that similar considerations apply to mental images of sounds, and especially speech sounds, has been developed in ingenious ways by H. Sachs in the above-mentioned work. Here too, the relationship of tones and sounds influences each other within memory images, and it is therefore likely that the reach of such relationships is linked to an acoustic motor projection field—corresponding to the oculomotor projection field. Only propagation of the aberrant activation from this supposed field to the acoustic perception field gives rise to the hallucination, and (since speech sounds are defined by a vast number of related variables) to the subjective quality of the speech sounds. In exceptional cases, where the acoustic perception field is primarily affected by such activation, there arise subjective sounds and tonal combinations of a random nature, which we earlier called acousmata. Because, unlike visual hallucinations, auditory hallucinations—especially phonemes—bear the full stamp of reality, we might expect the 'centre' [Ed] for word sound patterns to be unilateral, so that in phonemes, we are presented with an exquisite focal symptom of the left temporal lobe although the symptoms have limited value for localizing the symptoms. As is known, this value increases significantly as soon as deficit symptoms are mixed in with those of activation; and here we should recollect what I earlier called 'manic aphasia' [Ed] [5]. We will see later that this name may no longer apply, since it is more of a simultaneous hyper- and parakinetic symptom. This symptom itself, not uncommon among paralytics, is an impulse to paraphasic speech, specifically a symptom of *motor* [Ed] activation within which the deficit, a disturbance arising in the first left temporal convolution, manifests itself as paraphasically altered speech output. In contrast to such a deficit is a speech compulsion, commonly quite isolated, seen in paralytics, with no admixture of paraphasias. This is actually a symptom of mania, where compulsive speech, by its content, reveals mainly motor characteristics, based undoubtedly on activation whose starting point is the diseased left temporal lobe. We conclude from this that any activation in the left temporal lobe can develop along quite different lines, which are to some extent the opposite of those of the acoustic perception field, the activation then making use of the preformed pathway to Broca's convolution [6].

With similar focus on localizing points of activation, another fact deserves mention here: I mean the common cases of compulsive repetition of phonemes. This equally specific motor symptom, which under special circumstances can also be linked with paraphasias, indicates activation which strikes, one after the other, the two familiar pathways for spread. It has the peculiarity that the actual phonemes are often a memorized series of associations, otherwise lacking Affect, for example, the list of a series of numbers. Although this fact speaks for localization of activation closer to the temporal lobe itself, these cases in no way belong among paralyses, but among motility psychoses, the same being true of the compulsive speech, especially without prior hallucinatory speech sounds.

Gentlemen! You can see that just by getting to know all these internally-associated symptoms we see in the right light the significance of the first left temporal convolution as the site of 'phonemes' [Ed], the most common—and you could almost say, the most important—of all the psychotic symptoms. Nevertheless, we cannot doubt that, except for certain very special cases hinted at here, the left temporal lobe is not the actual seat of the disease process, the effects of whose activation are revealed to us. Phonemes are more commonly indirect effects, or side effects, and, in any case, are phenomena based on spreading, to be interpreted as disease processes—sejunction processes—whose localized origin is elsewhere. This is already proven by the admittedly fundamental fact that exactly the same types of disease can occur sometimes with, and sometimes without, phonemes. Phonemes then show up as replaced by corresponding thought content, although not assembled precisely in words. Furthermore, the phoneme content follows a set pattern, depending on the disease type, just as do the thought contents. We should look into this point immediately.

Gentlemen! You have found that any attempt to reach a deeper understanding of psychoses leads necessarily to some burning questions about brain pathology, such as the one just dealt with: the specific localization of memory images. In my opinion such a question, the so-called *asymbolia*, has now been closely studied—not only from the well-known theoretical side by H. Sachs, but also from the admittedly few observations into such cases, where more accurate post-mortem findings have been compiled. Three such cases from my clinic, including two with autopsy results, have recently been described by Heilbronner [7] in treatises on psychiatry published by myself; and according to these, asymbolia presents as a combined disorder, insofar as there are losses in identifying sensory impressions—which is in part secondary, and in part primary identification. The former can be explained by autopsy findings, namely bilateral damage to deep white matter of the cortical convexity between occipital-temporal lobe and the rest of the brain. Disturbance of primary identification, however, finds sufficient explanation in the partial destruction of occipital and temporal lobes themselves. Thus the clinical syndrome of asymbolia, with the integrity of the actual act of perceiving, is thereby also confirmed by autopsy findings—in that Sach's so-called light field of the occipital lobe and large parts of the temporal lobe are preserved and remain along with the projection fibres. To state my view on this unambiguity, I should explain that I take it that functional propagation from centres for perception to those for memory serves primary identification; and I understand that the transcortical conduction of the stimulus via the latter is needed only for secondary identification. Moreover, autopsy findings of a case of psychic blindness, accurately observed in the clinic by Lissauer [8] and anatomically studied by Hahn [9], support this view.

A second, equally-sharp question, mainly of interest in psychiatry, is whether thinking takes place in—or mainly in—words, or in concepts. As you may recall, I have previously expressed my view that thinking is not tied exclusively to existence of concepts as words, or even just word sound patterns, but rather that we recognize conceptual thinking as independent. However I did concede earlier that individual differences may exist in this respect, as 'brain habits' [Ed], so to speak, according to which, one person thinks predominantly in words, and another predominantly in concepts. I imagine also that predominantly conceptual thinking is a superior form, more closely matching reality and to some extent the more scientific. However, I cannot conceal the fact that outstanding brain experts like H. Sachs hold a different view and locate the entirety of logical thought in the site for sound patterns, that is, in the left temporal lobe. As I commented earlier, in my opinion, this is going too far, and is refuted by clinical experience of disorders of the left temporal lobe. However I must admit that, apart from any individual differences, various words may be connected mainly with the left temporal lobe as the site of word memory images; and that is because, in contrast to other words—notably all concrete concepts—the corresponding image of a word sound becomes the sole focal point of all its associative links, all of which links are acquired via language. Here, I do not mean expressions for states of inner experience that I mentioned earlier, but rather artificially learned concepts, acquired through instruction, and not only abstract concepts. Here belong, for example, series of numbers and their manipulations; concepts of historical data and personalities; and many abstractions attached to certain names. We can then envisage a thought which is independent of the left temporal lobe only when restricted to examples which are mainly concrete, with a somewhat simplified thought content. While clinical psychiatry takes motor behaviour under various external conditions as the focus of observation, it makes no extensive claims about this matter; the less so, the more colourful is the clinical picture, so that we really should take account of the proposed variation between individuals.

In any case, I know for a fact that there is a whole series of mental illnesses that occur sometimes with and sometimes without hallucinations—always involving mainly phonemes—and there is no other explanation than that there are individual differences in habits of thinking, which can easily clarify the increased excitability of word sound patterns, and thus the easier occurrence of hallucination, among those who think predominantly in words.

Gentlemen! If there is any possible doubt about whether thinking occurs exclusively as verbal memory images, it is impossible to deny that it occurs mainly through memory images, and that we do need a clear marker of the difference between a mental image and a visual image. However, the question is how might we judge mental images of varying intensity—and whether, in this respect, a more detailed analysis of elementary symptoms, as we envisaged them earlier, such as autochthonous thoughts, obsessions, and overvalued ideas might be possible. Of these three symptoms, obsessions appear to be best known and easiest to demarcate. However, they are of only minor significance in acute psychoses. Overvalued ideas, as we shall soon see, require a somewhat broader definition. It then turns out that they can claim a significance similar to hallucinations in the clinical picture of acute psychoses. As for autochthonous ideas, we saw earlier that they are closely related to phonemes: they can precede them or be transformed into them; and occasionally they are indistinguishable from them, in that patients themselves do not know whether or not thoughts that have come into their heads are based on an actual vocal sound. It may also happen that autochthonous ideas appear to focus consistently on certain words, and that, in their content, these have the same meaning, as shown most clearly when the content corresponds to a command or a prohibition, and has a decisive effect on actions of the patient.

The aspects listed allow us to interpret autochthonous ideas, just like phonemes, as symptoms of excitation of the temporal lobe; that is, they appear as very vivid *remembered images* [Ed] of word sounds, without the stimulation extending to actual auditory *sensations* [Ed]. Given the same strength of aberrant activation, the further assumption then necessarily arises: Activation extending back to the site of organ sensation, that is, the acoustic perception field, must have its origin lying functionally closer to one of the temporal lobes, than to the other, which had already exhausted itself at the site of where memory images are located. We thus come to conclude, as I suggested earlier, that differences in location of the sejunction process are the basis for differences between hallucinations and autochthonous ideas.

Gentlemen! I indicated earlier that primary identification can be affected in mentally ill people. The two symptoms to be considered here involve the borderline between secondary and primary identification, namely those actual sensations which are closely linked to 'perceptual cells' [W]; and it is probably no coincidence that they are observed mainly in disease states, which, in their entire character, are close to the so-called organic [W] brain—or neurological diseases.

Under *hypermetamorphosis* [W] we recognize an organically-produced compulsion to take note of sense impressions, and to fixate attention on them. This can usually be determined experimentally, by bringing favourite sensory stimuli into the vicinity of the patient: for example, pulling out a watch, a handkerchief, the stock market report, or noting how objects are casually played with, to give a sense of sight; producing a sound, making the clock strike, or making a suppressed comment to a third person, letting a tap run, and humming a melody in front of him, to produce auditory impressions; occasionally touching the patient, to produce tactile sensations; and placing scented materials nearby to give a person sensations of smell. Usually the whole deportment of the patient makes the symptom unambiguous, and immediately recognizable, and hospital procedures are especially likely to capture interest of such patients. There is often a difference in sensory areas affected, in that many patients are captivated more by mental impressions, and many others by auditory sensations, especially comments made by other patients. We find one explanation for the symptom if we assume an increased excitability of organ sensations, so that the intrinsic tendency for attention to be captured even by weak, otherwise imperceptible sensory stimuli is enhanced. It is self-evident that with such an increase of organ sensations, even the most peaceful wards, with the most monotonous activity, offer patients sufficiently extensive material for their sensory perceptions. The symptom has considerable practical implications, since it can evoke, maintain, and increase restlessness in such a patient, apart from the fact that other patients are usually affected, and disturbed; and so the most suitable place for such patients to stay is in an isolated room. The main consequence of hypermetamorphosis is absent-mindedness, that is, the intractable nature of thought processes, and inability to follow a closed train of thought. A patients' answers, disclosures that they share, and messages that they want to initiate can therefore give the appearance of incoherence, because they can be interrupted at any moment by each new sense impression. Hypermetamorphosis is therefore a key part of the complex of symptoms that we will come to know in more detail under the name 'confusion' [Ed]. In this symptom complex hypermetamorphosis can sometimes even be the decisive, dominant element, although it cannot constitute a disease in itself, but seems always to be just an accompaniment, though nevertheless an important symptom. (The discoverer of the symptom, H. Neumann, indeed proposed such a disease, but with such an admixture of so many other elements that it can support my opinion.)

Most closely related to hypermetamorphosis is the so-called *hyperaesthesia of the sense organs* [W], a symptom well known in many physical illnesses. Hyperaesthesia is by no means the same as hypermetamorphosis and should not be confused with it. Among mentally-ill persons it is of only minor significance, hardly ever occurring independently, and mostly found amongst those chronically mentally-ill persons, where it has to be seen as a transition to a hysterical personality, and is thus found almost exclusively amongst hysterical women. Furthermore, it is the possible cause of the symptom of startle responses in some semi-consciousness states in epileptics, when, because of apparent reduced activity of the sensorium and presence of stupor, it is very similar to known symptoms of organic brain disease (especially meningitis). The 'jumpiness' [Ed] of some of the most acute pictures of mental illness that we will get to know later probably has the same basis. Apart from this, hyperaesthesia of the sense organs is observed particularly in the initial stage of developing acute psychoses, and during convalescence from these, where it makes the patients more or less insufferable, discontented, or irritable, according to their personality, by the impressions made by their surroundings.

Gentlemen! You can hardly have missed the reminder that the last two symptoms gave you of earlier discussions, where we attempted to define mental illnesses as distinct from brain diseases. If hypermetamorphosis is based on increased excitability, as a sustained state of activation of the perceptual elements, namely perception cells as we called them, then they do not belong to the disturbances of secondary identification but have their site in the immediate destination after the projection system itself. The same applies to hyperaesthesia of sense organs even though the origin of such symptoms is to be sought more peripherally in the nervous system, a generalization that might apply equally to all cases of hyperaesthesia manifest in just a single sensory area. That is also why hyperaesthesia has, from time immemorial, been treated amongst the diseases of the peripheral nervous system. Hypermetamorphosis on the other hand has always been credited with having a central origin. Clinical observations confirm our opinion insofar as we meet this symptom mainly in severe disease conditions, other than its very common occurrence in agitated forms of paralytic psychoses. Amongst non-paralytic psychoses there are in particular the two clinical pictures of confused mania and hyperkinetic motility psychosis, where the symptom is almost never absent, and forms an essential part of the clinical picture.

Gentlemen! You must not be surprised that our *sAZm* schema also allows us to derive certain borderline cases, in which a disorder of secondary identification is the primary impairment, and a transition between primary and secondary disturbances of identification seems to occur. We will encounter the same experience in the area of motility, where we confront states of muscle rigidity accompanied by severe loss of consciousness, which form a transition to epileptic seizures, and yet, to judge from their development, can be considered only as a massive increase of hyper- and parakinetic motility symptoms in the course of severe motility psychoses. Moreover, we will often see actual contractures developing as a result of parakinetic disturbances of identification, which have become habitual in the psychomotor area. This demonstrates how, in our schema, as everywhere else in Nature, nature does not actually work schematically. We should always remember, simply, that any schema, ours included, has value merely of a means of teaching and understanding, and becomes superfluous as soon as a better, simpler, or more correct grouping of facts is found. Rest assured, gentlemen, nobody is more aware of this than I, and that respect for the facts when searching for a way to represent mental illness as seen in the clinic is my primary consideration.

You will now also understand that without risking the charge of inconsistency, we are entitled to amend our schema itself as needed. Here is probably the appropriate place to explore how far such a need exists.

I remind you once more of my introductory remarks on organ sensations and consciousness of corporeality. Back then we became familiar with certain ways in which movement was expressed, which we interpreted as protective measures for the body, and which could be traced back to preformed, probably hereditary mechanisms [1]. Some such movements, such as innate reflexes like the locating movement of the eyes, and the withdrawal of a limb from a painful stimulus, were of a simple nature; others were more complex patterning of movements, such as our recoil in terror, sideways leaping, and the like. Such movements have in common that they are reactions to vigorous organ sensations, and are indeed only half-conscious, or at any rate occur without any more complex mental activity. Amendment of our schema, as required here, needs to consider no more than that we have a type of cortical reflex, which, through a 'short-circuit' [Ed], seems to imply the shortest path between *s* and *m*, a path that still conveys full conscious awareness of corporeality, yet is relatively independent of other activity in the organ of consciousness. We thereby gain understanding of the variety of ways in which movements can be expressed, which, according to their form, are familiar to us in healthy mental life, as reactions to strong organ sensations, and are observed in mentally ill persons, under conditions indicative of major reduction in functions of the sensorium.

For example, wallowing or burrowing movements in many deep twilight states of epileptics and paralytics, reminiscent of jactation and often totally identical with it, sometimes continue unabated for several weeks, always executed in the same monotonous style. Sometimes the movements have a more definite configuration, such as writhing (in pain), or doubling-up, indicating vivid organ sensations in abdominal viscera leaving no doubt about their central origin. We can then presuppose the same mode of origin when patients are indeed conscious, but are also capable, at the time, or subsequently, of giving information about their organ sensations as the reason for their movements. Thus you will observe a patient's expressive movements of screaming and roaring, often at the top of his voice, due to the Affect of anxiety. Such movements may be modified when anxiety is expressed in specific locations, such as the throat, stomach, bladder, or uterus, usually accompanied by severe physical sensations in these organs, and utterance of grunts, and more or less animal-like sounds, with touching of the body regions in question, or tugging at them, etc. Moreover, the feeling of indefinite physical restlessness, combined with corresponding restless movement, often found during full awareness, which the patient traces back to indescribable uncomfortable sensations, would fairly be attributed to murky organ sensation, analogous to the jactation seen in unconscious states. As you can see, in these expressions of movement, induced purely in somatopsychic ways by short-circuit, consciousness need not be switched off; yet consciousness participates merely as a spectator to these processes, which play out partly at a deeper level, and sometimes even as an 'active' [Ed] spectator, when an Affect of disarray or certain explanatory delusions develop against this background.

Gentlemen! When you consider that paralytic weakness of hind limbs can be produced experimentally by crushing of internal organs such as the kidneys, you will also take into account the possibility that, in the same way, direct influence of aberrant organ sensations on motility (by short-circuit) can also bring about conditions of immobility, even of an akinetic type. Healthy mental life already provides analogies of this. When patients with renal or biliary colic cannot move because of pain, we take it as quite natural. Perhaps we should apply the same concept when a moderate state of general immobility is seen in a patient who complains of unbearable tickling sensations in his intestines, or when a female patient after emerging from a state of severe general immobility of several months' duration indicates that the reason for it was that she sensed that she had a bird within her body, and so on. In particular, we will then find that we can understand in this way the emergence of akinetic symptoms, when musculature itself is the site of aberrant organ feelings. I have repeatedly observed such cases, wherever more extensive passive movement is felt as pain, this going hand in hand with the most severe malaise and usually a complex of symptoms of melancholia.

References

1. Hirth GCLO. Energetische Epigenesis und epigenetische Energieformen, ins besondere Merksysteme und plastische Spiegelungen. Eine Programmschrift für Naturforscher und Aerzte. München und Leipzig: G Hirth; 1898.
2. Pick A. Uber die Beziehung der senilen Hirnatrophie zur Aphasie. Prag Med Wochenschr. 1892;17:165–7.
3. Pick A. Beiträge zur Pathologie und pathologischen Anatomie des Centralnervensystems. Mit Bemerkungen zur Normalen. Berlin: Karger; 1898.
4. Sachs H. Die Entstehung der Raumvorstellung aus Sinnesempfindungen. Breslau: Schlettersche Buchhandlung; 1897.
5. Wernicke C. Lehrbuch der Gehirnkrankheiten für Aerzte und Studirende, vol. 3. Berlin: Th Fischer; 1883. p. 551.
6. Broca PP. Nouvelle observation d'aphémie produite par une lésion de la moitié postérieure des deuxième et troisième circonvolution frontales gauches. Bull Soc Anat. 1861;36:398–407.
7. Heilbronner K. Über Asymbolie. Psych Abhandl. 1897;3/4:42.
8. Lissauer H. Ein Fall von Seelenblindheit, nebst einem Beitrag zur Theorie derselben. Arch Psychiatr Nervenkr. 1890;21(2):222–70.
9. Hahn E. Pathologisch-anatomische Untersuchung des Lissauerschen Falles von Seelenblindheit. Arbeiten aus der psychiatrischen Klinik in Breslau. Leipzig. 1895;2:105.

Lecture 21

21

- Disorientation: the fundamental symptom of every psychosis
- 'Disarray' [Ed] linked with conditions of acute origin
- Various types of disorientation and disarray
- Treatments arising from this
- Motor disorientation and disarray
- Transitivism

Lecture

Gentlemen!

Before we go any further, it would be advantageous for us to consider in greater detail the patient who is the most authentic example of all acute mental illnesses to whom we have access at present, our instructive case, the engineer K. The psychosis that Mr K. has experienced will not be looked at in any greater detail later, because it represents a very complex and as-yet little known form of illness. For this very reason the case is useful for our present purpose, because the patient not only has personal experience of most of the elementary symptoms that can be derived from our schema for problems of identification, but can also convey with eloquence the effects that they have produced in him. The best general term we have for this effect is *disorientation* [W]. In disorientation we come to see the real essence of any psychosis. Disorientation disorders included in our schema represent only the *route* [Ed] by which nature brings about such disorientation; but every psychiatric patient is in some way disoriented. If he is not, then he is not mentally ill in a strict sense. The actual damage that the still-largely-unknown disease process wreaks on mentally ill people is through such disorientation. All abnormal alterations in content of consciousness that occur temporarily or permanently in mental patients are included under this concept of disorientation. From my earlier explanations about our schema, namely the relationship between activity of consciousness and its actual content, these regular consequences of disorientation will appear just as natural aberrant modifications of the activity of consciousness. We are struck by the importance of this aspect all the more, as I already stressed, by the fact that the content of consciousness—and alterations to it—provides us with the most tangible, most obvious, and most easily assessed symptoms. Therefore we will derive our classification of acute psychoses from the material changes brought about by the illness, in exactly the same way as we did for chronic psychoses; and we will find that we obtain a basis for a natural system of classification, with room enough to accommodate all the facts. Corresponding to our classification of consciousness into the three areas—of corporeality, the outside world, and personhood—we will meet the clinical requirement of differentiating corresponding types of disorientation; and here

R. Miller, K.J. Dennison (eds.), *An Outline of Psychiatry in Clinical Lectures*,
DOI 10.1007/978-3-319-18051-9_21

we use the terms 'somatopsychically' [Ed], 'allopsychically' [Ed], and 'autopsychically' [Ed]. In addition, we will distinguish the domain of motility disturbances, which falls partly under the term 'somatopsychic' [Ed] and partly under 'autopsychic' [Ed], as a special type of disorientation. When disorientation irrupts acutely, as in acute psychoses, it is inherently connected with a vivid Affective response. For this Affective state, the German language offers us the pithy expression *Ratlosigkeit* [W], a term often used by mentally ill persons themselves. According to this, in what follows, we will also use precise expressions for various colorations of this Affect, with the words somatopsychic, allopsychic, autopsychic, and motor *disarray* [Ed].

Thus Mr K. spoke spontaneously of the disarray in which he had, for a long time, found himself: 'He had always wondered; he had not come out of the wonderment'. The sensory delusions to which he had been subjected, in particular, gave rise to this. Since he always remained, by and large, oriented about his whereabouts, and the people in his immediate surroundings, and had even preserved a degree of orientation towards the combined hallucinations, by conceiving them as dream images, we see from this example that the importance of the sensory delusions consists, as we suggested earlier (p. 69), of an image of the outside world exhibiting abnormal accretions, not corresponding to reality; but that reality is, in addition, recognized as such, and so allopsychic orientation can still, to a degree, be maintained. In another sense we must still regard this aberrant growth as disorientating. However orientation to the data actually presented from the outside world is not abolished by the hallucinations. I emphasize this because we will meet the same experience over and over again in acute mental illnesses: Patients cannot be deprived of their orientation by sensory deceptions alone, not even those combining different senses, unless there is a simultaneous state of significant drowsiness. On the other hand, a high degree of allopsychic disarray [Ed] can result. I recently had the opportunity to observe one of the most instructive examples of this principle on the ward. This was a 26-year-old serving maid W., suffering from epilepsy which had developed years previously; who, 1½ years ago in the eighth month of pregnancy, and following frequent epileptic seizures, underwent a brief period of psychosis lasting only 6 days, after which she has become imbecilic, and has since survived repeated shorter and longer bouts of severe, post-epileptic psychoses. Recently she again had four epileptic seizures in 1 day, fell ill with febrile angina the following day, but slept in the evening and the greater part of the night. Towards morning she woke up suddenly, in a state I was able to observe during a ward round 6 h later. She presented with a most Affect-laden picture of despair: fire, hell, and murder threatened her; she should be taken by the devil, torn to pieces, tortured, killed, broken on the wheel, burned, and thrown into water. The world would be destroyed by fire, the city burned, and the Kaiser would come. She heard all this through voices coming from all sides, which she sought to escape by furious attention-seeking, and the most desperate attempts at suicide and self-harm. A whole team of warders was needed to protect her from harm. At the same time she saw heads, shapes, flags, and soldiers at the windows. Despite this, she remained completely oriented, accessible to support and comfort by medical staff, recognized all of the people around her, and greedily took medication handed to her. At the same time she had extreme anxiety in her chest in relation to phonemes. Four grams of amyl hydrate had an immediate calming effect; and she herself said that the terrible speech had subsided, as had the nagging feeling of fear. The attack was thus initially controlled without putting her to sleep. However, similar bouts of lower intensity were repeated over the next 10 days, and only then did normal interictal behaviour occur. With this patient we found that bromide preparations, even in high dose, always failed to reduce her psychotic symptoms.

Incidentally, you cannot but recall that state that I previously referred to as the decay of the individuality, and explained using the sejunction process. Here too, two mutually-incompatible groups of ideas oppose each other in full consciousness, namely the correct notion of location and people, and on the other hand the fantastic threats which are just as readily conceived. The Affective coloration of the latter, it seems, cannot rise up against the former.

We will learn later about states of allopsychic disorientation, accompanied by vivid hallucinations. We will not be able to derive the fact of disorientation from experiences that you have just heard about, and they must be viewed as independent phenomena.

In this respect it is instructive that the same patient K., who has now almost recovered from a second bout of mental disorder, at the time of his first visit to the clinic 2 years ago, went through a state for several months of moderate allopsychic disorientation, and was totally free from hallucinations. During that period he was in a state of wonderment about everything he saw or experienced, and regarded everything as significant; for example, on one occasion, food was placed in his hands, another time beside his bed, and a third time handed to him from the other side of his bed; the ward doctor sat with his legs crossed on one occasion, another time with legs outstretched, then on the edge of the bed, and another time he sat on a chair. Once when a pile of laundry was being counted in the corridor the patient stood in wonderment, and declared that he would like to stay up all night to see what would become of the stacked laundry. At that time the patient did not notice his own compulsion to think about every little thing, which made him incapable of any organized activity, an incapacity about which he himself talked: 'He did not know the ropes about everything that was going on there; he did not know what he should do and should leave alone'. Since food intake also suffered, he was expressly ordered to eat, and then things went better.

In addition to states of allopsychic disarray and allopsychic disorientation, we also had to verify in our patient, with regard to autopsychic functioning, an 'errancy' [Ed] in his orientation. The patient told us that during his illness he was led to believe that in his earliest childhood he had been brought up not by his parents but in a diaconate institution, and only then had he been given into his parents' care. He claimed that he could remember entire scenes from his childhood that he interpreted in this way. We also learned that the idea came to him that he had to suffer for the sins of others, that this idea was transferred, so that others had to do the same (p. 114), and that also his family and the ward doctor had such an obligation. Also, the idea of being a saint, and that he had already existed several times, dominated him for a long time. Thus, his autopsychic orientation had suffered, without any loss of memory for his real, personal experiences. The frame of mind into which he was driven, due to the opposition of two mutually-incompatible series—of real and imagined facts—he described with the word 'disarray'. We can designate this as 'autopsychic' [Ed].

Obviously, the various abnormal sensations and disturbances of general feelings to which he had been subjected were likely to provoke an Affective response, a matter which leaves us with no room for doubt. We will see later that the most violent Affective reactions are linked specifically to perceived changes in the body. Affect will be influenced more strongly, depending on how far physical sensations and emerging feelings depart from what is familiar. Thus we heard the patient describe feeling as if his brain were soft, as if it had stretched itself out and contracted again, as if his head and body were hollow, as if his body was pulled in particular directions, and as if he were switched on in a magnetic field. Most of these expressions were evidently just comparisons, and were those still available to him, in his embarrassment. From the resulting setting of the Affective state of his mind, we can conclude that, when, at the time, he attempted to take his own life, he was motivated precisely by such feelings. *Somatopsychic disarray* [W] had apparently increased to the point of despair. As we learned, at the first outbreak of his illness, the patient also had strong feelings of anxiety. He localized the anxiety in the region of his heart, and distinguished it just as precisely from the feeling of heart spasm and cardiac arrest, just as he kept apart headaches from other abnormal sensations in his head. We will often encounter such localized fear, which we can perhaps understand as in part a manifestation of the *somatopsychic disarray* [W].

Gentlemen! We will not go far wrong if we regard the series of surprising actions, which we saw during this patient's severe illness, as outcomes of his prevailing mood of disarray; and we can try to understand them from this point of view. Thus he occasionally drank from a spittoon, and even emptied his bowel motions into the spittoon and into the living room; on another occasion he left urine in a mess tin, put his clothes on back to front, lay down on wet ground in the garden, and so on. Today we are hearing explanations of this from the patient; these are partly euphemisms. He suspects that he may suddenly have become very tired; or he explains that he had been surprised by the urgent need to defaecate or void urine; and he reacts with disbelief to any other explanation. He has also forgotten many other things, as you can imagine. From analogy with other patients however, we have no doubts that we are dealing here with *actions of disarray* [W].

Gentlemen! A series of other noteworthy expressions of movement in this patient should be judged from a totally different point of view. For example, from time to time he made apparent turning-movement exercises in his bed; for several days he sung single senseless syllables to himself, and accompanied them with beating movements of his arms. At the time, he had already made statements from which we gathered that in no way did he feel responsible for the corresponding merry mood he conveyed. Even now, he comes up with the same information. He might have sung, even though he would not have been aware of it later, and did not know how to explain it even now. However, upon questioning, we find out that both singing and beating time with the arms represented an accompaniment to voices, without being aware of his being subject to any direct constraint. In the same way he explains the fact that on one occasion, shortly before admission to hospital, he had thrown himself to the ground and rhythmically shouted with all his might. This too had been no more than a reaction to voices that had 'offered him blood' [W]. The patient explained the technical term, 'to offer blood' [W] that escaped from him on this occasion, as being the frequent repetition of the word 'blood' [W] on the part of the voices. We will later encounter the phenomenon that any kind of movement made with full awareness by a patient—but not deliberately—is analogous to autochthonous ideas, except that we are dealing with motor objectives or goals, so much so that it is already helpful to apply a name to such peculiar phenomena. I tend to designate them as 'pseudospontaneous' [Ed] movements. They are usually connected with explanatory delusions. If patients simply report the fact to us without adding any explanatory delusion, it is probably only because at the same time, they are far too distracted by his voices. Less accurate than the term 'pseudospontaneous movement' [Ed] is a patient's information about certain motor deficits that he had noticed in himself for a long time. Thus, the patient has not spoken on his own initiative for weeks ('initiative mutism' [Ed]) and only seldom, if at all, upon questioning ('reactive mutism' [Ed]). However the rest of his behaviour did not suggest that this was a conscious refusal: Often the patient was seen to make approaches, and to speak, and his lips were moving without any sound being uttered, and despite obvious efforts. The patient at present definitely concedes only so much: that there was no actual paralysis of the musculature that prevented him from speaking. As for the rest, he knows only that speaking was difficult, without being able to state the exact reason; he also expressly denies that speaking was forbidden by the voices. Here we hear of both hyper- (para-) kinetic and akinetic states (as disturbances of identification) in localized areas of musculature as described by the patient himself; he is able to do this because he can still remember it accurately. However, he cannot describe the state of mind in which he found himself producing this strange and incomprehensible phenomenon; he can only express his general amazement about it. Yet since he has perceived these phenomena in his own body when fully conscious—which is not always the case, because such states are often accompanied by clouding of the sensorium—we can also suspect that a corresponding Affective state has been produced, which we can call *motor disarray* [W]. This provides us with a term for a very complicated state of mind, involving autopsychic as much as somatopsychic areas of function: the former insofar as movements carried out with full awareness tend to emanate from the entire person, and the latter because involuntary movements must be perceived as alterations to the body (with respect to its position in space). Such motor disarray will, in general, necessarily lead to formation of explanatory delusions. If we wanted to believe only information provided by the patient, we would have entirely missed the point here. On the other hand, however, I rely on numerous other experiences that do not make it seem accidental that the patient, in discussing his autopsychic disorientation, has given us hints that we can now interpret in the context of reports of motor identification problems. He has already talked about believing that he had to suffer for others. These 'redeemer ideas' [W] as we can call them, occur often among mentally ill patients, commonly connected with motor symptoms as explanatory delusions, as described above, in that akinetic symptoms have to be interpreted as suffering imposed by God, the hyperkinetic ones, in the sense that the patient is an instrument of God.

Gentlemen! The Affective state of disarray, as you will realize, is a reactive phenomenon, in response to the 'errancy' [Ed] in the sense of orientation, limited to reported disturbances of secondary identification. It is therefore not strictly separate from disorientation, with which it is connected in various ways. However it can even occur, as you have seen, when a degree of orientation still exists, and in this way influences the contrast between reality and manifestations of disease in the patient. It is to be found only among acute psychoses; you will seek it in vain in wholly chronic psychoses. On the other hand, it reappears in the frequent, acute exacerbations of chronic psychoses, and gives them the distinct character of acute illnesses. In the case of very extensive disorientation, the Affective state may be absent for this very reason, and the picture of disorientation which confronts us will then become purer, whether it be allopsychic, autopsychic, or somatopsychic areas.

On the other hand, as is easily understandable, the Affective state can also be absent, because any ability to respond strongly to acute disturbances of identification is generally reduced, as occurs in deficit states, found in progressive paralysis, presbyophrenia, and hebephrenia. Here the lack of disarray is often just as distinctive as is its presence in the other cases. I mention here a symptom that is often combined with disarray, yet is entirely different, and is essentially a consequence of autopsychic disorientation: We shall call it *transitivism* [W]. It is based on patients who show no sign of psychological malaise, yet are so altered in their entire way of thinking and feeling that the assumption of identical trains of thought, which force us towards a correct conception of the behaviour and conduct for other people that no longer holds true for them. Preferably it is their own loved ones whose behaviour becomes so weird, strange, and incomprehensible to the patients that they come to suspect that the former must probably be mentally ill. In its purest form this symptom occurs in certain acute disease cases where a long preparatory stage is preceded by symptoms which are not actually psychotic. It culminates in instances I have encountered a few times, where a patient accompanies his family to a consultation, to introduce them to the doctor as supposedly mentally ill. In such incidences closer examination of the patient has always shown me that there have been preceding periods of intense Affect, connected with disorientation.

Gentlemen! With the above remarks, of course, I have not given a full description of the Affective states of acute psychoses, even less should it be said that every acute psychosis is invariably accompanied by the same Affects; but at least you have the material to hand that is essential so that we can focus on learning about illusions and the regularity in content of phonemes. It turns out that we need to return once more to the concept of the overvalued idea.

Lecture 22

22

- More about overvalued presentations
- The science of illusions
- Regular content of these
- Regular content of deceptive appearances generally

Lecture

Gentlemen!

In an earlier lecture we took frequent repetition to be the basis of the 'overvalued idea' [Ed] and, following from this, we even considered deliberate practice of certain trains of thought, a process which we must accept to have greatest influence in individual education, and for which the succinct expression 'channeling' [W] has recently been used. We need to make this concept more robust, insofar as channeling generally goes hand in hand with Affective coloration of the overvalued idea. Professional activities are particularly likely to generate overvaluation of certain ideas; their Affective coloration is an expression of the fact that a person's overwhelming interest is normally directed towards his professional activity. We then observe the extraordinary fact that sensitivity to certain very specific sensory perceptions is thereby heightened in a remarkable way. Choosing examples closest to hand, an experienced alienist is immediately aware during his rounds of the institution, of any disruption and neglect of clinical services; his attention and interest are directed to the matter in question without need for any conscious effort; in any professional capacity, what we call 'vigilance' [W] has just such a basis. Likewise, a visual artist quite automatically notices shapes; the tailor eyes up peoples' suits; the cobbler the shoes; and unmarried women observe the ring on a man's finger. Here, the increased arousal produced by certain sensory stimuli seems to depend on the increased value ascribed to particular complex mental processes. Under specific circumstances, when the attention of a Newton turns to such an everyday event as an apple falling from a tree, this is likewise no coincidence but is based on the increased interest shown to processes which were hitherto of no concern, as a consequence of ideas currently in ascendance. It is the same with all experiences and discoveries, insofar as they are linked to everyday observations. Just how selective this facility can be, for noticing specific sensory impressions as a result of the dominance of certain ideas and their Affective coloration, is shown by the example of the mother, who, in deep sleep, ignores every other sound, but awakens instantly at the slightest sound from the child. We will call this selective process intrapsychic hypermetamorphosis [Ed]. We can now consider that such Affective coloration, and therefore the distinct overvaluation of ideas, is the most common basis for illusions.

R. Miller, K.J. Dennison (eds.), *An Outline of Psychiatry in Clinical Lectures*,
DOI 10.1007/978-3-319-18051-9_22

The theory of illusions is based largely on experiences in the visual sense. The most familiar examples are the interpretation of vague, imprecise, and visual impressions as angst-ridden fantastic sensations, for instance a distant tree stump as a robber and fluttering laundry as a ghost. Evidently these are deliria of judgment, that is, clouding of judgment by Affects, such as fear or anxiety. Pragmatically we should distinguish firstly between two cases: clear versus indistinct sensory perceptions. Clouding of judgment in the latter case occurs as in the examples of visual illusions just given, and you can then take the Affective state to be the origin of the illusion. However, the question is as follows: By what process does Affect produce this influence? As we have seen we must attribute to Affective states the capacity to alter the normal value of ideas, in such a way that certain ideas are overvalued, while others, by comparison, are undervalued. In turn, overvalued ideas can be excited from the periphery more easily, and undervalued ones less easily than normal. Overvaluation of Affective concepts—a robber and a ghost in our example—therefore produces an abnormal facilitation of secondary identification, while undervaluation of remembered images in other sensory domains, or even in the same one, complicates any correction.

Now, that Affects can also take on different natures; or all manner of individualized processes of association can lead to overvaluation of ideas, which has precisely the same effect. I know the example of a young married man on a business trip in a foreign city, who made acquaintance with an easygoing woman, and visited a pleasure garden with her. Then he remembered that his wife had relatives in the same city; and that, by coincidence—as a less likely but still possible scenario—she might spontaneously decide to visit them, with the result that she might be in the same city, even conceivably at the same location. He looked around the people present, and was quickly so firmly convinced that a woman sitting in the distance was his wife that he did not dare convince himself of the truth of his belief by going closer, but preferred to get away from the place. I hardly know a better example to illustrate so succinctly the basic influence of individual, Affect-laden, coloured—and thus overvalued—perceptions for secondary identification in a normal person. Let us imagine the Affect level increasing by only a small amount, and thus clouding a person's discretion. This is an emotional state that we can assume without further ado, in many new patients brought to the clinic against their will; and a series of illusions, that we see frequently in such situations, then become completely understandable. Here, the obviously overvalued ideas are the fact of the patient's separation from his family, and pressures applied along with his becoming an inpatient. It is then not surprising that distant people, not clearly seen, are perceived as relatives; the doctor, as a prosecutor; and the clinic, as a prison. Such illusions are common in many acute mental illnesses. They are usually transitory in nature and easily corrected. In very severe cases, a degree of stupefaction and manifest inattentiveness may also occur, so that inaccurate sensory perception is replaced by a defective state of the sensorium. Then, so long as this situation holds, numerous other such illusions may arise which have in common that they change their content, depending on the usual rapid change of overvalued perceptions. States of delirium of most diverse origins provide common examples of this. It is no coincidence that the person with alcoholic delirium believes himself to be among his fellows, either in the tavern, or in his daily employment; he believes he recognizes in the doctor his haulage boss or his drinking companions: Such illusions match his overvalued perceptions. In such circumstances a good patriot probably considers the head warder to be the Kaiser or, if delirium is coloured by anxiety, he imagines the executioner and prosecutor. Perceptual inaccuracy, which favours the occurrence of illusions, can be made use of, if it is available, just as long as the patient is left to his own resources and is obviously in this so-called twilight state. The same condition leads to corresponding illusions in states of hysterical or epileptic delirium, and in the so-called delirium of exhaustion, etc.

Illusions are harder to understand when they occur in someone who appears to be in a totally level-headed state, with attentive behaviour, and demonstrable clarity of perception. Yet even in this situation the content of illusions is usually brought about by certain related, and Affect-laden ideas. In such cases, any kind of real-world event can determine what the patient has evaluated for his false identification. Thus it often happens that a mental patient comes to view the doctor, or a warder, or another specific patient as a close relative, because he sees some kind of existing affinity with him, for instance in his facial expression, body form, manner of movement, or vocal inflection. This confusion of persons appears to be stable, and is very difficult to correct. In one case of such 'person confusion' [Ed] cited by Kahlbaum [1], I suspect with a similar basis that the illusion was so firmly fixed that the patient failed to recognize genuine relatives who met him face to face, and he declared them to be imposters. This, incidentally, is quite a common experience amongst mental patients after prolonged stay in an institution. It is certainly no coincidence, and perhaps it is the longing for those nearest and dearest, brought about by stay in the institution that leads to such misjudgments. Apparently the abnormality consists of the fact that the conceptualization of relatives—perhaps a brother—becomes so overvalued that even partial identification, like the sound of a familiar voice, has the same effect as that of an impaired, and imprecise sensorium, whose function is diminished as in previously mentioned cases. Normally differences in shape, size, facial contour, or expression would hinder identification.

You will ask me: Is there not a deficit, or a weakness in replication in those partial representations belonging to the concept of the brother, relating to the shape, size, and in his facial contours or facial expressions—a weakness of cortical performance in Meynert's [2] sense, or of the 'critic' [Ed] in Neumann's sense? Well, gentleman, this assumption is quite unnecessary, if you recall the characteristics of overvalued perceptions discussed above. It is sufficient, as we saw in the case of hallucinations, for abnormal overvaluation of perceptions by themselves to call forth a process of identification; the more is this likely, when actually present (even though only partial) primary identification comes to assist this internal process! This reflects only the internal strength of the fabric of the once-acquired, but now-overvalued, concept: 'brother' [Ed]. We need not deny that in some circumstances even such a weakness in replication—even deficiencies in a specific concept in certain partial perceptions—may be present in mental patients. For instance paralytics and people with senile dementia might declare that straw—due to its yellow colour—is gold, or broken glass, due to its hardness and transparency, gemstones. But then such deficiencies should be evident elsewhere, and this is certainly not the case in the acute mental patients we discussed earlier. Gentlemen! You can see that in conceptualizing an illusion, which is now our task, the difference between clear and unclear sensory perceptions, which initially seemed essential and important for gaining understanding, loses its meaning. In just the same way, we lose the main difference between illusions and hallucinations. An illusion now appears to us as a hallucination, whose occurrence is facilitated by chance occurrence of external conditions, a conclusion which insightful older authors, such as Kahlbaum, reached long ago. Of course, we will accept this proposal only when illusions occur in mentally-ill people; and, for descriptive and practical purposes, we must maintain a strict difference between illusions and hallucinations amongst such people in our clinic. Similar reasoning also allows us to define those hallucinations mentioned previously, which are demonstrably peripheral, that is, formed in the sensory organs themselves—Kahlbaum's *phenazisma*—so that hallucinations of purely central origin can be given no other status. Such phenazisms have an important role, especially for taste and smell, where the foul taste of oral catarrh and the bad smell of nasal catarrh become misinterpreted as poisons. Again, as we shall see later, overvalued allopsychic perceptions of fear are the main feature.

Gentlemen! From conditions just discussed, we can readily understand why, as far as the frequency of hallucinations goes, the orderly relationship highlighted above prevails, according to which phonemes predominate by far, and often exist just by themselves. This is especially true for many chronic mental illnesses. In acute mental illnesses we often observe that only phonemes appear initially, and addition of hallucinations in other senses corresponds to the otherwise familiar increase of symptoms to a certain severity of illness. Given the intimate connection between the act of perception and the sensory field for speech, it is easy to understand that, in order to broadcast to projection fields of the other senses which word sounds can bring forth hallucinations, a greater spread of the stimulus is required. Admittedly, I know that there is a widespread belief, especially from the work of Charcot and his school [3], that thought processes play out in ways that differ between individuals, which go far beyond the individual differences I have proposed. It is alleged that thinking is carried out by many people only, or mainly in visual images, by others through acoustic images, and by others again as motor or word images. Without denying such possibilities, however, I consider them only as very rare exceptions, and therefore not to be used in the theory of hallucinations. Hallucinations of taste and smell are, after phonemes, the next most frequently observed, at least amongst those whose mental illnesses are exclusively acute, which is explained by their being based mainly on phenazisms, which must naturally arise more easily than hallucinations themselves.

Gentlemen! Only now, after having presented to you a particular theory of sensory deceptions of mental illnesses am I in a position, by way of a few examples, to comment briefly on the orderliness of their content (as I have repeatedly emphasized). The rule that we deal with here is that the content of sensory deceptions is determined by the Affective state that prevails at the time. Affective, and thus overvalued, perceptions are the ones which are most excitable at that time, and indeed, this applies not only for stimuli originating in the outside world, and initiated by the sense organs—as we saw previously—but also for *central* [Ed] aberrant stimuli connected with the sejunction process. In order to link this to something familiar, I remind you of the occurrence of hypochondriacal sensations of happiness (p. 107). Corresponding with this, overvalued ideas can appear, from which feelings of happiness may be expressed, and corresponding phonemes, containing grandiose ideas. Later we will become familiar with the abnormal euphoria of mania. If hallucinations occur here, these are likewise hallucinatory perceptions of grandiosity. In situations which are the opposite of mania, that is in melancholia, feelings of deep unhappiness develop. Corresponding to this are phonemes, which, if they arise, usually convey a 'delusion of belittlement' [Ed]. In this case, visions are most often perceptions of misfortune, assimilated as visual images. I have often mentioned anxiety psychoses, in paranoid states. The Affective state of fear leads, exactly according to rule, to certain perceptions of fear, which I differentiate as autopsychic, allopsychic, and somatopsychic. Of these the autopsychic are in part identical with the delusion of belittlement in melancholics; they therefore include self-recriminations, or, grouped as phonemes, words of accusation or insult. Allopsychic perceptions of fear contain themes of threat and injury. Corresponding to this, sick people hear that they would be killed, tortured, roasted, thrown to wild animals, hunted in the snow, or chased naked through the streets, and so on. Somatopsychic perceptions of fear may be the basis, for instance of a female patient who hears, through a voice, that her *globus pharyngis* [W] has cancer of the larynx—with a cough as a sure sign—or tuberculosis, or cool extremities, signifying that she is dying.

Gentlemen! The most common and most general Affect in this state you will encounter in new patients is that of 'disarray', evoked by moderate levels of disorientation. This corresponds to the most frequent content of phonemes. A patient's utterances convey this quite conspicuously—'where am I' [Ed]; 'what am I supposed to do' [Ed]; 'what is the matter with me' [Ed]; 'I do not even know' [Ed]—fragmentary utterances one hears over and over again. When a patient hears slanderous names and insults, or accusations of evil deeds allegedly committed, or notes about experiences that have never happened, these are outcomes of autopsychic disarray. Often one can do no more than trace back from the utterances of the patients to this type of phoneme, although this can be done with some certainty because such utterances allow no other interpretation. I introduce the following by way of example: 'I am not a thief' [Ed]; 'I have never poisoned anyone' [Ed]; 'I have not killed children' [Ed]—and so on. If the voices deny the patient's identity which leads to statements such as 'I am called so-and-so but I'm not a princess' [Ed], 'I am not married' [Ed], or 'I have no children' [Ed], these are obviously reactions to the Affective state of autopsychic disarray. Allopsychic disarray comes to be expressed in phonemes conveying the importance of location and environment. Patients might hear that they are in a penal institution, in Heaven, in an enchanted castle, on a ship, and so on; that the other patients are dressed up and belong to the opposite sex, or are policemen in disguise; that their bed is not a natural bed; that the bath tub is an instrument of torture; or that the food contains disgusting ingredients, or human flesh, etc. Somatopsychic disarray leads to emergence of phonemes such as the following: the intestinal tract has become overgrown; the body is full of faeces, or transformed into one solid mass; the heart is standing still; blood has stopped flowing; patients are paralyzed or dead; the head is separated from the body, or transformed into an ape's skull; their arms have been torn off, or are several times longer than previously, or instead of two, there are five arms, etc. Motor disarray too is very frequently manifest as phonemes. This emerges most clearly when a patient hears completely opposite commands, such as 'eat' [Ed] and 'don't eat' [Ed]. Moreover, commands to adopt a certain posture, to keep protruding the tongue, to walk on all fours like an animal are all hallucinatory manifestations of motor disarray, and likewise when patients are commanded not to swallow, not to speak, not to move their hands. Finally, a major part of the so-called impulsive actions, in reality brought about by phonemes, can be explained in the same way. Patients hear requests to free themselves; to smash the window; to go into the water; to hang themselves; to plunge headfirst; to tear out their tongues; to rip out their genitalia; and to drill out their eyes.

Gentlemen! I restrict myself to these examples which, I believe, are sufficiently conclusive to demonstrate how the content of phonemes depends on the most commonly encountered Affective states in acute mental illnesses. I would add that delusions of relatedness are also based on Affective conditions; in this regard I refer to remarks I made in my 13th lecture. While this covered mainly delusions of relatedness in enduring paranoid states, it will be readily understood that in acute psychoses, such delusions occur with far more Affect. In acute psychoses, it is the satisfaction of natural needs—intake of food, elimination of stools, and voiding of urine—which favours the appearance of phonemes whose content refers to delusions of relatedness, and—most often—disorientating phonemes, which take on the guise of the vocal inflections of those closest to hand, namely the staff in attendance or the doctors. Taunts and disapproving remarks naturally predominate such as 'Now he is eating again', or 'He can eat well, but not work'.

In all probability, not only phonemes but all hallucinations show an orderly dependence on the prevailing Affective state, such as is familiar to us in the case of phonemes. However much further evidence for this is still required before completion. That content is determined by the prevailing Affective state is known best for visions, where it applies especially to melancholia and fear psychoses. Corresponding with the prevailing feeling of unhappiness are hallucinatory corpses, coffins, eerie black figures, funereal proceedings, or, in more fantastic cases, demise of relatives when their house collapses or in drowning, fire, railway accidents, and so on, but usually in a more shadowy form, given that we are dealing with images. After all that has been said, it is easy to understand why ecstatic visions, corresponding to religious feelings of happiness, refer to the sky, and that they often concern more than visions, but rather dreamlike hallucinations.

References

1. Kahlbaum KL. Die Sinnesdelirien. Allg Ztschr Psych. 1886;23(1 and 2):1–86.
2. Meynert T. Amentia. Die Verwirrheit acuter Wahnsinn. In: Deutlicke F, editor. Jahrbücher für Psychiatrie, vol. 9. Wien: Braumüller; 1890. p. 1–112.
3. Charcot JM. Sur les divers états nerveux déterminés par l'hypnotisation chez les hystériques. Paris; 1882.

Lecture 23

23

- Presentation of a case of anxiety psychosis
- Clinical picture, course, diagnosis, prognosis, treatment
- Delimitation from the area of anxiety neuroses
- An example of hypochondriacal anxiety psychosis

Lecture

Gentlemen!

Patient Sch., who you see before you, came only reluctantly to the lecture theatre. He looks around anxiously, comes closer, but hesitantly, and then greets me as an acquaintance. You see him as a 55-year-old, heavily-built man of poor nutritional status, with somewhat cyanotic discoloration of face and hands, and cool extremities, fearful in posture and facial expression. Again and again, he repeats in a rhythmic manner a low moan, and also interrupts his speech every so often, when he shows a great need to express himself. When I interrupt him to give you information, he resents it. He gives correct answers to my questions about his age, family situation, and home town, but you will notice that due to his Affective state, his concentration is impaired; and he introduces pauses, during which he looks around absent-mindedly, so that his answers to simple questions, which would otherwise be quite prompt, sometimes take a long time to reach their conclusion. He also repeatedly suggests that it is difficult for him to concentrate. The impression we gain from his prevailing Affective state is one of bewilderment, anxiety, and disarray. The fact that such Affective states complicate an orderly train of thought has long been known, and has frequently been shown to you. On enquiry we learn that the patient complains of unceasing anxiety. If the seat of the anxiety is in his heart: 'It wants to crush him' [W]. He is also breathless, and therefore is sleepless at nights. The patient therefore wished to be examined by me, and in his anxious and overhasty manner, made arrangements to undress. When asked why he is afraid, he tells me of his fear of being beheaded; he had also heard that each day he would receive 50 lashes, counted-out; he would be expected to eat a roll that had lain in a fellow-patient's spitting glass. On questioning, we hear that other patients lying in the same room with him made these statements. Therefore the patient is well oriented and knows he is in a clinic for the mentally ill. However, he has not judged the current situation quite correctly; and presumably his viewpoint was already rather limited, as we often find among country folk from his region. He knows me; he recognizes the audience as students, and thinks that I have granted them 'an hour' [W], but he believes that all men there want to be ministers of religion, like his son, who is currently a theology student and accompanied him to the clinic. On the ward,

R. Miller, K.J. Dennison (eds.), *An Outline of Psychiatry in Clinical Lectures*,
DOI 10.1007/978-3-319-18051-9_23

the patient also claimed that they would cut off his head; he would be taken to the place where corpses were stored. Incidentally, it is not primarily fear from these threats that dominates this patient; rather, we usually hear from him his complaints about the fate of his family. He believes that all his possessions were gone: His son would no longer be able to study. He heard the voice of his young son saying: 'For three weeks we have had nothing reasonable to eat' [W]; he had also seen his son standing in front of him, with a pathetic gesture. He believes that his family will all die of hunger; the children are all sickly; his son, the student, was refused life insurance due to heart failure. It was his fault; he had shamed himself by an immoral lifestyle and secret sins of his youth. He had become lazy. He had also harmed himself by chewing a lot of tobacco. The patient tells of an assault, during which he recognized one of his attackers and reported him. He had probably committed perjury at the time, because it had been night, and he could not see clearly. Earlier, when his anxiety was even greater, he also complained that his two youngest children had been poisoned, and his wife had taken her life. At the same time this patient, who has suffered a hernia, eats only meagerly, and says that he gets abdominal pain after a meal.

Apart from the hernia, no organic disease can be found in this patient; and in no way does he look older than his age, but rather younger. He has now been in the clinic for more than a month, and was ill for about 3 months before that. The 'external cause' [Ed] of his illness was said to be that the patient, proprietor of a village smithy and associated farm holding, sold his plot of land and the blacksmith's workshop in order to retire. Although this transaction turned out to be quite advantageous for him, with a smooth transition, the idea gradually came to him that he had ruined his family and would impoverish them. Gradually this idea was joined by anxiety, self-blame in reference to alleged perjury (see above), and the idea that he was a great sinner and was being persecuted by Satan. These autopsychic ideas of anxiety existed on their own in the initial period of illness, and only shortly before his admission were they joined by those of fantastic threats; and at the same time, there was an increase in the patient's restlessness, which became so noticeable that it was inevitable that he be transferred to an institution. At this time, he seems to have reached the most critical point in his illness and even to have moved beyond it. This is supported by a reduction in his somatopsychic ideas of anxiety. Moreover, the phenomenon had been present, of which there is now no more than a hint; his rhythmic moans, which had been much more pronounced early in his stay, had risen from time to time to monotonous repetition of the same phrase, 'I, a poor sinner' [W]. This was occasionally accompanied by rhythmic movements of his arms. Also, anxiety seemed to have reached its peak at about this time. Eating became difficult only at the time when there were these somatopsychic ideas of anxiety; and sleep had to be induced mainly through sleeping pills. His body weight of 78 kg at the time of admission fell to 72 kg, where it is at present; so his food intake has usually been quite sufficient.

As for his prognosis, based on progress so far and other evidence, we are quite confident in viewing it favourably. The course of his illness showed an acute origin followed by increase in symptoms over about a week, in which parakinetic and hyperkinetic symptoms appeared in the form of verbigeration and rhythmic arm movements. This period corresponded with the height of his anxiety and production of somatopsychic ideas of anxiety. Since then independent motor symptoms and likewise his symptoms of hypochondria have ceased, and anxiety has subsided in intensity. Moreover delusions of relatedness, and disorientating phonemes with content to match have not increased. Thus the intensity of the basic phenomenon, namely anxiety, runs in parallel with the range of other symptoms; the decline of these phenomena is to be expected, in a similar sequence. (In fact the patient became healthy in the space of 3 months after the demonstration, and has remained so for 2 years since).

Gentlemen! This clinical picture described is typical of a large number of similar cases, given that we ignore a few anomalies which make this case not quite typical. Perhaps these are peculiar to this individual, as I have suggested. In general, we cannot deny that the elementary symptom of anxiety provides the exclusive source of a disease, which in many cases produces no symptoms other than ones attributable to anxiety. We can summarize all such cases of illness as *anxiety psychoses* [W]. The basic symptom is anxiety, usually localized in the chest, especially in the heart and epigastrium; next most commonly, in the head; next in frequency to the entire body; and regularly, it has a fluctuating character, and, at the beginning, or as the illness abates, an intermittent character. Such anxiety regularly leads to the emergence of various ideas, which therefore deserve to be called 'anxiety ideas' [Ed]. They show grades of intensity such that the autopsychic ideas of anxiety correspond to lower intensity, and the allopsychic and somatopsychic ones to more severe anxiety. Somatopsychic ideas can sometimes be missing or even, as here, emerge only temporarily at the peak of illness. When the disease starts, and as it subsides, only autopsychic ideas of anxiety are usually present. In some cases anxiety persists, accompanied just by such ideas; far more often the ideas are 'dressed up' [Ed] as phonemes. At the height of the anxiety state, hallucinations can also appear temporarily in other modalities and, in some of the most acute cases, as in the example of anxiety in a case of epilepsy described above, can occur simultaneously in all senses, as combined hallucinations. Often, only autopsychic ideas are present, at a moderate level; or there may even be a combination of autopsychic and allopsychic ideas of anxiety, with added phonemes only at times when anxiety intensifies. Allopsychic orientation is retained but autopsychic orientation is usually permanently altered, in the sense of delusions of belittlement. On the other hand, disarray can expand to include the allopsychic area. Hints of delusions of reference are often encountered at times of intense anxiety; also, disorientating phonemes with such content occur. Common contents of autopsychic ideas of anxiety and matching phonemes express concern for family members, for the financial situation, and challenges to personal honour, and there may be ideas of belittlement, and self-recrimination, with corresponding abusive phonemes. The content of allopsychic ideas of anxiety is usually a threat to life, or of ignominious disciplinary actions, abuse, etc. Delusions of reference operate in the same way. The hallucinations whose intensity is most prominently linked with very high levels of Affect are those of smell and taste, because they are usually interpreted in terms of poisoning and lead temporarily to rejection of food.

Amongst the aetiological factors are alcoholism, epilepsy, and climacteric; and anxiety psychosis seems to be closely related to growing old.

As for the duration of such psychoses, they may last anywhere from a week to several months. The shortest course is seen in 'abortive' [Ed] cases among epileptics and alcoholics. It sometimes happens that *Delirium tremens* [W] will be replaced by acute anxiety psychosis, with its characteristic intense Affect, and with predominantly autopsychic ideas of anxiety. The psychotic state is then correspondingly short in duration and accompanied by tremors and symptoms arising in the projection system, as discussed later. In terms of symptoms, anxiety psychosis is not rare, especially in cases of poorly resolved heart failure; its time course then tends to be bound up with this situation.

An actual paranoid stage, reaching the point where insight into the illness is lost for a long time, tends not to develop.

Motor behaviour of patients is generally determined purely in psychological ways through Affective states, or the content of ideas of anxiety and of hallucinations. Usually, most patients can be treated in bed; however, as anxiety increases, a degree of motor restlessness is produced, initially as movements expressing anxiety, such as crying, sobbing, wringing of hands, kneeling down, and praying, according to the patient's individual manner. In many cases it may lead to tremors, gnashing of teeth, and outbreaks of perspiration. Should anxiety undergo a further crescendo, patients leave their beds, and walk restlessly up and down, probably also forcing themselves. Some expressions of movement—or at least borderline motility symptoms—are not psychologically motivated, such as rhythmic moaning or rocking movements of the trunk (usually both together); endless uniform movements of hands, which are repetitive, if not rhythmical; fiddling around with the bed or pieces of clothing; rubbing the hands together, etc. There is almost always a strong suicidal tendency, or a wish to die, often expressed with comments such as 'Make an end to it. Strike me dead' [W]. At the height of the disease, even more severe motility symptoms are prone to occur, such as parakinetic behaviours, rhythmic movements, and verbigeration. On the other hand, at the peak of allopsychic disorientation, increase of sensory symptoms may occur, to the point of anxiety displayed even when approached, and as blind defensiveness.

As a particular form of anxiety psychosis, the so-called *Melancholia agitata* [W] deserves to be mentioned explicitly. In this condition, there is ever-present marked restlessness; movements are driven mostly, but not exclusively in psychological ways; sometimes, as described above, they are on the borderline of an actual motility disorder. Above all, increased production of anxiety ideas can lead surprisingly to pressured speech and flights of fancy, symptoms that we will encounter later in a very different clinical picture, where there can be no mistaking their sensory derivation. Also, it seems to be intrinsic to such cases of agitated melancholia that autopsychic ideas of anxiety outweigh by far any others in their content, even though allopsychic ideas may never be totally absent.

In *diagnostic* [W] terms, the assumption is that the illness will often develop further, forming no more than the initial stage of a more complex disease picture. Such development takes place in two ways: to a scenario of complex motility psychosis, characterized usually by the onset of akinetic symptoms, and to one of expanded sensory psychosis with disorientation. We should always suspect the latter when disorientating phonemes and delusions of reference make up more than a trivial part of the clinical picture.

Further development can also take place very quickly, so that the most acute medical conditions such as the so-called transitory psychoses [Ed] may result.

For differential diagnosis against Affective melancholia (see later), it is crucial to prove the presence of allopsychic ideas of anxiety or delusions of reference. Diagnosis of acute hallucinosis (see later) is likewise usually easily established. The symptom of anxiety predominates, from patients' accounts, and is also conspicuous objectively; and the dependence of phonemes on the fluctuations of anxiety, so often seen, is a usual characteristic. However, in acute hallucinosis a characteristic paranoid stage develops very early, which is not the case for simple anxiety psychosis. In the latter condition, allopsychic orientation remains intact, unlike the anxiety-laden state found in *delirium tremens* [W]. Likewise, disorientation tends to be found in generalized sensory psychoses. Therefore, many cases of anxiety psychosis are indistinguishable from progressive paralysis, because, from a clinical standpoint, one must accept the existence of a 'paralytic anxiety psychosis' [Ed]. While the Affective overlay often makes it difficult to establish those disturbances of thinking, judgment, and memory retention which can almost always be found in paralysis, the possibility nevertheless exists that key symptoms of paralysis or alcoholism, arising in the projection system, are still initially absent, only entering the picture later in the course.

Gentlemen! Very often you will come across cases of illness that you might call 'borderline' [Ed] cases, or cases of mixed *anxiety psychosis* [W] and *Affective melancholia* [W]. They are characterized by the fact that neither one nor the other clinical picture exists in pure or complete form. In their outward character, the picture of Affective melancholia is usually predominant, particularly because fluctuations based on anxiety are less pronounced, so that a more continuous and consistent clinical picture prevails. Subjective deficits, which befit Affective melancholia, are often absent, while prominent ideas of belittlement, self-recrimination, and other autopsychic ideas of anxiety are present. The dominant Affective state is a feeling of misfortune, but at the same time, a state of anxiety always exists, which can usually be localized. Expressions of anxiety usually restrict themselves to the simplest movements such as crying and occasional outbursts of despair, but agitation is generally missing. Allopsychic ideas of anxiety can almost always be detected, but remain isolated, their importance falling away, so that one must often actively search for them. Likewise delusions of reference emerge entirely on their own. Forebodings of misfortune prevailing along with wider perceptions of anxiety often remain limited to circumscribed areas, as is found with pure melancholia. Phonemes play only a minor role.

Thus a fairly common clinical picture can be characterized adequately in both directions. It seems to occur preferentially among very young persons and in old age. The diagnosis is therefore not unimportant, because the prognosis of this illness can be stated more securely not only than in cases of anxiety psychosis, but, in itself, is also far more favourable. Cases of this type that I know all had a favourable outcome.

The *prognosis* [W] of anxiety psychoses *per se* [W] would be designated as favourable, since by far the majority of cases such as those outlined above have progressed towards full health. This favourable judgment is hindered by the difficulty in making a firm diagnosis until some way into the course of the illness. Only when, as in the case I just presented to you, the patient has already gone through the critical point of the disease, can we assume it as likely that a transition of the clinical picture to a more complex one will no longer take place; and in this too, our hopes may sometimes be dashed, because, after a stage of apparent recovery, development of psychosis with a chronically progressive course may ensue. Such was the case, for example, in a case of senile anxiety psychosis in a 73-year-old woman who I could present to you after a 1½-year course, as a typical example of a chronic psychiatric patient with so-called hypochondriacal delusions of persecution [Ed], in the stage of allopsychic disorientation [1]. In this case the clinical picture was unfavourably clouded by numerous disorientating phonemes and delusions of relatedness.

Treatment [W] of anxiety psychoses has the special task of fighting the symptom of anxiety. We cannot humanely ask any patient simply to endure a high level of anxiety, any more than we can for analogous symptoms of pain. In general *Extractum Opii* [W], to be injected subcutaneously in doses of ½ to 1 dcg, is a reliable remedy. Along with this, a combination of hyoscine with morphine proves itself to be valuable: half as many milligrams of the former as centigrams of the latter. With that dosage one can increase the daily dose progressively from ¼ mg:½ cg up to ½ mg:1 cg. For anxiety attacks in epileptics it is preferable to administer a sleep-inducing dose of amyl hydrate internally or by enema. Incidentally, treatment of anxiety psychoses gives outcomes just the same as those for psychoses generally, so I refer you to my comments on the subject at the end of these lectures [2].

Gentlemen! In no other area of mental illness are there so many points of contact with the functional disorders of the nervous system as the one we deal with here. However common the anxiety psychoses may be, there can be no doubt that states of anxiety to be classed with the neuroses are far more frequent. This raises the following question: Are there any sure criteria by which one can distinguish *anxiety neurosis* [W] from an anxiety psychosis? This question is of great practical importance, for it is precisely anxiety psychoses for which doctors are obliged to provide timely security, by committal of patients to an institution, sometimes involuntarily. Such interference in the personal liberty of another fellow human would never be tolerated in the case of mere neurosis. Fortunately the clinical picture I described now offers more reliable and easily identifiable indicators in its complex of symptoms, such that a positive diagnosis of anxiety psychosis can be made easily, and any doubt about the appropriate course of action is thus excluded. However, without doubt, as everywhere else in Nature, there are borderline cases, where there is justified uncertainty about the wisdom of such a measure. Here, a physician will be tasked with ensuring the greatest possible reassurance while monitoring the patient privately. For this, there is no better way than strict adherence to bed rest. This is the way in which the symptom of anxiety itself, as shown above, is to be treated. The well-being of the patient precedes all other considerations, and so the focus must be on practical implications that the patient infers from his feelings of anxiety, and from subsequent unhappiness and anxiety about his own actions.

Always remember that although a single symptom such as anxiety is never sufficient to produce psychosis, nevertheless, at least as much value should always be placed on actions of patients, as on what they say. Where there are attempts at suicide, safeguarding a patient by internment in a lunatic asylum is imperative even in borderline cases.

Gentlemen! I have begun describing specific types of illness by choosing anxiety psychoses because, on the one hand, cases of such illness are relatively easy to understand, and on the other, because their points of contact with many other acute psychoses are so varied that they soon lead us right into the centre ground of our practical tasks. I need hardly point out that practical knowledge of mental illnesses in itself has nothing to do with theoretical assumptions. Therefore the series of our demonstrations is set up mainly for teaching purposes, these being subordinate to practical needs. The patient who I shall now present to you still belongs, in a practical sense, within the area of anxiety psychoses, but, as you will soon see, will continue into the topic of our next lecture.

This 69-year-old factory worker, Mrs L., as you can see, is a silver-haired woman, who walks with a slight stoop, with downcast, facial expression, easily made anxious, and with corresponding attitude. She answers questions that are directed to her promptly, albeit with a rather faint voice. She tells us her birthday, the date of her marriage, how long she has been married, the date of her husband's death, his illness, and the names of her children; she talks about her only surviving daughter, and tells of her grandchildren. Also, we learn directly from her the history of her illness. In the spring of 1896 she was diagnosed with a growth in her abdomen, which had subsequently been operated on. She had then spent 11 weeks in hospital and was subsequently quite weak but was otherwise healthy. In November she was diagnosed with shingles, and for 3 weeks was virtually unable to sleep. At the beginning of December the present illness started. She gives the duration of her stay in the clinic—from 24th February this year—which is roughly correct; she shows herself to be completely orientated about the way in which the institution functions, and about her fellow patients; and she knows that the gentlemen present are students who visit the clinic. I led her to a discussion of her illness. What kind of illness was it? She could not eat anything because her throat had 'grown over' [Ed] or, as she corrected herself, only very little would pass through. Her tongue had grown onto her palate. She felt with her hand, and also showed me that the upper surface of her tongue touched the palate. She also had a constant taste of 'bad luck' [W] in her mouth, and everything she ate lacked flavour. Anything she did swallow in her laborious way, she felt became stuck in her oesophagus. It piled up in the region of her stomach, and led to feelings of bloating. It had previously been impossible for her to pass any stools, and they now passed only by artificial means and insufficiently.

I asked whether things were not already improving, which she denied. I must comment here that she is actually already recovering well. She used to be so weak and feeble that she could answer only in a toneless, flat voice; and a demonstration like today's would have been totally impossible. Due to her severe malaise, at that time, she hardly ever spoke about herself, while now she sometimes does so; she had shown no interest in her environment, whereas now she takes some interest in it. At that time she also stated that the canal for passage of her food had grown over completely, and she had to be forcibly fed, whereas now she can take some nourishment spontaneously. We also learned, from her daughter, that she had earlier complained of not being able to breathe.

This patient cannot specify exactly the nature of her disease; at least it was something very bad, and totally hopeless. In the past she had given her view that it was plague, and that she was afraid of infecting others by contact. In this respect, too, she has clearly made progress because now she no longer believes this.

When we now ask the patient how satisfied she is with her treatment here, she replies: Good, but it is just not worth it. Why ever should she blame herself? She was bad and sinful through and through; she had already attempted to take her own life; she was a monster, a spectacle amongst men; she deserved to be discarded. Other patients shouted out about her. She had brought her illness on herself by starving herself; during her last illness she had been reckless in treatment of her mother. As a further sign of a fantastic delusion of belittlement, I want to mention that the patient refuses to go into the visitors' room, because she should not be seen by others. When preparations were being made for photography the photographer would be so frightened at the sight of her that he would drop down dead. Furthermore, she believes that she cannot die, because she is too bad; and yet now she says she wants to die and, prior to her admission, she had made two attempts to strangle herself because she could bear it no longer. As for her grandchildren, the patient believes that they are very ill, perhaps dead, and she previously gave us the opinion that they would die on her behalf. She even claimed to be the cause of all misfortune, from which she heard, as an example, when a friend had burnt her hand. She likewise expressed the fear that she would be admitted to hospital because she was too evil. Although she gives quite coherent information, and conveys no outward sign of anxiety, she says on questioning that she suffers constantly from anxiety. Where is the root of the anxiety? In my head. The anxiety is precisely differentiated from a feeling of excitement in her epigastrium; but according to earlier information, the anxiety had been temporarily localized in her chest. With regard to this patient's conduct on the ward, she has always shown herself conspicuous as accessible and trustworthy. She always keeps herself clean, and the only hindrance to this is on occasions when, as a consequence of her delusions, she attacks her anus or touches her faeces.

Gentlemen! No other symptoms have been found in this patient. There remain only her delusions based on the abnormal notion she describes, restricted just to her body and her personality, and which thereby determine her behaviour. With regard to the conceptualization of this illness, it is very instructive to provide an overview of its course. In fact it turns out, beyond doubt, that the hypochondriacal complaints which still exist had been present right from the beginning, and had led gradually to the most severe emaciation of the patient—her body mass was 31 kg at admission—which had precipitated the need for admission to the clinic.

The other unusual ideas were added only when her illness reached a certain level of severity, after the isolated hypochondriacal complaints had been present for weeks. Tests of memory retention and attentiveness gave normal results. The information that we received from the patient came only as short answers to the questions directed to her.

References

1. Wernicke C. Krankenvorstellungen aus der psychiatrischen Klinik in Breslau, vol. 1, Case 1. Breslau: Schletter, 1899.
2. Wernicke C. Krankenvorstellungen, vol. 1, Cases 3, 8, 9 and 12; vol.2 Cases 5, 21, 22 and 23 are examples of anxiety psychoses, 1899.

Lecture 24

24

- Intestinal, worsening, and diffuse somatopsychoses
- Hypochondriacal reflex psychoses
- Severe hypochondriacal psychosis in a drunkard
- Example of paralytic somatopsychosis
- Clinical picture
- Treatments of somatopsychic disarray
- Outcomes
- Overview of hypochondriacal symptoms

Lecture

Gentlemen!

Among the patients who have been briefly presented to you, you have become familiar with an example of those common cases that have earned the distinctive name of *hypochondriacal anxiety psychosis* [W]. Clearly, this is a localized intestinal somatopsychosis, based on abnormal bodily sensations in the area of the digestive tract, which can quickly lead to disorientation in a circumscribed area of consciousness of corporeality, specifically the intestines. The accompanying severe malaise is easily understood as a consequence of somatopsychic disturbance of identification. Our patient identified her state of mind as anxiety, but more often, corresponding with the main substantive alteration, the patient's Affective state is reported not as actual anxiety, but as something different, especially for patients who, by virtue of their educated linguistic expression, are more erudite. Apparently these are Affective states that we have already come to recognize as bodily or somatopsychic disarray. In addition, sometimes, we can distinguish a new component, something special, anxiety occurring in paroxysms.

This *circumscribed intestinal hypochondria* [W] is itself localized preferentially near either end of the digestive tract. Corresponding to this, complaints that stand out are firstly, a difficulty in swallowing—considered in the broadest sense, so that it covers the entire action of transporting food to the stomach—and then, difficulty in evacuating stools. In a case of the latter type, we could identify the starting point for hypochondriacal ideas, as a mucous rectal catarrh sustained by haemorrhoids; likewise, in female patients, a pre-existing global sensation could often be the starting point for such a symptom, attributed to swallowing difficulties.

As you can see from such examples, it is beyond doubt that we interpret this as a psychosensory disturbance of identification in organ sensations, although it is difficult—even impossible—to establish whether it is hyperaesthesia, paraesthesia, or anaesthesia which is present.

At a certain stage, emergence of these two different initial localizations comes to the same thing, that is a feeling of repletion or 'surfeit' [Ed] of food: on one hand, starting with food that is either laboriously swallowed or artificially

R. Miller, K.J. Dennison (eds.), *An Outline of Psychiatry in Clinical Lectures*,
DOI 10.1007/978-3-319-18051-9_24

introduced and accumulates in the stomach area; on the other, a faecal mass backs up from below, eventually right up as far as the pharynx. The most common and most important of these abnormal sensations is refusal of food, which in such cases almost always requires force-feeding by oesophageal tube. A heavy feeling of dolour is always present, quite understandably so, given the feeling of severe physical illness which predominates. This also affects patients' outlook on the future: They always believe themselves to be lost and quite without hope. In pure cases of this sort, actual perceptions of anxiety are restricted to the autopsychic area, often in a quite limited way, in that patients blame themselves for having brought about or aggravated their illness through neglect of medical advice and medical planning. In the case of a 60-year-old, unmarried woman, after a long career in nursing, combined with a sad Affective state, she quite suddenly she fell ill with this form of intestinal somatopsychosis and severe food refusal. After about 6 months of illness, the abnormal sensations in her pharynx diminished. However, the dolour and autopsychic focus of her anxiety remained, as did the somatopsychic perception of anxiety about having no bowel movements, and the illness eventually led to her death.

As far as motor behaviour is concerned, in such patients, in pure cases, its motivation remains entirely psychological. In one patient, more of an agitated state was observed: outbursts of whining and despair, lamentation, hand-wringing, etc.; while in others, perhaps based on individual differences, there was a moderate failure of motility, as we find clearly in evidence, when people feel severely ill. Either such behaviour can exist in the same way throughout the illness or one condition can replace the other, or even agitated behaviour can correspond to one of several peaks along the trajectory of the illness. Conversely, severe loss of motility, in other words an intrapsychic akinesia (with psychosensory relations), can appear, corresponding to an increasing range of symptoms; indeed I have seen this, for example in the case of *worsening somatopsychosis* [W], initially only intestinal. Here therefore, akinesia, derived, according to its severity, from an increase in the feeling of being ill, was the more severe event, for the patient then became unclean and claimed not to be able to stand, walk, or speak. In fact, these functions were preserved, as could be seen from her chance responses.

A 57-year-old female patient, who had struggled for years with severe food problems, was subsequently diagnosed as having sensations of intestinal obstruction. Six months later, at the height of her illness, she claimed to be full to the top with faecal matter, and unable either to breathe or to move. When her illness began, she had repeatedly expressed her fear of starvation, with despairing restlessness; but after an intercurrent bout of influenza she veered towards a severe state of fatigue, in which she also complained about slowness and difficulty in her thought processes. Subsequent infiltration of the upper lobes of both lungs seemed to make the prognosis totally hopeless; nevertheless, after several weeks in this condition, she started to convalesce, and after about a year was discharged to family care as improved. The disease trajectory in this case can be regarded as purely extensive, and the akinesia then corresponded to a peak in that curve. This case was interesting in that her anxiety, which focused on the heart, was always stated to be a separate phenomenon, and suggestions of ideas of autopsychic anxiety taking the form of self-recrimination were quite short-lived.

Even clearer than in the previous case, the worsening behaviour of a hypochondria with initial localization restricted to the genital organs was demonstrated in the case that I presented a few semesters ago. This was a 23-year-old Jewish lady, who had suffered psychotic attacks on several previous occasions, sometimes more melancholic, sometimes more manic in nature; her sister had been mentally disturbed in a similar way on two occasions. She had lived with her brother's family, and looked after his very sick child with utmost devotion. At the beginning of her own illness she complained of feeling a solid body in her genitals and was treated by the gynaecologist. The symptom was combined with a burning sensation, urinary tenesmus, and pressure, with failure of menstruation. There were no objective findings. When the sick child died about 2 months later, she began to take on the hardest work, in spite of which she soon declared that she was no good, could not work, was superfluous, and was a burden to her brother. About 2 months later she attempted suicide with chloroform and was unconscious for several hours. A foiled attempt at drowning provided the occasion 3 months later for her being transferred to the clinic, where the patient's delusions of belittlement have been intensely managed up until very recently. In the last 2 weeks prior to admission, and during the first months of her stay in the clinic, her physical ailments intensified to an extremely desperate state. She said that as a result of unsatisfactory stools, her food had accumulated inside her—not faeces, she explicitly stated—and had been transformed into a solid mass. This solid mass had penetrated every part of her body, disfiguring it; only her skin remained in its natural state. The patient had convinced herself of this because of feelings of internal heaviness, and from palpating herself with her hands. Her body felt dead, as if it had expired, and there was no longer any blood flowing through it, although the patient could feel her pulse and also hear her heart beating. This 'solidification' [Ed] extended also to her sense organs: Although she could hear with her ears, her eyes remained fixed within her head; she could not move them, nor open her eyelids. When she made eye movements during the examination, she assured us that this would not otherwise have occurred, and that she had to turn her head instead. She doubted whether she could smell, feel, touch, or taste; she tried it with milk, and found it to be so. However, she could swallow and move her tongue. The patient constantly refused food during this time, and had to be tube-fed. As for bowel movements, she claimed that they were insufficient, even though infusions or laxatives—which she willingly accepted by the way—had had an effect from which she felt instantly relieved. She constantly felt severely ill, with a sense of absolute hopelessness, and a correspondingly desperate mood in relation to her physical condition. However, she complained of anxiety only transitorily, at times of extreme excitement and despair, the anxious feelings then being localized to her breast.

As for this patient's motor behaviour, there were periods of outpouring of despair as a result of progressive decline of strength. There was her delusion of having sinned through having eaten too much; she was lost to all eternity; she deserved all the most severe punishments awaiting her, such as being consumed by fire. Similarly she regarded her stay in the clinic—where perforce she had to be kept at the monitoring station—as a well-deserved albeit minor punishment. Moreover her intelligence was intact, her orientation fully preserved; despite physical weakness there was no slowdown, nor hallucinations, nor delusion of relatedness. With continuing weight loss, death ensued after a 9-month stay in the clinic.

A modification of intestinal somatopsychoses, which is not rare, occurs in cases in which the aberrant sensation is localized more towards the airways. In one such case the nasal passages were the main site of this abnormal feeling, associated with fear of suffocation; in another case there was a feeling that the throat had dried up and the trachea was overgrown, although swallowing and nourishment continued undisturbed, and without any respiratory distress. Nevertheless, the patient, a 42-year-old farmer's wife, experienced a localized feeling of severe loading in the epigastrium, as if from a stone, which was so severe that she described it as a 'death feeling' [Ed]. Apparently this feeling climbed only gradually up to the pharynx. The patient tossed and turned with internal unrest, whined incessantly, and had most pronounced tendencies to suicide. Multiple attempts had already been thwarted. At the time of observation she had already been ill for a year and it was learned that during the first half of the year she had spoken in self-accusatory terms, and of fears for her family, with even more vehement anxiety. Her husky voice and occasional bouts of coughing led us to examine her larynx, and it turned out that, in addition to catarrh that had led to swelling of her vocal cords, one vocal cord was completely paralyzed. Although suspicion of tuberculosis of the larynx had arisen in this case, clearly this did not explain the paralysis of the vocal cord; and you could even ask whether it was more of a direct consequence of the hypochondriacal sensation arising in the laryngeal innervation, in other words, an effect of abnormally altered sensation in an organ which at the same time serves motility, in the sense of comments made earlier (p. 132). The possibility was then considered that the catarrh was only a consequence of deficient motor activation, as the end result of morbid sensation. I submit that the unilateral nature of the vocal cord paralysis does not support this explanation, and a different view of this rare condition is closer to the truth. Vocal cord paralysis and catarrh were perhaps the common outcome of a latent, undetectable cause, and only the paraesthesia of abnormal organ sensations was the starting point of circumscribed—and in due course, clearly symptomatic—intestinal somatopsychosis.

Gentlemen! In light of the above comments, symptoms of paralysis in cases of circumscribed bladder hypochondria are much more likely to be understood as psychosensorily induced akinesia. These cases mark a transition between hypochondriacal psychosis and neurosis, in that they encroach even less than the previously described ones on the rest of mental life. Moreover, treatment in our institution can often be avoided, the more so since the numerous subjective complaints associated with paralysis of the sphincter muscles are usually limited to certain times of the day, the rest being symptom-free. Particularly burdensome is the feeling of urinary pressure sometimes connected with a tendency to involuntary ejaculation: The latter are also able to occur without erections. Patients are therefore in constant fear of causing embarrassment; besides this, localized feelings of anxiety can exist in the epigastrium. Outside the spasm, the patient may appear mentally normal; however, during the attacks they suffer from more or less severe autopsychic notions of anxiety and despair to the point that they become tired of life, with a tendency to suicide. These patients usually organize their way of life so that incidents of the type described cannot arise; professional activity and dealings with other people suffer as a result. In one such case, treatment with several hours of warm baths, in which the patient felt relieved of every concern over unexpected moments of embarrassment, had a sustainable, long-term success. I need not emphasize that these cases are distinguished by absence of any local changes, and of any symptoms arising in sensory nerves or the spinal cord, while the patients' history of persisting cystitis or gonorrhoea is not without significance.

Certain cases of defaecation hypochondria are related to hypochondriacal neurosis in a similar way: The main burden on patients, and likewise the fear, with its sequelae, is similarly eliminated by controlling production of stools.

Gentlemen! Not unexpectedly, circumscribed intestinal hypochondria can also be localized in the female genitalia. A typical case of this kind, who I presented in the clinic, concerned a 22-year-old serving girl who, before her illness, was of normal intelligence, but always easily excited, and inclined to outbursts of anger; her brother was mentally ill when he died. After bouts of anger, she was said to have had repeated seizures of an unspecified nature. At the time she presented here, she had been suffering for about 2 years—though with several long intermissions—from a burning sensation, which was not directly painful but was yet described as quite unbearable, in the genitalia and internally in the lower abdomen. This burning was not continually present, but recurred persistently. It was worse towards evening, and was simultaneously associated with low back pain, headaches, dizziness, and nausea. At the same time she complained of anxiety in the epigastrium. The illness was accompanied by unhappiness, low mood, and hopelessness; and her facial expression, and her apathetic behaviour altogether, conformed to this mood. At the time of her menstruation, there were fewer complaints; before and after it, there was lower back pain and some discharge. Special mention must be made of the patient's motor behaviour. While she usually stayed in bed, depressed and apathetic, occasionally there were outbursts of totally unmotivated, senseless rage, when the patient screamed, lashed out, bit, and scratched, quite unaware of her surroundings.

The patient subsequently had no recollection of these instances, which did not last for hours; and each time, they were initiated by an increase in abnormal sensations in her genitalia; then came, like a type of aura, a feeling as if the body were dying, with consciousness fading. These motor expressions bear the stamp of senseless rage, and would be correctly understood as a type of reflex response to violently-increased organ sensations, and thus as hyperkinesia induced by psychosensory means, via a short circuit. At the time of observation she was suffering from ulceration of the cervix and vagina. The beginning of her illness was allegedly related to a delivery and subsequent metritis. As a result of her tantrums, this patient had to be transferred to a nursing home. Although the reported symptoms are close to the clinical picture of epilepsy, typical epileptic seizures were never observed.

Except for bouts of motor discharge just considered—attributable to twilight states in the so-called transitory psychoses, as discussed later—a circumscribed intestinal somatopsychosis, with its origin specifically in the genital organs, is featured in this case. It is correct to note the close relationship of tantrums with those of epileptic and hysterical twilight states, but this will not prevent it being suggested that permanent abnormality of intestinal sensation is also the starting point for the acute transitory seizures; and thus such seizures appear to derive from a reflex psychosis induced by the genital organs. However, in this transitory condition, disturbance of identification then spreads to all three areas of consciousness, while the motor discharge retains the character of a psychosensory condition, fully characterized as somatopsychic disarray. This approach has the advantage of providing a uniform view of the illness itself. It is supported mainly by the fact that an increase of localized complaints always preceded the tantrums, but also by experience in similar cases. For example, quite separately I observed a very similar tantrum in a 20-year-old girl who constantly brought to light severe unhappiness with suicidal tendencies; and when she once relaxed her guarded nature and expressed herself openly, remarked that, quite definitely, her abdominal pain was the cause of her behaviour. The pain generally fluctuated; and in the oft-repeated periods of several days' exacerbation, could be localized spasmodically in the region of the uterus and the parametrium, connected with terrible feelings of anxiety rising right up to the heart, which were described along with ideas of her being incurable, and with suicidal impulses. The patient screamed and moaned loudly, and required monitoring due to her outbreaks of despair. At one time she could be calmed with soothing words, but more often chloroform had to be administered. She did not come up with any fantastic names for her illness. Objective findings in the genital organs led to the conclusion of previous masturbation (erosion of the vulva and vagina with mild catarrh and bladder complaints). There was also slight retroversion of the uterus and chronic severe constipation. Sleep and food intake were continuously very disturbed. The patient, a sales assistant in a clothing store, was the daughter of a well-known eccentric father; and, after a severely hysterical attack of irritability, during which she struck out blindly and shouted fearfully, brought about by a dispute with her boss, she was admitted to hospital. Six months later, she too was moved to a nursing home, as permanent improvement could not be achieved. The tantrum that we observed occurred around the middle of her stay in the hospital, allegedly caused by anger. Here, too in my opinion we might be forced to interpret the short-duration transitory psychosis arising in the rest of the clinical picture as in no way different from the previous case, since the motor discharge again corresponded with widespread somatopsychic disarray. Incidentally, this patient was discharged from the nursing home after 6 weeks, allegedly completely recovered, probably as a result of the powerful impression that transfer there must have had on her.

Gentlemen! That idea that sense organs too can give rise to abnormal organ sensations and thereby to circumscribed hypochondriacal symptoms or somatopsychosis is shown by the following instructive case. A 71-year-old physically spry woman who, up to 9 months ago, had served as a nanny and on closer examination showed no signs of weakened intellect or senile mental disorder sought spontaneous admission to our hospital because she was afraid that she might commit suicide. During her stay in the clinic of more than 4 months, she always presented the same symptoms, right up to the time of her previous discharge: On admission, she moaned to herself about anxiety in her heart. Her chief complaint, however, was a noise in her head. The noise was constant; and increased at times of complete silence, so that she preferred to remain at the rather noisy monitoring station. This noise was subjectively extremely unpleasant, gave her no rest, interfered with her thinking, and compelled her attention. When the noise was bad, restlessness in her heart and anxiety also occurred. Also present were severe unhappiness, hopelessness, autopsychic ideas of anxiety with a self-accusatory content—which at the same time she rejected—insomnia, fear of silence at night when the noise increased, and thoughts of suicide. She had an attentive face, no deficits of any sort, and good retention in memory. She looks after herself, but sleeps with the aid of sleeping pills. According to the patient and her family, this condition had developed slowly over 4 months. Initially, only the noise in her ears was present, which is why she consulted several ear specialists. Then the restlessness and anxiety in her heart started. She ran back and forth a lot, and could stand it no longer. Finally, she deliberately reduced her food intake and had suicidal ideas. The condition was always worse in the evening, which was confirmed in the clinic. In the clinic, her food intake was good, and over the last 2 months her body weight has increased from 52 to 55 kg. Results from hearing tests and ear examination were interesting. There were old changes in both ears; constriction of the tympanic membrane more on the left than the right (old *Otitis media* [W]). On admission she understood speech whispered at 3–3½ m.; it was also shown that her hearing improved or worsened according to the intensity of the noise. Over the first 2 months there was a clear decrease in her auditory acuity. This was noticeable even at ordinary conversational levels; for whispered speech, auditory acuity decreased to 30 cm on the left and 20 cm on the right. Here, we discovered particularly poor bone conduction; against the skull or mastoid process the clock was not heard at all. An improvement of her mental condition in the last 2 months clearly ran parallel with favourable results of ear treatment using the *Politzer* [W] method. At the time of her discharge the noise was certainly still present; there was also a disproportionate feeling of illness in relation to this, and fear of recurrence of the old situation. However, anxiety, unhappiness, self-accusations, and suicidal ideas had been eliminated. She could hear whispered speech in both ears at five metres, and bone conduction also appeared to be improved, albeit worse in the right than the left.

I will try to describe to you one of the strangest cases of somatopsychosis, according to notes from my time employed in the Asylum Department of the Charité, this being pervasive and also acute (in terms of external configuration). The 46-year-old worker N. was admitted as a delirious patient to the Asylum Department of the Charité on 6 December 1876. He had previously been admitted on 8 March the same year into a secure unit and after 3 days was transferred to the Delirium Department, but was discharged from there on 31 March as recovered. The few data available from the time giving the diagnosis of *Delirium tremens* [W] seemed doubtful, but many things showed that he had severe hypochondriacal difficulties (semen flowed from him continually, he suffered burning in his mouth, his larynx had been removed); and, apart from marked tremor and other objective signs of alcohol abuse, he presented familiar visual hallucinations, amongst others. His restlessness and current delirious behaviour were put forward as the reason for his readmission. His alcohol consumption was only moderate, before which he was alleged to have had complete allopsychic orientation, and intact memory of his earlier stay. His face was deep-ridged and grief-stricken, with an anxious, yet sometimes still-smiling expression, an increased respiration rate due to his anxiety, no hand tremor, only a light lingual tremor, with perpetual moaning and talking to himself. Hypochondriacal offerings included that his brain could have been frozen; he couldn't speak; his jaws might have been so loose that his throat would be divided; to him, his tongue appeared to have grown and fell down outside; and he had lost his hearing. Such utterances were often made without apparent Affect in a peaceful, conversational tone. He does not answer for a start despite talking very loudly, but soon after, says, in a whisper 'He could hear already, but there was no tension in his ears', and grasps with his fingers in the external auditory meatus. He answered my question about headache in the affirmative. He poked his tongue out, after he had suggested that this would not work. For past medical history, he indicates only that it had been remarkable for him for some time, but up until recently he had acted as a house servant. His pupils were fairly narrow, equidistant, and widened only a little, when his eyes were shaded. He claimed that he had no face; his head was as hard as stone. Other complaints: his rectum had been torn out; his head was back-to-front with the face backwards. Similar complaints, shifting in content and temporarily corrected again during the whole duration of the illness, among them the delusion of the reversed position of the head being surprisingly fixed. Apparently there were no hallucinations, which he could speak of, accessible on first asking. Gradual refusal of food was motivated by the patient having no stomach, and he would get no air. Tube-feeding was often required. Sleep was achieved only with the aid of sleeping pills. Most striking motor behaviour occurred throughout the duration of his illness. Soon he used the side rails, separated by gaps between neighbouring beds, like the rungs of a ladder, so that he could get about; sometimes, standing in bed, he let himself topple over backwards, into and beyond the bed; at other times he violently threw himself out while rotating his torso, usually with the motivation that his head would turn right way round. Frequently, he expressed his discomfort by whining so disturbingly that he had to be kept in seclusion, and at other times strikingly stoic, even with a characteristically smiling manner, often monotonously recounting previous experiences—reminiscent of verbigeration: 'N., do you want to stay here?' 'No, sergeant' whereby he explained that he had been an NCO, and now very much regretted that he had refused the invitation to surrender. Often he piled himself into a corner, hiding, singing to himself of similar experiences, like those mentioned above, but never with actual motor symptoms. Gradual resistance and blind defence against any actions prevailed; a strait jacket became necessary; his cleanliness and strength declined. Multiple injuries were incurred from the movements described above, including his violent beating of his own face with a clenched fist, etc. Finally, refusal of food, alternating or simultaneous with his insisting that he could not swallow, he drove us away, in animal-like manner, with bared teeth, so that you were afraid of being bitten, and that he then swallowed whole what he had bitten. After a restless night, in a sudden moment of calm, he died, on 4 May 1877. The autopsy revealed, apart from a very strong, virtually unbroken thickening and opacity of the pia over the convexity, *Hydrocephalus*—both *internus* [W] and *externus* [W] as the main finding; countless calcified trichinae in all his muscles, especially those of the neck. Under the deep fascia of the supraclavicular region, an ill-defined, pus-soaked body was found, the size of a pigeon's egg, apparently corresponding to an abscessed lymph node, and continuing upward into the deep musculature and gradually disappearing. His intestines were unchanged, except for the signs of general marasmus.

Gentlemen! The expressions of somatopsychic disarray which showed up in this patient's motor behaviour were so strange that they have remained indelibly in my memory. In part they can be understood from the autopsy findings, and in particular, we can infer an internal connection between the pus focus in the deep muscles of the neck, and the peculiar—often perilous—jumps, by which he attempted to correct the supposed perverse orientation of his head. We are entitled here to interpret the underlying psychosensory disturbances of identification as abnormal paraesthesia of position sense for the head, induced psychotically.

Alteration to the external configuration of the body confronts us in no less instructive a manner, in a case that I would like to outline to you only briefly. It concerns a 35-year-old former officer of high nobility, with development of a marked organic syndrome. For 3 years now, his life has been temporarily in discord; over the last 6 months he has been in a bad way, which is when I got to know him. During that time he slept badly, with occasional bedwetting, along with *Impotentia coeundi* [W]. Apart from low-level ataxia of his legs when lying in bed, a dubious, but enduring speech disorder, and traces of a right-sided facial paralysis, there had been no detectable symptoms of paralysis, although there was an old infection. Specifically, attentiveness, memory, and judgment were good; there was no fainting, but frequent deep breathing. Unhappiness, subjective inability to work etc., matched these complaints, related exclusively to his own body, which he himself says he can no longer understand. His body itself has changed, becoming thick and foul-tasting, like a lump of dough, his nose has become a red cucumber, his tongue and mouth are swollen, and he could not open his mouth wide enough. His stools were quite inadequate—he was full right up to the middle of his trachea; eating and drinking were performed, without any sense of taste, merely out of a sense of duty; there was a constant unsavoury, slimy taste in the mouth; his neck and throat were hot and dry as though burned out. He denied any real feeling of anxiety. Due to the continuation of these complaints he had to be transferred to a mental institution because of his dangerous abuse of his caring, self-sacrificing wife; and he went there, and within a few months, a rapidly progressing paralysis developed.

Gentlemen! Those examples of hypochondriacal psychosis or somatopsychosis that I presented may suffice to show that we are dealing with an area where individual cases show very different characteristics. We want to try to summarise characteristics common to them all, in order to define their demarcation from other psychoses. Turning first to *aetiology* [W], we see that quite often the content of a disorder of aberrant identification is determined by a detectable physical illness. Nevertheless it may not be a simple cause-and-effect relationship, because the same diseases of organs can be seen countless times without resulting in any form of psychosis. On the other hand, it is permissible to regard such cases as regular examples of psychosensory paraesthesia of the organ systems involved. The old theory of positional changes in the colon as the cause of mental illnesses now appears to some extent understandable, and even, with the constraints just given, closer to reality in individual cases. The clinical picture is always determined essentially by psychosensory disturbance of identification of organ sensation, for which it is often uncertain whether paraesthesia, anaesthesia, or hyperaesthesia is present.

Localization of the morbid sensations [W] is often quite vague and diffuse, as is particularly common for example during initial stages of progressive paralysis, when severe malaise can be traced back to terrible, indescribable sensations throughout the body. Moreover, it can be very diverse, affecting almost all body areas, including sense organs. However, pure somatopsychosis can be identified when the resulting substantive change leaves the allopsychic area intact, in other words, the origins of the substantive changes cannot be found in the outside world—as for example, when the sensation of stabbing instruments, electric shocks, palpations, etc. always go beyond the range of pure somatopsychosis, or equally those of somatopsychic delusions of relatedness.

On the other hand, the autopsychic area shows itself always to be involved, to varying degrees, corresponding with the Affective state induced by anxiety or somatopsychic disarray. A despairing depressed mood, unhappiness, hopelessness, and autopsychic perceptions of anxiety of the most varied content are always to be found. Surprisingly phonemes are very often missing and, where they do occur, serve only to summarize in words the ideas of autopsychic anxiety and the bodily sensations. Explanatory delusions are usually, though not always, present. Through them, those sensations get their fantastic interpretations. Thus the concept of mental disorder is often already accessible to the layman, such as when there are complaints about worms in the brain, or a frog or bird in the body. Anxiety, with its favourite location in the chest, the head, or the entire body, is an almost invariable accompanying event. The more pronounced it is, the more actual ideas of anxiety assert themselves; and they can become so dominant that it is justifiable to separate certain cases of somatopsychosis as 'hypochondriacal anxiety psychosis' [Ed]. The recently introduced Mrs L. (p. 150 *seq*) was an example of this. Also, these cases remain well characterized, due to the absence of allopsychic anxiety ideas and delusions of relatedness.

The *motor behaviour* [W] of this patient can be understood in psychological terms, as dependent on his sensations and bodily malaise: at times, more agitated, at other times, reduced virtually to motionlessness; his speech follows a similar pattern. Those sensations that result from self-harm, through food refusal, suicidal impulses, and actions of somatopsychic disarray, assume special importance. Some such acts are specially emphasized, since they compel our interest by their enormity. Belonging among these are ripping out the tongue, tearing out the genitals, ripping the body orifices, boring out the eyes, and crawling into a fire hearth. Some abnormal movements can emerge from paræsthesia of the position sense, as we have just seen, in the example of patient N (p. 158).

It is a mistaken notion, although one held as authoritative, that the distinction of hypochondriacal mental illness from hypochondriacal neurosis is based on the fact that fantastic or explanatory delusional ideas are missing in the latter. In contrast the distinguishing feature here is whether or not the hypochondriacal feelings exert any influence on the patients' actions. Patients who, out of fear of succumbing to suicide, themselves seek out a mental institution, like the above-mentioned Mrs B., will have to be considered mentally ill, but without all the fantastic interpretation, just as do all those who refuse food. Otherwise the exclusive focus on morbid feelings can make patients unable to apply themselves to all manner of tasks, and, particularly, to their personal needs. The sensation that, in breathing, the lungs rub against each other, with vivid accompanying pain but with no objective findings, formed the main complaint of a patient, who made no fanciful interpretations, but was totally immersed in his severe feeling of illness, which made him incapable of any activity. You could fairly use this case to exemplify the difference between hypochondriacal psychosis and neurosis. However, another case, I would claim beyond doubt to be one of mental illness: a general failure of motility bordering on immobility, without any other disturbance of intelligence, driven by an unbearable tickling sensation in the intestine, again without fantastic interpretation.

Anxiety psychoses both in pure cases and in hypochondriacal anxiety psychosis and also the somatopsychoses are relatively simple types of illness, dominated in their entire course by the same complex of symptoms. The trajectory of their illnesses can often be constructed just as well from the intensity as from the range of their symptoms, for which the Affects of anxiety and motor disarray will be decisive factors in the intensity curve. Where the range of symptoms remains the same throughout the illness, which is often the case for localized intestinal somatopsychosis, the curve is purely one of intensity. Cases where there is a spread of abnormal feelings from one circumscribed region of the body towards additional organs result in a curve based on the range of symptoms, which may be independent of the intensity. The relationship of the two curves to each other may determine the *prognosis* [W], where an increase in range without any corresponding increase in Affective intensity seems to be an unfavourable pointer. Moreover, in all cases, prognosis depends primarily on a patient's nutritional status, but only in the sense that restoration of a certain body weight is a prerequisite for healing and averting a lethal outcome. Good nutritional status at the onset of the illness by no means guarantees a favourable course. Invariably, there is a threat to life. For paralytic and hebephrenic somatopsychosis, severe organic loading is taken to be prognostically unfavourable when the limits of hypochondriacal neurosis are exceeded and an undoubted mental illness is present. Nevertheless, overall, acute somatopsychoses must be included amongst treatable mental illnesses.

Whether a treatable paranoid stage occurs in pure somatopsychoses can be learned only from further clinical observations. On the other hand, in cases whose acute character is conditioned more by their Affective colouration than by their temporal course, progression to a chronic mental disorder seems to be quite common.

Gentlemen! I would like to mention briefly a common combination of localized intestinal hypochondria with the clinical picture of Affective melancholia, which I have yet to describe. The hypochondriacal sensation we deal with here is mostly intestinal or, in women, often stems from a global feeling, or from the sexual organs. These illnesses merit the name *Hypochondriacal melancholia* [W], a term otherwise much abused, characterized by very favourable prognosis once treatment is appropriate, that is, to be undertaken within an institution.

Gentlemen! According to our course curriculum, I now pass over to a brief description of hypochondriacal symptoms, whether or not they occur in isolation or combined with other symptoms, and whether or not explanatory delusions and other *sequelae* [Ed] are present. When the functioning of organs, which usually goes unnoticed, reaches perception and is accompanied by abnormal sensations, we have examples of *psychosensory hyperaesthesia* [Ed]. Digestive activity in the stomach or intestines after a meal belongs here. Increasing from a slight feeling of unease to totally fantastic ailments, this symptom is frequently found in mental illnesses, usually linked with explanatory delusional ideas, that harmful substances have been mixed in with the food. Often, a genuine gastritis is the starting point for aberrant identification, leading to complaints of a heavy feeling, as though a stone lay in the pit of the stomach. Localized anxiety in Affective melancholia often has such an origin. The feeling of burning, seething, tugging, smouldering in the gut, the chest, or in the abdominal cavities occurs commonly among the mentally ill. The heart is the starting point of many complaints: Sometimes it beats too violently, sometimes too little: It seems, to the patient, to stand still, with blood faltering in the veins. In one of Kahlbaum's patients a painful sensation in the heart was related to having seen a flame in the stove: Her heart might have 'burnt out' [Ed]. Muscle pains often underlie a very severe feeling of illness, as proven by occasional examples of rapid onset, resolved by relief of muscle pain. When moderate muscular exertion, as in standing, walking, and sitting, brings on a severe feeling of fatigue, and thereby ideas of complete loss of strength, and of approaching death, this is also based on hyperaesthesia. The notion of developing pulmonary phthisis and therefore being destined to die is likely to arise from muscle pains in the thoracic region. It may imply feelings originating more in the intestines, when the claim is made that the lungs are ulcerated or putrefied; sometimes there is also a misinterpretation of mucus, expectorated from the throat or nasal passages, often accompanied by a corresponding olfactory hallucination.

The brain is a particularly rich source for hypochondriacal sensations. Often you meet the idea that it moves about within the cranium: descriptions include sloshing, flowing, seeping, or trickling sensations. The feeling is often conveyed that the brain is shrinking, drying out, glowing, or being eaten away. A tingling, crawling sensation may be ascribed to the brain surface, and to small animals. The feeling that the brain is attracted to some external agency leads to the notion of apparatuses and persecutors. A patient described various nerves that 'straightened up' [Ed] within his brain; he compared them with wax candles of varying lengths and indicated the precise points where he felt them. A buzzing, roaring, or thundering is often said to arise inside the brain itself and not in the ears.

The feeling of hollowness must be based on very strange sensations, where patients specify that ingested food falls into the void. One patient expressed the idea that his diaphragm was broken, so that air reached the abdominal cavity with each breath. Such strong sensations are particularly common among paralytics.

It is a specific characteristic of paralytics, for patients to announce that workmen are sitting in their brains, carrying out a particular exercise, and dispatching fully laden vehicles; when patients assert that they have a regiment of soldiers, or a factory, or a church tower within their body, or a number of brandy barrels under their skin. Amongst very specific sensations, but ones that also occur normally, are announcements by mentally-ill women that they are pregnant, or have just given birth, or that they are suffering severe abdominal pain.

Moreover, alterations of their external features are commonly felt. Most often, the cranium is specified as being soft and yields to pressure; at other times you are told that the chest is sunken or misshapen; the shoulders are not in the right place—sometimes they are shoved upward and sometimes have slipped down; limbs are abnormally thick or long. A young lady believed that she was abnormally ugly and had been given an ape's skull. She gave an approximation of its form, with a midline sagittal crest, and she claimed that in the mirror she recognized an ape's face. An acutely ill patient claimed that he felt his left leg on his right side, and his right leg on his left; a female patient that she had more than four arms, of very different lengths. Another patient became ill in a most-acute manner, with bouts of extremely severe somatopsychic disarray and disorientation. Although restrained by several strong men, he could barely be prevented from boring out his eyes with his fists. The bruises, suffused with blood, remained after the attacks, covering the eyeballs, which, fortunately, were not injured, and showed the site of his worst sensations, which nevertheless the patient could not remember. However, he stated during a so-called lucid moment that the worst thing about his attack had been the indescribably horrible feeling of no longer knowing what position his head, trunk, and limbs were in relation to each other—whether above or below, right or left. A few attacks of this type left behind profound idiocy. Starting from a strong family taint, the patient perished within a year from progressive paralysis. The idea of being abnormally small or abnormally large recurs frequently, especially among paralytics. Also, the delusion of any kind of physical transformation, such as a woman changing into a man or being transformed into an animal, seems to be based in part on feeling of the body configuration to be modified.

When patients describe themselves as being blind and pretend not to be able to see, we have to interpret this as a psychosensory paraesthesia. We know for example of the insensitivity to pain from the above-mentioned patient, who slapped his own face to show that he felt no pain. Pains of hypochondriacal origin are common amongst mentally ill people. They complain that they are driven out of their beds, by the stabbing of sharp knives, that they are electrified, tormented, tortured, their limbs broken, etc. The pains are often described in greater detail as burning, glowing, piercing, ripping, and clubbing. Painful muscle tensions are explained as electric shocks. One of Kahlbaum's female patients complained, 'What are you drawing out of me?' when she saw a warder distributing soup. Undoubtedly, these are all examples of psychosensory hyperaesthesia of common sensation. I have heard, from patients who had the habit of holding themselves bent forward, in a lying position with their head raised from the pillow, that they felt that, without support, their head would sink too far backward. Remaining in an abnormal position—which we will often come across later in a particular group of patients—probably has its origin in disturbed position sense. Such behaviour might be similar to that in the so-called hypochondriacal paralyses, an example of which I recall from a right-sided hemiplegia with mutacismus from the Charité. Autopsy findings from this case were negative.

The feeling of cohabitation about which female mental patients very frequently complain should be viewed as a more complex form of psychosensory identification disturbance of common sensibility. Only occasionally can one obtain further details about this; and it is then either the sensation of a hard body moving up and down inside the vagina or a combination of dream-like hallucinations, where tactile and general sensations are combined in the whole experience of cohabitation. A similar process is described by male patients as 'palpation' [Ed] or 'envelopment' [Ed], and is then projected onto the outside world. Generally, complaints of sexual abuse are heard very frequently from male patients.

More indeterminate paraesthesias of common sensibility, probably combined with abnormal muscle and organ sensations, are those of 'being attracted' [Ed], that is with their entire body, in a particular direction—a sensation that occurred reflexively in a patient, when he looked at the gas lamp burning beneath the ceiling. Furthermore, there may be the feeling of floating, of being lifted up or falling, possibly to some extent as an abnormal manifestation of vertigo, and also the delusion of being able to fly. This was retained for months in one case that I observed in the Charité and led, among other things, to the awkward situation that the patient climbed a tree in the garden and rocked himself on branches that were far too weak, so that a dangerous fall seemed inevitable. Bringing in a fire engine only led him to shift his position, and therefore had to be abandoned as useless. However it all ended happily, because the patient climbed down by himself after he had been left completely alone, and the garden had been cleared.

Lecture 25

25

- Acute hallucinosis
- Presentation of a typical case during the healing process
- Aetiology
- Danger of relapse

Lecture

Gentlemen!

The patient I present to you today is the 32-year-old businessman K. As you see, he is a well-fed man, apparently totally level-headed, who can tell us himself why he has come to the clinic. He came to us in the evening 5 days ago, voluntarily, seeking refuge from alleged persecutors. He lives at the opposite end of the city and is the owner of a grocery shop, connected to a bar. Opposite him lives a watchmaker, who is probably to blame for the whole fracas. He presumes this, because the latter had spoken out shortly before, very unpleasantly, about the dismissal of a clerk by the patient, and because the watchmaker was the main spokesman for 'the whole group' [Ed]. While sitting quietly in his room that evening doing his books he suddenly heard their voices, 'Now he is reckoning the accounts'; then he also heard the total sum, which book-entry he should take in his hand, and what he would write. He concluded that someone was watching all his movements, and knew his thoughts, probably using some form of mirror system, because he believed that he had also noticed a light shining and could see his persecutors—although this was quite impossible because of the location of the windows—and he heard their voices—presumably they were using a telephone, installed without his knowledge. Moreover, since he also heard common swear words, he left the room to find a policeman, who would give him peace of mind. However, since he did not find one in the vicinity he went to a nearby tavern, and ate his supper there. Then he left the bar and met a policeman to whom he made his request. The policeman went with him and said that he saw nobody, nor did he hear anyone making scolding remarks; he advised him to go to sleep. Everything was peaceful as long as the policeman was there. He then went to bed, but soon noticed that the old game was starting up again. He now heard his thoughts repeated; thoughts were even intruding upon him, and indeed the chief of police seemed to want to 'extract' from him thoughts whose content was ridiculous, on the basis of which his punishment would be given. It seemed to him as though a telephone led into the garden, and his thoughts were being collected by people in this way. As he lay in bed, he felt as though his face was illuminated. As a result of hearing vulgar swear words, and life-threatening statements such as: 'The fellow has eaten supper and should be executed' or 'People were standing outside who wanted to beat him to death with stones', he was overwhelmed by

R. Miller, K.J. Dennison (eds.), *An Outline of Psychiatry in Clinical Lectures*,
DOI 10.1007/978-3-319-18051-9_25

terrible fear and got up from his bed to go and seek shelter. On the street he was greeted with 'Hello'; everybody seemed to know him, everybody ran after him, 'Here he comes, there he is, the scoundrel, the liquidator, into the Oder with him!' In his fear, he ran aimlessly through the streets, constantly hounded and persecuted by the crowd behind him, and at length, he went breathless and dripping with sweat into an alehouse near our clinic. There he bought a cognac and asked for a rope to hang himself. As a result, it was recognized that he was sick and was directed to our clinic. He spent the first night here for the most part sleepless. He well knew where he was and felt a little safer, but he could still hear the crowd screaming outside, wanting to drag him to the Oder and throw him in. At one point it seemed to him as though three elephants had come into the room, but he would probably have been deceived. A powder (Phenacetin 2.0) was then given him to sleep. Here in the clinic, he knew well that nothing would happen to him; however, he assumed that he would be handed over if people came to get him. On questioning, he indicated that he would still prefer to end his life in order to escape the fear of his impending fate. He gave clear information about his business affairs, but wished to meet his 'last orders', and he stated his intention to 'follow without resistance'. Fear is suffused throughout his body, accompanied only occasionally by heart palpitations and the feeling of pressure in the pit of his stomach. He explains the fear resulting from the voices, which he hears continually. Literally they declaim expressions such as: 'For God's sake. Is not executed. That's right, the ratbag; now he's laughing, the doctor is writing. That's just nonsense, that everything is written down (referring to management of medical history); that's a malingerer. Insane he may be, but he is also a malingerer. What do we think of such a malingerer? K. is a malingerer. K. you are not listening, you are a malingerer. What does it mean, that everything is written down? The doctor is a good man. The doctor is a fool. The doctor is an ass'. The patient has repeatedly heard the doctor's injunction: 'Beware, lest anyone is scolding outside'. Likewise questions were often addressed to him, and his own thoughts were repeated by the crowd of people. Derogatory judgments about doctors, about the Kaiser etc., who were a long way away from him, had been 'set in his head' in the first days; later he had heard corresponding voices. The foul language and vulgar words that he had heard on the way here were sometimes individual voices that he recognized, and sometimes were screaming in unison, as if on command. 'Now he will go in the moat'. But he thought, 'No, certainly not'. He heard of a dispatch from the Kaiser, 'Within eight days his head will fall'; saw the telegram handed over to the prosecutor. Several times the criminal bell had rung, as if he were now going to his death.

The patient showed that he was perfectly orientated, knew the doctors, each of the warders, and the other patients, and had never projected the voices onto any of these people known to him. It was always the crowd of people 'out there' [Ed] of whom he spoke. On questioning he stated that he had often seen the people outside, with the watchmaker included amongst them, who was always there. He was surprised that the people sometimes remained even during his meal times and did not keep their distance. He has heard voices: that there is poison in the food; that he should not eat, but nevertheless he did eat, admittedly in the hope of escaping a worse death in this way. The patient is uncertain that he has had sensations of taste and smell to match this content. When he was given paraldehyde in the evening as a sleeping aid, he heard a voice saying, 'This will please him, that he still gets cognac'. As for abnormal sensations, this patient declares that it often happened that he felt himself to be electrified; he also believes that there must be a powerful electrifying machine somewhere. Several details of this patient's auditory hallucinations are interesting. He complains of continual ringing and buzzing in his ears. These are joined by rhythmic ringing as soon as his head rests on the pillow, in the ear of the same side. He has repeatedly stated that the rhythm of the ringing has synchronized his pulse; and he then hears voices in the other ear. As for his behaviour on the ward, you often find him kneeling at the side of his bed; he offers up his last prayer, as he is soon to be 'taken away' [Ed].

He also often leaves his bed and stands listening at the doors. He never loses his focus, and encouragement always rapidly succeeds in calming him. Sleep is brought on only with a sleeping draft, or, as in many similar cases, a dose of 2 g of Phenacetin.

Let us summarize the essential features of the clinical picture: We have here a physically well-nourished, prosperous man, who is probably in a position to give information in a level-headed way. However, from his manner of speaking, he conveys restrained Affect; he is 'focused' [W], as he says himself, yet is tormented by perpetual fear. Also, his speech is sometimes hasty, and his vocal tone a little shaky. His outstretched hands soon start to tremble. The main symptom we know about are phonemes, whose content, corresponding with his anxious state, is partly of a threatening nature and partly expresses his reduced personal status (that is, part allopsychic part autopsychic notions of anxiety). He hears the most defamatory claims about him personally, shameful insults, and threats; he describes how he is being hounded to death, and even now awaits an ignominious death. He makes most definite comments about the fact that his medical condition has become very acute, and within a few hours has risen to a high level; furthermore, he has heard voices, and, as a result, is overcome by anxiety. When he first met all those people together on the street, and when, as though by agreement, he heard shameful suspicions screamed at him, that fixed in his mind the first comprehensive anxious idea: that it might all be over, for his business, if these people made him out to be so bad. The severe anxiety only came later, when he was chased down the street. Attempts made by the patient to provide an explanation are remarkable. He is convinced that a telephone had been placed in his home; he talks of a 'mind reader' and describes a corresponding apparatus that he has allegedly seen: a lamp with a mirror above it, trailing electric wires. He assumes that there is a specific starting point for these persecutions, where he refers to the watchmaker as the 'people's stirrer' [Ed], and implies that the latter's motive is wanting the patient to suffer for the dismissal of a clerk. In all these situations we see attempts to systematize towards a uniform explanation of the phenomena that frightens patients, and this, just a few days after the acute onset of psychosis. We shall soon see that this rapid systematization is quite characteristic of the current illness. It is based undoubtedly on the relative intactness of formal reasoning ability, as we have since seen; and that during the demonstration the patient was free from voices and was never distracted by them. Visual hallucinations take second place, appearing preferentially in combination with auditory hallucinations, and have a delirious quality. Other sensory delusions, with the exception of those of skin sense (as electricity!), did not occur. This patient is firmly convinced of the reality of his perceptions, although there is no loss of his orientation, and he assesses his current situation properly, while confined to the clinic. The contradiction arising from this is not lost on the patient, as is revealed even in the form of a phoneme which he tells us. Namely he has heard, 'If he were in prison, he could be taken by force; but because he is in the hospital, one must wait until he comes naturally'.

Gentlemen! This patient represents one of the best-defined forms of acute psychoses, which, if you follow the practical advice for clinical analysis, deserves the name *Acute hallucinosis* [W]. For some such cases the aetiology is well known: the *Abusus spirituosorum* [W] in the case of *Delirium tremens* [W] (see: the following lecture), and yet what a different clinical picture! We also learn from our patient that he had been drinking heavily for several years, as a result of anger about his business—in recent times mainly cognac. He had already long been suffering from headaches, dizziness, and restless sleep; and now there are the lawsuits, which he submits. However, the onset of psychosis was quite acute, as the patient himself portrayed so vividly. On the basis of experiences from similar cases we can suggest a favourable prognosis, and expect a complete recovery in the space of a few weeks. (The patient was discharged as recovered after a 10-week hospitalization, and since then - 4 years ago - he has remained healthy.) However this is definitive, only if there is steadfast avoidance of alcohol. Without this, we should expect, without hesitation, the occurrence of relapses of a gradually increasingly severity, with a final outcome of incurable chronic psychosis. Cases originating without alcoholism or other intoxicants, while in other ways quite analogous, do not appear to subject patients to risk of relapse.

To complete the clinical picture, I remind you of an example of such a relapsed acute hallucinosis, who I presented to you several semesters ago in the clinic. This patient, the 45-year-old trainee and hack lawyer W., now incurably mentally ill, has been transferred to the provincial secure unit at T., and was found, at the time of the demonstration, in the third relapse of his illness (over the course of 1½ years)—the last relapse from which he had been discharged as 'cured' [Ed]—while the fourth relapse, 1¼ years later, ended as an incurable mental illness. This patient W., a former elementary school teacher, had been sentenced to 3 years in prison for a crime against morality and had thereby been torn away from his normal life. Nevertheless since then, he had struggled through, as an honest and decent trainee, and had started a family. Gradually however, he developed problems in feeding, and succumbed to hard liquor, which, 2 years before the time of his clinical presentation, had led to onset of his first mental illness. This showed a clinical picture of acute hallucinosis similar to the one you have come to know through patient K. Six months after the first attack, he was released from a provincial lunatic asylum as 'recovered' [Ed]; but 9 months later, his first relapse occurred as suddenly as before, and he was treated in our clinic, for less than 3 months, before he recovered. Just over 3 months later came the second relapse, from which he was discharged as recovered after 2 months' treatment; the third deleterious relapse came, as already mentioned, 1¼ years later. During the intervening periods he always regained full insight into his illness. I now remind you of the clinical picture that we had before us at the time; it was significantly more difficult than that of patient K. This patient could also give us well-considered information about forthcoming events prior to his admission. But occasionally his level of Affect rose to such extremes of anxiety and discomposure that he fell to his knees and begged for his life. The tremor of his voice and lips when speaking, the tremor in his hands, and the bloated, pale, and sickly appearance of this excessively obese patient indicate a further advance in his state of alcoholic degeneration. In a hasty, precipitate manner he reported that, shortly before, he had moved into a new apartment. When he looked out of the window for the first time, he noticed that the people went to and fro in such a peculiar manner, and looked up towards him and made such remarks, that he was able to gather from this that his entire past had been made known to all these people. In the street people were then yelling out behind his back, singing satirical songs, and whistling at him, 'Lawyer of the right, lawyer of the left, people's advocate, villain of a trainee, scoundrel, rascal, the villain has raped his own daughter. The prosecutor will throw him out. Into the well, and under the water with him; he should be pumped full and cut open; then into the puddle with him; put him to death'. He heard the worst things about his wife and daughter as well. 'Bitch, old whore, procuress, taken away to the penitentiary. They should be sewn into a cowhide and sent out to beg'. Among the voices he recognized were, in particular, those of two policemen who lived in his house; but children's voices, animal sounds, and beating of drums were mixed in as well. Dogs barked, 'Wenceslas is coming, Wenceslas is coming, Wenceslas is already here'. In addition the patient complained that somebody had sprayed something in his face through the window and poured sulphuric acid into his cognac, so that his head was splitting apart—because he felt as though his head was swollen. This patient experienced the same hallucinations in the clinic: He heard voices, sometimes from the street, sometimes from openings in the air heating system; he believed that he had been sprayed with morphine from the latter. On the ward he lay quietly in bed most of the time, 'ready for anything' [W], because he anticipated at any moment to be taken for execution. Occasionally his anxiety increased with fear to the level of mild motor restlessness when people approached him, especially at night, and when he came out in a vigorous sweat. From the outset he had developed a 'tracking system' [Ed]: As a hack lawyer he had often pleaded for his clients in submissions to the state prosecutor; all his persecutions were as responses to this, and the police were involved as well. They wanted to ruin him in this way and deprive him of his livelihood. Despite the ferocity of the episode, it was only short-lived, because after 8 days, some reassurance developed, and gradually, over the following weeks, he gained perfect insight into his illness. It is noted that a characteristic feature was that he had come voluntarily to the institution because he felt unwell and feared the onset of *Delirium tremens* [W]; and in his preceding relapse, and even earlier, he had made suicide attempts. Moreover, this patient, despite firmly-held delusions, never lost his orientation about where he was staying and his surroundings. A marked stage of paranoia, which is of varying duration, usually lasting only a few weeks, always seems to be present in those cases where recovery occurs. Recovery involves elimination of the hallucinations, despite tenacious retention of the system of delusions already formed. Usually however, the Affective state of anxiety gradually recedes, while hallucinations remain. Nevertheless, as the general condition returns to normal, there may, as a façade, be a chronic state of physical persecution ideas, or of a 'tracking system' [Ed], which, after existing for weeks, may well astonish inexperienced onlookers, by its sudden disappearance. A patient of this type, having survived an acute stage, during which a suicide attempt had been made, could be looked after at his home, under supervision of a warder; yet he believed his house to be surrounded by police, and was under constant surveillance by telephones that had been installed, and by an optical apparatus.

Gentlemen! The clinical picture about which you have now learnt is so common that I have no doubt that it is already familiar to most alienists. Nevertheless, it has not been emphasized strongly enough that it is an independent clinical picture, to be distinguished from related conditions. I still find the best description to be that in Marcel's thesis [1] where, in particular, the following features apply to the clinical picture: the acute mode of origin, the prevalence of suicide attempts, the defamatory and fantastic threatening content of phonemes, and the preponderance of auditory hallucinations.

As regards the *aetiology* [W] of acute hallucinosis, chronic alcohol intoxication is established in the vast majority of cases. However, there are rare cases where alcohol abuse can definitely be ruled out; in one such case there was a strong family predisposition to mental illness. Where alcoholism is found to be the aetiology, the causal relationship is quite different from that in *Delirium tremens* [W], because acute hallucinosis occurs mainly after serious binge drinking; delirium on the other hand, as is well known, occurs after periods of abstinence.

Diagnostically [W] the clinical picture can be differentiated more precisely in three directions: namely from *Delirium tremens* [W], the most common form of alcoholic psychosis; from simple acute anxiety psychosis; and from cases which develop chronically from the outset, which I characterized earlier (pp. 102, 103) as chronic hallucinosis. The illness is easily differentiated from *Delirium tremens* [W] because of the point of difference from the former—the fundamental symptom of allopsychic disorientation in its strict sense. Yet occasionally transitional cases do occur: It may be that hallucinations in temporary combinations tarnish the image of acute hallucinosis and also temporarily evoke the restlessness associated *with Delirium tremens* [W]; alternatively, in otherwise well-characterized *Delirium tremens* [W], the clinical picture approaches that of acute hallucinosis, because of the preponderance of threatening phonemes. The differential diagnosis from acute anxiety psychosis can easily lead to confusion, because of the main point in common between the two, which we should acknowledge: the abusive and fantastically threatening character of phonemes, and that they arise out of ideas of anxiety of an autopsychic and allopsychic nature is undoubtedly common to both. But with anxiety psychoses, ideas of autopsychic anxiety namely those of belittlement quite often predominate, these being grouped not so often into phonemes, as here. Furthermore, the whole clinical picture of acute hallucinosis is less-powerfully influenced by fluctuations in the

Affective state than in the case of acute anxiety psychosis. In addition however, an indication that a patient is suffering acute hallucinosis is that the voices come first, and states of anxiety appear only later. However, although the claim is made that in anxiety psychosis the relationship is the opposite, this relationship may be reversed in acute hallucinosis too often for it to serve any practical use. A specific characteristic of acute hallucinosis seems to be the occurrence of phonemes on a grand scale, their content being autopsychic and allopsychic delusions of reference. Finally, the rapid, comprehensive, and indeed allopsychic falsification of content, and the emergence of a manner of being persecuted physically, and usually soon directed against specific persons of groups of persons, are highly characteristic of acute hallucinosis, while in acute anxiety psychosis, except for certain less common cases with chronic progression (see: notes, p. 149), this is absent. The separation from chronic hallucinosis based on the clinical picture is always easy [2], as soon as the acute mode of origin has been established securely from the case history. The only reason for confusion here could be the fact that an aetiology of alcoholism also frequently applies to chronic hallucinosis, while the systematic character of physical persecution mania—which, according to a currently widely held opinion, should happen only in chronic and incurable cases—is also a feature in acute hallucinosis. Incidentally, cases of chronic alcohol-based hallucinosis seem to obtain their special character when combined with definite signs of degeneration, which are always in the context of chronic psychosis.

The *course of the illness* [W] is satisfactorily characterized by the purely acute and rapid rise followed by the descending path of the disease curve.

Treatment [W] of acute hallucinosis, at least during the period of the acute symptoms, is possible only within a mental institution. This has been repeatedly pointed out, because of the risk of suicide. As an exception, in the paranoid stage, treatment is possible in private situations, but with very careful monitoring. A strict bed regime must then be imposed, to ensure adequate sleep and nutrition, and to alleviate occasional fits of anxiety, using opium. In alcoholics, absolute abstinence is required—a mere *restriction* [Ed] of use of alcohol is usually not enough to prevent occasional excesses and consequent relapses.

The *prognosis* [W] seems to be most favourable after the first attacks of this illness, apart from exceptions, which are soon to be discussed. The more relapses that have occurred, the more doubtful does a favourable outcome become in the strikingly colourful clinical picture, and eventually a relapse is transformed into an incurable chronic hallucinosis. It always seems that the relapse can be blamed on continuing alcohol abuse. As we will come to know from most simple psychoses, acute hallucinosis is often just the initial, more-or-less 'pure' [Ed] stage of a rapidly accelerating sensory psychosis, which deserves the name *acute progressive hallucinosis* [W]. Mostly, such cases of illness already show more ominous characteristics from the outset: The patients behave more adversely, are less accessible to treatment, and are fearful of being approached, without any admixtures of delirium to explain this. Phonemes are not so predominant, but tactile, olfactory, and particularly taste hallucinations play a major role; and, correspondingly, the notion of poisoning is prominent, which, in practice, makes this so dangerous. Nevertheless, the predominant features of acute hallucinosis, the preserved allopsychic orientation, and the absence of any formal thought disorder can persist for weeks, until an increase in defensive reactions and the occurrence of new symptoms marks the progression of the illness. In these cases motor symptoms always seem to appear quickly, along with a state of severe confusion with disorientation in all three areas of consciousness.

References

1. Marcel CNS. De la folie causée par l'abus des boissons alcoholiques [dissertation]. Paris: Imp. Rignoux; 1847
2. Wernicke C. Krankenvorstellungen vol.1, Cases 10, vol.3 Case 3, on the other hand.

Lecture 26

26

- Presentation of a patient with alcoholic delirium
- Clinical picture
- Aetiology
- Diagnosis
- Treatment
- Post-mortem findings

Lecture

Gentlemen!

The 35-year-old plumber H. (discharged as recovered 8 days after the presentation) who you see before you initially makes an orderly, sober impression. He answers questions put to him promptly and apparently deliberately. When asked, he gives an outline of his life story, talks about his life in the military and where he served, how he fared, the name of his captain, the commissioned officers, a number of his comrades, where he later found civilian work, the company he now works for, when and who he married, how many children he has, their names, and where he now lives. He has ready access to commonly accepted knowledge. He knows the key dates of the last war; knows about Bismarck, Moltke, and the three Kaisers; his participation in the election; shows himself to be well orientated about city streets; can describe the course of the Oder, etc. From his quiet way of speaking and the attentive nature of his answers the only surprise is that he does not know how he came to be here. He believes he has been here only today, whereas he was admitted in the evening, of the day before yesterday. What is this place? An office of the Upper Silesian Railway Station? Does he know me? Yes, I am the chief stationmaster or station inspector. Why is he here? To provide information about his identity and possibly to be put to service. He promises faithfully to do his full duty. Who is this audience? Office assistants, scheduled to start the negotiations. The ward doctor, who has treated him so far, is shown to him: 'He knows the gentleman very well; he is the station doctor, who treated him for rheumatism some time ago, and had always warned him against drinking'. The patient is made aware of his hospital garb: 'These are hospital clothes prescribed by the doctor because the smell of liquor permeated his ordinary clothes, which would hinder his working'. On questioning about liquor consumption, he says that he spends 50 Pf a day on drink, but, conniving, he denies that he is a drinker.

Examination of the patient therefore reveals total misjudgement of the immediate situation, his understanding being replaced by terms for the most common ideas in his daily life. Results of the clinical examination so far can be summarized as saying that we are dealing with a patient who, in contrast to near-completely preserved autopsychic orientation—up to the last 2 days—presents severe allopsychic disorientation.

R. Miller, K.J. Dennison (eds.), *An Outline of Psychiatry in Clinical Lectures*,
DOI 10.1007/978-3-319-18051-9_26

You will notice, as soon as we leave him to himself, how his attentive, collected, and fully alert nature changes: He begins with his eyes wandering about, he stands up, bends down as though he were looking for something, appears to pick up objects, goes to the wall and manipulates it with his hands, braces himself against it; in short, he seems to be completely 'absent-minded' [W] and in a delirium. A spoken word suffices to bring him back to an attentive state and makes him return to his seat.

We ask him whether he recognizes the picture on the wall (a portrait of Th. Meynert with his signature beneath); he responds promptly that it is Kaiser Friedrich, and the signature

> 'Theodor Meynert (autograph)
> Med. Dr. Theodor Meynert.
> k. k. Hofrat o. ö. Professor a. d. Universität Wien etc.
> gestorben den 31. Mai 1892.'

is read as follows:

> "Theodor Mehlquot
> Paul Theodor Theodor Mehlquot
> k. k. Kauf . u. k. k. Prcesser a. d. Unterurdish in Wunde.
> abgeordnenedeten.
> gesalbten 31. Mai 1892."

We encourage him to fixate his gaze again on the wall, and then ask him what he sees: 'Military, the Kaiser is there, they are at drill'. Does he hear anything: 'They are shouting Hurrah'. On questioning, and while he continues to fixate on the wall he describes all the infantry formations that should be practised. Suddenly he begins to laugh: 'Bismarck is riding on a porcupine'. Now we draw the patient's attention to the floor. He is to see what is moving down there: He bends and begins to collect ants and mites, which he then empties out of his hands and onto the table. Since his attention is now directed to the table top, he claims that there are also horses and Krupp's cannons there, but in tiny form. From his movements it can be inferred with certainty that he believes in the reality of events he describes. He disregards any contradictions which might occur to a healthy person, with remarkable lack of judgment. Thus, when asked in relation to the military drill how far apart the soldiers should stand, he gives a prompt reply of 'about eight metres' [Ed]. He approaches a wall about two metres distant, and on being invited to go up close, he then stops, because he can go no further. About the nature of the obstacle, we can learn nothing more definite from him.

If we want to characterize the singular nature of the hallucinations that we see him experiencing, we recognize at once their similarity to dream experiences. As in dreams, the hallucinations are not limited to a single modality, but combine hallucinations in several senses, such that entire experiences giving a full impression of reality are thereby witnessed, heard, and felt by the patient. We have referred to this type of experience as 'dream-like hallucinations' (p. 122) [Ed], because of their similarity to dream experiences, noting that they occur in cases where a sleep-related clouding of the sensorium occurs, which is why they can be summarized under the name of 'twilight conditions' [Ed]. Does such a twilight condition exist in our patient? Given the periods when the patient, left to himself, forages, you must answer in the affirmative, despite his eyes being open, and retaining their ability to move; but the answer is very different for those times when the patient, fully awake and attentive, answers every question directed to him and—as he assures on questioning—experiences no hallucinations. In such periods, which can be extended at will, he still completely misunderstands the situation, which, quite logically, leads us to reject the obvious assumption that his disorientation is a by-product of hallucinations, especially when we take note of the fact that his misjudgment of the situation is a very stable characteristic, remaining the same in its content for hours and days, while hallucinations are subject to continual change. One might also think that there is impaired function in the sense organs themselves, for instance, as a detectable disturbance of vision and hearing that could bring about his disorientation. But apart from the fact that we see no analogous impairment in any other mental patients in suitable cases, we are led to a direct proof that no such disorder is present, our patient having normal visual and auditory acuity. So this patient gives us an instructive example of disturbed secondary identification, a relatively rare opportunity to observe, as a spectator, the very process of this identification disorder.

What we see here in uncommonly pure form should be classed as psychosensory anaesthesia or paraesthesia. The allopsychic disorientation can be understood easily as a necessary consequence of the disturbance of identification. His failure to recognize people and situations happens according to principles emphasized earlier (pp. 140, 141), and undoubtedly falls under the heading of optical illusions. However, this failure—his non-recognition—remains as a very remarkable feature, because concepts such as the hospital, the clinic, and the auditorium are well known and familiar to him—as could be shown in a later experiment.

Gentlemen! As you will have noticed we are dealing here with a typical case of *Delirium tremens* [W]. We will therefore not go wrong if we attribute such symptoms to the toxic effects of alcohol. This toxic effect can, of course, become manifest only by either irritating or paralyzing the nerve elements. Apparently we see in his allopsychic disorientation a failure corresponding to paralysis; and we may assume that those complicated arrangements of mutually associated memory images which allow recognition of the immediate situation have become paralyzed or inexcitable. It is then perhaps not accidental that the irritant effect becomes so clear, in that analogous arrays of memory images, corresponding to whole situations and experiences, emerge spontaneously, and with abnormal clarity. When such paralysis and irritation combine to influence—as we say—these allopsychic elements of consciousness, we see the specific peculiarity of this illness.

It is almost pathognomonic for *Delirium tremens* [W] that we find, in sharp contrast, well-preserved autopsychic orientation. Only at the time of crisis is there any autopsychic deficit.

Incidentally, the above features do not exhaust the symptoms of *Delirium tremens* [W]. In fact, right now, during my discussion of this case you have the opportunity to observe another important primary symptom, namely the peculiar restlessness of this patient. Left to himself, he is constantly doing something: He looks around, fumbles with his clothing, begins to undress, knocks on the wall, braces himself against it, rubs and polishes it, and is constantly busy. All such movements are indeed accompanied by tremors, but they are functional and coordinated, and obviously adapted to certain situations in which the patient believes he has found himself. They stop instantly, as soon as we call him, and with sharp questioning he is brought back to full consciousness. As you know, people tend to designate this physical restlessness as 'occupational delirium' [Ed], which is thus fully explained by the ever-changing combined hallucinations. Motor symptoms occurring independently are foreign to typical *Delirium tremens* [W].

Also, we are entitled to attribute another main symptom of *Delirium tremens* [W]—total insomnia—to the stimulating effect of the dream-like hallucinations. At least the onset of spontaneous sleep defines, quite literally, the period when the combined hallucinations cease, while the allopsychic disorientation and belief in the reality of the dream-like experiences may continue for days—but of course with cessation of pre-existing restlessness.

We now return to our patient again, to demonstrate several other important symptoms. On our very first examination you will have been surprised by the quavering, uneven tone of his voice; likewise, you will probably have noticed during his occupational delirium the conspicuous tremor in his movements. When he speaks, that same tremor becomes noticeable in his lips, and all over his face. As you can see, when his tongue is protruded, there is also a marked tremor. But this is not the only speech disorder: We also notice that, with all the more difficult words, there is a coarser type of speech disorder, normally found only in two other well-known diseases, meningitis and progressive paralysis. This is called syllable-stumbling. In order to establish this symptom we use certain test words, in an expedient manner, such as 'civilization' [Ed], 'army reorganization' [Ed], 'Guiglelminetti' [Ed], and 'extraterritoriality' [Ed]. Also, we encounter hints of paraphasias in our patient, as soon as we subject him to a reading test; and the writing test gives a very similar result, as with many paralytics, namely 'paragraphia' [Ed]. Finally, I must mention that many patients, when protruding their tongue, are clumsy and awkward in a manner that is otherwise intrinsic only to the above-mentioned severe illnesses. As you will have seen, the patient has a somewhat wry face: The right Facialis muscle at rest has less tone than the left, and tests of function also reveal a sag of cheek musculature on the right side. Not infrequently, deviation of the tongue is also observed, indicating unilateral hypoglossal paresis.

In addition to these direct symptoms of paralysis, the general frailty of the patient catches our attention. Since he has served in the army, we make him perform an about-turn and note that he staggers. Likewise, his movements when performing more complex tasks, such as climbing on a chair, are awkward and clumsy. The hallmark of a more severe clinical picture is then confirmed by his accelerated pulse (120), which is small and soft, with a demonstrable fever (temperature of 38.5°), a heavily coated tongue, and slight tenderness in the stomach region. Since all other organs were found to be healthy and the stools showed no abnormal constituents, we settle on the presence of a febrile gastric catarrh. Because of the conspicuous heart failure due to the patient's nutritional status, we must regard the prognosis as doubtful. However, we will attempt to strengthen his cardiac function by administering camphor and counter any imminent collapse from strong liquor.

The clinical picture presented by our patient is related to his predominantly cheerful, jovial, and jocular mood—the same character we saw in his combined hallucinations: Think no further than 'Bismarck on a porcupine' [Ed]. This predominantly bright colouration indeed seems to fit the majority of cases, but is certainly not universal. In a large minority of cases, especially—so it seems—those with a severe course, fearful ideas and hallucinations outweigh the others: the devil, hangman, black men, robbers, wild animals are hallucinated, and matching fearful scenes are experienced, or even the walls closing together or threatening to collapse, water rising higher and higher, and so on. Combined tactile and auditory hallucinations, such as a fire, an approaching and haunting pursuer, the rising and rushing water, snakes, crabs, rats, and other disgusting vermin, are often the origin of ruthless attempts to escape or become inducements to suicide attempts. When alcohol abuse deserves to be punished, it is bestowed in abundance, which leads to delirium with such fearful colouring.

The patient's restlessness is then transferred with similar characteristics to these hallucinations: rats, snakes, and toads are warded off, thrown out, stripped; sitting and swimming movements are made, any obstacle in the way of his attempts is moved with the utmost effort, or the patient slaves away—lying exposed in bed—to rip or slough off any alleged fetters he feels. Such anxious deliria are accompanied by profuse perspiration, as an easily understandable consequence of purposeless muscular work.

In general, such delirious patients only rarely express themselves verbally. In most cases patients limit themselves to slight murmurs or remain in complete silence, giving voice only occasionally, with commands or cries for help, showing that they are not mere spectators but are themselves acting within their pseudo-experiences.

The redeeming approach of sleep thus tends to signify that the Affects of such pseudo-experiences, as well as the restlessness, gradually subside, and moments appear when a patient is clearly drowsy, until, finally he is overwhelmed by real deep sleep, often in very uncomfortable positions, a sleep in which there may be some initial twitching movements, but which gradually becomes of such depth that even the most frightening noises and intense shaking fail to rouse him; and then, any necessary moving or change of position can be undertaken without affecting his sleep. The duration of the sleep is often quite extraordinary—up to 24 h or more. Light rhonchi and stertorous sounds when breathing do not disturb him, if no other signs of danger are present.

Gentlemen! In the patient just presented, you are witness to a typical example of that acute mental illness that bears the name *Delirium tremens* [W] or *Delirium potatorum* [W]. Prevalent as this illness is, there is a complete lack of any accurate description of its essential features [1].

Therefore, let us pause for a moment on this subject. The fundamental importance of *Delirium tremens* [W] is based in part on its well-known aetiology. *Delirium tremens* [W] can be classed aetiologically as the most common form of acute alcoholic intoxication psychosis, amongst which you should also include the most acute form of alcoholic psychosis: a pathological state of intoxication.

This latter pathological state, a special form of transitory psychoses, should undoubtedly be construed as an actual psychosis; however, it differs from *Delirium tremens* [W], only in its duration of no more than a few hours, compared to the latter which always lasts for at least several days. I will find an opportunity later to return to the matching symptoms of pathological intoxication when I take the opportunity of talking about similar transitory psychoses. However, apart from such transitory psychoses and *Delirium tremens* [W], the same poison produces two quite different illnesses, namely acute hallucinosis (see: the previous lecture) and the so-called polyneuritic psychosis, two acute mental illnesses where we cannot deny the aetiological connection with chronic alcohol poisoning, any more than we can deny the other fact, that the same illnesses can be seen with totally different aetiology. We will see later, when discussing polyneuritic psychosis, that this illness coincides with *Delirium tremens* [W] in terms of its respective allopsychic disorientation. You might want to conclude from this that allopsychic disorientation and the toxic effects of alcohol have an unconditional cause-and-effect relationship to each other. However, such a conclusion would not be justified because on the one hand acute hallucinosis, even if of alcoholic aetiology, lacks this symptom, and, on the other hand, the symptom is present in a pronounced way in presbyophrenia, the mental illness whose aetiology is specific to senility. These remarks may show you how wrong it is to attempt to classify mental illnesses purely on their aetiological basis (p. 104). The accuracy of this view is proven most clearly by the fact that even *Delirium tremens* [W] is not exclusively alcoholic in origin. At least, to reinforce the facts, if you wanted to deny the occurrence of the same mental illness picture under very different conditions, consider the following:

1. In meningitis with its main focus on the convexity of the hemispheres: Here it is indeed usually found, as in febrile delirium of infectious diseases, that when the above picture of psychosis is reached, an increase of bodily symptoms is also required in order to enable the diagnosis of meningitis to be made; however, in exceptional cases, where these other symptoms are not recognized for weeks, the clinical picture of *Delirium tremens* [W] is all that exists, while autopsy reveals clear findings of meningitis on the convexity of the brain. In one case of this kind, diagnosis was finally made, shortly before death, by the finding of a blood-red discolouration of the *Papilla optica* [W].
2. Furthermore, the picture of *Delirium tremens* [W] can be produced by other intoxicants, such as chloroform, ether, and belladonna.
3. Every stage of progressive paralysis can taken on the appearance of *Delirium tremens* [W].
4. Sometimes acute presbyophrenia (see: the following lecture) cannot be distinguished from *Delirium* [W].
5. In very rare cases *Delirium tremens* [W] occurs as the first acute episode of a subsequent chronically progressive psychosis characterized by grandiose followed by persecutory delusions with intact formal logic.

Let us return to the specific aetiology of *Delirium tremens* [W]: You are well aware that the present illness occurs only as a consequence of long-continued alcohol abuse and can itself thus be considered as a sign of alcoholic degeneration. In this regard, *Delirium tremens* [W] seemingly lays claim to being a symptom of degeneration, in a more exclusive way than conditions of pathological intoxication occurring occasionally in individuals prone to nervous diseases, after a single session of drinking unaccustomed quantities of alcohol. A second factor, taken to have a significance similar to alcohol abuse, applies quite generally, when any kind of external condition—usually illness, or surgical intervention—brings about forced abstinence from alcohol. This is generally taken as the usual cause of the outbreak of such a disorder, and it is customary to take this into account; so that moderate further liquor consumption is prescribed whenever injuries or intercurrent illnesses occur in alcoholics. In my experience however, such an opportunistic precursor is often absent, and we encounter many cases where *Delirium tremens* [W] occurs unrelated to any complication, not even gastritis. On the other hand such a complication, when detected, does not always lead us to permit continued consumption of liquor in the habitual drunkard. Even so the damage done by enforced abstinence applies in the majority of cases. That this is quite different from acute hallucinosis in alcoholics has been emphasized previously (p. 170).

Regarding *complications,* [W] epilepsy requires special mention. Epileptic seizures in tipplers are a sign of alcohol-induced degeneration in the brain, just as is *Delirium tremens* [W]. According to experiences in our clinic, there is a certain regularity in their timing, since they tend to occur 36–48 h before the outbreak of delirium following an excess; but if complete abstinence has been achieved, seizures are permanently avoided. In the clinic itself, alcohol-related epileptic seizures are always limited to the first few days following admission. If, as often happens, we therefore have to document during admission the aftermath of an epileptic process—the tongue-biting etc.—then we have the task, if at all possible, of ensuring complete abstinence. Bonhöffer has pointed this out, as almost routine practice.

I need not point out the myriad other random complications or incidental causes which come into question when treating *Delirium tremens* [W]. Amongst the top few here is pneumonia, a particularly dangerous development at times of critical deterioration. Whether the course is favourable or unfavourable in such cases depends critically on the behaviour of cardiac muscle. If, as is common, this reaches a severe grade, as a result of the prevailing degeneration in a drunkard, then fatal pulmonary oedema is often unavoidable despite all stimulants. But apart from this, the condition of the heart should also be identified as a principal factor, even in uncomplicated delirium, for, in a not-insignificant fraction of such cases, after apparently good general findings, the end is a sudden, quite unpredicted collapse. Then, when the autopsy fails to show major degeneration of the heart—which sometimes happens—the only assumption we have left is that of an effective envenomation of the heart.

Diagnosis [W] is easy if you have the whole picture to survey, as just described. The picture is so characteristic that experienced clinicians would hardly ever go wrong in making the correct diagnosis from the overall impression given by patients. However, only a detailed analysis would give you a more secure grasp, and here it is particularly the contrast between well-preserved autopsychic orientation and severe allopsychic disorientation that provides a decisive criterion. No other illness that I know provides such a striking contrast. Change in the state of consciousness provides an immediate differentiation, according to whether patients are left to themselves, or their attention is held by talking with them, asking questions, or while examining them. Their facility for quite prompt, attentive dialogue might be found in no other condition where there is equally deep, dream-like fogging of consciousness. In post-epileptic twilight states, this facility is particularly absent. Finally, the tremor and its admixture with the above-mentioned signs of the involvement of the projection system, namely the speech disorder, can be used for diagnosis.

For differential diagnosis, the conditions mentioned above (p. 174) come into play, especially the rare cases of meningitis of the convexity and the far more common progressive paralysis.

Gentlemen! *Treatment* [W] of *Delirium tremens* [W] provides a physician with the most diverse tasks, depending on the type of complication or their occasioning causes. I will have to neglect further comment here, restricting myself just to answering the following fundamental questions: When, and based on what indications, is it necessary: (1) to administer sleeping aids, and (2) to isolate patients? We need not discuss that coercive methods should not be used on delirious patients, or on other mental patients; surgical complications alone justify this prohibition, yet some circumstances may make it mandatory to break this rule.

Gentlemen! Administration of hypnotics in our clinic happens, as I already mentioned, only as an exception, because we have learned that prematurely induced sleep completely lacks the effectiveness of naturally occurring sleep and does not prevent delirium following its usual course. We have even seen interruptions by sleep being ineffective in this. If everything takes its usual course, we wait until spontaneous sleep occurs. But in the case of patients who come into treatment with their strength or nutritional status already reduced, we induce sleep as often as deemed necessary, according to their status; and we prefer to use paraldehyde (dose 3–6 g), and under some circumstances also chloral hydrate (1.5–3 g) or opium or morphine injections (on average 0.1 of the former, 0.01 of morphine). If the delirium becomes prolonged, without the normal fatigue setting in, or the pulse begins to become soft and small, or other signs of exhaustion appear, we see this as an indication for administering paraldehyde, and have never seen an adverse effect, even with larger doses of this agent, up to 10 g. Depending on this, morphine or opium may be indicated while chloral, due to its hypotensive effect, will naturally tend to be avoided. Rather, in particularly difficult situations, inhalation of pure ether can be appropriate to achieve sedation and sleep.

If we now turn to the second question, that of seclusion, under some circumstances the answer may depend on whether a suitable seclusion room is available. It cannot be sufficiently stressed that any risk of suicide or self-harm inherent to the seclusion room must be avoided, so that not just any room, but only one provided with all safeguards against this danger must be chosen, such as those available in every lunatic institution. In general, seclusion comes into question only with delirium coloured by anxiety; and it is then required if the anxiety increases substantially or is maintained, due to misunderstandings on the part of the ward staff, or when patients—supposedly defending themselves—make sudden attacks on their surroundings. But even in the latter case, an experienced warder permanently stationed by the bed is often preferable to seclusion. For the vast majority of patients, bed treatment at a nursing station is the only proper method, and at a moment's notice, can be stopped, and shifted to seclusion if you are satisfied that calm will prevail, which is currently delayed or prevented just by effects of the surroundings. Most patients sleep, as mentioned above, at the monitoring station and continue to sleep despite all the disturbances [2].

Pathological findings [W] in *Delirium tremens* [W] point to a certain kinship, according to clinical symptoms, between this illness and progressive paralysis. This similarity is claimed because in *Delirium tremens* [W] the projection system is also affected, as it is in progressive paralysis. Resulting symptoms include tremor in the vocal and speech musculature, stumbling over syllables, hints of paraphasias, awkwardness of tongue and mouth movements, the often-present deviation of the tongue, and the awkwardness of more complex movements.

Gentlemen! If you remember our first clinical meetings, when I sought to give you an idea of the possible localization of mental illnesses (p. 7), you will know that such a mixture of symptoms points to the involvement of the projection system, which, for us, was the characteristic of progressive paralysis. We now recognize in *Delirium tremens* [W] an illness that in this regard is similar to progressive paralysis. Accordingly, it is also possible at *post-mortem* [W] to detect the disease in the projection system. This is seen at least in those severe cases, where there are no other complications, and lead to death. In the cortex of the central gyrus and in Broca's gyrus, abundant signs can be found of incipient white matter atrophy, which are also restricted to the radial fibres from the cortex becoming thicker towards the medullary pyramid, leaving the tangentially running ones within the cortex intact. A similar medullary degeneration has become apparent in the vermiform process of the cerebellum, indeed exclusively in the white matter layer. More sparse but nevertheless undoubted signs of medullary decay are then found in the pyramidal tracts and dorsal columns of the spinal cord. It is thanks to Bonhöffer [3] that such important findings have been made, and their significance appreciated.

Bonhöffer's findings have been raised in a few particularly difficult cases that also distinguished themselves clinically, where the patients appeared to have lost the spatial orientation of their body. You can read the relevant description in the original. Bonhöffer suspected that this phenomenon was related to an alteration in the cerebellum. In any case, it remains extremely instructive that the actual sensory projection fields present no such changes of this kind, a finding which can be generalized without compunction from the type of cases that have come to autopsy. This applies however, insofar as we quite generally have to expect tangible pathological findings from chronic malfunction symptoms, not stimulus symptoms. However, the combined hallucinations seem to refer to stimulus events in the sensory projection fields. Broca's gyrus and central sulci, as known sources of the motor projection system, revealed the expected changes, according to the observed symptoms of paralysis.

References

1. Bonhöffer K. Der Geisteszustand des Alkoholdeliranten. Psych Abhandl 6 Breslau: Schletter; 1898.
2. Wernicke C. Krankenvorstellung vol. 1, Case 4 is also an example of *Delirium tremens*.
3. Bonhöffer K. Klinische und anatomische Beiträge zur Kenntnis der Alkoholdelirien. Monatsschr Psychiatr Neurol. 1897;1:229–51.

Lecture 27

27

- Chronic and protracted alcoholic delirium
- Polyneuritic psychosis
- Presbyophrenia
- A case of acute asymbolic allopsychosis

Lecture

Gentlemen!

I have already mentioned that a short-lived paranoid stage is often observed after a person in an alcoholic delirium wakes from the critical sleep. This phase seldom lasts longer than hours, or 2 days at most, and is well characterized by continued impairment of orientation and falsification of consciousness, and by belief in the lived reality of the dream experiences. However, in exceptional cases, even after an intervening stage of sleep, a state essentially the same as this paranoid stage can persist for weeks, months, and beyond—cases that can be described as 'chronic alcoholic delirium' [Ed] [1]. *Chronic alcoholic delirium* [W] develops either in the manner of an acute *Delirium tremens* [W] or as such a state which does not proceed with a distinct form, but more often as repeated abortive episodes limited to shorter periods of a few hours or less. An initial stage occurs, of variable duration, mixed in with traces to varying degrees of acute delirium, which never seem to be totally absent in cases of chronic alcoholic delirium. Furthermore, the chronic nature of these cases shows certain features that can probably be put down to an added component of alcoholic degeneration. These features include very severe loss of memory retention (but with a relatively intact store of past memory), disorientation—probably derived from this with respect to the immediate situation, and occurrence of confabulations, whether these are reported spontaneously, or are invented by the patients themselves to fill in noticeable lapses in memory for the recent past. It has already been emphasized that acute symptoms—hallucinations, and resulting restlessness and insomnia—are absent from this chronic delirium. It is still possible, even in chronic alcoholic delirium, for health to be restored if the patient's general condition can be improved, and, with continued abstinence, other signs of cachexia and degeneration can be reduced. If this favourable outcome cannot be achieved, dementia ensues, with progressive dwindling of memory content and gradual loss of initiative.

Protracted Delirium tremens [W] is to be distinguished from chronic delirium, and is similarly curable. Here, acute symptoms of combined hallucinations and restlessness can often persist for several weeks. Any debilitating factor, such as chronic suppurations, tuberculous bone processes, chronic pulmonary tuberculosis, or even cirrhosis of the liver, can form the basis for such a protracted course. An alternative outcome for this protracted delirium, as seen in such cases, is

R. Miller, K.J. Dennison (eds.), *An Outline of Psychiatry in Clinical Lectures*,
DOI 10.1007/978-3-319-18051-9_27

often death resulting from the underlying debilitating diseases. Protracted delirium can form a transition to so-called inanition deliria [Ed], but is usually differentiated from these.

Gentlemen! Our knowledge of chronic *Delirium tremens* [W] prepares us to learn about two further well-characterized types of illness, without my having to present you with examples. It will suffice to remind you of two earlier patients. You will remember the 41-year-old wife of a master tailor S., who I presented to you some time ago as an example of *polyneuritic psychosis* [W], and who had to be carried to bed because she was unable to walk, due to an atrophic paralysis of her legs of a polyneuritic nature. It was easy to gather psychological evidence from her because she showed herself to be completely level-headed and attentive, and examining her level of attentiveness by testing her domains of experience gave normal findings. More surprisingly, we soon encountered a combination of four familiar psychotic symptoms. The first was allopsychic disorientation: The patient had no idea where she was; she believed that she was a subject of an earlier fiefdom, and in the country as a temporary assistant; looking out of the window she recognized the towers of the neighbouring town of R.; she mistook me for the family doctor, the attendant nurse as his maid, and the medical assistant as the son of her sovereign. She regarded the current scenario as the session in a law court where she was to be heard; in the auditorium she believed that she recognized members of the court familiar to her from R., and several youthful acquaintances. She instantly recognized all other concrete objects and utensils. Her second symptom was a highly significant deficit in memory retention. The patient forgot in a moment what she had just said. A three-digit number, a foreign-sounding word which she should have retained after interposing a short question, was already forgotten, and a little while later, she had even forgotten that such a task had been set up. When she was shown an ophthalmoscope—an instrument unknown to her—a short time later, she looked at it with the same interest that she had been shown on the first occasion, and declared that she had never seen anything like it before. In like manner, neither did she know how she had come to the auditorium, and that she had been carried up two stories, nor did she know the time of day and whether she had had lunch or not. However, she thought that the latter was possible because she did not feel hungry. When I asked what she had done yesterday, she declared initially that she would have to think about this, but then recounted with all certainty and detail about an excursion with the family of the feudal estate to a local brewery and park in a neighbouring village. She also recounted various experiences from past days. She remembered precisely having put the children to bed the night before. She had been with this feudal lord for 16 years and had gone back temporarily because the lord was unhappy with his staff and she was unable to help her husband during the time of unemployment. Here we encountered the third conspicuous symptom: confabulation, or accretions of falsified memory. You will recall that I alluded to the connection of this symptom with thought deficits. However, the extent of this memory loss surprised us, for it extended far beyond the period of acute illness, going back years. There could be no doubt about the fact that such a deficit existed—as revealed most strikingly when I pointed out to the patient the contradiction between the paralysis of her legs and that she claimed to have gone for a walk for several hours yesterday. The origin of the paralysis was a total mystery to her.

Gentlemen! As you will remember, I have pointed out that such a loss of memory for the duration of her illness, that is, for the period when her retentiveness in memory had been lost, appeared easily understandable (p. 48), but also that a so-called retroactive amnesia (p. 40) was evident in this case. The patient still believed that, as before, she lived in R., whereas she had actually moved to Breslau with her husband several years ago. She remembered all too well her marriage and her maintaining friendly relations with her former community of R. Likewise, she gave entirely correct information from further back in her past life. She could easily prove that she still retained knowledge learned at school, insofar as could be expected of people of her age and circumstances. Admittedly, in mental arithmetic she failed completely, because, despite reliable multiplication of one number, she always forgot the other; however, working on paper she could solve arithmetic problems with several-digit numbers properly.

As for the case history, we learned that at the time she presented, this very ill, almost waxy-looking woman had suffered for 6 months from frequent uterine bleeding. A particularly heavy blood loss over 4 weeks had preceded the acute outbreak of her illness. Weakness in her legs had started earlier, with pain and paraesthesia. We obtained a report of the exact time of onset of her acute mental disorder, which was very inaccurate. Apparently, a short-lived state of mental disorder had occurred, at times even of delirious excitement, especially at night. Here, only in the first few days did she show an exquisitely coloured motor restlessness (with simultaneous mytacism!) Then, gradually, the state that I could demonstrate to you began to emerge; and it has now existed virtually unchanged for months, but has gradually merged into an acceptable level of recovery, since, 6 months later, the patient could be discharged back home as 'improved' [Ed].

As for the aetiology of the case, we initially emphasized mainly the patient's repeated blood loss. This was supported not only by her medical history and appearance but also by the blood test, for we could determine a haemoglobin content (Gowers) [2] of only 55 %. Later however, we gained useful information from the patient that over the last couple of years she had been drinking a lot of Bavarian beer, and also, in recent times, large quantities of corn schnapps and cognac.

Gentlemen! As you can see, we are dealing with a clinical picture that, despite its acute development, has seen subsequent addition of certain deficit symptoms. I mean the loss of retentiveness in memory, the retroactive amnesia, and the severe memory impairment. Therefore you probably cannot speak of actual dementia, if you want to be strict with this term. The animated face, the attentive character, and the demonstrably well-preserved attention are conclusive proof in this regard. Nonetheless, the existing deficit will explain the fact that no trace of disarray was present, in obvious contrast to the severe allopsychic disorientation. However, a mood of fear can be inferred from her misjudgment of the surroundings as a local court, this being easily understood, given the circumstances of a clinical presentation. Similarly, the totally apathetic and impassive behaviour of the patient in the ward, without Affect, indicates a certain mental deficit.

It remains only to say a few words on the precise time of origin of the illness. In our case, we lacked sufficient information about it; and, to judge solely from our own observations, the typical clinical picture of a hyperkinetic motility psychosis had been occurring intermittently. From experience of other similar cases, it seems as though, most often, a form of twilight state exists, with motor restlessness and hallucinations, mostly reminiscent of *delirium tremens* [W], but not following the typical course; that is, a delirious stage occurred in the acute phase of illness, to which is added the more chronic state as described, usually of much longer duration. This then decays more gradually. In my opinion, this latter stage alone is characteristic and decisive in making a diagnosis, due to its specific make-up from the above definitely observable symptoms. Regarding the 'polyneuritic' [Ed] symptoms of the illness, in our case they were very pronounced and had led to a total inability to walk and to stand. The paralysis was flaccid, tendon reflexes were absent, and musculature was universally very pressure, sensitive—with quadriceps and peroneus muscles predominantly affected, bilaterally. In the muscles most affected there were degenerative changes, and everywhere marked reduction in electrical excitability. Sensitivity was seen most clearly at the terminal phalanges, and position sense was also particularly involved. On discharge from the hospital, restoration of function was already so far advanced that she could stand and walk without support.

The picture of polyneuritis is not always as pronounced as in this case; more commonly there is only a diffuse wasting of muscles, slight reduction of electrical excitability and tendon reflexes, slight tenderness of the muscles, and a tendency to spasm. In other cases, even the polyneuritis, from where we get the name, is completely absent from the presenting psychosis, a point to which I will return. For the time being, let us hold fast to the disease concept of 'polyneuritic psychosis' [Ed], since, if the harmful causative agent is removed, the prognosis is generally favourable. In the vast majority of cases, restitution develops, even if only very slowly. However, a proportion of cases do become lethal within a few weeks. Without doubt, this course of events depends on the causative agent responsible, and it is precisely in this respect that alcoholic poisoning seems to herald a relatively favourable outcome. Here it seems to follow a course similar to that of the polyneuritis itself, which, as you know, most often underlies the deleterious clinical picture of acute worsening paralysis or Landry's [3] paralysis. Oddly enough, I have never seen such severe cases of polyneuritis accompanied by polyneuritic psychosis. Incidentally, given the number of cases, alcohol poisoning is probably the first to be considered, followed by the metallic poisons, namely lead and arsenic [4].

Gentlemen! I have repeatedly pointed out that, in psychiatry, correlations between the clinical picture and aetiology are recognizable only to the extent that certain clinical conditions have a *tendency* [Ed] to follow certain harmful agents. On the other hand an *exclusive* [Ed] association of this nature is refuted by daily experience. So it is with the building up of the clinical picture of polyneuritic psychosis, which is initially purely empirical. Granted, this very naming is inclusive, in that very different noxious agents can be considered to be the aetiology, just as for polyneuritis. However, we again see certain proof of the correctness of our position on this, because exactly the same clinical picture can be encountered without polyneuritis, as I already mentioned. This is especially true of the variety where delirium is manifest. I recall such a case, involving a doctor's wife, whose child was leaning against the compartment door during a train journey - the door not being completely closed - and the child fell out; while she, in her fear, could do nothing better than leap after him. She suffered a serious head injury and, after she regained consciousness, presented the typical picture of the delirious form of polyneuritic psychosis. On examination it was revealed that the four symptoms peculiar to the chronic stage were simultaneously present. A similar case, still under my care, had been combined with major surgery, a gastroenterostomosis that had been successful, and is currently convalescent. As in these two cases, an association of severe psychic effects and physical interventions triggered the onset of illness; thus, a proportion of cases characterized as so-called symptomatic [Ed] or inanition psychoses [Ed] offers the same clinical picture as polyneuritic psychosis. However the most convincing example of our viewpoint on polyneuritic psychosis is the virtually identical clinical picture of presbyophrenia.

Presbyophrenia [W] is a specific mental illness of old age, in the sense and with the restriction with which we recognize aetiological classification of mental illnesses. That is, if we differentiate it from polyneuritic psychosis, it is encountered exclusively among the elderly, and in many cases, no alternative aetiology can be found. However, it makes up but a substantial fraction of the psychoses associated with senescence. Like polyneuritic psychosis it occurs in two forms: an acute delirious form, and a chronic one. The latter consists of the same components as the above-described picture of polyneuritic psychosis; we can consider it to be incurable, even after long-persisting treatment. You encounter the same symptoms of allopsychic disorientation without disarray and loss of ability to retain memory, but with retained attentiveness, confabulation, and retroactive amnesia. In addition there are often changes of mood, especially of two varieties: One consists of euphoria, which is incongruent in relation to reality, and the other a 'choleric' [Ed] mood, these two being permanently intermingled. You will remember the two examples that I demonstrated to you. One was 78-year-old Mrs H., who expressed her well-being by a certain talkativeness and, because she still considered herself to be a young girl, showed fits of bashfulness, which was comic in effect, given her age. The other, 84-year-old Mrs K., is memorable to you as markedly loudmouthed, who projected herself with the filthiest manner of speech, and accused her neighbourhood of the most fantastic mistreatment. Apparently these were confabulated memories, based on misinterpreted experiences and hypochondriacal sensations. Both patients had in common the fact that, by their facial expression, gestures, verbal utterances, and their energy, any suspicion of pre-existing dementia is immediately refuted. The acute or delirious form of presbyophrenia was essentially the same as the chronic form, with the possible exception of retroactive amnesia. However, there is also a moderate degree of restlessness, insomnia, and intermittent hallucinations, especially in the visual sense. On the whole, it suggests a significantly attenuated and correspondingly long-drawn-out *Delirium tremens* [W]. I remember a case of this sort, where, in a 76-year-old woman—previously very active—the illness proceeded so favourably that the patient could continue a very extensive business for many years. In cases that recover, which occurs frequently, the duration of the illness is from 4 to 8 weeks. In other cases it merges imperceptibly into the chronic form, or it remains as a simple senile dementia, which is also always the end stage of the chronic form.

Gentlemen! The cases of disease that you have come to know so far have the common feature of allopsychic disorientation and therefore deserve the name acute allopsychoses. Among these, acute hallucinosis stands out by the fact that it is the process of activation by hallucinations, which, over time, leads to disorientation, so that the initial paranoid stage allows disorientation to emerge in a pure form. On the other hand, in *Delirium tremens* [W], polyneuritic psychosis, and presbyophrenia, allopsychic disorientation from here on appears as a symptom of the actual breakdown. I refer you to earlier presentations with regard to *delirium tremens* [W]. Regarding polyneuritic psychosis and presbyophrenia, one is tempted to incorporate general ability to retain memory loss along with allopsychic disorientation for both illnesses. We learn that this is, unequivocally, *not* [Ed] the case (for example) in a case of post-epileptic allopsychosis [5] with good memory retention. Also, it sometimes happens that the allopsychic disorientation seems to be aggravated to the point of 'asymbolia' [6] [Ed]. Thus, I could demonstrate a patient who had previously presented only an average picture of polyneuritic psychosis, but on a second occasion as asymbolia. However, an independent asymbolic form of acute allopsychosis *does* [Ed] occur, albeit very rarely, as the following case shows. It involves a 43-year-old teacher, N., who was admitted to the clinic on 10 February 1887 and 7 weeks later (29 March) was discharged as recovered. The outbreak of his illness occurred extremely acutely, after the eventful nursing and then death of his wife, which had severely affected the patient. For several days subsequently he had wandered around neighbouring villages totally disorientated, with vivid hallucinations; and he was brought to the clinic by his village friends bound hand and foot. In the clinic he behaved quite badly, only rarely and unwillingly giving us any information, and apparently misjudging the staff and the situation. This could be seen not only from his sparse answers, but also mainly from his behaviour. While he apparently saw and heard adequately, presented no neurological symptoms, and had full control over his movements, use of the most common objects appeared totally unfamiliar to him. He put his head into the food bowl, tried to put his pants on as a shirt, and did not know what to do with a knife, fork, and spoon. Later he learned to recognize the food bowl, and held it in his hands. He found himself constantly in an Affective state of allopsychic disarray, which stayed within moderate limits. However, because it usually led to difficult behavior in this patient, it hindered detailed examination of his mental condition. This much can nevertheless be said with certainty, that not even traces of aphasia were ever seen. From his occasional responses it could also be concluded that for simpler questions his comprehension of speech remained intact. With regard to motor behaviour a corresponding state of moderate restlessness prevailed, without addition of any actual motor symptoms, but mostly matching the idea of helpless motor impulses. He shifted back and forth in his bed, adopted the strangest positions, built a kind of cage with pieces of mattress, fumbled with his shirt, took it off, twisted the blankets together, etc. It was very difficult to move him when getting him out of bed, apparently because he had become familiar with this abode. A pronounced anxious Affective state was seen only when a change of his situation was brought about, while at other times, a moderate state of disarrayed Affect, or even an air of flattened Affect, was all that could be seen. The patient had to be coerced into looking after his bodily needs; otherwise he soiled himself, apparently the result of disorientation. Hallucinations could not be ruled out completely, although they were certainly not abundant, and in no way the forerunner of his periods of restlessness. With remission of such symptoms, this patient started to convalesce.

References

1. Kiefer E. Über einige Falle von chronischen Alkoholdelirien [dissertation]. Breslau; 1890.
2. Gowers WR. Apparatus for the clinical estimation of haemoglobin. Trans Clin Soc Lond. 1879;12: 64–7.
3. Landry de Thézillat JBO. Paralysies. Gaz Hebd de Méd 1859;6:472–4.
4. Wernicke C. Krankenvorstellungen aus der psychiatrischen Klinik in Breslau. Breslau: Schletter; 1899. vol. 1, Case 17, and vol.2 Case 9 are cases of polyneuritic psychoses.
5. Wernicke C. Krankenvorstellung vol. 2, Case 7.
6. Wernicke C. Krankenvorstellung vol. 2, Case 9.

Lecture 28

28

- A case of acute autopsychosis based on hysteria.
- Description of autopsychic disarray.
- Examples of alternating consciousness, the 'second state' of French authors.
- Episodic drinker.
- Cure of one such by bromide treatment.
- Acquired moral insanity, a special form of autopsychosis.
- Example of one such case of recurrent behaviour.

Lecture

Gentlemen!

The examples of acute mental illness that I have presented to you so far can be regarded as relatively pure and simple cases of acute somatopsychosis and acute allopsychosis, since the main elementary symptoms in the first consisted of disturbances of secondary identification in perception of physicality; and in the second in perception of the outside world. These disturbances of identification themselves involved exclusively the sensory domain, that is the relationship of *s* to *A* in our schema, even if, in detail, the subgrouping of symptoms as either anaesthesia, paraesthesia, or hyperaesthesia was often left in doubt, and open to discretion. If we are to pursue previously developed ideas about psychological mechanisms in a consistent fashion, we come to the question: Are there analogous disturbances of secondary identification in the third area of consciousness that we differentiated—that of personhood. In other words, just as our schema assumed centripetal conduction extending via the next sensory projection field into associated projection fields, can it also apply to interrelationships forming much more complicated associative complexes? Clearly an answer can be provided only from experiences in the clinic, since our whole schema can claim to be no more than a convenient aid for representing symptoms objectively, which is so extraordinarily difficult in our field. You will have already gathered from introductory comments at the beginning of our demonstrations that it has become necessary, just as with somatopsychic and allopsychic disorientation and disarray—and we had also got to know of motor disorientation and disarray—that we acknowledge autopsychic disorientation and disarray as effects of acute psychoses (p. 135). Disturbances of identification, analogous to those in the fields of physicality and of the outside world, *can* [Ed] also be found in the autopsychic field; and this enables us to differentiate a special group among the acute psychoses: the acute autopsychoses.

I have repeatedly stressed that, in the area of consciousness of personhood, it is no longer possible to use any spatial concept of eligible pathways. However, naturally, that will not stop us from recognizing that, in the overall complex concept of personhood—the sum of all memories

R. Miller, K.J. Dennison (eds.), *An Outline of Psychiatry in Clinical Lectures*,
DOI 10.1007/978-3-319-18051-9_28

as I defined it earlier—if all contrasts with the two other areas of consciousness (as the sum of all memory images) are to emerge correctly, subdivisions can be made, which are feasible, genuine, and determined empirically. They should therefore be recognized. Examples of this are character, and personal areas of interest—like professional and family interests—that are quite often independent of one another. Furthermore, we have to assume that, contained within the sum of all memories is a more limited complex, which appears to each person as 'personality' [Ed] in a narrower sense, and which is experienced as a unit. Disturbed identification with respect to this complex can come about without any demonstrable impairment of memory, in the sense I defined earlier. It must then remain in doubt whether diagnoses applied to sensory perceptions—hyperaesthesia, paraesthesia, and anaesthesia—still have a place. I would rather avoid attempting such distinctions. Expressions such as 'psychic anaesthesia' [Ed] and 'psychic hyperaesthesia' [Ed] etc., that you will find in other authors (I mean Griesinger [1] and Emminghaus [2] in particular), naturally have quite different meanings; but also, because of their subjective implications, in my view, they are not appropriate choices. In what follows, I see a most instructive example of highly acute autopsychosis, almost apoplectic in nature, in which both the Affect of autopsychic disarray, and the aberration in autopsychic orientation are seen in very pure form. In places I use actual recorded words and oral accounts of this highly educated and uncommonly expressive female patient.

Miss v. F., currently aged 50, was in my care for several years, and can now probably be considered as recovered, apart from certain subjective complaints. Until the start of her illness, she had suffered only mild hysterical manifestations, namely tension headaches, unexplained bouts of weeping, and a feeling of great fatigue. During the unusually hot summer of 1886 she was detained for 2 months in a charitable institution in a big city, because she was hyperactive, and suffered a great deal from the heat. Not until July could she go into the countryside to a family friend, where she recovered over the first 2 weeks, slept well and lost her headaches. One evening, after working hard in the garden, she felt upset, sensitive, annoyed by everything. Next day she was still morose, and felt so nervous that several times she had to hold back tears: 'Withal a thunderstorm hovered in Nature.' The following night she awoke suddenly, after a vivid dream with a feeling of anxiety, and such a strong heartbeat that she had to press her hands 'firmly over her heart to stop it from springing out.' She felt dizzy, and had the feeling that her mind was fading, and as if her head was covered by felt. She tried to open the door or window to escape, but found that everything was locked and had to restrict herself to putting cold compresses on her head. 'So she felt like a prisoner and wandered to and fro for hours in the confined space, sometimes looking out letters from her family, at other times holding up a mirror *in order to reassure herself of her own identity* [W].' Next morning she felt very ill, still almost totally sleepless, and suffered particularly from an hourly, violent fear. The thought that she would lose her mind did not leave her the following day, and made her insensitive to everything, everywhere seeming too confining for her, and she had to get outside as much as possible. Moreover, being left alone led her to a state of fear, and the journey home in a railway compartment was particularly terrible; she felt that she had to leap out of the compartment. However, the night after she came home, she had her first good night's sleep. Then her condition stabilized, and continued throughout the years with minor variations in intensity; and I will attempt to describe it to you in the patient's own words.

To this end I quote some diary notes, recorded at my request from the summer of the year following her illness.

'After my sad experience the matter rests, that I am constantly beset by an intellectual inability to grasp my own being, mentally and physically. Efforts to achieve this cause me unending torment, and I have to give up the attempt to find the key to the enigmatic intellectual phenomenon, in which I am repeatedly unsuccessful. *I am not aware of myself, must always prompt myself who I am, what my name is* [W]. I try to be self-aware from the inside out, all in vain; and likewise looking at my outer person, and this is completely foreign to me and beyond my consciousness; and so this condition has caused terrible torment. The same thing happens for my past. I know that all the events, my experiences, did happen to me, but it is as though another, a stranger to me, had experienced it. My speech is mostly also totally foreign to me, as if another person were speaking out of me; yet this symptom began only towards the end of winter. Familiar old intimate relationships with family and enjoyments seem intangible, and far removed from me; the dearest, best-known people often seem foreign and strange to me. For a time, I felt identical to my sister Olga. Strangers and new people are not so scary to me, and they can temporarily bring me out of myself.'

'By looking at my limbs I always hoped to regain my consciousness, but this effort always ended with the feeling of having seen something familiar, without being able to be conscious of the unity of my body and mind. When taking a walk, especially in winter, I wandered around often in a state of utter unconsciousness. Then again, I have been transformed into a totally foreign being. Terrible were the days—which all seemed turned into weeks during the winter—when I was so nervous that I did not move, did not even dare turn over in bed, because the level of consciousness required for this caused me such anguish. This went so far that I always had to sit with my back leaning against something, because I could not have my back free without the question arising whether it still belonged to me. I am sensitive and irritable to a high degree; often obnoxious and unbearable, despite self-control. Probably I want to discover something that is unfathomable … for I have always felt as though I were composed of several people, none of whom was the right one, that is I myself. It is best that I live quite mechanically, or suppress as much as possible my quest to find myself. The worst days are those where restlessness and anxiety join me in this search.' In addition the patient describes severe headaches, sometimes as pressure in the middle of the head, at other times as throbbing in the temples, and also backache. These always brought a feeling of coercion. It was often as if her head were being compressed, or everything was contracting internally.

Only after several years of what she perceived to be a wholly intolerable state, was there gradual improvement, and in 1890 she felt almost well again. Following the menopause a relapse occurred in 1894, but not nearly as violent as during the first episode; and, even now, 3 years later, she is not fully recovered. However, her general condition is only slightly disturbed, and she appears to be thriving, and is still remarkably youthful.

To leave no doubt about the importance of this case, I have to pass the following comments: Although her self-control towards the doctor always remained adequately preserved so that she always seemed competent socially, her feeling of unhappiness often rose to unbearable heights, with reckless outbursts of despair towards her relatives. For years there was the most profound world-weariness, and our fear of imminent suicide was allayed, not just because of its being forbidden by her religious convictions: Religion gave her a certain solace. She had cut herself off from dealing with people for years, not only by her own wish, but also because her situation required it; and it was only because of the great sacrifice and personal attachment of an older sister who shared her isolation, that made it possible for the patient's treatment to be carried out outside a mental institution. From all of this it appears that her clinical state was an actual mental illness; and, notwithstanding the well-preserved formal mental activity, in no way could she be construed as a 'borderline' [Ed] case better classed amongst the neuroses.

From our point of view the case is also very clear, because it presents a typical example of autopsychic disarray and disorientation. Addition of somatopsychic disarray and disorientation should not distract us from this view, but will, on the contrary, strengthen it. Manifold abnormal sensations of which she complained belong here only in part; in other ways their importance is probably that of independent, hysterical concomitants.

With regard to the aetiology of this case, you will not complain about its being placed with the multiform picture of 'hysterical psychoses' [Ed]. A decisive criterion here would be the internal relationship between the symptom picture and other undoubted hysterical mental illnesses, about which I speak soon. With regard to the present case, given that the course of illness was continual and, taking a long-term view, it was clearly abating. Periodic fluctuations in its intensity were indeed felt very strongly in subjective terms, but remained quite mild in objective assessments. There was never any talk of 'exchange' [Ed] of symptoms as is alleged to be characteristic of hysteria; and there were no actual hysterical stigmata such as fainting, sensory disturbances, ovarian neuralgia, etc.

Gentlemen! In the literature—indeed not only the psychiatric but also the scientific literature—you will already have encountered cases which bear a certain internal relationship with the one I just described; I mean the states of dual, or alternating consciousness, from the psychiatric side, often unwisely described as 'twilight states' [Ed]. However, the latter name should be reserved solely for those acute psychoses where there is stupefaction of the sensorium *per se* [W], and therefore an actual clouding of consciousness to an appreciable degree. This is not the situation in cases hitherto described—the sensorium is apparently well-preserved; on the other hand, to some extent, there is a break in continuity in consciousness of personhood, such that two personalities, very different from each other, override each other, the one appearing in place of the other. In this case, memory of the abnormally modified personality, that is the experiences, actions, and thoughts are either completely lost—as an autopsychic memory deficit for the time in question—or remains just as a synoptic, blurred memory, or one extending only to individual actions and experiences during this time. What interests us here, however, is not the memory deficit, but the state of mind at the time to which the memory deficit refers which, on account of its significant deviation from consciousness of personhood in the normal state, has been called the 'second state', *état second* [W] of French authors. Such changing states (which, at the same time remain steady in themselves), one of which is normal, the other aberrant, can follow each other in multiple successions; and memory will then always reach back just to the same-sense phases, so that consciousness of personhood actually breaks up into two—and in rare cases more—such groupings. These groupings, being independent of one another, owe their co-existence in a brain to some extent merely to chance. Independence of one personage from another is thereby defined not just by the selection of certain memories, but also by the fields of interest, likes and dislikes, personality traits, etc. A previously irreproachable character can, in the 'second state' [Ed], adopt the state of mind of a bestial criminal [3]. Although I do not deny the theoretical interest in these most enigmatic states, this should not affect their factual status. However, they appear to be partly artifacts of hypnotic suggestion, and are also so rare—I have, for example, never been faced with such a case—that they need not detain us, given the urgent requirements of the clinic. It is sufficient to have mentioned it.

On the other hand, rather more often, we see sporadic bouts of such an *état second* [W], and indeed, it seems, exclusively in the context of hysteria, epilepsy or degenerative conditions due to alcohol. Over the course of a year no fewer than four such cases were admitted to our clinic. Perhaps only one of them belongs in the 'twilight state' [Ed] category.

On the night of 11 June, 1896, a 23-year-old businessman was admitted. He complained of anxiety, gave vent to allopsychic delusions of reference and allopsychic ideas, was poorly orientated, and felt that he was being persecuted. It was learned that on 31 May he had had an 'absence' [Ed] lasting half a minute, accompanied by peculiar disorders of movement. On 1 June he had left home where he lived with his parents, and had not returned since. A scab on the left edge of his tongue suggested that he has recovered from a recent seizure. By 14 June, there had been complete calming, and the beginnings of insight into his illness, but an almost total loss of memory for the period between 1 and 12 June, except for very sporadic fragments of memory. At the end of July he was discharged as recovered. He was not a drinker; had no significant burden of epilepsy, and had never before suffered an epileptic attack. Up to the time of admission he had not been regarded as ill. During this time he had rented his own apartment, and had stayed for 2 days with a girl with whom he had a relationship. In any event, a number of very complicated events occurred during this time, which led to much deliberation; a mental illness noticeable to lay people would have come to the surface only shortly before his admission. This seems to highlight the period of transition to the abnormal second state from his normal personality. Complete restitution of the memory deficit never occurred. (Readmission of the same patient on 3 January 1898 followed a suicide attempt on the open street. His memory deficit lasted 3 days, a period for suspected tongue-biting. Meanwhile he has been healthy.)

A second case involved a 26-year-old Jewish businessman from Alsace. He was admitted on 19 September 1896 in a slightly dazed, and severely exhausted state; he claimed to be Felix Faure, President of France, and 3 weeks before, he had set out with his bicycle on a tour from Paris to Lille–Luxembourg–Basel–Constance–Ragaz–Innsbruck–Vienna–Warsaw–Breslau. After a deep sleep, the following day, he had full insight into his illness. He was discharged home on 14 October. Of his tour he stated that he had covered it 'half in a daze' [W], and for some stretches had also used the train. His recollection of it was a blur. Nevertheless, one must assume that this profoundly deaf, and visually impaired man had completed his tour without harm; that he has carried out a series of complex actions apparently in a conscious state; and apparent signs of mental illness have come to light only as a result of excessive strain. According to his statement, he came from a problem family; he often drank absinthe to excess, and following binge drinking had even had to spend 10 days in St Anne 6 years ago. The delusion of being President of France and of his being appointed to Warsaw by the Tsar first came to him in Vienna. He had good recollection of the period prior to his departure from Paris.

A 44-year-old businessman, who for many years had suffered bouts of drunkenness, the so-called *Semmelwochen* [W], was admitted on 1 September 1896 and, on admission, presented with mild motor restlessness, slight tremor, insomnia, complaints of anxiety, tension headache, and traces of acute alcohol intoxication. He could go back in memory only until 18 August, at which time he had left Wolgast to take up another position in Breslau. For the time between he had total amnesia. On the ward he appeared apathetic, indifferent, without any need to busy himself, and with a subjective difficulty in thinking through complex tasks, while his retention memory, attentiveness, and judgment about his fellow-patients, were fairly normal.

The fourth case involved a 19-year-old maid, whose father was epileptic, who had herself suffered sporadic epileptic attacks over the last 1½ years, and had left her employment before a series of epileptic attacks, and then wandered round for hours. Recollection returned only for the start of this pre-epileptic twilight; while, for everything subsequent to that, nothing.

Naef [4] describes a quite remarkable and instructive case from Forel's observation. This involved a 32-year-old educated man with a severe hereditary affliction, who was himself always extremely nervous, who had held a position in the Australian civil service for several months, travelled on official business to a town in the interior, and became acutely ill, probably from an attack of dengue fever. To return to his normal place of residence he sets out by railway; but arriving there after a 36-h journey, knows nothing further about his intentions; believes that he is in a strange town; is seen by a lady who he knows, without recognizing her; travels on to a second harbour town that must have been familiar to him from his inward journey, but does not recognize this either; and travels back to Europe, where he stays for several aimless weeks in Zürich; and only from a newspaper article reporting the conspicuous disappearance of the functionary in question, does he reach the assumption that this report might concern him. When he comes to the attention of Forel [5], he has an almost total memory deficit for a period of about 8 months, which includes not only his experiences in Australia and the outward and return journeys, but also the time of applying for the position and his preparation for the application. In a highly ingenious manner, with the aid of hypnotic suggestion, Forel succeeds, over several months' treatment—admittedly including an attack of hysteria—to fill in the memory gaps. Evidence was put forward that the so-called twilight condition dated back only to the attack of fever, and that the memory deficit reaching further back is therefore to be regarded as the so-called retroactive amnesia. The details that interest us more here, are mainly the description of the 'second state' [Ed], still present at the time of observation, although in the process of abating. Certainly, a thorough investigation along lines that were not considered would have been highly desirable, yet we can still extract much of value. Immediately after starting the return trip, he may well have been mostly in a state of stupor; later, during the entire, complicated journey and during his stay in Zürich, he must have made a relatively normal impression. On the ship he presumably used a false name; perhaps at the time an even greater part of his personality had disappeared. Memory of the travel experiences, which, it turned out, he could still recall under Forel's treatment, was in very summary fashion, limited to a loose juxtaposition of the most striking incidents, without his being consciously aware of motives for his actions, except for the one obscure objective, to reach his home country. In this case he spent his time aboard ship in walking and reading; for example he read Dickens' novels. He led a similar, but more vegetative life in Zürich, where he stayed for several weeks, without considering that he had relatives and a home country nearby. It was only the newspaper article that awakened in him the Affective state of autopsychic disarray, and which prompted him to seek medical help. According to his description, his memory retention in this 'second state' [Ed] must have been greatly impaired. Attentiveness was not specifically tested, although amnesia for the period of the second state can be understood as a consequence of impaired attentiveness, and was interpreted as such by Forel. It is also worth mentioning that there was a temporary disturbance of sleep, all kinds of hypochondriacal sensations, and a nervous twitching of the eyelids in the poorly-nourished patient.

You see, gentlemen, that cases of the so-called 'second state' [Ed] can be very different, one from another. In duration they may last only a few hours, or sometimes several months. They are usually initiated by an epileptic, hysterical or hystero-epileptic, or cataleptic attack, or an actual twilight state, be it of hysterical or of alcoholic origin. Only heavily afflicted people, the so-called degenerates, are exposed to this disease. What remains is a memory deficit that is either total, or permits only cursory recall, sometimes including as an added deficit, a form of retroactive amnesia. As with all mental illnesses, recovery is marked by insight into the illness; recovery of the memory deficit, important though it may be in practical matters, is therefore without significance. If we look to give it a closer clinical definition, it is the sudden appearance of altered content of consciousness in the domain of personhood, undoubtedly signifying an acute autopsychosis. Interrupted continuity in consciousness of personality is totally lacking here, and appears only temporarily during the recovery period. Such total autopsychic disorientation, with which would come the possibility of a new personality different from the earlier one, also implies the Affective state of autopsychic disarray, so characteristic of the illness described first, and which is totally lacking here or only appears temporarily during restitution. Even when there is such loss of continuity, there is an underlying deficit condition. We can sense this as a type of 'levelling' [Ed] of ideas, a lack of the more sophisticated ideas making up the normal personality, resulting in a modified and easily understandable, but diminished character. Motives for action always seem to be directed just towards specific situations, as the simplest selfish motives (Compare this with the above-cited dissertation from my clinic.). Detailed knowledge of the symptomatology is, unfortunately, very incomplete and complicated by the fact that patients of this type, who convince lay people as being healthy, do not come under expert observation at the time of their illness. In any case this type of illness can be distinguished rigorously from actual twilight states, which are easily recognizable by stupor, and some degree of allopsychic disorientation. Twilight states always offer more than the manifest symptom complex; often, as I like to point out, they may represent an intensified version of the same, this coinciding largely with their aetiology. I suspect that relatively good attentiveness and poor memory retention may be found in all relevant cases, perhaps also with concentric narrowing of the visual fields. Corresponding to the 'mental narrowing' [Ed] of the personality to a mainly selfish set of ideas, there usually seems to be slight lifting of mood, and an unusually flippant view of the situation, if not a tendency to brutality. Accordingly, fleeting grandiose ideas can appear. Therefore, there is an undeniable kinship with the picture of mania in which, however, you should recognize a totally different illness.

These are cases of the so-called 'reasoning mania,' [Ed] which may belong here, a type of mania that is manifest only from a patient's so-called manic discourse. If such states recur frequently, people may speak of 'periodic mania' [Ed], a doubly erroneous term, since there is no question of either periodicity or of real mania. In these so-called periodic manias, it is often found, especially in reports from French authors, that, in attacks, the same conceptual content always recurs; and, resulting from this, likewise, the same behaviour, often matching in detail. I recall a case of this kind in which a clerk pretended to be a doctor; and he apparently repeatedly carried out sophisticated fraud; and always acted in the same manner, so that the police eventually recognized the perpetrator of this type of fraud. Later, the case became clearer, when the patient lapsed into epileptic idiocy. It is therefore regrettable that clinical knowledge of the so-called 'second state' [Ed] still leaves so much to be desired, precisely because of the importance of such cases in practical forensic situations; and it is obvious that forensic cases are not suitable material from which to derive the symptomatology of particular mental illnesses. Simulation of a memory deficit as such suggests itself to criminals of any kind, and is easily accomplished.

Conditions are just as complicated in the case of the so-called drunkards ('*Semmelwochen*' [W]) but do not include the vast majority of cases here. Grounds for grouping these amongst periodic manias, a view which is widely accepted in current psychiatric nomenclature, are totally lacking, especially since actual periodicity is detected in very few cases; and, if you want to validate the popular expression 'drunkard' [Ed], note simply that, through external circumstances, the opportunity to drink alcohol and seek out like-minded company, is repeated each quarter year, in certain social classes. In many cases it is just that the first glass of alcoholic beverage becomes no more than a challenge to exceed it. Most likely, the periodicity may apply to those cases for whom alcohol is used to mitigate anxious feelings; yet the number of such cases is exaggerated.

Thus when questioned on this point, the above-mentioned (p. 190) patient from our clinic gave the following response: 'I cannot say that I have ever had the feeling of being *forced* [Ed] at this or that time of day to drink a glass of beer or a brandy; I do not have such a feeling even over a period of months. However, it does happen that, when in I am energized by strong liquor, I hanker after another drink. In several cases I found myself in social groups which I would have never sought out, had not my healthy thought processes been subverted by consumption of such strong drink. I have never been able to see clearly the beginning and the end of such situations; and it is only later, when friends tell me of incidents in which I did the most childish things, that it appeared almost incomprehensible that I, as a decent and—in my opinion—mentally healthy man, had got into such situations. Thus, clarification of these matters later on has been totally impossible for me.' This man admitted that he was a nervous, obstinate and irritable individual, suffered heart palpitations at times, and was easily infuriated by business annoyances. He had once stayed away from his business for 14 days, yet, in spite of this, was given high credit from his superior, who had been affected by this. Even more unambiguous is the information that I received from a high-ranking judicial official about his status related in this field. This 47-year-old gentleman from a heavily-afflicted noble family had, 16 years earlier, experienced *Status epilepticus* [W] for several hours. For 5 or 6 years he had occasionally suffered periods of agitation, initiated by restlessness and heart anxiety, where he spent 2 or 3 days away from home, hung around several taverns, showed off, made riot and outrage, and was careless in the company he chose. He had only a very sketchy memory of these times when he felt ill. This was repeated at irregular intervals. Since he was obviously overworked in his profession and his dietary intake had reduced, I initially recommended him to take a break for recovery on the Riviera, with the result that he remained clear of such attacks for a year. After this, there were 6 months of growing excesses, and occasional states of nocturnal anxiety in between. As a result, he was recommended systematic bromide treatment, initially with large doses and later with diminishing ones. In the early days of this treatment, small bruises could be detected repeatedly on his tongue, pointing to previous probable, but very mild—and therefore overlooked—nocturnal seizures. The favourable outcome of this treatment confirmed the conjecture that the condition was a form of epilepsy.

The pathological intoxication that was mentioned earlier does not belong here, but rather in the actual twilight state, as do most of the short-lived pre- and post-epileptic psychoses.

Gentlemen! You will notice that the cases belonging to our group of illnesses have not yet been brought together is a unified way. There can hardly be a greater contrast than that between the twilight states and real mania: Nevertheless, you will find in the literature cases which seem to belong in our present group of illnesses, that are sometimes associated with one, and sometimes with the other of these opposing terms. If you are surprised by such a proof of the prevailing confusion of terminology, sad to say, this is not an isolated example: We come across this in almost all areas of our discipline, for lack of robust definitions. Hence, as I constantly regret, it is impossible for me to recommend to you one of the best-known textbooks of psychiatry for your private studies. This digression, gentlemen, is not superfluous: It shows us rather that we need to keep looking for an appropriate name for our illness. In my opinion the same should be related to the concept of the second state, which is unambiguous in itself—yet currently always too narrowly defined—I am unable to find a better, equally descriptive, short name. I have already emphasized that in our sense it involves acute, disorientating autopsychosis, including a deficit which has a specific degenerative basis.

This might be the place for me to respond to an objection that you could easily make. Is the sudden onset of such a deficit, where personal identity is so totally modified, even possible, unless memory of the normal state, at least of the recent past as in Naef's case, has been completely erased? Retroactive amnesia would then have to be proven in any event, as a necessary precondition for our illness. However, already we note that the above case of the bicycle tourist lacked this symptom; and in general we can only say that it is so difficult to understand that such a changed personality can exist along with at least a tolerable recollection of the normal—yet it is an indisputable fact. The so-called 'drunkards' [Ed] are proof of this. One such patient can be the best father of a family; but in his altered state he can, without hesitation, leave his family in need, knowing exactly the position in which he left them. His mistake is based on his having concluded by analogy that his family takes life easily, just as he does himself, and that God will provide at times of need. A vivid description of this altered concept in a drunkard, is to be found in Dostoevsky's Raskolnikov. The judicial officer mentioned above had so little memory deficit for the immediate past that he might even be aware of dates falling within this time period; and throughout the duration he was fairly proficient. One explanation for this remarkable contrast between the sick personality, and simultaneously, the remembered healthy one, can also be found by assuming a toxic effect, which is indeed very close to the concept of a drunkard, though not actually found. At such times one can speak of a 'split personality' [Ed], a case analogous to my earlier description of the state of decay of individuality, which can be explained by assuming the process of sejunction.

Gentlemen! It is likely to astonish you beyond measure if I were at this moment to remind you of cases of the so-called acquired 'moral insanity' [Ed] or 'moral madness' [Ed], and likewise to bring this into consideration here. You know that this is about cases of illness which lawyers, unfortunately supported by clashing opinions, have been particularly reluctant to recognize, which, in our own view, has diverted attention from much of both the factual reality of these aberrant conditions and their theoretical basis. Unfortunately, it must be admitted that the tendency to make the cases conform to a particular scheme has also seduced individual professional colleagues to ignore certain facts and to defend the view that a state of deficit in the 'moral' [Ed] area must be connected with one in the intellectual area, which is to be recognized as aberrant. However, this assertion does not hold a candle compared to the facts; it can probably only come from the misconception that one has transferred the characteristics of chronic—and especially the cases of innate—so-called moral idiocy to those which are more-or-less acute in origin. On the other hand, the latter often lack so much as a trace of intellectual disorder. It becomes understandable to us, if we consider the above-indicated (p. 191) elementary symptom of 'levelling of ideas' [Ed] as their basis. In fact, almost all other elementary symptoms can be missing, including even, in most cases, internal restlessness and irritable mood. This levelling of ideas is what gives it a certain similarity to mania, for we shall see later that it accounts for a major symptom of the latter illness; however, what is missing here are all the other equally important symptoms belonging to this clinical picture, such as flight of ideas, pressured speech, abnormal euphoria etc. If you remember, the normal superior status of certain ideas forms the basis of character and morality; that likes and dislikes have the same origin; that therein we find the only inhibition to set limits on the predominant selfishness which drives people in their natural state; then you will understand that elimination of such higher values produces a change of personality which, when extended to the realm of morality of likes and dislikes towards certain people, reveals ruthless, egotistic drives with great clarity. Explanatory delusions arising from resistance on the part of family or wider society to the changed moral behaviour may come next, in the form of delusions of persecution.

A description of these states in detail would lead us too far astray; but I want to touch briefly on the aetiology. In this respect, a connection between processes of development and recovery in the organism is quite unmistakable. If we decide to call these cases *moral autopsychosis* [W], we can distinguish a 'hebephrenic' [Ed], a 'climacteric' [Ed], and a 'senile' [Ed] form of moral autopsychosis. Soon a menstrual form, usually lasting only a few days, might be recognized. Incidentally, I do not doubt that other aetiological factors, hereditary and degenerative in nature may also play a role in this, and that other harmful effects that can otherwise lead to onset of acute psychoses, such as head trauma, can have the same effect, in exceptional cases. That this concerns actual psychosis, or, in other words, an expression of abnormal brain activity, and not just persisting moral aberration, is proven for some such cases by the fact of their curability. However, the climacteric form seems predominantly—and the senile form invariably—unfavourable, the latter eventually blending gradually into senile dementia. The clinical picture described by Kahlbaum of heboids or heboidophrenia based purely on empirical criteria, seems to me to belong with some of the cases here. The relative curability of the illness has already been pointed out by Kahlbaum.

With regard to the course of the disease, it is likely to depend on the aetiology. For example, I saw a highly acute outbreak in a 15-year-old girl, below average intelligence, who had been afflicted by her father's drunkenness. The later course developed as a certain period of prominent illness (lasting 7 weeks), and then abating towards a basic insight of the illness over the next few months. Over the course of 3 years there were three subsequent recurrences, of slightly lower intensity and somewhat shorter duration, following the same course. Melancholy moods occurred during intervening free periods, so that, for a time the thought of a 'circular psychosis' [Ed] was entertained. However, this idea soon had to be abandoned, when people wanted to define 'circular psychosis' [Ed] as a regular alternation between mania and melancholia. On the one hand, a melancholy 'phase' [Ed] was out of the question, since it was usually a mere temporary, transient fit of melancholy mood, which could as well be really the impact of insights into the illness. On the other hand, there was the abnormal condition, connected with excitement, albeit temporarily, but certainly not manic. This was rather outweighed by the moral deficiencies, lack of obedience, lack of respect for ward staff and doctors, and even for the older fellow patients; above all, the lack of discipline; the most pronounced individualism; lack of appreciation for any kindness shown to her; lack of shame or feelings of civility; propensity for foul-mouthed and obscene language, with corresponding behaviour to the point of gross uncleanliness. Actual pressured speech, flights of fancy, and hyperactivity never existed. In fact, even the patient's condition, initially presumed to be a congenital deficit that would have increased by the time of puberty, was interpreted as a 'moral degeneration' [Ed]; and even a stay in a correctional facility was considered. The mother's testimony, according to which she had been a good-natured and well mannered child until the outbreak of her illness, was initially given scant credence because of the apparent shortcomings of the mother. Characteristically, there was absolutely no trace of shame during a pelvic exam, to which her gross uncleanliness had given rise. However, it was the total change that occurred later in her behaviour, when she became a modest, demure girl, and was diligent and helpful at the monitoring station, which taught us about our misconception. As for the intellectual development of the girl, her judgment and store of school knowledge at age of 18 years lagged somewhat behind expectations, similar to that of a 14-year-old girl in the same situation. In her physical development on the other hand, she had not lagged behind, and during the entire time of observation she menstruated regularly.

Gentlemen! If we take a look back at cases of illness classed as acute psychoses, we can bring them together in as much as they are all characterized as deficits in the autopsychic area. Even the state of mind presented by Miss v. F., who I described first, showed us the failure of secondary identification, autopsychic disorientation, and the Affective state of autopsychic disarray that derived from it. Then we had states of interrupted continuity of personal identity; and we recognized the so-called 'second state' [Ed] of French authors; and likewise we perceived a state of deficit as not contrasting with the healthy condition and therefore lacking the Affective state of autopsychic disarray. The common, severely-neurotic degenerative aetiology formed a mediating state between these two states, which are otherwise so different. Furthermore, we learned to recognize cases of the so-called periodic drunkenness, in which sudden occurrence of a changed, always diminished personality was assumed to be due to internal aberrant processes, as was the so-called second state. I mentioned that people had tended to attribute these cases to periodic mania. Finally we found that the acquired moral insanity represented a totally analogous deficit state in the autopsychic area, such that one can validly admit the existence of an acute 'moral psychosis' [Ed], and subsume amongst its cases some of the so-called periodic mania, but also the so-called 'reasoning mania' [Ed]. For this latter category, physical changes accompanying onset and loss of sexual maturity, and of senile involution, prove to be decisive influences. In the next patient demonstrations, in contrast to these deficits, we will deal with certain irritative phenomena in the autopsychic area.

References

1. Griesinger W. Die Pathologie und Therapie der psychischen Krankheiten für Ärzte und Studierende. 3rd ed. Braunschweig: F Wreden; 1871.
2. Emminghaus H. Allgemeine Psychopathologie zur Einführung in das Studium der Geistesstörung. Leipzig: FCW Vogel; 1878.
3. Bohn RWT. Ein Fall von doppeltem Bewußtsein [dissertation]. Universität Breslau; 1898.
4. Naef M. Ein Fall von temporärer totaler teilweiser retrograder Amnesie. [dissertation]. Universität Zürich; 1898.
5. Forel A. Untersuchungen über die Haubenregion und ihre oberen Verknüpfungen im Gehirne des Menschen und einiger Säugethiere, mit Beiträgen zu den Methoden der Gehirnuntersuchung. Arch Psychiatr Nervenkr. 1877;7(3):393–495.

Lecture 29

29

- Acute expansive autopsychosis due to autochthonous ideas
- Disappearance of thoughts as an elementary symptom
- Obsessive neurosis
- Obsessive psychosis
- Audible thoughts as the basis of an ascending form of acute autopsychosis

Lecture

Gentlemen!

The 38-year-old municipal secretary we examine today has been difficult to motivate, and to bring to the lecture theatre, but eventually he declared his willingness, as he says, to provide a service to science. You see a thriving, seemingly healthy man with impeccable manners and intelligence manifest in his facial expression and speech. Given his situation, the unusual level of general education, which he soon betrays, is explained by the fact that he had studied philology; and, very shortly before his *Staatsexamen* [W] had to take a different career path for health reasons. There is no sign of formal thought disorder from him. He feels healthy. Nevertheless, the need to detain him here in the clinic, despite his objections is based on the fact that we have reason to fear that, as soon as he is free, he will go to Berlin and seek out the Kaiser; for he feels it his duty and his task to remove from the Kaiser a part of his government. Accordingly, he considers that his being detained here is an injustice and an act of deprivation of liberty. Despite this, you can see how soberly and considerately he passes judgment, from the fact that in no way does he put our behaviour down to 'bad faith' [Ed], but suggests a mistake on our part only with the politest warning to us not to approach too closely. I drew his attention to the fact that when he entered the hospital 3 months ago he came voluntarily, and felt ill; therefore as we hear, he was probably well aware of the purpose and provision of the institution. He has to admit that fact, but now vividly regrets having done it, because he is sure that he was wrong to have done so. Rather when he had been ill earlier, he had been nervous, but was now so healthy, so strong, and more efficient in every way than before. On questioning, we still hear that, up to the time of his being detained, he felt completely happy, and did not doubt that the doctors would gradually see the error of their ways. I must acknowledge, moreover, that his general health has been excellent in the last few weeks. During his stay his body weight increased from 63 to 70 kg. He has no doubt that the Kaiser will receive him with open arms. How does he know this? An inner voice tells him. As we see from a piece of paper, this inner voice compares the patient with the *daimonion* [W] of Socrates, 'who people have also now declared insane' as the patient casually

R. Miller, K.J. Dennison (eds.), *An Outline of Psychiatry in Clinical Lectures*,
DOI 10.1007/978-3-319-18051-9_29

remarks. From more detailed characteristics of this voice we learn that it is not localized, has no particular vocal quality, but might include certain words from time to time, and—which is the main thing—is based on divine inspiration. The patient also harbours fears that we doctors are heading towards severe divine punishment because of our delusion. He does not doubt—and this is also evident from his documents—that he is placed in direct communication with God, and receives revelations and enlightenments from Him. He denies hearing voices, as do other mental patients, nor has he ever experienced face-to-face apparitions. I argue with him that, if injustice is being done to him here, this does not lead to the conclusion of a special providence from God. Then he explains that it is quite likely that the thought has been assimilated here, and had in due course been given to him by an evil spirit. He could only regard his time here as probation imposed upon him; he nods approvingly when I remind him of an analogy with other heroes and prophets. As you have already heard, he has no grudge against us doctors, yet is convinced that we believe that we have our duty to do; but he emphasizes the difference between his spiritual concept and our materialistic one, which of course would exclude belief in God and spirits. The patient is confirmed in his belief by an experience from childhood, in which one night, as his grandfather lay seriously ill, he awoke to see a woman clad all in grey, disappearing through a half-open double door. His mother had seen the same phenomenon and could confirm it, and at that very moment his grandfather had died. When we attempt a psychological account of this well-known type of half-wakeful hallucination, he just smiles. He is weighed down, as we have seen, by his writing and, he confirms, with his big plans for the future. As soon as he gets to government, he intends to bless all the world; to install the senior physician with 30,000 Marks as his personal physician; to build a golden bridge over the Rhine near the Niederwald monument as a symbol of peoples' eternal freedom—the gold represents the purity of the mind—and take the money for this from the Julian Tower. Certainly he carries a whole series of nonsensical fantastic ideas that he is concealing from us.

Gentlemen! The illness that we are concerned with here arose very acutely, yet the day before his admission, he was carrying out his office work satisfactorily. We learned that the patient, whose mentally ill father had died in a mental institution, had for years expressed his fear of becoming mentally ill. A brief bout of severe nervous agitation had occurred 17 years ago, just before an exam, and had impelled him to give up philological study, as being too strenuous. However, he was said to have been very capable mentally. When the patient himself sought admission to the clinic he was agitated, as the delusions of grandeur appeared, which he himself acknowledged as being abnormal, and he asked for help so that he did not become insane. His face was markedly congested; the skin of his entire body was cyanotically discoloured; a rapid pulse of 120, small and soft, not quite regular; subjective complaints of heart palpitations; and objective evidence of a right ventricular enlargement reaching to a finger's breadth to the right of the right sternal margin. Examination of the nervous system revealed no pathological findings, other than when he articulated more difficult words, his speech stumbling a little and rather flat—matters of which he himself was well aware. However, that was never seen later. Moreover, the feeling of illness was not constant, but so irregular that, soon after, he declared that he *was* [Ed] the Kaiser; demanded to be addressed as 'Wilhelm' [Ed]; and even in the admission room itself wrote a note with the words: 'To arrest. Wilhelm.' During the course of the day he repeatedly asked to be released, because he was not sick and not until evening did he definitely let his grandiose ideas drop. Despite 3 g. potassium bromide he spent the night in sleeplessness. The following day he had full insight, and only occasionally complained that such foolish thoughts were troubling him. The nights became better and the palpitations subsided. On the evening of the fifth day he was temporarily restless again, demanding his discharge in order to go to Berlin; but soon after, he confided again his great distress that the unhealthy ideas had returned. At the same time there was an increase in cyanosis, with pulse increasing up to 130, with return of palpitations. Over the following days there was improvement and the pulse dropped back to 88.

However, with the least effort, palpitations and cyanosis returned. Treatment with digitalis, prolonged bed rest, and regulation of sleep by paraldehyde and trional had such a favourable effect and the patient's condition improved to such an extent that thought was given to his being discharged. His body weight had increased by about 6 kg. Six weeks after admission, one evening, there was a sudden relapse, initiated by an anxious, bewildered facial expression and a plaintive cry: 'The ideas have come back'; and after a few minutes, again he had the intention of going to Berlin to see the Kaiser, along with vehement demands for him to be discharged. He was hurried and anxious in his nature; in visible discomfort; occasional gesticulating towards his heart; complaining of palpitations; his pulse up to 128; a congested face; and general cyanosis. The disturbances of his general condition subsided again after a few days, but the grandiose ideas remained, and seemed to gradually assert themselves more strongly. At the time he felt he could rejoice over the abundance of his ideas; at times he could not sleep; he showed, what he called a 'freshness of his mind'; and he boasted about his possession of total self-control. In the week of the relapse he lost about 1½ kg in weight, but since then, gradually made up this loss, and has now increased it by a further kilogram (The patient recovered 8 weeks later and was discharged with normal heart limits.).

Gentlemen! Those of you who heard me earlier will remember a very similar case of illness that I presented 1½ years ago. At that time it involved a young 22-year-old mechanic named Sch., who was discharged as recovered after a 4-month stay with us. He also came to the clinic as a voluntary patient, because he thought he was mentally ill. In his opinion he had been ill for about 10 weeks, and this matched details from his acquaintances. At the time of admission his complaints were: a headache; a feeling in his head as though he were drunk; palpitations which occurred during attacks; also dizziness in his head and inability to think, 'he feels so jaded.' Objectively: He had a congested face, reddened conjunctiva, and a slight cyanosis, the latter exacerbated by walking around his room. Pulse not accelerated, cardiac findings normal. He was evidently in remission from his illness and presented with no psychotic symptoms, apart from increased need for sleep; but he described with great precision the phenomena of the illness from which he was recovering, and that was the reason I presented him here. However, 14 days later a state of excitement ensued, which, as the patient later stated when his judgment had returned to normal, was a repetition of his earlier state, but at a much lower intensity. This brought about a few sleepless nights, and the state completely subsided in about 8 days. This second burst was also connected with striking vasomotor disturbances, congested face, cyanosis of the extremities, increased perspiration, and increased heart rate. From then on, full insight into the illness quickly returned, so that he could be discharged as recovered after 3 months; and, up to now, 1¼ years after discharge, he has remained in good health and is again active in his previous occupation. We learned from him that his first attack, of 10 weeks duration, began with poor sleep and irritable mood. Then a feeling of anxiety appeared in the cardiac region, lasted for 2 days, and put him in state of fearful agitation, 'as if he should go into the Oder.' After about 4 days, this feeling gave place to another mood, 'the opposite of the previous one,' such a happy feeling 'as if the Holy Spirit were within him.' This was located at the self-same spot as the feeling of anxiety that preceded it. The patient found it difficult to give a more detailed description of this feeling: Sometimes he described it as 'ramparts in his chest' [Ed] and sometimes as unusually light, free breathing. At the same time 'strange thoughts' [W] came to him and he realized that he had become another person, as he suspected, enlightened by the Holy Spirit. He noticed that he had acquired special abilities, believed that he had invented a machine for perpetual motion; believed that he had the ability to immediately distinguish 'noble and ignoble people' [W]; believed that he was able to influence people in the manner of a hypnotist, so that they would do what he wanted; and made a plan to transform his employer's business into a corporation. At the same time he appreciated that he was not doing well at his work, and that his thoughts were not well focused on the matter; and that those around were making fun of him, declared his plans to be nonsense, or told him they did not understand him. For 3 weeks, these were the only strange thoughts of which he was aware, and then he heard them taken over, and pronounced by a fine female voice; and then the 'rampart' [Ed] existed again in his chest. Consciousness of his being inspired by the Holy Spirit now overcame him more clearly. The voice also let him know of the attitude people took towards his plans, whether, for example, they wanted to join the corporation or not. At night, the voice spoke to him, and often continuously disturbed him in his sleep. Once he heard three voices, coming out of his chest, and simultaneously saying good night: two strong voices and one finer voice. After that, he had become tired and went to sleep. An unusual abundance of words came over him; the words presented themselves 'involuntarily' [W], and it seemed to him as though the Holy Spirit were speaking 'out of' [Ed] him. He preached for hours; on one occasion, he spoke in verse, and finally, a few days before his admission he went home in order to be blessed by the priest of the place, as a court preacher. Through diligent reading of the Bible, he had come to believe that he was one of the two witnesses that appear in the Revelation of John. The patient had told us all this in the clinical presentation a few days after his admission, with full insight into the abnormality of the experiences he described. The second, short-duration attack was also preceded by fear and anxious ideas, the anxiety again being localized in his heart—and the content of the fearful ideas was that he would not come out of here, that he would die here, and his body would be handed over for anatomy, etc. He impetuously demanded his discharge, but could be appeased. Over the next few days he showed only a haughty, demanding manner; he sought to instruct the doctor, but yet remained open to encouragement. He wrote a guide for the physician to examine mentally ill people; spoke of his 'great abundance of ideas' [W], his 'death-defying courage' [W], and his ability to excel. He retained a certain degree of insight into his sickness and of the vast multitude of thoughts that came to him, even though he did not regard their content as being abnormal. Yet even in this respect insight into illness rapidly returned, and the only complaint, which was lost over the course of the next week, was that so many thoughts came to him. At times of greatest excitement the localized feeling of happiness was again present; however, the patient did not hear a voice during this second attack. Of importance is the fact that this patient grew up with orthodox religious views, as evidenced by letters from his parents, and by the fact that his calling to the priesthood had initially been recognized by them; and moreover there was violent opposition to his being admitted voluntarily into the clinic. We learned later that he had always been somewhat peculiar, and that during his illness, fantastically grandiose ideas had beset him, for instance that he had offered millions to his colleagues. Up to the time of his discharge, his bodyweight had increased from 56 to 65 kg.

Gentlemen! The two patients that you have come to know apparently have this in common: that their autochthonous ideas, about which you learned earlier, formed acutely and then became the basis of their illness. All other symptoms can be considered as consequences or companion phenomena of this single main symptom. This includes phonemes, whose internal connection with the autochthonous ideas stand out particularly clearly in these cases; and likewise the explanatory delusions, which depend on the content. Ideas of happiness observed in the first patient, stand in strange contrast with the Affect of anxiety, which, albeit mild, was dominant at the same time. The 'hypochondriacal feeling of happiness' [Ed], which is peculiar to the second case, has been mentioned already (p. 107); it is a quite rare phenomenon. We shall characterize the illness as an independent form of autopsychosis, recognized by acute onset of autochthonous ideas with prominent participation of the vasomotor nervous system, through a course in short bursts that follow one another in rapid succession, and then through to the surprisingly favourable outcome within several months. The spotlight therefore falls on the independent significance of the autochthonous ideas. Provisionally, I would like to propose the name of *acute expansive autopsychosis mediated by autochthonous ideas* [W].

In addition to these two cases, whose diagnoses are sufficiently secure, I know of another one that I would like to refer to as 'abortive' [Ed], and not really belonging amongst the psychoses, because the elementary symptom of an autochthonous idea remained isolated, without leading even to any relatively fixed delusional explanatory ideas. I have seen casual mention of this case once before (p. 69, note). This was a 52-year-old lady, the wife of a high-ranking military officer, who had suffered from diarrhoea for years, and was quite 'run down' [Ed], forever telling of all manner of hypochondriacal complaints, particularly during the last few months. Quite suddenly, she showed a striking urge to communicate, as a result of thoughts that were 'talking' [Ed] within her, but which were expressly not described as voices. 'These can only be my own thoughts or inspirations.' At times she showed a feeling of anxiety, which, severely disturbed her sleep because of her thoughts. Attempts to provide an explanatory delusion were linked to a personage who the patient had met shortly before, a dealer in magnetic cures; their content being the possibility of her being affected by this person. By improving her diet, bed rest, care with sleeping, complete restitution within 8 weeks.

While autochthonous ideas all too often constitute a separate clinical picture as just described, this is not the case with the opposite elementary symptom. (I touch here, on a point that could already have been mentioned in the context of paranoid states, since only the combined explanatory delusion is obvious.) Just as *emergence* [Ed] of thoughts by local abnormal irritation is usually attributed to an external influence, so can momentary *disappearance* [Ed] of thoughts occur as a symptom of illness, to be interpreted in a similar way by a sick person. The complaint by certain patients, often heard in mental institutions, that thoughts were 'drawn out of' [W] them, usually seems to refer to this symptom. A further explanatory delusion is often linked with this, that medical measures are to blame, and that the thoughts in question are known to the physician. I have quite recently received secure information, which excludes any doubt as to the meaning of the symptom.

Gentlemen! We have concerned ourselves earlier with overvalued ideas, but if we consider just the time course to be the decisive factor, we often have to attribute new stages of these to acute autopsychoses, occurring during a chronic course of illness.

Here it might also be the place to discuss briefly the not infrequent cases of *psychoses by obsessions* [W]. In no other area is it more difficult to separate psychosis from neurosis: Thus, to identify both the degenerative aetiology as well as elementary symptoms as lying within the normal mental range, it might be fitting to speak solely of *obsessional neurosis* [1]. [W] This term might be the more suitable, since the analogous name of 'anxiety neurosis' [Ed] has already long become familiar. In general we can propose that obsessions fall within the neuroses, as long as they remain isolated, and are not followed or accompanied by other psychotic symptoms. (For these cases Westphal has proposed the name 'abortive insanity' [W] for these cases. However, it is inadvisable in any direction.). However, an exception to this criterion should be expressly stated, namely for mild anxiety, which often accompanies obsessions which are otherwise isolated. A criterion that is reliable in most cases might be found in the oft-stated question of how far a patient's irresistible obsessions might affect their treatment: The content and richness of the obsessions undoubtedly have an influence, in that in individual cases, the limits of neurosis are exceeded. This seems to be a very rare instance, where, with great richness and abundant change of obsessions, it is not so much the content of thoughts, but the compulsion to be continually thinking, which is perceived to be so distressing. In general, this falls amongst the type of brooding-addiction described by O. Berger [2]. If you remember the schema presented in the introduction to these lectures, you will tend to class such brooding addictions amongst ideas registered as a result of abnormal stimulation. That compulsion is transferred by the patient to vivid registration, which then impels achievement of goals. The *maladie du doute avec délire de toucher* [W] described by the French [3] is likely to be only a special case of the brooding-addiction. However,

I do not doubt that in some cases, the state of general brooding addiction can be so agonizing that it leads to psychotic acts, including suicide. Those cases of limited but repetitious, and thus markedly Affect-laden content often reach psychotic proportions. Sometimes the content is motor in nature, where patients complain of their being compelled to carry out certain actions that they know to be unreasonable or unjust. An accompaniment of anxious feelings tends only to soften the action carried out. Cases of arson by young epileptics, and the irresistible desire to steal—the so-called kleptomania—at the time of menstruation are best known here.

In our clinic we most commonly observe obsessions whose content is limited to religion, leading to delusions of belittlement. I want to outline briefly a typical example of this. A 43-year-old single woman, well endowed, without hereditary affliction but always very religious, was admitted as a voluntary patient on 31 August 1891, because she was afraid of committing suicide. She had already been treated for 3 months in 1881 for 'religious mania' [Ed], had made a suicide attempt at the time, and had been discharged completely recovered. She dated her current illness from the spring, but it had been especially bad over the last 14 days, along with insomnia and periods of despair. She knows that she is mentally ill and had appealed to a clergyman for comfort, who has however encouraged her in her delusions. When she prays, the worst blasphemies come into her head; that she must curse the risen God, Jesus Christ, and the Virgin Mary, belabour them with the worst epithets, and utter indecent phrases against them. She cannot help these thoughts: They come against her will, but they are her own thoughts. How bad must she be that she, hitherto always pious, should have such thoughts! The clergyman also said that to her. Thus, she knew that she was mentally ill; and she had also previously turned to the panel doctor, who had sent her here. Her explanatory delusion, that she was wholly and eternally lost, was maintained at first, despite partial insight into her illness. Linked to this was the idea that she had brought the illness on herself; that she had lived too much on her own; that she should have arranged her whole life differently; and that she could no longer live. It was only fear of shame that had held her back from 'going into the water' [Ed]. Her obsessions came in bouts, connected with a lively fear 'inside' [W], in the heart. After each bout, she felt generally weak, particularly with trembling in her legs, feet, and hands. It was as if her eyes were dim; she feels unable to read or to perform any work. Depressed mood continually; also a sense of subjective inefficiency. Admission into the institution resulted immediately in significant improvement; the attacks became less frequent and less severe; insight into the illness gradually prevailed; and there was complete healing, with steady weight gain (4 kg) up to the time of her discharge on 15 November of this year. A hint of autopsychic delusions of reference should also be mentioned, in which, during the initial stage of her stay, a triple murder was reported in the newspaper, for which she felt a sense of self-blame. Furthermore, she had frequent complaints about her head, about tinnitus, and a feeling that her head would spring off, etc. Objectively, she experienced no disturbance of intelligence, memory, or attentiveness, etc. The same patient was again admitted with a relapse of a much lesser severity, although similar in content, in 1898, and, after a short period, she was again discharged. I have seen a similar favourable course in a 20-year-old hereditarily afflicted journeyman. In him too the feeling of unhappiness, the suicidal tendency, and the inability to work, were so pronounced, in spite of insight into his illness, that the only place of refuge for him was the mental asylum. Moreover, there were a number of accompanying physical symptoms, such as palpitations, headaches, and hypochondriacal sensations. Outbreak rather sudden, after a shock. Content: blasphemies when praying; recovered within 9 months. Years ago, during the evening meal, similar obsessions had surfaced quite temporarily [4].

Gentlemen! The strange phenomena that, in themselves, are personal thoughts totally free from Affect, are transformed into phonemes through which explanatory delusions arise. The thoughts then become known to others, and can similarly be seen as the main component of a particular, worsening form of acute autopsychosis. As you will recall, we reserved the term *thought echo* [W] used by Cramer [5] (notes to pages 69 and 88) expressly for cases of this sort. Patients first notice that what they read and write, and later also what they speak, is repeated as voices. Soon, every intention to do anything is heard as a voice. The resulting disturbance in thought, when established, is experienced as painful, and attention is forcibly drawn towards it. The anxiety that accompanies it is localized to the head, and is stated explicitly to be its consequence. Hypochondriacal sensations of a minor nature, such as general lassitude, headache, dyspnoea, paraesthesia of the limbs, in the mouth, and in the abdomen etc., are initially disregarded in the delusion, but nevertheless create the external impression of a depressed, melancholic state. I recall two cases of this kind, involving a 22-year-old maid and a 30-year-old woman telegraphist, with acute onset; and, within a year, rapid development to the point of persecutory and consequent grandiose delusions, and pervading falsification of content. In one case the thought echo occurred only during seizures, initially only for hours, but then lasting for days. With gradual habituation to the echo, the depressive impact faded and attentiveness became freer. Only in the depressive phase of the illness was the elementary symptom present in isolation, but later the voices occurred independently. Not only that, but the voices also commented on what the patient was thinking, and initially did so in a hostile manner, so that the voices were ascribed to certain persecutors; yet later they commented in a joyful way, so that, for example, voices are interpreted as a royal court. In addition, everything that people in the neighbourhood say or do is assessed as if those people know the patient's thoughts; and so it reaches the point, symptomatically, of generalized autopsychic delusions of reference, with corresponding reinterpretation of the outside world. Allopsychic orientation will then also be impaired.

'Thought echo' [Ed] is the fact that the voices are explicitly described as loudly resonant personal thoughts, this being adequately distinguished from autochthonous ideas. However, we need to add an internal relationship between these two elementary symptoms, which will seem much more plausible to you, if you remember my remarks on the importance of the left temporal lobe in my twentieth lecture (p. 129). In this sense we should regard thought echo as a special form of functional disturbance of the left temporal lobe. Moreover, the relationship with obsessions is itself made clinically valid, in that, in the one case, at the time when the voices had already become independent, for a brief period there was also a compulsion to repeat the voice content, and, if the voices are questioning, to give an answer.

It seems almost as if thought echo, in the narrow sense that we can understand, could lay claim to a particularly serious and fatal import. In addition, more complicated cases of illness in which it has occurred are striking in their severity and rapidly progressing course.

Gentlemen! In the above, I have paid considerable attention to cases of special theoretical or practical significance. However, with this, we are far from having exhausted the topic of acute autopsychoses. Rather, it seems to be a particularly rich field, and some differentiation is needed if we are to include a great number of cases of illness. Thus you recently became familiar with a case of acute traumatic autopsychosis [6], which besides showing severe autopsychic disarray and disorientation, also presented an autopsychic deficit of retroactive amnesia extending back to childhood. In terms of disarray and disorientation this case was quite reminiscent of Miss v. F. described in the last lecture. Furthermore, we have seen [7] that, in a chronic residual case, a delusional system existed that could be attributed almost exclusively to the elementary symptom of a generalized autopsychic delusion of reference. All events in the environment seemed to the patient to be related to her thoughts, or to depend on them. Moreover, she assumed that her thoughts were known to everybody else, although she never experienced thought echo. Rather, these were autochthonous ideas which could be identified here as the source of her generalized autopsychic delusion of reference.

We will learn about still other cases of acute autopsychoses in the next few lectures.

References

1. Westphal CFO. Über Zwangsvorstellungen. Arch Psychiatr Nervenkr. 1878;8:734–50.
2. Berger O. Die Grübelsucht, ein pathologisches symptom. Arch Psychiatr Nervenkr. 1876;6:217–48.
3. Le Grand du Saulle H. La folie du doute (avec délire de toucher). Paris: V. Adrien Delahaye; 1875.
4. Wernicke C. Krankenvorstellungen aus der psychiatrischen Klinik in Breslau. Breslau: Schletter; 1899. vol. 2 Case 27 is a case of autopsychosis due to obsessions.
5. Cramer A. Die Hallucinationen im Muskelsinn bei Geisteskranken und ihre klinische Bedeutung, ein Beitrag zur Kenntniss der Paranoia. Freiburg im Breisgau: P. Siebeck; 1889.
6. Wernicke C. Krankenvorstellungen vol. 1, Case 22.
7. Wernicke C. Krankenvorstellungen vol. 1, Case 13.

Lecture 30

30

- Presentation of two opposite types of illness
- Digression on volition
- Clinical picture of Affective melancholia
- Risk of suicide due to this
- Fantastic delusions of belittlement
- Phonemes and visions
- Course, frequency of the illness
- Diagnosis
- Treatment
- Prognosis

Lecture

Gentlemen!

In the 43-year-old patient, Mrs H. [1], who I present to you today, you will notice, from her posture and facial expression, the deeply depressed mood. When she notices me speaking of her bad mood, she bursts into tears. When I ask the reason, she replies that she feels unhappy.

'Why unhappy?'

'You cannot do anything more; you are physically tired and always prefer just to sleep.'

'What about thinking?'

Thinking strains her.

How about memory?

This too has become worse. To test her memory retention, she is given the unfamiliar word 'Antananarivo' [Ed] to remember. It turns out that comprehension of a foreign word is more difficult for her and slower than normal, whilst her answers are otherwise prompt. What job did she do? She helped with housework in her parents' inn; something that was hitherto not difficult for her. Once she became ill, she could do this no longer, could not settle down to anything. Even getting up in the morning was an effort for her. Everything that she had to do seemed terribly difficult; and she was terrified of the coming days. Thoughts of the future frightened her, and brought her to thoughts of suicide.

By what method?

She wanted to go into the nearby pond, but was thwarted, because she was not allowed to be left alone.

Was she afraid of anything else?

No, just the thought of the future.

Where was anxiety located?

In her breast and head.

Returning to the question of which word she had been given to remember, it turns out that she had forgotten it after a few minutes, and knows only that it began with 'A' [Ed]. However, she recognized it again amongst a number of words spoken to her. Does she have any other reason to take her own life, such as a physical ailment?

No, she was in good standing with her loved ones, but everything was indifferent to her, even as far as her parents and siblings. Whether her siblings came to visit her in the clinic or not, even were war to be declared, or the Kaiser should die, this would not affect her. She could feel neither

R. Miller, K.J. Dennison (eds.), *An Outline of Psychiatry in Clinical Lectures*,
DOI 10.1007/978-3-319-18051-9_30

joy nor grief; her heart was turned to stone. In fact she was constantly confined to bed, taking no part in the events around her; takes no notice of visits by her relatives; and never expresses any wishes. This even includes care of her body, satisfaction of her needs, making beds, and the like. She shows no initiative at all for chores undertaken at certain times by all patients on the ward, and generally does not speak about herself except when asked—yet this, as has been noted, is always prompt, provided the question makes no hard demands. When asked whether she thinks of anything at all, she replies that she goes over and over an agonizing thought, namely that, after the death of her husband (a year before), she has felt so alone and abandoned.

She is fully orientated as to her situation, feels sick, and has total confidence in what the doctors have arranged; and she came to the clinic voluntarily, to protect herself from suicide. Her spirits are brightened by encouragement, but she can never overcome her doubts of ever being healthy again. She is physically healthy and reasonably well fed. However, her appetite is very poor; she eats enough only at the behest of others. Despite her need for sleep, it occurs only with the aid of sleeping pills. Fifteen years ago she suffered an attack of melancholia, from which she recovered. For many years she was then one of the best female warders at hospital X. She was married for 6 years and, since the death of her husband, just a year ago, she has several times suffered bouts of an illness similar to that she presents with today; their duration is usually about 4 weeks, with intervals of similar length in between. She describes healthy times as feeling totally comfortable, sleeping well, eating well, and enjoying hard work. The abnormal state always comes on fairly quickly, within 1 or 2 days, its arrival being preceded by cessation of her usual copious armpit perspiration. Such dryness in her armpits remains throughout the period of illness. Perimetric examination produced results of great interest for the concept of this illness state. This revealed concentric narrowing of the visual fields in both eyes, which, in the horizontal meridian, went laterally up to 50°, and medially up to 40°, and, in fatigue tests could be increased by a further 8–10°. (The visual field examination in the healthy state shows itself normal.)

Presentation of our second patient, the 24-year-old shop assistant Bertha Pr. [2], as expected, takes the form of a dialogue.

The patient enters the auditorium convulsed with laughter, and greets those present in a loud, somewhat imperious voice (imitating a lieutenant).

'Good morning, gentlemen, good morning Storch, good morning Liepmann, how's the little woman doing? Ah, good morning Professor, I am very pleased to see you. How are you? Better every day? Right? I'm always a bit funny, but that doesn't hurt, right? Why shouldn't I be funny?'

Me: 'Now, just quieten down a bit; and sit down; I want to say something to the gentlemen and then you can talk again.'

The patient sits down quite unabashed, legs outstretched, supporting her face in her hands, turned towards the audience.

'Of course, I will be very quiet. Only you will speak. I won't say a word. Ah, what is that?' (upon seeing the water pipe with a basin). 'You have a nice closet,' goes closer, 'Ah, a basin, a fine basin, and soap, and such a clean towel.'

'I think you want to be quiet?'

'Yes, I am too, but ugh, this is dirty' (runs her finger over the basin, shakes it in disgust and then sticks her finger in her mouth).

'Now, just sit down again. Are you Bertha Przytek?'

'Yes, but we have known each other for such a long time, Professor. Oh, what a fine frock coat you have; you are a very handsome man, Professor.' Grabbing me by the hand and posing herself with me after the style of song-and-dance people, in a *pas de deux* [W], she sings as off-key as possible in a loud, harsh voice:

Wir sind zwei Wunderkinder
Wie so Kinder sind,
Das sieht sogar ein Blinder,
Und wäre er ganz blind.

[We are two Wunderkinder]
[Like such children]
[That even a blind man can see]
[Even though he is totally blind.]

Then in another corresponding theatrical position:

'The wedding will be within a year.' She then says with a comical, languishing glance: 'Finally alone.'

Me: 'Now be reasonable for once, Bertha, and let me say something.'

'Indeed, I am always reasonable, that is my strong point! You too, what? Now I am perfectly quiet.'

Nevertheless, she continues to talk, taking up everything she sees and hears and using it in her stream of words. As she hears the word hypermetamorphosis, she says, for example, 'Yes, Meta, who has given me too much morphine.' Catching the word Wesen, she says: 'I have been on the Weser.'

'How old are you?'

'I am now exactly 16 years 2 min old.'

'But how can that be?'

'Believe me, I am 16 years 2 min.'

'Where are you now?'

'In the insane asylum on Göpperstraße.'

'How are you treated?'

'Oh, let bygones be bygones.'

'Good or bad?'

'Bad? There's no word for it.'

'Then you aren't pleased to be here?'

'I will go away. Why should I be here among thieves, whores, pickpockets and murderers?'

'Whores? How do you come to be among whores?'

'How did you find *me* [Ed], Professor?'

'What are the gentlemen here for, Bertha?'

'Ugh, they are old gentlemen, last time they were handsome young men.'

'You once said that you were a daughter of the Empress. How is that?'

'Oh, nonsense. I have never been an Empress, I am a Bofel.'

'Adieu, Bertha, you may go now.'

Nodding familiarly to everyone, she departs, laughing loudly, as she came. 'Adieu, Liepmann, remember me to the little woman. Adieu, gentlemen.'

Gentlemen! The main point in presenting these two patients is their entirely opposite mental state, and their equally contrasting conduct. I shall soon point out that I consider them to be relatively pure examples of those alterations derived from our scheme which I have designated as 'intrapsychic loss of function' [Ed] (or 'hypofunction') [Ed], and 'intrapsychic hyperfunction' [Ed], that is, expressing abnormally reduced and, by contrast, abnormally increased activity of intrapsychic pathways. However, our experience so far is that disturbances of conscious activity, derived from our scheme *sAZm*, always lead to changes in content of consciousness, mainly in one of the three areas of consciousness we have differentiated; and this is also confirmed here. We will find that autopsychic orientation is disturbed in both cases, and accordingly intrapsychic loss of function is shifted towards belittlement, and in hyperfunction towards grandiosity. Functions of consciousness also include that act, which constitutes self-awareness of the mental condition, which, momentarily, we are in. This fact led Griesinger [3] to speak of a 'psychic tonus' [W], and to clarify the abnormally exalted mood from a release of—and the depressed mood from an inhibition of—movements occurring in the 'psychic reflex arc' [W]. However, changed mental states, as the fundamental deviation of intrapsychic function, are, to an equal extent, essential qualities of personality or individuality. Therefore it is hardly surprising that an active consciousness notices such changes in personality and reacts to it. This results in an autopsychic disturbance of identification in the sense of my introductory comments in Lecture 28 (p. 185). In transferring such a disorder of identification, assumed to occur in psychosensory areas, to consciousness of personality, it should be seen as a 'paraesthesia' [Ed], according to our schema. Since we learn from experience that there are numerous relatively pure cases in which the totality of symptoms are to be derived from hypothetical states, such as we assume, for intrapsychic loss of function and hyperfunction, we therefore have a way to define two sharply differentiated forms of autopsychosis, which we can call 'melancholia' [Ed] and 'mania' [Ed].

Let us first consider *melancholia* [W], for which Mrs H. gives us a good example.

We cannot avoid here some brief detail about what we understand by *will* [W] from our standpoint. For anyone to 'will' [Ed] a certain action presumes making a decision, unquestionably an action of pure thought (even if not totally pure: the reduction in memory retentiveness and the concentric narrowing of the visual field are admixtures, which are not present in the majority of cases and possibly belong to a particular, very rare, recurrent form.). In content, this implies that two or more, possibilities have been weighed against each other. It is only natural that in normal situations, *one* [W] possibility easily wins a victory, having gained its advantage through habit and usage. Making a decision is then a normal process, through evaluation of ideas and trains of thought. Let us take a simple example. I wake up in the morning and have to get up and dress, which requires a decision. The two possibilities are to get up and to stay in bed; nothing is more natural than to get up promptly if one has done this all one's life. But then—getting up may depend on other factors. For instance the time: a glance at the clock makes you decide to stay in bed; or, I have spent a restless night, or believe I have a fever and feel sick, and so decide to stay in bed. Clearly the decision is only correct and rational when a large number of cooperating ideas have their normal value; and it becomes abnormal when the value of these ideas changes as a result of a mental illness. Thus a hypochondriacal patient does not get up, perhaps because of the abnormal physical sensations arising from the mental illness make him feel physically ill and too weak to rise.

If, as in this example, only two possibilities are to be weighed up, either to do or not do something, it would be thought that only the first case concludes an action, and that therefore the conditions for *its* [Ed] occurrence are always harder than for the second case. That would in itself probably be correct, as we shall see soon. However, for this partially 'prepared' [Ed] state of consciousness in an awake person, the 'value' [Ed] a certain idea has attained by usage, training and habit becomes decisive; and in comparison to this, it is fairly irrelevant whether 'to do' [Ed] or 'not to do' [Ed], forms the essence of the idea. If we assume that, over a long period, ideas have come to possess a certain 'value' [Ed], which is then lost or greatly reduced, a more severe dementia occurs, for example in a paralytic patient. Then this habitual relation will be validated; and for the simplest of all reasons, he decides to stay in bed. However, under certain circumstances, *inaction* [Ed], the refraining from action, requires a greater effort of will. Think, for example, of a conscientious mother, accustomed to getting up at a certain time to care for her child: In the case of severe physical illness, she will need all her self-control to obey the physician, and refrain from her accustomed activity.

We can now define as 'will' [Ed] that more or less complex idea which has proceeded from a resolution; and in turn 'resolution' [Ed] can be defined as the 'weighing-up' [Ed] ('contest' [Ed] would be more accurate) of two or more ideas, or series of ideas, of which at least one fulfills the condition that it has a motor content, and can therefore at the same time form the point for initiating motor processes. 'Freedom of will' [Ed] presupposes freedom of determination, in other words, the normal value of all ideas which have cooperated in reaching the resolution. We do no violence to language if the act of determination is included in 'will' [Ed], which term may then be defined thus: Will is the result of the competition of different groups of ideas, of which at least one is the idea of a motor goal, and has access to the point for initiating activity in the centrifugal projection system. From such a conceptualization, we can understand that the 'will' [Ed] represents, to some extent, an index of the intrapsychic function connected to the *AZ* path of our scheme.

Our consciousness must have a rough knowledge of the resistances in this centrifugal tract *Zm*, and of the necessary expenditure of energy to overcome these resistances, since we learn by experience that it is harder to resolve to do something, the more difficult is the task. Things that are new, unknown, and hitherto untried, always seem the hardest, even when the difficulty is only an apparent one, based on our misjudgement of our own ability. Thus, for an inexperienced person, a strong 'will' [Ed], or an unaccustomed 'effort of will' [Ed] as people say, is necessary to jump on to a snow-bridge in crossing a crevasse, even when the leap is quite easy, and presents no real danger. If this example seems too complicated, it is much the same when one pronounces a difficult word in a foreign language: A timid scholar gives up pronouncing the word right away, and makes no attempt.

Many actions have mutual dependence on one another, in such a cogent manner that one of them, once begun, forms the initial link in a whole chain of subsequent actions. Likewise, our consciousness is aware that much greater effort is required under these circumstances, and therefore requires especially strong motivation to reach a resolution in our will for such an undertaking. These undertakings, in contrast to the simple actions just described, are rare ones which require a person to climb a mountain, learn a foreign language, or take an examination.

These few considerations suffice to help us understand symptoms which are based on reduction of 'will power' [Ed] by loss of function [Ed] at intrapsychic levels. The onset of *Affective melancholia* [W] is often manifested by inability to carry out some very easy tasks. The tradesman for whom a new project is required every day, fails in his tasks; the student refuses to enter an examination, although earlier he had been quite sure of his success; and for another, it becomes quite impossible to make a decision on some matter, etc. Here we can see the mildest form of intrapsychic akinesia. (Many suicides among young men can be traced back to their inability to decide to sit an examination).

At first, individual actions which run along the familiar tracks of daily life can continue with few problems; yet gradually the difficulty of thought processes increases, and then even a simple action appears to be a major undertaking. The patient himself notices that, for him, any resolution to act creates major difficulties. The difficulty increases with the complexity of the task: Initially it is manifest on every occasion which falls outside the scope of routine activities of life, such as when a judicial matter has to be attended to, a journey has to be made, or a person has to act in support, or in the interests of other people. Chiefly these are all the more important decisions.

Consequently it is hard for a patient to make decisions about necessary actions of everyday life, and eventually, about any action at all. In this phase of illness we often hear the complaint that a patient cannot get up and leave his beds without overcoming his very self.

The effect of this condition is manifested in different ways according to the personality of the individual afflicted. In personalities who are more highly esteemed socially, who consider that carrying out necessary actions of daily life to be a duty, the feeling of failure, exacerbated carrying out those duties, leads to the idea of 'neglect of duty' [Ed], wickedness, or accordingly, iniquity; that is, it becomes the source of delusions of guilt, or of belittlement. At the very least, developing from this is a *fear of the future* [W], which always seems to impose new tasks on performance of duty; and this fear of the future is often synonymous with a dread of living longer. Any incidental factor which complicates such tasks, even if it falls within the range of habitual duties, readily leads to a feeling of catastrophe in conscientious persons. In this regard, 1 can never forget the case of a colleague at Charité who, on return from leave of absence after an attack of Affective melancholia, was given charge of the ward for syphilitic women, and who could not get over the painful impressions of this service. He shot himself on the day he was to begin the service, and left a note bearing the significant words: 'I am absolutely unable to live any longer.' Prior to this he had left no stone unturned, to get transferred to another ward. There are numerous suicides which, in origin, take this form, and in most cases the motives come to be understood only after they have happened; for the conditions surrounding these acts are such that the individuals concerned tend not to express their feelings, and it is only later, usually when half-automatic utterances are seen in their proper light, that any conclusion can be reached about the mental state of the suicide victim.

The self-knowledge that there are obstructions to 'acts of will' [Ed], the *subjective feeling of inadequacy* [W], is perhaps the most significant and characteristic symptom of Affective melancholia. It is often described by patients in very practical terms, and forms the very core of their intense feeling of misery.

A blunting of psychic feelings goes hand in hand with the difficulty in decision-making. When I speak of 'psychic feelings' [Ed] I refer to another sort of feeling about which you already know: the 'organ feelings' [Ed], which I have contrasted with the 'quality of sensations' [Ed], endowing the latter with the so-called 'tone of feeling' [Ed]. These psychic feelings have nothing in common with such sensations; rather, they show themselves to depend on prolific intrapsychic activity, encompassing a plethora of associative connections. We understand by them some of the following ideas: love, hate, like, dislike, friendship, sorrow, worry, etc., all of which are verbal expressions for certain internal experiences which, with some justification, are assumed to be the same in all persons. While the psychic feelings mentioned usually refer to relations with *persons* [Ed],we understand by the term 'interest' [Ed] a similar Affective state in relation to *things* [Ed] and *conditions* [Ed], and so we can speak of an interest in art, science, in politics, in following some occupation, especially business, etc. As is seen, 'interest' [Ed] really belongs amongst the psychic feelings, and it is only in practice that it is split off from them, as an oversight. Both are states of the individual, derived exclusively from intrapsychic activity. When they are compromised and distorted, the patient notices a blunting and a cooling of his feelings, for instance in his closeness to his nearest relatives, with lessening of interest, for example in business, public affairs, and his usual diversions. The consequence of self-knowledge of this is a state of abnormal indifference and inner emptiness, whose prototype is the blasé attitude, the renowned 'spleen' [W] of the English. For more refined individuals who are not satisfied by gross sensual pleasures, the charm of life then ceases, and thoughts of suicide, at first indefinite, gradually take on a more tangible form. This thought becomes a real danger when the patients have resolved upon a way to carry it out.

The other consequence is delusions of belittlement, or 'self-accusatory delirium' [Ed]. As a consequence of the error, promulgated by the scholastics, that a person can control his thoughts and feelings, whereas actually the thoughts control the person, there arises the idea of neglect of duty, wickedness, and unworthiness, which itself can become the starting point for the idea of suicide: 'I no longer deserve to live, I no longer deserve the love of relatives' [Ed], etc., are expressions often heard from these patients. All in all, the mental state of these patients may be described most accurately as a feeling of misery. However, this feeling of misery, as just analysed, has a very different origin from that mentioned earlier, which has its source in hypochondria. It is based on awareness of an aberrant change in personality, and may thus be regarded as a special type of autopsychic disarray.

Gentlemen! As you see, these are essentially *subjective* [Ed] troubles which define Affective melancholia. *Objective* [Ed] symptoms are first noticeable when the illness reaches a certain level of intensity, but may easily be overlooked or misinterpreted. These are the signs of intrapsychic akinesia, which are thus essentially negative symptoms: Patients gradually cease to talk about themselves, or to do anything. That was also seen in our patient, Mrs. H. However, a noticeable retardation and severe limitation in her reaction to external promptings exceeds the narrower perspective on our illness. The reason lies in the following condition: The absence of reactions—reactive akinesia—always corresponds to a relatively severe attenuation of intrapsychic function, which will likewise inhibit occurrence of the fundamental symptom of subjective insufficiency. We have seen such severe loss of intrapsychic function and akinesia—characterized mainly by objective symptoms of deficit—often enough, that it can be separated totally from Affective melancholia—a condition which we shall call *depressive melancholia* [W]. We will have much more to say on this later. Here I merely raise the question whether depressive melancholia can be regarded as a special mental illness. For Affective melancholia, in our limited perspective, no such doubts exist.

For completion of our clinical picture, a few more symptoms are still to be mentioned. These are so frequent that we must conclude that there is some internal connection between the symptoms. Most of these patients complain of anxiety; and this has the hallmark of a physical anxiety, localized by far most frequently in the thoracic region, followed by the head. 'Sad thoughts' [W], a frequent expression of suicidal ideas, are manifest especially as seizures or as an increase in anxiety. Such anxiety can only be seen as a direct consequence of inhibition of intrapsychic function. It is the same with a further symptom, the monotonous persistence of certain nagging, obtruding ideas which the patient cannot dispel. In content, these ideas are of two kinds, referring either to experiences in the past going along with the notions of the self-accusations, or of a hypochondriacal nature: Slight muscular pains lead to ideas of being permanently paralyzed; a globus sensation in the neck is interpreted as a cancerous growth; *Molimina uterina* [W] or *Molimina alvi* [W] as degrading sexual diseases. Patients' feelings of misery and hopelessness are thus increased. Emergence of such 'overvalued' [W] ideas seems to be a plausible secondary effect of the same process, by which the illness is aggravated, and associative activity is reduced. Finally, certain general symptoms need to be sought. Many patients have a coated tongue, or more obvious symptoms of gastritis, and all have poor appetites, which may reach the level of a pronounced aversion to eating. The majority have cold—often even cyanotic—extremities.

Affective melancholia usually develops quite slowly, over the course of weeks or months, from almost imperceptible beginnings. It therefore first becomes evident to patients themselves and to their relatives when the above symptoms have already become clear, and the diagnosis is then made easily, on the basis of suitable leading questions. The clinical picture may itself be coloured in individual ways, depending on whether self-accusation, feelings of misery, or the blasé attitude are more prominent. Self-accusation is occasionally limited to the idea of being to blame for the illness, by having incorrectly understood or neglected some activities. Otherwise, its content varies according to the patient's personality. The delusion of being to blame for the death of some deceased relative is particularly common, in that they could have been saved had different approaches to care, or other measures been taken; and each person's occupation provides the content for more-or-less fanciful self-accusations: a merchant says he is a swindler; an officer, that he is dishonourable, and so on. Secret sins of youth and sexual excesses are very common self-accusations.

Affective melancholia can develop progressively so that the intensity of symptoms depicted reaches particularly severe levels. In this situation a patient's complaints, which heretofore have not exceeded the bounds of possibility, take on a fanciful, and manifestly unlikely direction, resulting in *fanciful delusions of belittlement* [W]. The patient accuses himself of being to blame for the fact that there are so many sick people, that people must starve, that the world is coming to an end. The fanciful element appears also in assertions which reveal, in content, a failure of processes of association, for example, 'I am no longer a person,' 'I can never die,' 'Evening will never come again,' and finally 'Nothing exists anymore.' Such assertions can only be interpreted as the patient's becoming consciously aware of the failure of association pathways to render possible an image of the world, of their own personhood, and of their body.

From the same belittling delusional idea, namely of unworthiness to live—and especially to eat—a persistent refusal of food may arise, with violent resistance to all attempts to feed.

Ideas of belittlement may also take on the guise of voices. Patients hear themselves being charged with most hideous misdeeds; they hear words like: 'murderer, adultress, whore' and, as expressions of hopelessness, words like: 'eternally damned' or 'eternally lost.' However, such phonemes are always isolated and sporadic, remaining confined in their content to ideas of autopsychic anxiety, even when anxiety is severe.

Visual hallucinations of more-or-less confused form occur in milder forms of melancholia. These generally appear under favourable conditions—at twilight or at night—and relate to the sad thought content which preoccupies the patient. Patients see coffins, corpses, or an entire funeral, people in mourning, or deceased relatives. They usually expressly state that these are 'images' [Ed] or 'shadows' [Ed].

More severe forms of such illness may arise from milder ones, as a worsening; but they may also develop independently, and then usually much more acutely than the mild forms.

The *course* [W] of Affective melancholia may be represented purely in the form of an 'intensity' [Ed] curve, that is, the grouping of symptoms summarizing the clinical picture, which itself remains the same throughout the duration of the illness; and it is only their intensity which shows some variation. As already stated, the illness generally develops slowly to its full intensity over a few weeks, then remains at this level, usually only for weeks, occasionally for months, and then, just as gradually or even more slowly than it developed, moves towards convalescence, and finally, to recovery. Slight variations in intensity may be manifested at the time of the height of the illness, but, overall the course is continuous.

After the illness has ended, a phase of mild manic exaltation is seen quite regularly, lasting only a few days or weeks; and it is always ill-advised to discharge the patient before this. The curve of body weight is an exact mirror image of the illness curve, and impending return to health is revealed by the fact that no further weight increase occurs. Gaining insight into the illness, the criterion generally required for every recovery, is therefore harder to evaluate in the present illness, because, for Affective melancholia, literally by definition, insight must be present to a certain degree through the whole duration of illness; at least a certain 'feeling of being ill' [Ed] always exists, or else real insight into being ill is lost only occasionally, and then at the height of the illness, when influenced by ideas of belittlement.

Prognosis [W] of the illness is generally favourable, provided the ever-present danger of suicide can be excluded, or is known to have been averted. However, there are rare cases where Affective melancholia becomes chronic, and only some years later does a slow decline emerge in intensity of symptoms, without it ever merging into either recovery or actual dementia. In their clinical picture, such cases show some relationship to depressive melancholia, while the Affective coloration corresponds more to milder grades of Affective melancholia.

Gentlemen! The clinical picture that I have outlined for you is not identical with the melancholia of some other authors, nor with the illness designated as 'melancholia' [Ed] by Meynert [4], which he identifies with 'micromania' [Ed]. We have already seen, and will be even more convinced later, that this form of belittlement has an entirely different aetiology, and therefore must be regarded differently. I have no reason to go into greater detail about the clinical pictures set forth as 'melancholia' [Ed] by other authors, and I say no more than that they usually include far too much. Nevertheless, an old tenet deserves mention here, the more so as it appears perfectly comprehensible to us from the little clinical knowledge that we have so far acquired. At the time when a prevailing unpleasant, painful mental state, so diverse in its coloration in cases of illnesses, was called 'melancholia' [Ed]—a time which, for many authors, has not yet passed—the proposition was advanced, and always fought for since then, that all mental illnesses should begin with melancholia. An exception has been recognized only in certain cases of chronic mental illness, the so-called 'primary paranoia' [Ed]. On the other hand, if we consider that the painful mental state of disarray, in its various colorations, forms the necessary attendant symptom of most acute psychoses, we can understand the meaning of this old maxim, and find in it the expression of a clinical observation that is correct in itself, even if very vague in content.

Gentlemen! If we want to understand by Affective melancholia [Ed] simply the clinical picture that I have outlined and traced back to the hypothetical state of loss of intrapsychic function, so setting the greatest possible limitation on the number of cases, you will still discover that it is one of the most common mental illnesses. Understandably, this opinion can depend on estimates which are only approximate, and on purely personal experiences; yet I do not doubt that all experienced alienists will agree with me, once they go beyond the statistics of actual institutions, to consider the experiences in private consultations.

In fact the vast majority of such patients go to a doctor's consulting room, and only a small number reach any mental institution, which, as the sad outcome often reveals, is greatly to be regretted. This fact cannot be taken as accidental: A natural explanation can be found in the feeling of illness that has often given rise to real insight. Much as such patients are willing to concede that their mind is affected, their 'irresolution' [Ed] stands in the way of any decision, when they are advised to go to an enclosed institution. Relatives are rarely so understanding that they see how much this measure is needed, for the general view is that only the insane belong in institutions. Hence every alienist will have cases where his warnings have been all in vain, and he must limit himself to prophesying suicide. On the other hand, 1 will soon explain how, under favourable conditions, real treatment in an institution can actually be avoided.

Gentlemen! It is the facts just mentioned, namely the frequency of the illness, the danger such patients always face, and the almost guaranteed benefits of appropriate medical measures, which will keep you constantly aware of the importance of an accurate *diagnosis* [W] of this illness. In this respect there is only one serious difficulty, differentiating it from the large group of anxiety psychoses in general, and specifically from anxiety neurosis with hysterical or neurasthenic bases. The differential diagnosis between Affective melancholia and anxiety psychoses depends essentially on the following criteria: A group of ideas is common to both illnesses, if the latter occur to a marked degree: those of autopsychic anxiety and especially those of belittlement. In both conditions there are complaints of anxiety, even though in melancholia these do not have such a primary status, and lack fluctuations characteristic of most anxiety psychoses. In contrast, subjective feeling of inadequacy the fundamental symptom of our illness, is missing in the anxiety psychoses, or is revealed only as an easily recognizable variant of belittlement, and thus takes on the form of autopsychic anxiety. On the other hand, Affective melancholia totally lacks ideas of allopsychic anxiety so typical of most cases of anxiety psychosis. Thus, the two illnesses are differentiated from one another by very definite 'pluses' [Ed] or 'minuses' [Ed] of symptoms. This must be the main principal to guide us. Of no less significance practically, is the fact that most patients with anxiety psychosis experience numerous phonemes, with contents corresponding to both groups of ideas just mentioned; whereas the melancholic has no sensory deceptions of any kind, at least, when he seeks medical advice. A further reference point in diagnosis is given by the internal relationship between Affective melancholia and depressive melancholia, namely signs of retarded thought and speech, and the inactivity, occasionally seen in patients—symptoms all totally foreign to anxiety psychoses. And so in most cases it is easy to exclude anxiety psychoses, and thus to confirm the positive symptoms of Affective melancholia.

It is often much more difficult to differentiate anxiety neuroses—whether hysterical or neurasthenic—from anxiety melancholia. The difficulty is obvious, and factually substantiated, in that subjective feelings of inadequacy may be prominent in anxiety neurosis, and can actually arise from attacks of anxiety; and further, on examining a patient—a process essentially aiming to elicit their subjective symptoms—has, in neurotics, a mildly suggestive effect, which brings to light troubles which, in reality, do not exist, and which are affirmed only momentarily by the patient, under the influence of the examination; and finally, the feeling of misery, and the fact that formal thought activity is intact, and may occur in both illnesses in the same way. In such cases, the chief consideration is that Affective melancholia is a *continuous* [Ed] illness from the outset, the anxiety being only an accompanying symptom not one which determines the essence of the illness as it does in anxiety neuroses. In contrast, anxiety neuroses always occur as isolated attacks, in which anxiety is the principal symptom; belittlement and ideas of actual anxiety, even autopsychic anxiety, are usually absent, and if suicidal ideas occasionally emerge, they are driven by motives entirely different from those in melancholia. If an opportunity is presented to observe an actual attack of anxiety, dyspnoea and the symptom of phrenic nerve insufficiency [5] will usually be encountered. Finally, careful history-taking will, in most cases, disclose previous hysterical or neurasthenic problems of other kinds. There are always borderline cases in which the differential diagnosis between Affective melancholia and anxiety neuroses remains unresolved, especially when impulsive suicidal tendencies are prominent. These are usually cases with the strongest hereditary affliction and neurotic degeneration, which are otherwise inaccessible to any kind of medical treatment. I know of a case where a patient, the young wife of a lawyer, after treatment in institutions with no benefit, and then being discharged home on a trial basis, locked herself in the closet for a moment, drenched her hair and clothing in petrol, and set it alight. Her maid, who had looked after her as best she could, but at the moment of that act was preoccupied with the children, was admitted to the clinic about a year later with the overvalued idea that she must take her own life, after she had actually jumped into the river.

Gentlemen! As mentioned above, an overvalued idea is usually a component of the symptom complex of Affective melancholia. Its content is generally derived from what Meynert [4] called self-accusatory delirium; and I have already said that it may have been based on actual experiences. Therefore, under certain conditions, cases of limited autopsychosis arising from an overvalued idea may show outward similarity to Affective melancholia, in that the overvalued idea, through its content, may approximate those of Affective melancholia. I mentioned cases earlier where another person's suicide, the accidental death of relatives, or the memory of some wrong committed, has led to the development of an overvalued idea, with which, naturally, there may be combined feelings of intense misery, feelings of anxiety, and suicidal tendencies. Absence of other symptoms characteristic of Affective melancholia, and presence of a circumscribed delusion of reference in such cases, prevent an incorrect diagnosis. Similarly, autopsychoses arising, through their content, from compulsive ideas, commonly result in self-accusatory delirium and delusions of belittlement. For example, in the briefly reported case (p. 200), of compulsive ideas of blasphemous content which appeared especially while praying, feelings of misery were very prominent, interest in other people and objects blunted, and belittling delusions of depravity, and often also anxiety, were present. Nevertheless, the origin of the trouble, and especially the exact description which the patient gave of her compulsive ideas, seem to exclude any confusion with Affective melancholia.

Gentlemen! *Treatment* [W] of Affective melancholia is one of the most gratifying tasks of our calling, for this condition almost always has a good outcome, the dangers well-known, and therefore relatively easy to avoid. In many cases the regime of a well-run institution is essential, and you should keep uppermost in your mind the transfer of a patient to a suitable institution as soon as you have made the diagnosis. Only an experienced specialist should make the definite decision that institutional treatment is *un*necessary [Ed]. In the latter case, arrangements must be set in place which are otherwise provided only in an institution; and these can be readily defined. They consist of provision of total physical and mental quiet, good food, sleep and completely reliable supervision. It is easily seen that these conditions are hard to secure in a private home, while relatively easily met in any hospital. If then a patient's family—for the patient's wishes cannot be the determining factor—does not consent to institutional treatment, whatever your advice, you must at least make sure that the aforementioned requirements are complied with, and bed-rest and isolation for the patient implemented. You must be ever conscious of the great responsibility that you shoulder with such an approach.

The principle of treatment is, moreover, relatively simple and consists of sparing the patient everything requiring a decision, which arouses psychic feelings, or makes a demand on their interest. Everything must be presented to the patient as self-evident and related to the treatment, and no independent action of any kind must be expected of them. They must be washed, combed, kept clean; food and drink must be brought to them, all these measures to be continued until the patients themselves regard them as purely mechanical, habitual actions, and participate in them of their own initiative. An attendant must, of course, always be present, but speaking to patients or exciting them in any way is to be avoided. Under such treatment, feelings of misery rapidly decline in intensity; patients soon sense it to be extremely beneficial. Nevertheless, it often occurs that, quite soon, patients show signs of impatience, and long for their occupation or return to their family, whether from years of habit, or from anxiety about the relatives. This desire must not be made possible: The phase of such premature requests ceases of its own accord, and then gives place to the insight that judgment of the proper time be left to the physician. Food, must, of course, be abundant and easily digestible; as soon as possible the patient is to become accustomed to overfeeding, by frequently taking small quantities of milk between meals. Any gastric troubles and disorders of digestion naturally require careful consideration. When convalescing, complaints of boredom and the need to be occupied are best allayed by such measures that require only the patient's passive cooperation, like wet packs, friction rubs, massage, and lukewarm baths. Thereby premature activity can be prevented.

Gentlemen! 1 have repeatedly stated that *prognosis* [W] of this illness is generally extremely favourable. However, naturally, this applies only to the sharply defined clinical picture we understand by the term 'Affective melancholia' [Ed]; and I must emphasize this all the more, because in the majority of textbooks, and in those most widely used in our discipline, you will come across quite different opinions. This comes about mainly because essentially different cases, for example ones of anxiety psychoses or even ones of a more complex nature, are thrown together with the Affective melancholia as we know it. Even in the clinical lectures of Meynert, to whom we owe so much, you will find this clinical picture defined far too broadly. The teachings of Kräpelin [6], are particularly widespread; and he deals with melancholia according to his mainly aetiological principle of classification in two entirely different places: first, as a specific psychosis of 'age-related degeneration,' in other words senile involution, which has a generally poor prognosis. In fact, you will learn that, in most cases, there can be recovery from Affective melancholia in old age, even though, on average, it seems to last longer, and the risk of relapse is higher than in melancholia of adolescence and middle age. In addition, according to Kräpelin, there is a form of melancholia which is more restricted and nearer to our clinical picture, but which he places amongst illnesses arising as constitutional traits; these are not regarded an independent illness, but rather as a component of a periodic mental illness conceived as 'manic-depressive' [Ed], or more recently as 'circular psychosis' [Ed]. From my own experiences, I must totally contradict this concept, according to which we should always expect recurrence, at least of the same disease. Affective melancholia does show a tendency to recur, but this is not an essential feature, and is, at any rate, a much less pronounced tendency than for many other mental illnesses. If circular mental illness is disregarded, and is not extended at will to include isolated attacks of melancholia or mania, as Kräpelin does, then his claim, advanced with so much certainty, can be explained only by the fact that he had in mind the cases of 'vicarious melancholia' [Ed]—which I will mention later—that is cases in which an attack of recurrent mania is replaced by one of Affective melancholia. Recurrent Affective melancholia, which occurs in a rapid succession of attacks, as does recurrent mania, admittedly does exist, but is one of the greatest rarities. Mrs H. is an example. These cases, by their rapid onset and decline, all seem to have a distinct status, compared with the great majority.

With respect to the *aetiology* [W] of the illness, most cases occurring during adolescence and most commonly among women are to be differentiated from the others; the former group of cases occurs almost exclusively in individuals who have severe hereditary loading.

References

1. Wernicke C. Krankenvorstellungen aus der psychiatrischen Klinik in Breslau. Breslau: Schletter; 1899. vol 1, Case 7.
2. Wernicke C. Krankenvorstellungen vol 1 Case 5.
3. Griesinger W. Die Pathologie und Therapie der psychischen Krankheiten für Ärzte und Studierende. Stuttgart: A Krabbe; 1845.
4. Meynert T. Melancholie, Kleinheitswahn, Selbstanklagewahn. Wien klin Wochenschr. 1889;11(39–42):745–47. 767–70, 783–86, 803–7.
5. Wernicke C. Die Insuffizienz der Nervi phrenici und ihre Behandlung. Monatsschr Psychiat Neurol. 1897;2:200–4.
6. Kraepelin E. Die klinische Stellung der Melancholie. Monatsschr Psychiatr Neurol. 1899;6:325–35.

Lecture 31

31

- Clinical picture of pure mania
- Levelling of ideas
- Course interruption through clear intervals
- Tendency to recurrence
- Diagnosis
- Paralytic mania
- Paralytic grandiose delusions without mania
- Kahlbaum's *Progressiva divergens* [W]
- Combinations with melancholia
- Circular mental illness
- Chronic mania

Lecture

Gentlemen!

Just as the clinical picture of Affective melancholia—which we derived from experience—is fully explained by assuming an intrapsychic *loss* [Ed] of function, so we also encounter, albeit less frequently, an acute mental illness that, in all its symptoms, may be derived from an opposite state—of intrapsychic *hyper*function [Ed]. We call it mania, and have an example in the recently presented patient Pr. Let us now consider its individual symptoms more closely.

Aberrant facilitation and acceleration of ideation, corresponding to the concept of intrapsychic hyperfunction, is manifested chiefly as *flights of ideas* [W]. It is not merely a more rapid flow of the chain of thought between *A* and *Z*; for such would not seem to us aberrant and would indicate, rather, a desirable increase of psychic ability. The prerogative of mental giftedness or of genius depends essentially on the unusually rapid and more extensive thoughts within the same timespace than is available to mediocrity. We describe wit, speed of repartee, presence of mind, versatility of interests, and other valued attributes of prominent people in this way. In contrast aberrant facilitation of 'acts of association' [Ed] produces the inconvenience that the train of thought is no longer strictly closed, as it is in the normal state, as represented by the well-worn path *AZ*, but that each link of the association chain extending from *A* to *Z* may afford the starting point for trains of thought, which correspond to secondary associations, which are normally suppressed. In my introduction, I developed the idea that a strictly terminated train of thought is the result of practice and training, that is, of functional acquisition. In general, however, where more complicated trains of thought are being modified, a degree of self-control or collectedness is needed to suppress all secondary associations which might disturb the main one. As long as this 'circumspect collectedness' [Ed] is not lost, secondary associations may be noticed to an intensified degree, and yet the main association is retained. This possibility exists particularly in highly trained minds. This results in a greater abundance of thoughts, a state of increased productivity, and eventually actual improved ability, as can occasionally be seen in initial stages of the abnormal state to be described

R. Miller, K.J. Dennison (eds.), *An Outline of Psychiatry in Clinical Lectures*,
DOI 10.1007/978-3-319-18051-9_31

here. Particularly in *Homo tardus* [W], a mentally sluggish, and unproductive individual, a beneficial change in the whole personality may be produced in this way for a short time. We could then speak of a 'coordinated flight of ideas' [Ed].

Usually, however, the flight of ideas reduces an individual's ability, in that it robs him, or limits his ability to retain the main association. The flight of ideas then becomes uncoordinated. Thus rational judgment of actual ability is lost, and a feeling of increased capacity arises, the counterpart of the subjective feelings of inadequacy in melancholia. While the latter leads to feelings of misery, here it induces feelings of happiness, to the point of abnormal euphoria; but here too, assuming that some degree of psychic ability prevails, self-awareness of the change in personality may be enabled—an autopsychic paraesthesia in the above sense. Consequently, the Affective state of abnormal euphoria which determines the clinical picture often shows up as transitions to autopsychic disarray. If the patient can be stabilized, at least for a moment, it may be possible for closed trains of thought to occur, perhaps by dint of strong efforts on attentiveness, and when requirements are not too difficult. If the disturbance exceeds such limits, the flight of ideas becomes not only uncoordinated, but incoherent. The result is a disconnected jumble, so that any possibility of intense Affective states is abolished. Flight of ideas in severe degree—the counterpart of depressive melancholia—leads to a state of confusion, without a definite, controlling Affective state, the 'flight-of-ideas confusion' [W] according to some authors, to be met again under the heading of 'confused mania' [W]. It is an intensified mania, a clinical picture that exceeds 'Affective mania' [W]. The justification for making this distinction, as much as any practical requirements, meets the needs of our theoretical derivation, demonstrably so, in that, in mania, we often observe transition of one state into the other. The connection is much more certain here than in melancholia, where I suggest that the depressive form, as a symptom complex, may be independent of the Affective form, and needs to be considered separately. However, mania is often limited just to the milder form, without progressing to the point of incoherence; and in what follows I will always have in mind just this, when I speak simply of 'mania' [Ed]. 'Confused mania' [Ed] will be given separate consideration.

Certain other symptoms are closely connected with abnormal euphoria: These include increased self-assurance, manifest in a pretentious appearance, a domineering manner, or a sense of superior knowledge and understanding. A degree of intrapsychic hyperkinesia is the counterpart of akinesia in Affective melancholia. In fact everything seems just as easy for a person who is manic as it is hard for one who is melancholic. Autopsychic disorientation takes the form of grandiose delusions, and a patient claims for himself attributes, property, offices, and functions which do not match reality. Nevertheless, such manifestations of grandiosity usually remain within limits not far removed from what is possible, or which are manifest only conditionally, as opinions and expectations, or which are expressed ironically, as though the patient were joking, and indulging in 'make-believe' [Ed]. Not uncommonly however, grandiosity reaches excessive proportions, and even fantastically grandiose ideas, arise sporadically, yet never fixed, changing from day to day.

Abnormal euphoria is sometimes permanently combined with a tendency to irascibility. At other times it may be interrupted by irascible Affects. Both of these are understandable, in that the exacting, obstinate, and domineering characteristics of this illness naturally arouse people's opposition, which enhances anger. If the irascible Affect does become permanent, it seems to be due either to physical maladies, or to long-continued, improper treatment by other people.

Increased activity in the process of association brings two other *sequelae* [W] to the fore, which show plainly the contrast with melancholia. A patient's interest in all events they witness, and their readiness to follow up on any outside suggestion is increased. Growing out of the increased thought activity, is to some extent the need to sustain stimulation. This mental disposition may be confused with hypermetamorphosis, but is entirely different, as we will see later. Similarly with the second *sequela*, the increased ease in taking decisions, and the tendency to transform decisions rapidly into action. The consequences of this are enterprise, drive, and interference in affairs of others. On the ward, these two attributes in combination are enough to produce the greatest uproar.

Patients are no less disturbing as a result of two other symptoms, which fall wholly within the range of intrapsychic hyperkinesia—the 'urge to be active' [Ed], and the 'urge to speak' [Ed]. The phrase 'urge to be active' expresses the idea that hyperkinesia, defined elsewhere as 'motor impulse', has a special content here, namely a drive to activity, or, better perhaps the *need* [Ed] for activity; in other words, a compulsion to act rather than merely to move. Hyperkinesia thus involves those types of initiative movement which are more complex. The impulse depends on the increased rapidity and readiness to make decisions, and increased interest in things, which lead patients to get up to all sorts of mischief: to throw furniture about, spill food, throw bedclothes around, take over the ward staff's duties, and to make suggestions correcting patients and staff, whether on proper or improper occasions, or even to attack them. In all severe cases, this urge deteriorates still further: Patients demolish everything which is not screwed or nailed down, destroy linen and bedding, paint the walls with improvised colours, not hesitating to use their own urine and faeces, or, each according to his own style, to write, compose poetry, draw, and in this way consume huge quantities of paper. Besides this, patients' movements usually manage to convey their exalted, happy, boisterous, or occasionally irascible mood: They dance, hop, jump, laugh, make faces, make teasing gestures, and—quite seriously—threatening and menacing ones etc. Many observations lead us to the view that motor strength and shrewdness of such patients may actually be increased; at least their performances are often surprising in their strength and shrewdness.

Loquacity seems to be an ever-present symptom of intrapsychic hyperfunction, matching our experience that mental activity is always accompanied by communication. How much more so in the boisterous, exalted mood of such patients! Only when an irascible tone prevails may this be missing, and probably then with comprehensible psychological motives. The verbal content of that loquacity always betrays increased mental productiveness, even if this is of highly varied quality, each according to his individual style. As the Affect tends towards an elevation of mood, it is readily understood how irritating and annoying such patients, with all their loquacity, can be.

Gentlemen! I should now speak of an important symptom, whose derivation from general intrapsychic hyperfunction is not immediately comprehensible, but which is constantly found in mania, and is of special interest to us, in that an opposite symptom occurs in melancholia. It is based on the levelling of groups of normally overvalued ideas. Manic patients all seem to undergo damage to their character. It never occurs to any such patient to express sympathy for other patients, when the latter arouse so many feelings of compassion. On the contrary, he only complains of the disturbance that he thereby sometimes experiences, and hits back at every interference. Thus, a certain brutality, or inconsiderate egotism, is manifest. The manic lies, cheats, and steals without compunction. He claims everything he is allowed, while criticizing this trait in others. Similarly, displays of sexual desire, which is usually increased, appear inconsiderate and shameless. No manic woman, who might previously have been the most innocent and modest of girls, holds back with her opinions and knowledge. Similarly, I have never seen a manic woman who would have considered it at all out of the ordinary to be in the bath when the physician came, and the tendency of these patients to undress and to use obscene language is well known. At a clinical presentation, despite its powerful effect encouraging a patient to exercise self-control, her free, uninhibited behaviour—quite uncalled-for in a girl—and the way she expresses herself, attract attention as being abnormal, without further comment. No officer who is manic takes the decent course, but breaks his word of honour not once, but ten times. All opinions on matters which had previously included the most sacred of feelings, are utterly transformed into cynicism. There are abundant extensive examples, by which patients show adherence to their convictions, disregarding all consideration for family, religion, honour, country, etc. We take this quite regular change in character as being due to the normal value of ideas having suffered. However, whereas in melancholia the way this happens is of a definite, narrow circle of ideas becoming overvalued and dominant by themselves, in mania we observe a suppression and levelling of the normal range of overvalued ideas that are decisive in attitude and action, and which also determine every person's character. It must be expected, and is confirmed by clinical observation, that such a levelling of ideas in persons whose character already left much to be desired, must be especially ugly, and imprints on them the stamp of vulgarity even more sharply than in other patients.

We can understand this *levelling of ideas* [W], which is one of the most important symptoms of mania, when we take intrapsychic hyperfunction to be a *general* [Ed] increase in excitability of intrapsychic paths. On the other hand, the normal overvaluation of ideas is to be explained by the physiological (functionally acquired) increase in excitability of *specific* [Ed], chosen paths. A general increase in excitability can then easily eliminate the difference in excitability that leads to overvaluation of specific pathways, a concept that also accounts for flight of ideas and failure to bring thought processes to an end-point.

Gentlemen! The clinical picture of pure mania is thus fully outlined. There is only one subsidiary point to be made, namely the occasional occurrence of phonemes, which then seem to be the only way in which grandiose ideas can be experienced. They are usually only isolated ones, present at the height of the illness, consisting of words like 'prophet' [W], 'Hohenzoller' [W], or even 'God' [W]. Numerous hallucinations of various senses occur only in confused mania, but of this, more later.

It is very striking, and different from all other acute mental illnesses, that, in most new cases of mania, general health is relatively unaffected. The longer the duration of illness, and with it the loss of muscular strength, the more it leads to objectively visible loss of vigour, and more severe decline of nutritional status. In part, we must trace this symptom back to the favourable influence that elevated mood normally has on food intake. The single deleterious effect which opposes it, is insomnia or, at least the reduced desire for sleep in these patients; for appetite tends to be increased, and influence on metabolism and circulation is always beneficial. Here we find the diametrical opposite of Affective melancholia, in which gastric and digestive disorders, as well as depressed circulation, are familiar and frequent symptoms. This contrast is shown most strikingly in cases of circular psychoses, where the transformation of the one clinical picture into the other may occur in days, occasionally even within hours.

Mania is usually an illness with acute-onset and rapid progression. It is then stable for a few weeks, occasionally months, at a certain intensity of illness, and then subsides, usually more slowly than it rose. It is the most curable of all mental illnesses, but not without danger. Mention should be made here of a tendency to suicide, which is not rare, its motive lying in overpowering moments of autopsychic disarray, which may also be accompanied by anxiety; and the ease of execution made possible by the rapidity of decision-making and unrestrained energy. In manic individuals I have often come across severe self-inflicted stab wounds in the region of the heart.

In its course mania is often interrupted by the so-called lucid intervals which, for a short time, may simulate the onset of recovery. Usually, a quick shift into what appears to be health is striking, but should always arouse suspicion of early relapse. Lucid intervals may last only hours, sometimes several days, and may recur frequently during the course of the illness. They are usually accompanied by fatigue and exhaustion, the consequence of the restlessness which preceded them. Alternatively, a state of profound moral depression may take place instead, especially in the rare cases where there is full insight into the illness during such intervals. Shame over their conduct during times of illness may even lead to suicide.

Gentlemen! *Diagnosis* [W] of mania in the narrowly confined sense that I have given it here, is made with ease. Where you find the above-mentioned symptoms all together, corresponding to intrapsychic hyperfunction, a manic condition can be diagnosed. If these symptoms are found exclusively, and no others, it is certainly a case of pure mania. As you can see, the disorder is mainly one of form. You can speak of delusion formation only in so far as subjective feelings of increased capability are related from the outset to grandiosity, which, in the course of the illness, occasionally leads to actual grandiose delusions. In new cases, where your advice and opinion are sought, you will hardly ever encounter actual grandiose delusions. However, there is an exception here, which I want to go into more fully, relating to the question of aetiology. In general, pure mania, like Affective melancholia—but possibly to a greater degree—is included among those psychoses often arising from a background of hereditary affliction and neurotic degeneration. This is especially true of mania in adolescence, but occasionally also in later decades. However, in the latter case another aetiology—namely paralytic—must always be considered first. *Paralytic mania* [W] is a relatively common illness, usually presenting with features that ensure diagnosis at the outset. These characteristics are so familiar to you, that I need only briefly recapitulate them: They are symptoms related to the projection system, recognizable as early dementia, but chiefly as impairment of attentiveness. However, there are also cases—none too rare—where there is no sign of such symptoms, yet which should still be viewed as paralytic mania. These cases otherwise correspond to the picture of pure mania just described, but where grandiose delusions are quite clear from the beginning. This grandiose delusional state has its special signature, for it belongs to the category of 'fantastic or demented state of grandiosity' [Ed], which is specific to progressive paralysis. Thus an expert member of railway management believed he had made an epoch-making discovery regarding the problem of central arrangements for points-switching. After his recovery he conceded that it represented no more than a totally insignificant change in the set-up used everywhere. He further expressed his conviction that, without difficulty, he could marry another wife in addition to his current one. Here, flight of ideas and loquacity only rarely go outside a degree of well-ordering. Eight weeks of bed treatment in a hospital, and subsequent travel were enough to restore him to good health. Two years later, after the patient had been steadily engaged in a responsible position, a relapse occurred, with far more fantastic grandiose delusions, and rapid progression to confused mania, and only at this stage did we notice symptoms related to the projection system. I need not say that reduced attentiveness and other symptoms of dementia were carefully sought, without finding anything. Only the placid, less-animated facial expression gave any reason for doubt in this regard. The further course unquestionably confirmed the diagnosis. I have come across many instances with a similar course [1].

I might emphasize at this point, that there are also cases of this type of fantastic grandiose delusion starting acutely, but without mania—cases that may initially be free from any symptoms of deficit, or ones implicating the projection system, and which later prove to be paralytic, a so-called paranoid form of progressive paralysis, probably already recognized by most specialists [2]. In our sense we claim them as an acute, expansive autopsychosis of specific paralytic aetiology. Since there is no evidence of real mania, there is no diagnostic difficulty. On the other hand I recall the form of *Progressiva divergens* [W] instituted by Kahlbaum [3]—divergence here is in the figurative sense of progressive disorientation or alienation from reality—which in its entire course, in addition to the rapidly expanding, fantastic grandiose delusions, may present symptoms of pure mania, albeit never leading to paralysis or mental deterioration. Yet these cases are very rare, and in my entire experience, which is quite extensive I have seen only a few.

Gentlemen! From these remarks you may get the idea that, for practical purposes, it is always a collection of manifestations which determines whether or not a case is pure mania. It requires no special mention that any additional disorders of content exclude a diagnosis of mania. Real motor symptoms, that is, hyperkinetic in the narrow sense (see our schema) have a similar significance. In addition, the symptom of hypermetamorphosis needs special mention. It likewise excludes pure mania, but is often encountered in confused mania, as we shall see.

Gentlemen! I have already said that besides pure mania, manic states of many other sorts occur, and are to be evaluated in an entirely different way. They are either manic phases of composite psychoses occurring episodically, or combinations of two or more fundamental forms. Of the latter type, the so-called irascible form of mania will be discussed shortly. I will come back to all the combinations later.

The relationship of pure mania to melancholia is remarkable. Both illnesses reveal an internal relationship, in that they are combined in the following three ways:

1. A mild form of one illness generally tends to appear during convalescence from the others and signals its termination. The duration of this switch, which often appears after the patient's condition has become apparently normal, sometimes amounts to a few days, sometimes a few weeks.
2. Mania is the one illness which, of all psychoses, is most likely to recur. Between individual attacks, at first a period of years usually elapses. Later, the interval is shortened, so that finally, the periods of illness may exceed those of health. Something similar, but only very rarely, is seen in melancholia. Clinical experience teaches us that, now and then, recurrence of mania is replaced by a period of melancholia, which is then a blessed portent of a better prognosis for the mania; and the same relation may also occur inversely. This is the *substitutional melancholia* [W] mentioned above (p. 213).
3. Finally, a combination of the two illnesses occurs quite often, in the way that one supersedes the other. They are separated by an interval of apparent health which may amount to days or even weeks, or sometimes is only very brief, and may even escape observation. Since Falret [4] and Baillarger [5] in 1854, this illness has long been known by the name of *circular mental illness* [6] [W], or *folie à double forme* [W], noted for its poor prognosis. In fact, prominent cases seem to be quite incurable.

Despite this, we must take note that a single episode of the sort occurs quite often, without implying a bad prognosis. It is probably a variant of the relationship described under 1. It is to be further noted, that this often applies to the mildest grade of both illnesses, which occasionally do not impair an individual's social ability at all, or, more often, do so only temporarily. I know of instances of the kind, which have never interfered with responsible business activity, while others needed to go into an institution only at times of greatest loquacity. With regard to prognosis, it should also be stated that dementia never arises from the circular form of mental disturbance, in the narrow sense, where it consists of alternating phases of Affective melancholia and pure mania. The attacks always tend to occur in the same way, whether the illness has existed for 2 or 20 years. These cases are, however, relatively rare. (In the broader sense, circular mental illness includes all psychoses that present a regular alternation of manic and melancholic conditions [3].) Duration of individual attacks varies, amounting on average to a few months. A special peculiarity of circular psychoses might be, that their individual phases develop more rapidly and especially decline much more rapidly than in the case of melancholia or mania alone. Duration of manic or melancholic phase need not always be the same. I shall return later to changes in body weight in this illness, which L. Meyer regarded as characteristic features [7].

While circular mental disorder in the narrower sense always develops the same pure forms of melancholia and mania, this does not apply to recurrent mania. Rather—and the experience is very general—it is transformed progressively into the more severe clinical picture of confused mania, with new foreign elements occasionally being added.

It should also be said that mania rarely remains pure over a long period, but that at the height of the illness a condition of confusion is readily established, which, in most favourable cases is based purely on flight of ideas, while in more severe cases other elements are added.

Treatment [W] of mania is generally only possible inside a mental institution.

Apart from acute mania, there is a special form of illness which deserves the name of *chronic mania* [W]. I can say nothing definite as to its origin, and only one thing seems to me to be established: that acute, pure mania never turns into chronic mania. When attacks of recurrent mania finally outweigh in duration the lucid intervals, they do not turn into a chronic mania, at least not in the strict meaning of the term, a point that I alone can defend. Chronic mania has all essential attributes of acute mania, modified only in that it brings with it prerequisites of any chronic, stable condition. Accordingly, the flight of ideas continues within moderate limits, still limited by a degree of discretion and self-control. Consequently the exaltation is less pronounced, but still occasionally breaks out. On the other hand, inevitable 'collisions' [Ed] in society tend to sustain irascible mental states. Elevated egotism, which does not reach a level of frank grandiose delusions, is still very noticeable, giving the individuals concerned a prominence which, in combination with their undeniable mental productivity, enables them to advance. Thus they constantly create various difficulties and collisions, by disregarding all the norms and considerations imposed by law and custom. They make no allowances, yet demand greatest forebearance. Suggestions of formal thought disorder need not be present in this condition. One case of this kind was preceded by severe psychosis of many years standing, for which no fuller reports were obtainable, but which was certainly not pure mania. The patient lacked any insight into his illness, and it was probably justifiable to regard his condition just as 'recovery with deficit' [Ed], or, if one takes objection to that, as a deficit state acquired through a psychosis.

References

1. Wernicke C. Krankenvorstellungen aus der psychiatrischen Klinik in Breslau. Breslau: Schletter; 1899. vol 2, Case 8 is an example of paralytic mania.
2. Wernicke C. Krankenvorstellungen. vol 2, Case 12.
3. Kahlbaum KL. Die Gruppierung der psychischen Krankheiten und die Eintheilung der Seelenstörungen. Danzig: AW Kafemann; 1863.
4. Falret JP. De la folie circulaire ou forme de maladie mentale caracterisée par alternative régulière de la manie et de la melancholie. Bull Acad Med. 1851;19:382–400.
5. Baillarger JGF. Folie à double forme. Ann Med Psychol (Paris). 1854;18:369–91.
6. Wernicke C. Krankenvorstellungen. vol 1, Case 5, and vol 2, Case 15.
7. Meyer L. Über circuläre Geisteskrankheiten. Arch Psychiatr Nervenkr. 1874;4:139–58.

Lecture 32

32

- Clinical presentations of a puerperally-induced and a menstrually-induced hyperkinetic motility psychosis
- Pseudospontaneous movements
- Idiosyncrasy of the movement
- Absence of compulsive speech in this
- Psychomotor compulsive speech
- Description of a case of jacktatoid compulsive movement
- Verbigeration in compulsive speech
- Choreatic compulsive movement
- Impulsive actions
- Disarrayed restless movement
- Hypermetamorphotic compulsive movement
- Periodic recurrent course of the illness
- Prognosis and treatment

Lecture

Gentlemen!

The patient who you see looks feeble, pale, and exhausted. In fact, for 4 weeks she has been in a severe state of arousal, in which she has produced an excess of movements, which probably explains why all her energy has been quite used up. To our great surprise, a turn-around occurred from yesterday, after she had been in constant motion the day before, mostly with histrionic-melodramatic expressive movements, and had been singing virtually without ever stopping. The way she carried out her singing was certainly surprising: It was accompanied by a fine tremor of her lower lip and the whole of her lower jaw, a movement akin to that of chattering teeth, but without the teeth ever occluding. Her voice thus attained a regular, tremulous character, reminiscent of many barrel organ performances, the more so as she sung only the notes, without accompanying words—evidently a wholly invented, sustained hymn, almost always at very high pitch—with steady, quiet 'conducting' [Ed] movements.

This singing, which, along with the patient's troubled, perplexed and unhappy facial expression, gave her a 'constrained' [Ed] look, hindered her eating food; and it ceased only in the evening, when, after of an injection of hyoscine and morphine, sleep ensued for several hours.

Firstly, convince yourselves of the extreme exhaustion and frailty of this patient. When she is raised to her feet, she sways and needs support; seated on a chair, she occasionally lets her head fall back, apparently in extreme fatigue; and she appears distracted when enquiries are made, or begins to answer, but soon loses the thought and stares into space. Evidently, she is able to follow only with effort, and I could not ask more of her, because she really is very much in need of rest and protection. Yet her perverse facial expression is remarkable to us: Firstly, she opens her eyes so wide that the whites can be seen above the cornea; then she wrinkles her forehead as if in anger, and again protrudes her lower lip and lower jaw.

R. Miller, K.J. Dennison (eds.), *An Outline of Psychiatry in Clinical Lectures*,
DOI 10.1007/978-3-319-18051-9_32

Further, at times, we see marked impediments in her speech: she forces out a single word like a stutterer, labouring a long time over initial consonants; or occasionally, she utters gurgling, inarticulate sounds; and she is unable to show her tongue when requested, but only opens her mouth in an awkward manner. Words are often toneless, and therefore unintelligible. Yet at other times she speaks with no trouble, and in this way tells us how her illness started. She is able to give her name correctly, her age, and the date of a previous confinement; she also expresses her feeling of being ill, that she feels dizzy, and cannot breathe properly. She also admits that the clinical examination took its toll on her. Now and then she turns her head and listens, evidently attracted by phonemes. She often turns to the female attendant beside her, as if for help, and it can be seen how hard it is for her to stay attentive. Yet familiar things, like the Lord's Prayer, seem to give her no trouble; she repeats it in a devout tone, with folded hands. She then voluntarily repeats Luther's exposition on one of the Ten Commandments, and begins to sing a chorale, with faultless words and melody. I then raise her right arm to a horizontal position; she permits this without resisting, and holds the position for a short time, before letting her arm sink. Bending her head forwards produces pain, and is met with mild resistance. When she stands to leave the auditorium, she spreads her arms sideways, palms supine, and makes a theatrical gesture, but then follows the attendant in the normal way.

Gentlemen! As you have seen the patient's mental state was not normal. First of all, apathy equating to exhaustion seemed to prevail, then moods of euphoria or irritation appeared, all within moderate limits, and always combined with expressions of helplessness and disarray. She was not visibly, or not adequately orientated to her surroundings and situation, and made the strangest statements about her own body: Last night she had a 'hump' [Ed], which has gone away again, and her 'eyes have been slashed' [Ed]. Any explanations we could obtain about the cause of her movements were quite incomplete; a few isolated statements seemed to show that she had been 'compelled' [Ed] to sing and dance.

Gentlemen! As I soon concluded, our patient has suffered a pronounced hyperkinetic motility psychosis over 4 weeks, and we see the subsequent state of exhaustion clearly showing signs of this illness, which are largely motor in character. Her facial expression conveys no psychological motivation; and the occasional protrusion of the lower jaw and lips, the peculiar impediment of speech, the fluctuating inability to protrude her tongue, the pseudoflexibility, unmotivated histrionic gestures, and equally motiveless singing are all distinct remnants of the preceding motility psychosis, to be interpreted partly as parakinetic, partly as akinetic symptoms.

With regard to the aetiology of our case, we know only that the illness developed acutely over the course of a few days, after the patient, a 27-year-old potter's wife, married for 9 months, had experienced her first- and normal-delivery at the women's clinic, and had remained psychically normal for 10 days. She had breastfed another child besides her own, and was thus somewhat debilitated. At home she was greatly worried about her child, listening to every breath, expressed fear that he might die; and on the second night after that, she began to sing, to dance around the room and to talk about angels, who she could hear singing. The next day she mistook her husband for a physician she knew. The hyperkinetic motility psychosis has developed, as it often does at the end of the puerperium, which, as we learn, is perfectly normal; and the patient is therefore an example of the falsely named 'puerperal mania' [Ed], which in reality covers all manner of acute psychoses, pure mania being the least common.

Gentlemen! Chance has favoured us, in that I can present another patient, in whom you will see the florid stage of a hyperkinetic motility psychosis. You witness the patient entering, dancing a waltz step and singing a waltz melody. She then taps the crown of her head with the flat of her hand and says 'Holy water', bows, and repeats the word and the same gesture five more times. She correctly interprets the gesture I make with my hand, inviting her to take a seat, and suddenly sits down in the chair. However, she soon stands up again, bends forward, and throws her head forward so that her loosened hair falls over her face. She repeats this rhythmically about 20 times. Then she walks round, her body bending and swaying, busily gesticulating and talking incessantly, with regularly accentuated steps, reminiscent of the enforced exaggeration in the expressive movements of a minuet. The rhythm of such dancing, hopping, and jumping whole-body movements is remarkably exact, when pushed to the limit and, in their execution may indicate great expenditure of energy. They are accompanied by movements of the arms, expressive and correspondingly energetic. Her face also displays an exaggerated countenance; she rolls her eyes, makes an angry face, and then a haughtily repellant, or comical one. She makes threatening movements, attempting to strike—but not in earnest—these being deflected immediately by herself. At the same time she makes several interconnected assertions, at one point: 'They (or you? not decided) must be chopped up at the stake'. On the whole, her mental state, like her movements, seems to be very unstable, sometimes extremely happy, then haughty or irritable. In general she cannot remain in one place, or can do so only for a moment; at one point, when asked "Why do you dance? Are you happy?" she promptly answers in the affirmative. Then, when asked 'Do you know who these gentlemen are?' she begins to sing, 'So might Heaven forgive you'.

The connection between her spontaneous, almost-continuous speech movements and her other movements is most extraordinary. It is shown in that her voice is often raised, matching the rhythm of her general movements; and, this happens to a greatly exaggerated degree, as are her movements. Thus, much of what she says is incomprehensible, or she gives voice to no more than fragmentary sentences or isolated words or syllables. Furthermore, the content of these isolated fragments of speech is often connected conspicuously with the movements. Thus, she adopts a military bearing, makes the movement of stroking a moustache with her right hand, and says in a gutteral tone 'Lieutenant of the guard'. On another occasion she raises her arm, bent at a right angle, opposes the tips of thumb and index finger with the gesture of the gourmet, and says 'Roast pork'; or she extends her arms and hands and says 'I still have ten healthy fingers'; or, while she has her arms outstretched and sways her torso: 'How can the tailoress balance?' Evidently these movements completely divert her attention, so that only momentarily can it become focused. Moreover, you have seen that incidental sensory impressions divert her, and lead to movements, although mainly she ignores my questions and requests. Nonetheless, when she has been enticed to sit down, limiting herself, in silence, to theatrical hand movements, and I say to her 'she can go now' [Ed], she at once comprehends this correctly, and stands up.

Gentlemen! This patient, a 36-year-old unmarried tailoress, also looks pale, emaciated and worn out, quite a natural consequence of the effort she has expended in almost-continual, unchosen movements. She has been in this same state for 5 weeks, varying now and then only in intensity. Sleep can be induced only by hypnotics, of which hyoscine seems especially effective; food intake is inadequate, and is disrupted by her motor restlessness.

With regard to this patient's clinical history we have learned the following. Psychoses or severe neuroses have not occurred before in her family; her father died of consumption at age 52. She had been a poor student at school, but was industrious, very honest, and had led an orderly life. She carried on a tailoring business with her sister, and has probably overworked; and over recent years she also suffered from *menstruatio nimia* [W]. Eight years ago, she had been depressed for 3 months, probably with melancholia; at any rate, she conveyed feelings of unhappiness, spoke with self-reproach, and at the time her relatives had noticed peculiar 'knotting' [W] movements of her hands. Afterwards she had been healthy, except at the times of her menses, when she always became markedly irritable and sensitive. Eight weeks prior to admission she had a 2-day premenstrual attack of 'frenzy' [Ed], in which she talked and sang constantly, always in motion, throwing furniture about, and had terrifying visual and auditory hallucinations, with verbigeration, occasionally mistaking people and her surroundings. From the family's description, she had very prominent hypermetamorphosis at this time. With onset of menstruation she quickly became quiet, and slept spontaneously. Four weeks later, menstruation passed without disturbance. Two days before the next menstruation, which was exactly 4 weeks later, admission to the clinic became necessary because of a fresh attack of frenzy, after having spent 2 days at home in this state. This time, appearance of her period had no influence on the illness. To-day, at this demonstration, she should have menstruated again, for it is 5 days over the 4 weeks since her last period, but this time, menstruation seems delayed or not to be happening at all.

Gentlemen! These data are of special value, because they show us a definite, though rather imprecise, influence of menstruation upon the origin and decline of psychoses, and—I must note here—that this is not an isolated experience, but recurs so often in hyperkinetic motility psychoses that we need to recognize it as, by far, the most common type of menstrual psychosis. In particular, hyperkinetic motility psychosis is more often of menstrual than of puerperal origin. I return to these aetiological circumstances later.

Gentlemen! Strange and outlandish as are the movements that you have seen in our patient, they might leave you suspecting that they are—in part at least—voluntary productions of a hysterical-histrionic personality. Admittedly, there are no hysterical antecedents, and the fact that being left alone has no influence also contradicts this, for it is not clear why a hysteric should continue such performances when there are no witnesses. Finally, there are patients' own statements made after they have recovered—or when they become calm just for a while—that these movements are independent of their volition, the result of some incomprehensible kind of coercion interpreted in various ways. However, you will reasonably ask for positive signs, to allow such *pseudospontaneous movements* [W] to be differentiated from deliberate productions. There actually are such signs, as you have seen in our patients. A certain uniformity and monotony of these movements, their tendency to recur with the same pattern of movement, perhaps increasing to rhythmical repetition, will be especially striking to you. It is manifest also in verbal performance, and has repeatedly led to verbigeration in our patient. Second, you will not have missed the exaggerated, violent, and to some extent affected character of these movements, along with the unusual muscular effort with which they are connected, giving some of the movements a grotesquely graceful appearance. In our patients this is also noticeable in their speech movements; and this is not always limited to pseudospontaneous movements, being occasionally incorporated into expressive ones, like laughing, crying, and singing. You will probably remember the patient (p. 75) who apologized for her song, irreproachable in itself, that she had to sing, a production in itself perfectly proper; but she had to sing it, even though she did not want to. Finally the evident aimlessness—and absurdity—in the form of her movements, must be emphasized, for instance, when the patient repeatedly placed the flat of her hand on the crown of her head, or spread her fingers, or rhythmically bent her body forward, or balanced on one leg, etc. This aimlessness differentiates pseudospontaneous movements from the so-called 'occupational deliria' [Ed], usually connected with compound hallucinations, repetitive to the point of perfection, and also from a psychosensory component of conditioned reactive movements (as in alcoholic delirium) driven especially by cutaneous hallucinations. However, when the movements resemble gymnastic exercises, as we often saw in the past semester, you find them here, in our clinical demonstration, totally out of place and evidently aimless.

Gentlemen! Closer analysis of the pseudospontaneous movements brings anecdotal evidence to our notice, namely that the movements are not psychologically motivated, but are a consequence of disordered identification between *Z* and *m*, that is, on a psychomotor pathway. Items of clinical evidence, which are only occasionally prominent in our case, lead to the same conclusion, in so far as the patient spoke a lot—although in many cases of hyperkinetic motility psychoses, this will confirm the diagnosis almost at first sight. The evidence is that the motor impulse of hyperkinetic motility psychosis is accompanied not by corresponding loquacity, but often by the opposite symptom in the speech domain, namely mutism. A striking contrast always exists, a lack of proportionality between the mild degree of loquacity and the severely affected motor impulse. As you can see, this is the direct opposite of mania, where loquacity predominates and the motor impulse retreats in proportion, or is manifest more as a 'desire' [Ed] for activity. But if pronounced loquacity exists, which is commonly the case, the changed form of speech shows that it originates from a psychomotor disorder of identification. Its undifferentiated form leads to verbigeration, or at least to conspicuous repetition of the same words or common phrases; excessive expenditure of effort leads to unmotivated crying or howling; the aimlessness in gratifying the vocal motor impulse leads to senseless stringing together of words, and of words or syllables not even related by sound. In general the signs of psychomotor loquacity—unlike those of an intrapsychic disorder—are monotony and incoherence rather than flight of ideas. A further sign referring to content is provided by the hypermetamorphosis which is hardly ever absent in hyperkinetic motility psychosis. The following reproduction of the spontaneous utterances of a patient may illustrate what has been said:

> Scullion or bubble, then it begins to bubble or to burn, or with others, ah, Jesus, says my Mutho, always from the beginning, if she was so small, ah so, ah, Anna, a, n, a, in the height, or so much drops from above, ah, Jesus, I findest thou, ah, Jesus and hence because she scullion, getel or gattel or Philadelphia or America or in Tyrol or the or doubles, ah, pocket pistol with and without a bang, since the matter is so, oh, Jesus, Jesus, it goes once, 2, 4 therefore so much even as one once goes to me so, so straight out, then 2, 3, ah, Jesus, ah indeed, that is very fine, that is called counting, the first, the first little song, oh Jesus, consequently one says work or destroying angel [strangling movements!] [to the attendant:] I might take away the cushions, for so many things, ah, Jesus, little star, her little child, come oh, come, oh not yet, just the same. Stop, what is it, what is it that comes from my home, ah, Jesus, ah, ah, ah, or from my school friend from the beginning either from Hanke, Anke, kekeke…

Difficulties in diagnosis are created only by milder or mildest grades of such pseudospontaneous *psychomotor loquacity* [W]. Any intention to continue with a coordinated form of speech then opposes the psychomotor impulse, with results which are very characteristic for specialists. Falsely placed pathos, singing, or declaiming, or an unctuous tone of speech with frequent elevation and lowering of pitch, and an increased rhythmic tendency, might lead one to ascribe such productions to a 'pulpit orator' [Ed] with their marked impact—even as far as the content. However, the content also shows itself to be influenced, apparently by the altered form of speech, just as the form of the motor impulse in our patients shows an influence on its ideation; for it is pre-eminently biblical, or at least is connected to passages from the Bible, verses of hymns, explanations of catechisms, remembered sermons, etc. A patient of this type found that her talk 'dripped from her lips like honey' [W]. For the sake of completeness I should mention that the monotony of content, the tendency to repeat the same words or phrases, also hold true. You see, gentlemen, that psychomotor loquacity in each case presents signs enough for it to be readily identified as such.

Gentlemen! The importance of this subject requires us to examine in greater depth the sort of movement executed in hyperkinetic motility psychoses. In general, movements range between two extremes, at one time appearing totally deliberate, yet in contrast, also totally involuntary, evidently occurring as an imposition on the patient's intention. As an example of the former type, I remind you of the acutely ill young man, who I presented in the previous semester, mute, with a congested face, who, with visible effort, performed regular gymnastic movements of arms and trunk for 10 min. These movements were so precise and apparently purposeful that you might doubt that they were involuntary performances by the patient. After a few weeks in this hyperkinetic state, which was sometimes replaced by akinetic phases of apparent exhaustion, he became calm, but at the same time with rapid increase of feeble-mindedness, while his greatly-reduced nutritional status gave way to a rapid increase in body weight. At present, you would scarcely recognize this ruddy, apparently profoundly demented patient, instantly refusing—and unbiddable towards—any demand to think. The contrast is provided by evidently *un*intentional [Ed] movements, reminiscent of the familiar jactation of unconscious states. Common to both is only the monotonous recurrence of the same form of movement. I was able to present a remarkably pure case of the latter in the winter semester of 1891. This moderately well-nourished, perfectly self-possessed, and thoroughly attentive and oriented 79-year-old patient, Mrs. W., claimed that her illness was constituted entirely by a peculiar motor restlessness. On awakening each morning this was only slight, but it increased slowly during the day, reaching its high-point in the evening, so that the patient could not rest for half the night—until finally she fell asleep from sheer exhaustion. My *Assistent* [W] at the time, Dr. Kemmler, left me with a splendid description of the style of her motor impulse. I want to convey only the essentials here:

> Patient sits in bed, but constantly changes her position; first she tries to move to the upper edge of the bed, then to the lower, or tries a position on the side, or raises herself up as if she would try to stand, then tries to get out of bed. These movements follow one another in extreme haste, usually one movement is not completed before the next begins, often a movement entirely contradictory in nature. Pauses for rest hardly ever happen. In her haste she always and incessantly makes the same futile efforts and the same movements. The patient's assertions, which accompany her restless impulses, confirm our assumption that she can find no position or posture in which she feels comfortable, as though every attempt to take a certain position evokes an unpleasant feeling, of which she would pay any price to rid herself. She is forever trying all possible means. Assertions such as: "I do not lie right like this, I cannot remain so; I must lie quite differently; I cannot remain sitting like this; I can't abide this; I must get some rest; if I could only stand up; if I could only lie down; but it doesn't do, perhaps it would if I don't lie down at all", etc. In her helplessness, she appeals to everyone for help, and finally moans like a person in despair. If anyone approaches her, she immediately claims their assistance. For example, she grasps the doctor's hands, lets go of them, immediately grabs them again, supports herself on his arm, clings firmly to his sleeve, and promptly ceases from every attempt. "Ah no. It doesn't work like this. You must help me differently. You are doing it wrong. If you would hold me like this", are characteristic comments. If you ask the patient how you should help her, she replies, "That's just it, I can't find out". The presence of the doctor or attendant always has a somewhat calming effect. Patient begs that someone should always be there, then it would be better for her. It is noticeable that the patient very often makes a movement entirely contrary to her stated intention. Thus for example, she decides that she should be laid down, and then always raises herself on the arm of the person who would help her. Or she wants to stand up, and makes no effort to rise. Her corresponding assertions leave us in no doubt about this: "Ah, that is not what I wanted at all; it should have been something totally different. I would gladly lie down so that I can sleep, but I do not know how to begin to go about it. For God's sake, what should I do to sit down?" She sometimes struggles directly against the very help for which she has asked. To a spirited, earnest request to desist from her movements, she is quiet for a time and feels visibly relieved. Likewise, it is seen that she can voluntarily perform all movements on request. However, a few minutes later her old movements begin. At the height of her motor restlessness she is entirely absorbed in her movements, and it is hard to fixate her attention. She then repeats the question instead of answering it, or uses rambling speech and thus loses the sentence construction, or leaves the sentence unfinished. In between times assertions like: "I will tell you afterwards what I cannot think of at the moment", etc. On one occasion the patient was even unable to give her name; on such occasions she shows her annoyance: "I know it perfectly well, but because of my restlessness I cannot speak it now". A portion of the patient's movements resemble a familiar example of so-called occupation delirium [Lecture 26]. Thus for example she occupies herself constantly with the bedding, pushes the covers off, pulls them up, covers herself, then uncovers herself. She also busies herself with her items of clothing; she puts it all on, or puts some of it on, and takes it off again, often with the wholly unplanned result, so that she sits there naked, and then complains, because it was so improper. While she utters a certain intention, she quite often does the opposite. One night she was very restless, constantly pushed the covers off and then expressed the desire to be covered, because it was so cold. When she was assisted and covered, she suddenly became perfectly quiet and soon went to sleep. Evidently she was unable to start the sequence of actions—sit up, grasp the covers, lie down, and draw the covers up—in order to unite them into a single action. Given a pencil and paper to write, she was able to accomplish just as little.

As already mentioned, restlessness ceases when she is earnestly admonished; similarly, when she performs some complicated movement on command—in which she is always successful—or when she is keyed-up to be attentive and impart certain information. Patient shows that she is talkative, in part garrulous, but without real loquacity. Now and then an expression fails her, especially in finding the word for verbs and abstract ideas, her prolixity then often serving to circumscribe or seek out the correct expression. When she is asked the reason for her aimless movements, she showed a certain insight: "That must lie in the nature in such a way that is just a misfortune. I do not know what it is for". Patient denied many movements after she had performed them. For example, she speedily pulls off her jacket and then claims that she could not have done it at all; another time, "that can only have been an accident". She puts a stocking around her neck and says that it is not a proper necktie. She turns the second stocking inside out and suddenly pulls it over her head like a cap; she is herself astonished at this moment, and pulls it on properly, over her foot. On request, she protrudes her tongue hesitatingly and spasmodically. Frequent verbigerating repetition of the same phrases, e.g. "Oh God, pity me. Please help me do right". Never hypochondriacal sensations, always perfect orientation, good memory and ability to be attentive.

After becoming quiet, a good disclosure: An uncomfortable feeling might have caused the movements, they could not have been voluntary. The uncomfortable feeling was located in the chest and gradually affected the whole body. At the time when the motor restlessness abated, indications of delusions of relatedness: Another female patient had behaved so peculiarly, that one could not get any rest—she must probably have lain on the bed, so that she could get no rest. In the morning she begged for a hypnotic, but immediately said she did not want it at all. Claimed that she was cold; at once asserted the opposite. Once said, quite aimlessly: "Can I sit up now, or can I eat something first?"

Female patient, previously healthy, had been in the public hospital. The last four weeks before her admission (on 12 September, 1891) often sleepless and complaints of headache and increasing weakness; a few days before admission the 'twitching' [W] began, as she called it. That she therefore had been considered mentally ill and brought to the lunatic asylum displeased her greatly. Motor restlessness soon attained the severity just described, and continued, except for a slight remission between 21–25 September, until the beginning of October, to be replaced in a few days by complete quiescence until 6 October. A relapse began 27 October, and increased in range and intensity until 17 November. On 18 November the severely-exhausted patient presented fever and symptoms of pneumonia, and died 22 November. An influenza epidemic prevailed at that time. The relapse then began, repeated assertions that the patient herself did not know what she really wanted, and that this might be just as remarkable. Soon again great helplessness in the choice of motor means. Transitory and half-corrected negative-impact ideas: She was being jeered at, laughed at, tormented, also mistrustful of those around, fretful, irritable in mood. Initially, only the impulse to get out of bed; later, motor impulse of the hands; and loquacity only after increase of the motor impulse from 1 November. This time, modification of respiration, which was of a gasping character as in extreme anxiety. Yet anxiety itself was always denied. Paraphasia in loquacity this time more pronounced; nutrition more impaired; the whole attack more severe and increased to temporary fear of approach. Never hallucinations; hypermetamorphosis never marked. Allopsychic orientation only temporarily disordered during extreme restlessness. In the last days before the rapid decline of the illness, flinging, twitching of the arms, which disturbed even voluntary movements. Otherwise, forcible attraction of her attention had a quietening influence similar to that in the first attack. The following sample of her loquacity, from 4 November, shows that ideas of anxiety did exist: "My dear doctor, I am entirely wrong; oh, God in Heaven pity me; Father in Heaven, pity me. Good doctor, help me. Let me out. Heavenly Father, do not forsake me. I am not able. I am perfectly right. You are compassionate. I cannot do differently, oh, dear God. No, no, no, I must go, be merciful. Doctor, you are merciful. Ah, Jesus Christ, pity me. I fail in everything. I have a false judgement. Further on nothing is important. Be merciful to me a sinner. Oh, doctor, forgive me. 1 will gladly follow, here I am damned. You do me great wrong, pity me. Now I stay. Yes, oh, my God and Father, do not forsake me. Doctor, I am unable to save myself. I earnestly pray, do what you will. I am entirely innocent. Thou all good God, pity me. Heavenly Father, pity me. Dear, good doctor, listen to me. Good God, stand by me; pity and be gracious to me. I am a sinful person. Oh pity me, Lord, pity me", etc.

This case is so instructive in many ways that we must linger with it awhile. First of all, it is extremely rare, that a hyperkinetic disorder of identification in the psychomotor tracts is so pure, and uncomplicated by other symptoms. I remember a similar case of a clerk K., 21 years old, who was admitted 27 December, 1894, and released to a provincial mental institution on

21 March, 1895. He had previously manifested a hyperkinetic state for several days, after a spree of excessive drinking, with explanatory delusions of being a gymnast; and he was therefore treated by us for 17 days in November, 1894. It was noticeable that, in this patient, there was no recurrence of rhythmical movements; he was perfectly oriented and no explanatory ideas accompanied with his movements; and he was so conscious of the fact that his attention had been engaged coercively by the movements, that he often answered questions: 'At once', or 'wait', or 'I must first…' In this patient we deal with the same sort of movements to be described in greater detail later. However, this condition intensified further, to a peak of complete confusion, during which he was incapable of remaining fixed in any one place. This was also always accompanied by very severe hypermetamorphosis, unlike the patient previously described. Here the course was not continuous, but the patient had a perfectly lucid interval, with insight into his illness, and signs of exhaustion from 17 to 26 January, 1895, and a second such spell, for just 1 day, with extreme exhaustion on 6 February. We found out later that this patient, after staying for a year in the mental institution, was discharged home. I am indebted to my colleagues for the following information: His illness was recognized in the institution as remitting mania (naturally not mania in our sense); periods of manic, even stormy excitement alternated with ones of calm, where he was still more-or-less confused. Later, the manic paroxysms became shorter and less intense; in periods of quiet his 'presence of mind' [Ed] gradually increased; and insight into his illness developed; the patient improved physically, with a marked increase in weight. From November, 1895 he could be regarded as convalescent, but as a precaution, his being detained in the institution continued during the winter months.

This is the same patient, moreover, from whom the examples of motor loquacity, given earlier in this lecture (p. 227), were obtained.

As for the type of movements, the motor impulse in both the last two patients can be characterized as reactive, while the patients presented first were shown to be executing essentially initiative and expressive motor impulses, just as in gymnastics. The movements in patient W. probably resulted reactively from uncomfortable muscular sensations; this was also largely the case in patient K., although, according to his assertions, there were additional abnormal physical sensations, including a 'tingling' [Ed] throughout the body and pressure in his throat. Transitory panting, blowing and emitting of inarticulate sounds can probably be traced to that statement. In any case, these are aberrant organ feelings, which are the basis of the reactive movements. The similarity to occupational deliria, an intrinsic part of the movements seen, can be easily understood from this point of view, because occupational deliria also arise as reactive movements. However, we will not go wrong, if, in our cases (in contrast to *Delirium tremens* [W]) we interpret the patients' manipulation with randomly presented objects as not actually being induced by these objects, but rather, assume that patients merely take the opportunity that they offer, to discharge their motor impulses in relation to these objects.

The name *jactatoid motor impulse* [W] might be applied in these cases. The similarity of the movements described to those of jactation in an unconscious state is evidently based on the fact, that jactation also is produced by unpleasant organ sensations.

The Affective state was much clearer in patient W. than in the other patients. It is that of 'motor disarray' [Ed], admittedly increased transiently to the point of actual anxiety and despair. Ideas expressing anxiety dated from this time of maximum intensity. We should also regard the temporary occurrence of random, uncoordinated movements as signs of increased intensity of the disease process, while on the other hand, when the illness was significantly abating, an undoubted contradiction was seen with the volitional intentions of patients, which were always soon able to correct the uncoordinated movements.

Gentlemen! It might not be superfluous at this time to mention that severe generalized chorea, which we usually place among the functional nervous diseases, is not so far removed from our topic. Of course, chorea can no longer be understood as a disorder of psychomotor identification, since it exceeds this by far, in that it may exhibit random performance of individual movements, and thus impairment in innate muscular coordination. From the perspective of differential diagnosis I should not omit brief mention of the signs otherwise linked to cases of severe generalized chorea. Corresponding to such discharge of muscular coordinations, patients with chorea also show symptoms of severe paralysis: during pauses in involuntary movement, the head usually drops in a quite unrestrained manner; the trunk can show the same instability, so that standing, walking, and sitting become impossible. If these patients are raised to their feet, they present a picture of most severe ataxia in their every effort to move. Moreover, in such cases, speech generally gives way to stammering and becomes unintelligible, and swallowing may be impossible at times due to paralytic lack of coordination of the tongue. On the other hand, a choreic impulse to crying and uttering of stammering sounds is occasionally manifest. It should be generally known that such cases of severe chorea are very commonly attended by certain manic symptoms: loquacity, flight of ideas, notable lack of embarrassment and thoughtlessness, for instance on matters of seemliness, etc. On the other hand, an abnormally irritable mood and irascibility may prevail [1].

Gentlemen! Knowledge of descriptions of severe generalized chorea, known for example as a dangerous complication of pregnancy, is all the more important in differential diagnosis between it and hyperkinetic motility psychoses, since transitions between the two states occur quite often, as our Case W. proves. We can then designate the form of hyperkinesia observed there, as a *choreic motor impulse* [W]. We can characterize it as an increase in hyperkinesia or, in other words, an overlap of the domains of primary identification. The combined magnitude of motor manifestations (pp. 32, 33) shows itself to be a threat to survival. Such a choreic motor impulse, which actually goes beyond the concept of hyperkinesia, is seen particularly in epileptics and paralytics: In the former it is a component symptom of profoundly dazed conditions, usually post-epileptic and of short duration, lasting a few days at most. In paralytics it is seen in two opposing states, depending on whether it is the initial or terminal stage of the illness. In initial stages of paralysis it corresponds to a mild degree of choreic motor restlessness, which may be largely unilateral, resembling Chorea minor. In terminal stages it is usually a matter of blind rage continuing for weeks; generally movements of the torso, usually performed mutely, apparently in a dazed condition.

Certain *impulsive actions* [W], evidently provide contrasts within these irritative states, and encroach on the motor projection field; their hyperkinetic mode of origin is beyond doubt, according to patients' statements, but also derived from the context of the whole illness. I observed a disease in a 28-year-old, unmarried woman, who presented the same condition unchanged for about 2 years, with certain remissions. During this period, she required constant supervision because, totally without provocation, she was inclined to violent acts—would strike out, throw knives and forks, or pull hair—usually against her female companions, towards whom she was, in fact, well intentioned. These impulsive acts occurred repeatedly, without any external provocation and wholly unexpectedly, and were therefore dangerous. Apart from that, in intervening periods she was perfectly calm and rational, could always be kept in her home, and only occasionally presented smacking movements of her lips, and another symptom that was particularly offensive to her and her relatives, the involuntary utterance of obscene words (*Coprolalia* of other authors). The patient was unable to suppress this, but was able to utter them half-audibly, or her attention could be diverted. This patient suffered an exacerbation of her condition over 8 days, in which a severe choreic motor impulse, as we defined it above, was continuously present. She usually muttered half-audibly and unintelligibly, then suddenly and spontaneously would raise her voice to hurl some insult or obscene expression. Just as suddenly and impulsively, the motor impulse was also interrupted by coordinated actions, in which she suddenly struck, scratched, and pulled the hair of people round about.

The state of exhaustion following this acute attack led to an improvement, which gradually passed into complete recovery.

In this case the impulsive actions, like the speech movements, plainly showed their origin as purposive schemata arising during aberrant irritation, and the patient herself stated later that she had definitely never heard voices or commands. We would do well only to differentiate this type of action, arising within psychomotor functions. Actions brought on by hallucinations or other sensory drives, even if they also occur spontaneously, evidently do not belong here. Especially characteristic of these impulsive actions however, is their kinship with the course of a definite state of psychosis. They then readily become the source of complex explanatory delusions. Thus the first attack of patient K., mentioned above (p. 230), which lasted only 3 days, consisted essentially of his performing gymnastic movements, which led him to imagine being a gymnast, and to develop a sort of grandiose delirium in respect to his personal capacity. Another patient, a 17-year-old baker's apprentice who had always been very pious, suddenly felt the need to kneel down and pray, and he interpreted this as a direct influence from God. A sort of religious grandiosity developed from this, with the admixture of other motility symptoms. He recovered completely. However, it became difficult for him to regain insight into his illness with respect to the first events, and this was delayed, so that such occurrences were still familiar to the patient at the time of complete recovery. Finally I call to mind the doctor of philosophy, who so drastically described to you the events that had taken place prior to his admission. He had suddenly knocked the hat off a totally unknown gentleman, with his cane. This gentleman, a perfect stranger, actually had nothing to do with him, but Dr Sch. claimed that the gentleman must have been a real blackguard, for the dear Lord had suddenly brought about an unpremeditated movement by the patient, raising his cane against him. This topic was on the mind of one of the patients, who believed himself to be continuously hypnotized in the institution (p. 86).

The jactatoid motor impulse of Mrs W. might remind casual observers of cases of disease that bear a superficial resemblance to hers, but are totally different in character. Perhaps we can differentiate a disarrayed motor impulse more correctly by designating it as *disarrayed motor restlessness* [W]. In such cases an intense Affective state of disarray leads to various movements, such as changes of location, restless wandering around, movements of embarrassment and despondency, and to monotonous moaning, clinging to others, etc. These movements have all the signs of psychological motivation, even though they are mediated by an Affective state that may be foreign to normal mental life, as, for example, in somatopsychic disorientation.

Earlier (p. 157) we became acquainted with motor discharges that bore the stamp of senseless rage, as an expression of somatopsychic disarray. The life-threatening movements, motivated in the strange ways of hypochondriacal patient N (p. 159) belong here.

This aimless motor impulse therefore has a basis totally different from that described above (p. 157). In the latter, movements are primary and lead then to disarray. This relationship is also fully expressed in the type of movements. On the other hand, in motor impulses with disarray, the relationship is the other way round: If disarray increases to the point of anxiety and despair, as it does in acute psychoses with an entirely sensory basis, resulting motor manifestations can be understood psychologically, presenting even fewer difficulties.

Gentlemen! For the sake of completeness, I want finally to discuss a type of motor impulse, which is furthest removed from the motor domain, although it is often observed in hyperkinetic motility psychoses. We can indicate it as *hypermetamorphotic motor impulse* [W]. The same process, which directs attention to immediate sensory impressions in an imperative way must, of course, often lead to movements matching these sensory impressions. Thus for example sight of a washing jug and bowl, or a slate brings patients to wash themselves, or to write on the slate. In this way rapid alternation of different actions may be produced, giving the appearance of independent motor impulses. Hyperkinetic motility psychoses, which as already mentioned, are almost always accompanied by hypermetamorphosis, occur in rich combinations with such movements, but also with various states of delirium, as for example in those of progressive paralysis. If sources of hypermetamorphosis are removed by seclusion of patients, such motor impulses subside quite predictably.

Gentlemen! I might use this occasion to set before you the wide diversity of conditions which can induce excesses of movement amongst mentally ill people. You know that more-or-less frenzied behaviour is very common among those who are acutely mentally ill, and may be due to most varied causes. Yet the term 'frenzy' [Ed] implies no kind of diagnosis: It is merely the broadest, best-known, popular expression for a state of restlessness.

Gentlemen! A review of all conditions that may lead to frenzied behaviour amongst mentally ill people will have shown you that concise definition of hyperkinetic motility psychoses faces some difficulties. Therefore I have presented detailed examples of several cases of special 'purity' [Ed]. Always the primary fact, that the movements are not motivated psychologically, and that a manifest impulse to such movements exists, must provide us with the main criterion. But it is in the nature of things, that illness, especially if it is severe, greatly interferes with any closer analysis of how far falsifications of content of consciousness extend, and are not mere consequences of movements; and even the information patients give us subsequently about their condition is often insufficient, because memory deficits may obscure part of the period of a patient's illness. It should then be expected that some cases belonging here are more than pure hyperkinetic motility psychosis, although they are understood in this way, according to signs described above.

If the purest cases possible are taken for guidance, the following may be said about the *course* [W] of the illness. The disease seems to be distinguished by the fact, that it recurs over a number of periods—four, in patients previously mentioned—and then exhausts itself and ends in full recovery. The course is, therefore, periodic and intermittent, with a very rapid sequence and at least short periods of remission. This periodicity is not perfectly regular. One attack, usually the first or the second, is more protracted than the others, and may be brought about by coincidence of two attacks. Prodromes often precede the first attack. These may consist of subjective troubles of various sorts, such as headaches, disturbed sleep, periods of anxiety, and inner restlessness; vasomotor troubles are especially common. The attack itself tends to begin quite suddenly, especially when periods of illness have preceded it. The duration of an individual attack is usually less than a month, except for protracted attacks, which usually correspond to the peak of the illness. Here I want particularly to emphasize that the so-called 'periodic mania' [Ed] of some authors belongs, in most cases, amongst the hyperkinetic motility psychoses.

Aetiologically, the periodic event of menstruation bears the closest relationship to our illness. Next most often, it is found among postpartum women, as the 'puerperal mania' [Ed] of other authors. This corresponds to the fact that the majority of persons so affected are women, and are young. If however the illness occurs in males, it shows a similar periodic, intermittent character, which therefore cannot be exclusively of menstrual aetiology. Common cases with paralytic aetiology provide an exception to the periodic course.

For *differential diagnosis* [W], in essence, we need consider only 'confused mania' [Ed], which usually is similarly periodic and recurrent; and this is to be studied in more detail later. In favour of the latter, a decisive fact is when the hyperkinetic clinical picture is merely an augmentation of pure mania and has demonstrably risen out of it. Moreover, mania is the only illness that presents an actual transition to hyperkinetic motility psychoses, and thus has an internal relationship with the latter. As a consequence of this relationship, differential diagnosis between the two diseases is sometimes impossible. We shall deal with this further when discussing confused mania. Later, we will get to know hyperkinetic motility psychoses as a phase of cyclic motility psychosis, and of periodical hyperkinetic states in the course of a total motility psychosis.

The *prognosis* [W] of the disease is generally favourable, and, as I must state, at odds with most authors, since, with careful treatment, after a number of periods, most cases end in complete recovery. The hereditary or degenerative predisposition which is usually present does not alter this view. Corresponding to preceding ill-health, puerperal hyperkinetic motility psychoses are usually more severe than the menstrual ones. Bromide treatment, as recommended by Krafft-Ebing [2], has never achieved anything substantial in my experience, nor has it in cases of menstrual psychoses. Moreover, the special aetiology is thoroughly decisive for the prognosis, so that the paralytic form here leads to dementia, as it does in other paralytic psychoses. This is true in cases of hyperkinetic motility psychoses, which occur in the course of a real hebephrenia or other chronic, hebephrenic degenerative psychoses. The dangers of hyperkinetic motility psychoses are chiefly the loss of energy from the continued muscular exertion, and the ever-present insomnia; and the continuous motor impulse adds essential impairment to nutritional status. States of sudden collapse are therefore commonly seen. Furthermore, there are injuries that patients incur through their violent movements; in particular, there is difficulty in carrying out aseptic treatment of these injuries.

Only in rare cases can *treatment* [W] be based on aetiology. I remember a case of this kind, corresponding to the boundary between our disease and confused mania. It was that of a 15-year-old girl, who had not yet menstruated, but repeatedly presented vasomotor symptoms of a worrisome nature. Periodical recurrence of attacks about every 4 weeks and the added vasomotor symptoms in these attacks persuaded me to apply leeches to the inner surfaces of both thighs during the third intermission, whereby the first menstrual flow was actually established, and further attacks prevented. The girl has remained healthy since then (about 8 years ago). Use of narcotics in the hyperkinetic motility psychoses is generally contraindicated. Almost all sleeping pills fail. Hyoscine seems to have a specific action on motor hyperkinesia, often in surprisingly small doses of ¼–½ mg. administered subcutaneously. Owing to this sedative action hyoscine is also the best hypnotic in these cases. Apart from bed rest, in so far as it is practical—use of warm baths, prolonged over several hours, and permanent under certain conditions, usually has a favourable effect. Hospital treatment can only very rarely be dispensed with.

References

1. Wernicke C. Krankenvorstellungen aus der psychiatrischen Klinik in Breslau. Breslau: Schletter; 1899. vol 2, Case 13 is a typical example of severe chorea.
2. von Krafft-Ebing R. Lehrbuch der Psychiatrie auf klinischer Grundlage für praktische Ärzte und Studierende. 4th ed. Stuttgart: Enke; 1890. p. 572–3.

Lecture 33

33

- Confused mania or agitated confusion
- Escalation of intrapsychic hyperfunction to confusion
- Different grades of flight of ideas
- Admixture of sensory and motor excitatory symptoms
- Clinical picture
- Meynert's *Amentia*
- Asthenic confusion as a phase of confused mania and as a stand-alone illness

Lecture

Gentlemen!

By *confused mania* [W] we wish to identify a clinical picture that is manifest as an exaggeration, imposed at a peak of mania, and presenting as its external signs a motor impulse and conspicuous loquacity with confused content; but, in addition, as soon as we analyze its individual symptoms, it can certainly present with entirely different components. Crucial to our approach is therefore the practical and clinical perspective, that this is an acute psychosis, which can begin and end as mania, but in intervals between peaks of illness, which may predominate overwhelmingly, it often loses some typical features of mania and, in their place, acquires all manner of strange admixtures. In this complex clinical picture, the chief signs derived from mania, are flight of ideas, loquacity, and motor impulse. The foreign elements that are added range between two extremes, sometimes in pure form, usually in combination, are either psychosensory or psychomotor disorders of identification, dominated by symptoms of irritation. If confused mania is to be regarded as an independent illness, as is often in fact justified, when the initial or end stages of pure mania are only very short in duration, it could be called *agitated confusion* [W], and its subdivisions could be differentiated as confusion with sensory or motor agitation. In the first case agitation is based on an essentially reactive motor and speech impulse, that is, on those that can be traced back to sensory states of irritation; in the second case it takes on the guise of a hyperkinetic motility psychosis. In the vast majority of cases these two contrasting sets of phenomena occur in combination. The rarer exceptions are mainly purely sensory cases; existence of purely hyperkinetic ones must remain questionable.

The preceding brief empirical principles may indicate to you the range within which we can manoeuvre. Such defining of boundaries is essential, because frequently you will find 'confusion' [Ed] described under the headings of 'primary confusion' [Ed] or 'dissociative confusion' [Ed] (according to Ziehen) [1], as an actual illness. Usually all that is thus designated is the respective state of a patient, in whom we always still have the task of determining the individual elements that lead to the state of confusion. In so

R. Miller, K.J. Dennison (eds.), *An Outline of Psychiatry in Clinical Lectures*,
DOI 10.1007/978-3-319-18051-9_33

doing we will at least have to raise the claim that confusion, as a symptom of stimulation—that is, one connected to flight of ideas and loquacity—is separated in principal from the corresponding state of deficit—that is simple incoherence by sejunction (dissociation). Only the first case would call for special consideration, in the task before us.

You may thus conclude that, despite this difficulty, I am motivated purely by empirical considerations, because generally, with a consensus all too rare in our discipline, the internal connection between mania and confusion, and the frequent transition of one into the other, has been accepted and is taught. I refer only to Meynert, who earlier (that is before the appearance of his clinical lectures) had even gone so far as to see every acute psychosis that we would call mania arising from a state of confusion, by way of weakened associations, leading to the clinical picture of Amentia, which he himself analyzed so masterfully; while later he designated under mania cases of illness that differ not significantly from our 'pure mania' [Ed]. What Meynert has expressed on this occasion about flight of ideas and associative weaknesses belongs among the most extreme views written by this thinker on psychological questions. Without being able to follow him completely, I would still try to shell out the kernel of this and make it useful for our purpose. My comments about the flight of ideas in mania summarized above—all too briefly—will thereby be complete. I disregard the fact that the basis will be vasomotor flux, or functional hyperaemia, a consequence of nutritive attraction as Meynert expresses it, an action produced by association fibres, corresponding to the 'closed thought pathway' between an idea being registered—Meynert's 'attack idea' [W]—and the idea of its 'objective' [Ed]. For our purpose, we may disregard vasomotor influences and be satisfied that, also according to Meynert, the closed train of thought is a functional acquisition pointing towards a most minute localization in definite anatomical elements. We rely upon the fact of pathways well-worn by use, which consequently have become more ready to respond and more excitable, in comparison to the others. Overvaluation of certain ideas—accepted by us—and the 'closed train of thought' [Ed], also have a definite internal connection, according to Meynert's formulation [2]. The majority of associations, are located within ordered thought processes characterized by Meynert as 'large, widely branched, long, profoundly and strongly coordinated', [W] and find their counterpart in simply coordinated 'narrow, brief, unbranched, weakly and shallowly ordered, aimless' [W] associations. 'The association intensity corresponds to the molecular tissue attraction as a source of strength. The mass of arching fibres, within which two sources of force, that of the idea of an "objective" and that of the initial idea, tend towards each other, as it were, in the act of thinking, always attaining vital force for elevation above the threshold of consciousness from two ideally centralized cortical areas; but the secondary association arises from only one of these areas: either that of the "objective" [Ed] or that of the initial idea, according to whether for example the rhyme fits its word picture. Functional attraction is the weaker here, and is inhibited by the stronger.' What is here called 'tissue attraction' [Ed], we again designate as increased excitability. If we disregard such functional differences of excitability in the functions of the organ of association, the primordial condition of the childlike brain—Meynert's 'genetic confusion' [W]), in which any given association is possible—reappears to some extent, and may be retained for a while, because anatomically preformed combinations exist between any two given cortical areas. Different gradations of 'flight of ideas' [Ed] can then increase to the highest grade, which, for us, represents disjointedness or incoherence, when, after uniform and general increase of excitability, individual differences between various association pathways are largely obliterated. It is such confusion, arising from an exaggeration of mania that we have in mind when we recognize the clinical picture of confused mania. A decisive criterion for this is the state of irritation evidently present, seen as loquacity and motor impulse, and—in the absence of any actual deficit—in the breakdown of associations. Therefore it remains possible for patients to fixate their attention momentarily, when they are given external stimulation, and likewise by their being given increased motor force; and they may even occasionally be amenable to more complex trains of thought. In other words, previously acquired contents of consciousness remain essentially untouched.

We must thereby return to the difference between activity and content of consciousness. Yet every ordering in contents of consciousness consists of gradations of excitability acquired by practice, in which total dissolution would have to occur of the contents of consciousness into their simplest elements, that is, into fragments. The immediate consequence of this must be total disorientation in all three domains of consciousness, which should appear in the same way in the contents of the loquacity, as it does in the way a patient's motor impulse becomes manifest. However, in confused mania we require that the levelling of ideas does not go beyond the autopsychic domain: No actual symptoms of deficit should appear with regard to the external world and to corporeality; yet even in the autopsychic domain we will no longer include in confused mania those states of the so-called confusion in which real deficits in contents of consciousness are demonstrable as reactions, such as when time is no longer correctly perceived, or when a person fails to be able to make a tally of different coins, even when given sufficient attention. These must be classed amongst the more severe clinical pictures.

In a word, we must try to confine the clinical picture of confused mania to those cases which do not actually show a close connection in their course with mania, but also, according to the degree of confusion, which appear just as a further increase of intrapsychic hyperfunction; that is, the incoherence, to whatever degree it reaches, remains largely a formal disturbance, without resulting in more severe deficit states for contents of consciousness. Evidence that such deficits do not exist can be gained from the fact that it is sometimes possible to elicit reactive statements from patients, showing their retaining the possibility of ordered trains of thought, albeit only exceptionally, and with special efforts to sustain attention (by the influence of the process which Meynert calls 'partial wakefulness' [Ed]). No firmer view can therefore be gained from the fact of incoherence in the flight of ideas, seen in the spontaneous loquacity of these patients; yet the patients' reactive statements can then themselves be judged correctly only when the fact of their constant diversion by internal irritation is taken into account.

If we recapitulate our views about the flight of ideas as expressing intrapsychic hyperfunction, we can differentiate three grades: The first and the second, the ordered and the disordered flight of ideas, are both peculiar to mania and determined more fully by accompanying abnormal euphoria. Moreover, the contained, closed train of thought—the *ordered* [Ed] flight of ideas—has the characteristic that it is organized essentially by its content, whereas the disordered flight is determined more by similarity of word sound, rhyme, assonances, sequences, etc. In the incoherent form—or flight of ideas of the third grade—which characterizes confused mania, word similarity and sequences likewise play a large part, but this can also extend to every comprehensible connection of the sequence of words brought up during loquacity, or only fragments of words, which are lost to us. An example of disordered flight of ideas is taken from a later demonstration [3] of one of our cases of mania, Miss P. To my question: 'Was your admission necessary?[she replied literally: '*Was it* necessary Professor? *Am I* the girl from *Wahrendorf*? *Were you then* in the village or in the city? Are you educated, reared, trained in the village? Or are you a *relic piece*, or what are you really, or *which piece* will you have? A rib, liver, a pair of feet or a couple of pickled ham hocks, brawn, ah, brawn perhaps? A bit of jelly perhaps?' In this example the jump to the relic piece is confined to incoherence, while we are well able to follow the mechanism of the combination of ideas.

Gentlemen! Confused mania in our strict sense occurs in rare cases as the acme of a single attack of pure mania and is then usually of shorter duration than the pure mania. It is encountered much more often in recurrent mania, and especially in cases of periodical mania, that is those cases in which relapses follow one another with actual periodicity. Most often, we encounter menstrually related periodic mania, usually appearing pre-menstrually, which we may certainly regard literally as a type of 'periodic' [Ed] mania. As an example of an irregularly-recurrent confused mania, I remind you of the case of Miss F., 37 years old, presented some time ago, who passed through her 23rd attack since age 20, and is now held in a provincial secure unit, where she is generally free from relapses. At the time of presentation she appeared to be extremely buoyant in her mood, but still irritable: she could not stop laughing; overwhelmed me with reproaches; uttered a stream of verbiage, which could hardly be interrupted; and her loquacity, unintelligible as it was, seemed to be determined in part by similarities of its content. Her motor impulse was largely manifest as an excess of expressive movements, used in part to express her dislike for me. With arms akimbo, body bent forward like a scolding door-to-door saleswoman, she made various grimaces towards me, stuck out her tongue, first approached, then stepped back; in short she enacted a sort of domestic scene with me, in which she did not spare her filthy remarks. She seemed to correctly recognize place and persons, although her conduct seemed to be controlled by some grandiose ideas, without confused loquacity providing any fuller explanation. Usually isolated, she became inaccessible to physical examination. She stripped off her clothing and was usually found naked, untidy, smeared food about, refused it in part, and occasionally showed a fear of being approached. Occasionally it was noticed that she started singing when under evident stress, for she had become hoarse because of her loquacity. Furthermore, there were many aimless movements, for example violent clapping of her hands and peculiar twisting movements of her torso. This condition had developed over the course of a few days from a form of pure mania, continued for about 14 days and then gradually passed into a state of calm, but also of exhaustion, after which the patient was able to impart intelligent information to us. You will remember the astonishing, unexpected content she gave us of her experiences. She felt that she was filled with supernatural strength and a feeling of happiness, which only occasionally gave way to anxious ideas. The strength of all departed souls was in her, and it was an abundance of thoughts which prompted her to talk. At first the situation seemed to her to be the time of resurrection, then to be a religious war, in which she believed that, by her intercession, she was called upon to decide the fight between good and evil. Her present experiences seemed to her to correspond with certain prophecies in the Bible. Innumerable voices of relatives, former pupils and their mothers, who she recognized by the sound of their voices, though unseen, were standing by her side to fight for her. She saw deceased persons as skeletons that moved, as well as dark forms whose likeness she had never seen before. All these could not harm her. She knew quite well where she was, yet she saw heaven and enlarged stars, saw angels, and could reach the sky with her hand. On the other hand, she often saw an entirely strange country in front of her, an unknown part of the earth, probably where evil spirits lived. She believed that she recognized relatives in fellow patients. Physicians and attendants, recognized as such, were representations of evil; she believed that I was the incarnation of evil; to fight against her I would kill her brothers. Also, gentlemen, she ascribed a hostile intent to you. She often believed that her food contained poison. Occasionally, she was anxious and had to sing. Her movements were such that she felt there was a snake in her body; its head stuck into her. When she closed her eyes she saw the snake, slender and glistening. She often put bread into her ears to feed the snake. She stripped off her clothes because they were poisoned by contact with the snake. One day, the snake was voided with her stool, and then calm prevailed. She poured milk into the toilet bowl to feed the snake. The snake was Eve's serpent and signified Original Sin. By suggestive questions it was ascertained that she believed that she was the Virgin Mary, made pregnant by the Holy Ghost.

At the time of these communications she had complete insight into her illness, and for a long time, she was then free from recurrences. Apart from recurrences, there had been representative 'vicarious melancholias' [Ed]. The connection of this clinical picture with mania is evident, even if only the beginning, but not the end of the recurrence corresponded to mania. Previous attacks of the illness, especially the first, which appeared along with menstruation, were pure manias. Actual disorientation in the allopsychic area never occurred; in the autopsychic area it had characteristics of grandiose delirium, understandable in the context of mania—this having religious coloration, corresponding with the patient's personality; and in the somatic domain, disorientation consisted essentially of abnormal sensations, perhaps linked with menstruation, and an explanatory delusion for the pseudospontaneous movements, particularly of her trunk. That this delusional explanation took on the form of a sensation and a vision, has numerous analogies elsewhere.

Another example of confused mania of which I remind you, was the case of Miss B., a periodic menstrual psychosis, which recurred six times in all, but then declined, never to return over the next 4 years. The regularity with which the manic attacks always heralded approaching menstruation, and the prevailing opinion that such cases were incurable, led us to propose removing her ovaries as a remedy, a procedure thwarted essentially by opposition from her relatives. The patient has now recovered without such an intervention, permanently I hope, for I have often had the same experience, that periodic mania, as we understand it, exhausts itself after three to eight recurrences, like the periodically-recurrent hyperkinetic motility psychoses. At the time she presented during the second attack, she showed a largely manic picture: confused loquacity, arising from incoherent flight of ideas, only a moderate motor impulse, but a very changeable mood, often suddenly transformed to dejection or anxiety, and certainly with anxious phonemes. Moreover, hyperkinetic symptoms were added more prominently than in the previous case, consisting of expressive movements of anxiety and despair, unmotivated raising of the voice, etc. In addition, a very marked hypermetamorphosis existed. Recovery in this case was accomplished, and in that the last attacks acquired a form more of pure mania, while the first attack, even more than the second just described, bore an overwhelming stamp of hyperkinetic motility psychosis. Allopsychic orientation in this case was completely intact. The course of periodic puerperal mania in Mrs. Cz., who I presented to you in her fifth attack, was similar. The main features of the clinical pictures consisted of incoherent flight of ideas manifested in occasional repartee; unrestrained, exalted mood, and correspondingly exaggerated expressive movements, desire for action expressed by tearing and smearing, unrestrained conduct, with addition of motor hyperkinesia, acting like a chansonette artist; and hypermetamorphosis. Preceding attacks had a form more akin to hyperkinetic motility psychoses, while the following sixth attack and last attack was purely manic followed by permanent restitution, once a stage of exhaustion had passed. This patient always remained perfectly orientated in the allopsychic domain.

Confused mania, in the sense we give to the name, does not by any means embrace all cases of the so-called periodic mania. Quite often, attacks of periodic mania do indeed correspond to the clinical picture outlined, yet allopsychic disorientation is also present, manifested as failure to recognize—or mistaking—the place of a situation or persons, often even objects. The three cases just described teach us that such allopsychic disorientation need not follow from marked incoherence in the flight of ideas. We will therefore proceed correctly, if we regard such cases not as confused mania, but as *periodic manic allopsychosis* [W]—and they are often also totally sensory psychoses.

Gentlemen! Permit me at this time to make a few comments on the clinical picture of Amentia, or acute confusion, outlined by Meynert. I have repeatedly indicated how important I consider Meynert's clinical lectures to be; in my opinion, they have provided the foundation for better understanding of the symptomatology of acute mental illnesses. However, it must be expressly stated that Meynert also succumbed to the general fate of other authors, who have laboured hard in their monographs in certain provinces in our discipline: He has embraced, under the term 'amentia' [Ed], a great number of acute psychoses that are fundamentally different. This is already intimated in the title of the section, where we find, as synonyms of amentia, the terms: 'acute insanity, general insanity, mania, frenzy, melancholia with excitement, melancholia with apathy of other authors'. However, you will also find transitory psychoses, the so-called twilight states and other conditions discussed in this chapter. Apart from amentia, Meynert then differentiates only melancholia and mania as specially acute psychoses. Nevertheless, the chapter on amentia is of lasting value for all time, and indicates the greatest advance psychiatry has made clinically since Kahlbaum's work on catatonia, since it contains the first real theory of mental illnesses and especially of acute psychoses, founded on hypotheses derived entirely from the condition of the affected organ. You can judge how far Meynert approximates the standpoint that I have always advocated in these demonstrations, from the fact that he always places in the foreground symptoms of functional deficit, that is the different grades of weakening of associations, and he considers symptoms of irritation to be a consequence of these. In just the same way, I have represented sejunction as the fundamental process, and derived symptoms of irritation from this. If I have often differed in detail from Meynert in how I carry out of this principle, the future will reveal how far this has been justified, and was required, unconditionally, in relation to clinical facts. I might emphasize specifically only that Meynert's amentia, according to his own description, may embrace all cases of illness that I described as acute autopsychosis, allopsychosis, somatopsychosis, motility psychosis, and their combinations; and that, from a clinical standpoint, it is necessary to postulate corresponding degrees of weakening of associations in Meynert's sense. The situation may arise, that the firmest associative links exist in the domain of consciousness of the body, the next firmest in consciousness of the environment, and the loosest—and likewise the latest to be acquired, with the greatest individual differences—in consciousness of personhood. Correspondingly, a similar measure of severity of illness, or, according to Meynert's concept, of general weakness of association, is always manifested first in the autopsychic region, and second and third in allopsychic and somatopsychic domains. If the phenomenon of confusion alone is kept in mind, this idea would correspond in some measure to the facts.

Gentlemen! I can accept a clinical picture of primary confusion only to a limited degree, when confusion consists of a deficit state shown as actual incoherence. We should have to consider as its signs the demonstrable exhaustibility of ideation either in absolute failure of flight of ideas, or at times when failure of flight of ideas is appearing. Doubtless there are those conditions, in which patients can occasionally fixate momentarily, and can be motivated to produce reactive movements or expressions; but these are always those of the simplest kind or are responses to intense impulses, by a sort of 'whipping-up' [Ed] of attentiveness. Incoherence in spontaneous expressions of these patients shows itself to be independent of loquacity and motor impulse. More complex questions and commands remain evidently not understood, without degradation of the sensorium being responsible. These patients always tend to be disorientated in allopsychic terms. Significant Affective reactions are absent. In consequence of the evident failure of associative activity—so that, apparently, the excitatory stimulus could be conducted to the more remote links of the association chain only with difficulty or not at all; and—to express the contrast with agitated confusion—these conditions might be called *asthenic confusion* [W]. Actually, they are usually accompanied by other symptoms of weakness, attention being captured only with difficulty, with considerable degradation of memory retention, along with general physical weakness and reduced state of nutrition. Such a picture of asthenic confusion, which can be accompanied by all manner of symptoms of sensory irritation, is often found to be a consequence of other acute exhaustive psychoses, or phases of such, but could not be referred to as primary confusion.

Gentlemen! If, to do justice to clinical facts, we must acknowledge confused mania as an independent clinical picture, and find its essential sign as an increase of the intrapsychic hyperfunction to the point of *incoherent* [Ed] flight of ideas, we cannot consider it accidental, that such conditions tend to occur especially after severe attacks of confused mania or agitated confusion. I might assign such cases to the highest grade of weakened association described by Meynert, which he compares to genetic confusion (see above). Two cases of this sort, for which more precise data exist, presented with asthenically recognizable signs, and with physical decline as well: That is, there was a completely quiet, affectless state of mind, and only occasional unmotivated grimacing, and absence of spontaneous utterances or movements. Simple commands, like raising the hand, poking out the tongue, standing up, and so on, are understood and obeyed. Likewise, simple questions such as name, age and other personal details were answered promptly. On the other hand, going beyond this, some tasks requiring combination could not be performed. For instance, numbers to which the big and little hands of the clock point are given correctly, yet the time is not known. Coins are named correctly, accurately counted, yet their value could not be computed. A simple route, through different streets which are perfectly familiar to the patient, cannot be described. However, enumeration of serial associations or simple, memorized material, like the Lord's Prayer, is carried out well. Attentiveness is relatively good; memory retention badly impaired. Places and situations are not recognized, and neither are persons, who would have been known before the illness. This goes so far that the physician, for instance, is claimed to be the mother, while later, when the state of weakness has abated, other more subtle mistakes come to the fore. Hence, there is no subjective feeling of inadequacy, not even a sufficient sense of physical weakness, no insight into the illness in the preceding attack of mania. For the latter, mainly, there is amnesia. With respect to the decline, over time, this state of weakness exists at a severe degree only for a few days, followed then by gradual restoration, along with simultaneous increase in strength and weight. Admittedly, the condition of apparent recovery lasted for only a few days, because a very acute relapse then occurred. In the menstrual psychosis of Miss B, described above, states of exhaustion after the first and second relapse occurred on two occasions in almost identical manner.

It is easy to interpret the allopsychic disorientation in such a case as a symptom of exhaustion, occurring in an area of content of consciousness that had previously exhibited active irritation, shown as hallucinations; so the disturbance of identification, the psychosensory paraesthesia and anaesthesia could be traced back to defective excitability of allopsychic contents of consciousness. At any rate it would be justifiable for us to regard the demonstrable weakness of association as a state of exhaustion of the intrapsychic pathways, a transformation of heightened excitability into a lowering of excitability. Thereby the weakness of association postulated by Meynert (see p. 236 above) would turn out to belong not to mania itself, but to be a consequence of mania appearing only during an unusually severe abnormal process.

Gentlemen! You have seen the internal connection of such inter-dependent clinical pictures, and I certainly believe that the stages of exhaustion substitute for confused mania. My views are less certain in support of a *primary asthenic confusion* [W], which can occur as an independent illness for many months, and can then be followed by complete recovery. In one case of this kind, the principal characteristics of the state of exhaustion were found as previously described, namely a certain defect in spontaneity; failure of ideation in more complex demands; attentiveness retained just through excitement; but very poor memory retention and simultaneous allopsychic disorientation, accompanied by symptoms of motor and sensory irritation of moderate nature. In other words, pseudospontaneous movements occurred that were monotonous but not rhythmic, along with phonemes and hypermetamorphosis. Significant Affective reactions were absent. The course was remitting, combined with akinetic symptoms for a few days at the height of the illness. The patient, a poorly developed, 20-year-old youth, has not had a relapse for 4 years. I might confine myself to mentioning such cases here, emphasizing only that precisely the same symptom complex should be called 'acute primary asthenic confusion' [Ed], and understood as such.

Gentlemen! To demarcate such cases it would be well to remember the old differentiation between habitual forms and actual illnesses advocated especially by Kahlbaum [4]. The state of exhaustion described above is evidently not to be regarded as an actual illness, but shows us asthenic confusion as a habitual form or, as recently termed, a disorder. Cases of the last-described kind are, on the other hand, examples of an independent and primary exhausting *illness* [Ed], certainly in the state of asthenic confusion.

The condition—or habitual form—of asthenic confusion could also be further conceived, as it has been here. I have often seen cases of weakened association, with autopsychic and allopsychic deficit symptoms, but no motor excitatory symptoms (therefore: 'asthenic autoallopsychoses' [Ed]) in very acutely ill young girls; and furthermore, whose outcome is always one of complete recovery, even if only after a long-lasting paranoid state. However, these cases had the peculiarity, that in contrast to a relatively poor attentiveness, which was hard to capture, memory retention was surprisingly good.

References

1. Ziehen GT. Neurol Centralbl. 1891;10:644.
2. Meynert T. Klinische Vorlesungen über Psychiatrie auf wissenschaftlichen Grundlagen für Studierende und Aerzte, Juristen und Psychologen. Vienna: Braumüller; 1890.
3. Wernicke C. Krankenvorstellungen aus der psychiatrischen Klinik in Breslau. Breslau: Schletter; 1899. vol 1, Case 5.
4. Kahlbaum KL. Die Katatonie oder das Spannungsirresein. Berlin: A Hirschwald; 1874.

Lecture 34

34

- Examples of akinetic motility psychosis
- General impassivity
- Negativism
- *Flexibilitas cerea*
- Muscular rigidity
- Persistence in positions
- Parakinetic behaviour in standing and walking
- Verbigeration
- Pseudo-flexibilitas
- Behaviour of the sensorium
- Catalepsy
- *Melancholia attonita* or *cum stupore*
- Kahlbaum's catatonia
- Course of the illness
- Outcomes

Lecture

Gentlemen!

When any impairment in motility—in other words, any state of general immobility—is manifest, we can learn nothing from this fact about the patient's internal processes, his state of mind, and current ideation. Facial expressions leaves us none the wiser, for akinesia often extends through this aspect of expressive movements, so that a simple 'demented' [Ed] expression may be the result of the *absence* [Ed] of any expression. As a consequence, it is not possible to present a pure case of akinetic motility psychosis from the clinic; or at least, we cannot be sure that the case is pure, until the patient returns from a motionless state to give us information about his internal processes. This awkward position is, of course, merely the result of our lack of knowledge, and we must not despair of succeeding later on in recognizing, from its own definite and specific signs, a pure akinetic state. At the time of when immobility actually exists from its own definite and specific signs. However, at present I must limit myself to singling out a few examples of akinetic motility psychosis, as can best be used for teaching purposes. For this it might be most suitable to report on Frau K. (p. 223 *seq*), who I presented to you in a stage of remission from a hyperkinetic motility psychosis. This patient then progressed to a state of general immobility, interrupted by only brief periods of hyperkinesia; the immobility has been presented as permanent, because a loss of basic strength indicated that an unfavourable outcome was likely, and yet, it was actually transitory. She is therefore an example of the akinetic phase of a 'cyclical motility psychosis' [Ed], in which both phases are involved, rather than the motility phase alone. The report of the demonstration runs as follows:

The patient is brought in on a portable bed and placed at the front of the auditorium.

The patient is left to her own devices: She lies on her back in bed, with head raised a little on her

R. Miller, K.J. Dennison (eds.), *An Outline of Psychiatry in Clinical Lectures*,
DOI 10.1007/978-3-319-18051-9_34

pillow. Her eyes are rigid without fixating on anything; blinking is rare. Facial features are flat, corresponding to a state of exhaustion, somewhat distorted by a half-open mouth, lowered at its corners.

Behaviour on external stimulation: When the patient's name is called repeatedly and loudly, and even when she is grasped by the arm, the sole reaction to be seen is an increased frequency of blinking. Her eyes remain unchanging, continuing to stare into space, and not directed towards the examiner.

Maintenance of imposed postures: When I elevate her right arm, there is very marked resistance, which gradually subsides to become more pliable ('waxy flexibility' [Ed]). Her arms remain in any position given to them, even if these are uncomfortable, until they are put in some other position. It is especially surprising that this patient, despite her evident weakness, holds her elbow fixed at a right angle and somewhat abducted at the shoulder, for a long time, totally without support.

Another behaviour can be seen in her lower limbs: As the lower leg is grasped and moved back and forth, the entire pelvis moves as well (that is, muscular rigidity of the pelvis–thigh muscles, as in spastic spinal paralysis). In addition, her legs are perfectly flaccid, and, when elevated, fall immediately under gravity. Her head is also freely and easily moveable in all directions. On the other hand, attempts to prise apart her mandible from her upper jaw meets with very stiff resistance, and similarly, later on, it is impossible to separate her eyelids, when they are kept closed after her outbreak of crying.

Reflex behaviour: Tendon reflexes in her legs are normal; those in her arms definitely exaggerated. Reflex excitability of cutaneous capillaries is normal.

On pricking the soles of her feet with a needle, the patient reacts promptly by dorsiflexion of the toes, then of the whole foot. On *repeated* [Ed] pricking she turns and twists it back and forth, and finally withdraws it by flexing her knees. As she does so, she wrinkles her eyebrows somewhat, and her face betrays the hint of a painful expression.

On pricking her hands, very similar behaviour is seen. Initially they are turned back and forth, but are not withdrawn, although they are in no way restrained, being allowed to rest freely on the open palms of the examiner. The right hand in particular is not withdrawn.

On pricking her cheeks, nose, and lips with a needle, she contorts her face in a markedly painful way and starts to cry with suppressed sobs. Thus, reactive akinesia can be interrupted by painful irritation.

The patient is requested to sit up, but remains immobile, so she is raised up in bed.

Reaction of the patient to incentives for activating movement: When requested to stand up, she moves her legs a little as though attempting it, but falls backward with her trunk in a recumbent posture. She is then raised up again to a sitting position, whereupon, in spite of a proven good intention, she crosses her legs in a totally inappropriate manner. On further encouragement she attempts to get up, but succeeds only with considerable assistance. She is now taken by the hand and led around the room, offering no resistance, although at each step she must be given a slight tug on the hand. Her gait is of a clockwork character, individual steps being separated by marked pauses. In standing, her knees are slightly bent, feet together, and she sways back and forth, but does not adopt a stable position on her feet.

When she is requested over and over again to walk, she begins to lean forward slowly; but, once her centre of gravity is outside her centre of balance, suddenly, and unexpectedly, she begins to run. This movement accelerates in a manner similar to propulsion in *Paralysis agitans* [W], and is clearly interpreted as preventing a forward fall, threatened by her initial inclination. In her path she reaches her bed, lets herself fall onto it, and lies, with proper decorum, on her side.

When once again, she is stood up, the patient, who has not stopped sobbing since being pricked with the needle, sways markedly, yet is supported by a female attendant, and apart from blinking more often, does not react in any way to demands made of her. She has to be put back to bed again, and is carried out.

It had been established in this patient, that during the hyperkinetic phase and in transitional periods between the opposite phases, in addition to motility, her orientation was affected by the disease, in all three areas of consciousness. I therefore chose the next case chiefly because she represents an unusually pure example of akinetic—or rather parakinetic—symptoms by themselves, while orientation remains quite normal; and not so much as a hint could be found in this female patient - who readily provided us with any information we required - of any explanatory delusions. Apart from headaches, any abnormal sensations about which the patient complained were probably exclusively aberrant ones from muscles, or ones of position, therefore to be classed amongst disorders of psychomotor identification (see later). The case involved a 47-year-old spinster, sister of a physician, so that her retrospective statements are unusually reliable.

Until the beginning of her illness, she had been a science teacher in a middle school, had no heredity taint, was formerly in good health, and became ill in September, 1897, in connection with menstruation. Her difficulties were thought initially to be hysterical, but increased over a few weeks to a state of general immobility. Tube feeding was needed for some weeks. Akinesia gradually remitted but stereotyped movements appeared. In place of mutism, there was verbigeration, but no real hyperkinesia. Encouragement and verbal suggestion led to improvement in her speech. There was then a cessation of all symptoms, giving us hope of full restitution. However, a relapse occurred in October 1898, similar to the present one, but worse, according to the patient's own statement. Her left hand became constantly clenched into a fist. After a few weeks, there was another remission, with progressive improvement almost to the point of free mobility. According to her physician brother she was then apparently normal for a few weeks. Three to four weeks ago, another relapse took place, again coinciding with onset of menstruation. According to the patient, it is now becoming worse, day by day.

Condition on 8 May, 1899: Nutrition level good, distorted features; organs and bodily functions in good order. Patient sits in a fixed position, left hand on the crown of her head, eyes straight ahead, paper and pencil lying on the table in front of her. Expression unhappy, perplexed; outburst of tears on seeing her brother. Facial expression not fixed, changing in comprehensible ways during the course of the examination. Patient stands up spontaneously, seizes paper and pencil in the right hand, indicates that she wants to go to the next room, her usual abode, sits there in her accustomed place, eyes directed to a fixed place on the opposite wall. This gaze is maintained forcibly, so that she looks neither at the questioner, nor down when she is writing. All answers are in writing, hastily written with the lead pencil in abbreviated form: For instance, to the question, 'why so excited?' [Ed]:—'Can't help it'. Complete mutism, yet, with urging, she attempts to repeat, but with evident effort. Instead of pronouncing the auditioned word 'Anna', prolonged verbigeration took place of the syllable 'ruh-ruh…', finally to be lost in toneless, rhythmic repetition of 'r-r'. She denies that she can poke out her tongue; but then, after several attempts, succeeds spasmodically for an instant. Instead of written answers, often makes intelligent gestures, which she otherwise prefers to employ. However, both hands are usually occupied: one is always pressed to the back part of the crown of her head, the other, with its index finger extended, rhythmically taps some part of the body, face, trunk, or thighs.

Q: What is on the head?
'Inside'; 'now pricks many times', 'fine nerves', 'sickness', 'worse every day', 'worse after eating'.
Q: Why is your hand held there?
'Not let loose, otherwise falls back', 'as if it breaks'.
Q: Can she otherwise move freely?
'Fingers held to a point'.
Q: What are your other complaints?
'Great restlessness when eating', 'nerve weakness', 'restlessness during the day', 'must often pass water', 'no will power', 'no help'.

Stress and many sleeping drugs were given as the cause of the illness. Had been worse in October. The following are excerpts from the patient's written statements: She must cry, is confused, complains of restlessness, but not of anxiety, knows and understands everything, can write, but the examination strains her, it is hard for her to keep her eyes open. The brain is sound, only the brain nerves are sick. Writes name, age; that she has menstruated every 3 weeks. She definitely denies external influences, electricity, secret forces, and voices. When she closes her eyes, she sees bright colours. She must be watched, when she closes her eyes.

She leans back as if exhausted, closes her eyes, lets her right hand fall over the arm of the sofa, the left remaining on her head. The right hand now makes rhythmical convulsive movements. On my remarking that this is involuntary, a fleeting look of thanks, patient grasps my hand with her right and carries it to her mouth to kiss it. On passive removal of the left hand from her head—but at times spontaneously also—the right hand replaces the left on her head. However, the right hand is always used for any activities, although the left is freely movable. However, she is unable to offer me her right hand on leaving, making helpless gestures instead. Spontaneous gestures are few, then hasty, most often changing location as a result of inner restlessness. No flexibility. Patient must be waited upon, but is tidy, and willingly fed with a spoon. Sleep and nutrition good. Full understanding of the situation, becoming dependent on her 'care-giver', satisfactory interest and memory of daily events.

With some resistance the patient is brought to sit in a chair by the window and to fixate on a finger held before her; and for a moment she seems able to move her eyes voluntarily, yet the haste with which she strives to return her gaze to their former direction prevents a definite statement. As for the relationship that a certain spot on the wall has with her eye movements, it is impossible to learn anything positive despite all efforts. She tries to convey by various gestures that such a relationship does indeed exist; but she definitely denies that it is a command, electricity, magnetism, or some secret force.

It is very rare that such good information can be obtained in akinetic motility psychosis during its actual presence. Evidently it is possible only when the area of akinesia is as circumscribed as in this patient. However, this circumscribed condition is correspondingly rare amongst acutely ill cases.

Several more examples of akinetic motility psychoses provide us with further information about the quintessential symptoms belonging here. The first comes from my time in Berlin:

This 33-year-old university Professor B. had suffered severe articular rheumatism 3 years before, then remained healthy, and had no familial tendency to nervous disorders. For 2 years he has laboured beyond his strength on a scientific project. Three days prior to his mental illness he had an attack of dysentery with bloody stools, marked meteorism, and very intense pain. He is markedly run down physically, became delirious, mistook people's identities, had visions, saw devils, and heard voices. This condition worsened, and, simultaneously a general muscular rigidity set in, at first in paroxysms, and then with longer duration. After 2 days of being almost motionless, he held a crucifix in his hand, convulsively, for half a day; raved excitedly about the devil; uttered inarticulate sounds, especially at night. Then these reactions to aberrant sensations ceased, and he remained in a perfectly motionless state for 8 days, usually accompanied by muscular rigidity, generally keeping his eyes tightly closed. He could swallow fluids occasionally, while at other times he spat out everything, and voided excreta into his clothes. In this condition he was taken by carriage to a mental institution, but because of his rigidity, could be transferred in and out of the carriage only with difficulty, and sat leaning back, poorly supported, with arms and legs stiffly extended. He could then be led into his room, or—actually—was slowly pushed. Absolute mutism prevailed, interrupted only from the third day of his stay in the institution by several hours of inarticulate outcries. Witless facial expression. On the 11th day of illness muscular rigidity ceased. On being addressed, lip movements but no sound; however, occasionally opens his eyes. Marked frailty during the following days, generally perfectly motionless, but occasional outcries. Patient then began to leave his bed occasionally; stood at the window for prolonged periods with raised, outstretched arms, and cried out several times. Went into the corridor in his night dress, once answered very slowly and softly: 'I do not know'. On the 14th day, the first spontaneous utterance: Patient said to his attendant: 'Look, Carl, see how I am'. The following day it was learned that the patient had pain over his entire body; does not know who he is, where he is, claims he has no head, and has been quartered. Speech is slow and childlike. Every request is felt to be arduous. On the 19th day, with his hand grasping his head: 'This is not my head, my head has been exchanged, I have a strange head, I am perfectly hollow'. From the 22 day on: marked improvement, better statements; patient is tidy. Feeling in his head as though it were sore—a confused feeling, patient feels that he is very severely ill, and asks for reports. Then continued improvement, tries to orientate himself; provides information on his thoughts during the severe illness. He sometimes felt that his brain consisted of many parts, which moved up and down; at other times as if he had no brain, but a piece of ice in his head. Patient remembers that he had considered himself to be a steamship (an explanatory delusion), that he did believe that he has been the undoing of navigation on the Rhine, in that he has twisted all the rudders. He has believed the world would be separated and has been able to bring it back together, has been in the royal palace, destroyed the floor there, and then tried to replace it with tile; Prince Bismarck came and gave him a malicious look. Patient wonders how such perverse ideas can arise in a person. He knows no reason for the muscular rigidity. Progressive increase in insight into the illness, sleep and appetite good, appearance improved. A few complaints of an uncomfortable feeling of pressure at a certain place in the left parietal region, which later occurred only intermittently. Six weeks after onset of the illness, in full convalescence. After a consultation and a bad night following this, a state of mild excitement occurred, in which the patient accused himself of an indiscretion the day before, talked hurriedly in a tremulous voice, trembled all over, made nervous movements with his hands, began to cry. He was pacified by encouragement, later was in a stable mood, only occasionally complains of pressure in the head as described above, or of a pulsation in the head: a feeling as if the brain were moving back and forth. These troubles gradually disappeared, and about 6 months after the outbreak of his illness the patient was discharged from the institution, fully recovered. Since then 12 years have raced by, during which time, the patient, an honoured professor, has been functioning perfectly well in his former position.

An even more acute type of illness is presented by the 26-year-old Doctor of Laws, of Jewish descent, who I was able to present to you a few days ago. He had become acutely ill with anxious ideas and most profoundly disarrayed, had refused food for several days and made four suicide attempts, all of which, fortunately, had been averted. We found him sitting in bed with congested face, hot head, feverish appearance, his pulse was not accelerated, yet remarkably weak. His facial expression was somewhat rigid and immobile. Patient did not answer any questions, but followed the questioner with his eyes. He did not comply with any requests, did not show his tongue, or open his mouth. Our efforts to prise apart his lips brought about rather the opposite effect—involuntary closure; the grasped hand was held as though it raised his hackles. Otherwise, the patient sat quite immovable, in a normal posture, except that, from time to time, slight shivering and trembling movements occurred, as if a cold shiver were passing over his body. If the patient was taken out of bed—to which he offered no, or only slight resistance—it was noticed that he tottered, and did not have full command of his movements. Finally he succeeded in standing alone, and then, it was striking that he held his right leg half-bent, resting only the outer border of his foot on the floor, while the left leg gave support to his body. He remained unsupported in this position for several minutes, with the same immobile facial expression. We now attempted to put his head into another position, by bending his neck. This was met with considerable resistance, which continued beyond the medium position, so that finally he stood with head and trunk bent forward. He never used his hand to defend himself. Meanwhile, during these imposed movements he could not regain his old position, and was swaying; in this new position he shifted from one leg to another, now standing on the right, with the left half-bent and resting it only slightly on the outer border of the foot. Next day we found him squatting in bed with his legs under him; the flaccid positioning of his legs was noticeable. Today, approach of a hand triggers the withdrawal of the upper limb on approach, and of the trunk on the same side, while touching the legs has no such effect. Not a trace of any real defensive movements can be seen. I now place my right hand in the patient's right palm; his hand then closes, while I begin to execute a slow tug with my hooked fingers. The more I pull, the more firmly he clamps his fingers against it, and so I could draw his upper body into a leaning position over the edge of the bed. He remains in this position as long as I pull, and gradually returns to his former position, once I stop pulling. This patient is now taken out of bed, and seems about to collapse, as though his lower extremities have failed him completely. But if one proceeds cautiously and supports him on both sides, we see that he can use them well; yet, owing to their abnormal position, an unusual amount of force must be employed. He remains in a squatting, almost sitting posture, with legs crossed, and is thus able to move forward unsupported, and to regain his balance when he loses it. It seems as if he might fall at any moment, yet he actually keeps himself securely on his legs. (The patient passes his excrement into his clothing, absolutely refuses food, and was tube-fed several times during the narcosis. Death from pneumonia after a few days.)

Another patient, who has also been taken ill very recently, has lain in bed groaning, answering requests very rarely, and usually seems preoccupied first in pursing her mouth, and then in everting it in snout-like fashion; she is taken out of bed and made to walk; then plants one foot before the other slowly and cautiously at definite distances in a dancing manner, somewhat like a tightrope walker. When she is left to stand quietly for a while, she rests on one leg and flexes the other, so that she touches the floor only with her toes; indeed, she also lifts it completely off the floor.

All these peculiar expressions of movement are devoid of any purpose that we can see, lack any change in facial expression, and without patients being able to provide any motive, when they are able to speak, as in this last case. When resting, whether in bed or sitting on a chair, some of these patients assume a *fixed abnormal position* [W], for instance, by flexing the cervical vertebrae forward, so that in reclining, the head is always raised from the pillow, or a squatting position is taken, like that of the male patient described above.

A localized tonic muscle spasm may occur in the context of such generalized immobility, with a predilection for it affecting the muscles of speech. I remind you of the patient Kl, who became very acutely ill with turbulent symptoms, and the next day was admitted to the clinic. He appeared to be conscious, and followed the examiner with his eyes. His tongue, maximally protruded, lay between firmly closed jaws; it was greatly swollen, cyanotic, and gangrenous near the teeth which had sunk deep into it. He was unable to utter even a sound or to swallow fluids, and had to be fed via nasogastric tube. Pain sensation and reflexes seemed generally to be markedly blunted. After I had waited the greater part of a day for the muscle tension to abate, I decided on 're-positioning' [Ed] under chloroform anaesthesia, and fixed his jaw in a half-open position. There followed a semi-somnolent state, lasting many days, and only very gradually was the protruded tongue withdrawn back into his mouth; then he started to convalescence, and, within a short time, could be discharged, recovered. The peculiarity of this case was that the patient, at a time when he still controlled his other movements, had to keep his tongue in this forcibly protruded position. The patient, a 32-year-old draughtsman, gave definite information as soon as he could speak, that he had always remained well orientated, maintaining full consciousness throughout the period of general immobility.

Gentlemen! These cases of illness, sometimes presented to you directly, sometimes only reported to you, show that 'akinetic motility psychosis' [Ed] encompasses some very different clinical pictures: They have in common as the most striking symptom, only the akinetic state, which differs in degree and extent during a period of continuous illness, and also varies greatly in duration. Later we shall be able to make a rather sharper differentiation. For the time being, we focus particularly on the different motor symptoms.

We call akinesia extending over most of the musculature by the name *immobility* [W]. It varies, as our cases show, according to its severity, in that sometimes it is so marked that it leads to cessation of almost all reactions, producing a condition apparently similar to death. In fact, confusion between such cases, with actual death must have occurred repeatedly, and is to be explained by the fact that respiration and the circulation in such cases may be greatly reduced, and a condition akin to syncope may sometimes exist. I shall return to this. Apart from such cases, we are dealing with somnolent states, which cannot be confused with actual death—at least, not by physicians—for the heart sounds, the respiratory murmur and pulse, albeit weakened, are plainly detectable. Extremities are usually cool, occasionally cyanotic, and body temperature may be considerably lowered. These are cases which appear from time to time, sensationally, in the daily press, with great regularity, as the 'sleeping uhlan' [W] or 'apparent death of a prisoner for weeks' [W]. In fact, in a portion of these cases, every reaction to painful stimuli is lost, due either to stupefaction of the sensorium, actual analgesia, or real loss of reflex action. Nevertheless, in the majority of cases, a reflex response to a needle prick can be demonstrated, if only as a twitching of the eyelids, or on applying the needle to the most sensitive parts of the face, or even to the eyes. Reduced tendon reflexes, especially the patellar reflex, can unquestionably occur sometimes, but not in conditions of longer duration discussed here. On the other hand, more commonly, tendon reflexes are exaggerated, so that patellar clonus and even foot clonus may occur. Faeces are usually voided in bed; at other times bladder catheterization and attention to bowel evacuation become necessary. Swallowing is usually markedly disturbed, so that prolonged artificial feeding may be needed. Nonetheless, it is rare for accumulated saliva not to be spontaneously swallowed, and real paralysis of the swallowing reflex is demonstrable. However, this undoubtedly can occur in more-acute, short-lived states, often with increased secretion of saliva. Of course, this condition includes cessation of all initiative movements, so including complete mutism. Remnants of reactions, such as tremor of the eyelids, are usually present. In the eyelids, one can almost always see noticeable reactions to passive movements, even when passive motility fully resembles that of a lifeless body, in which case, they may not only be retained but augmented. This is not the usual behaviour in persisting immobility, but corresponds rather to the more acute phases of akinesia. Reduction of passive motility is encountered more often, a symptom that can similarly assume very different levels of severity. Most commonly with this type of inert patient, only the excessive imposed movements meet with resistance, or only certain groups of muscles present resistance. Muscles for closing the eyes, mouth, and jaws are primarily involved. Grouped with such localized resistance, there can also be those symptoms often called 'negativity' [Ed] or 'negativism' [Ed]. *Negativism* [W] is shown in the eyelids when an attempt to open them is met by apparently active resistance, leading to even firmer eye closure; likewise, in the lips, attempts to separate them are met with closure of the mouth; and in the jaws, by a resistance which becomes stronger the greater the attempt to force down the lower jaw. Masseters and temporal muscles are then hard and tight to the touch. Such firm clenching of the jaws usually hinders introduction of a feeding tube by mouth, so this method of nourishment is only possible in exceptional cases; and hence a nasal tube is preferable. After the sites just described, negativism is most commonly encountered in muscles of the neck, in such a way that passive raising of the head from the pillow not only meets with resistance, but is responded to by vigorous backward bending of the head—a state of neck rigidity which ceases as soon as the effort is discontinued. Altogether, the symptom of negativism has the characteristic that it seems to follow passive muscle stretch in a reflex manner, and is increased in proportion to the force imposed. In the extremities, it therefore occasionally occurs only when movement is performed rapidly and with large excursions, whereas slow, less extensive movements often meet with no resistance. If generalized immobility is not very severe, such attempts can produce signs of pain, such as facial distortion, or flow of tears; in such cases, painful stiffness of the joints may be assumed, owing to the maintained fixation in one position. Meanwhile, I must return to cases characterized by a diffuse tenderness of the muscles.

Very often tests of passive motility lead to the finding of *waxy flexibility* [W], *Flexibilitas cerea* [W]: Every passive movement meets a moderate, and equal resistance in all joints involved. It results in maintenance of imposed positions. Most pronounced is *Flexibilitas cerea* [W] always occurring in the extremities; in the neck region there is instead mainly a degree of negativism. Positions that can be imposed on patients with *Flexibilitas cerea* [Ed] can be very uncomfortable and yet are maintained for a long time. Thus, lying in bed, all limbs may be raised nearly vertically, this position being maintained. When patients sit on a chair, the trunk may be bent to one side, arms outstretched, one leg elevated, thereby putting the patients in a position that, for normal persons, could be maintained for a long time only with great effort. If a patient is stood upright, one leg may be flexed at its joints in such a way that only tips of the toes touch the floor, or the trunk is bent so that the arms touch the floor. Under these conditions, patients often seem to have a special facility for preserving their balance, so that comparison with Goltz's [1] decapitated frogs springs to mind. In all these experiments the patient takes no part; even in moderate immobility there is no distortion of his features, no glance directed at the examiner. Maintenance of uncomfortable positions may be observed for 5, 10 min or longer, according to the degree of immobility; and in the end, and most often, limbs yield to gravity, and uncomfortable postures of the trunk are corrected. An exception to this is to be found only in the rare cases of continued muscular rigidity.

Muscular rigidity [W] is a manifestation usually occurring only as paroxysms in the context of more general immobility. I have never seen it continue uninterrupted for days; but occasional attacks are seen in almost every case. They occur either spontaneously, or from trivial provocations, usually consisting of attempts to get the patient into an upright position, or to impose passive movements. In the warder's notes the statement is often found that patients had held themselves rigid. Not uncommonly profuse perspiration follows, or the face becomes congested. Such attacks usually last for only a few minutes, but for hours in severe cases. In these attacks, patients may be suspended, supported only at head and foot, as in a hypnotic experiment, and may even also be weighed down. As in tetanus, it is a matter of a tonic muscle spasm—and often no less powerful—with involvement of masseters and facial muscles, but remissions, and ever-returning sudden paroxysms, characteristic of tetanus, are absent: The whole condition is always a continuous one, and usually less-stormy in character. We saw, in the case of one patient, that these states of rigidity may interfere with the patient being transferred. You will remember that this patient, Mrs. K., presented with moderate localized rigidity limited to pelvic–thigh muscles; yet this condition might have another significance, to be regarded merely as a mechanical consequence of prolonged immobility, analogous to the muscular stiffness in paralyzed limbs.

If we encounter a patient with generalized immobility, it is always advisable to get him out of bed and stand him on his feet. It is then usually found that this person—appearing to be dead—can stand and walk, provided some care is taken, and the patient sufficiently supported. I recall one patient I presented, whose knees gave away, but was then in a position to walk and stand, albeit in a strikingly changed way. Total failure of the legs, as found in flaccid paralysis, occurs only temporarily, in more acute states. On the other hand, lack of spontaneity in these patients is always very noticeable. They remain standing *ad infinitum* [W] wherever and however they are placed, and any shift in their position can be achieved only when they are pushed, or a change in balance requires them to move. In this regard, the behaviour of Mrs. K. was characteristic. Lack of spontaneity can be understood when we observe the conduct of patients, once a milder grade of immobility prevails, so that somewhat more complex experiments can be set up. Under certain conditions it is possible, under certain conditions, to help such patients, for example, to get up onto a chair, but they then show themselves to be quite incapable of getting down and, if forced, may finally fall in an awkward way. Similarly, patients plainly show that they have understood a request to get in or out of bed, yet they make futile attempts to comply, for they cannot recruit the necessary muscular coordination. Evidently in such cases the motor system is not freely at their disposal as it is in normal persons, one consequence being akinesia for initiative movements. Another symptom, which is often seen, is the Affective state of motor disarray—I remind you of our patient, Mrs. W.

Disturbance of the motor system is also suggested by parakinetic symptoms, which appear usually when a patient's location is changed for external reasons. We can only assume that any change in position adopted by a patient must be based on some abnormality of position sense, or some other constituent in the complex sum of motor concepts, despite general mechanisms of walking and standing remaining intact. Since balance evidently cannot be maintained on the basis of a particular level of mental ability, the only possibility remaining is unconscious compensation, in other words, adjustment acting exclusively within consciousness of corporeality. *Shift of the form of movement* [W] away from the norm may vary greatly from one case to another. Thus, one example is the peculiar gait of the tightrope walker who, cautiously balancing, places one foot exactly in front of the other, or of one who walks wholly on their heels, or on the edge of their foot, and so on. It is improbable, as Cramer [2] assumes, that this is a case of hallucination in muscle sense, because—apart from inappropriate use of the term hallucination—the abnormal position must be viewed as a compensation for certain deficit symptoms. You will remember, gentlemen, that I always explicitly emphasized that motility is represented along with consciousness of corporeality. You see how far I was justified in this, from what I have just said.

Certain parakinetic symptoms, in hyperkinetic motility psychosis, about which we have already had a chance to learn, give us a better hope of their being traced back to processes of irritation. In fact, it is impossible to draw a sharp boundary here between hyperkinesia and parakinesia. In most cases of less severe, yet more extensive akinesia, as in our patient Miss M. (p. 245), this takes the form of *verbigeration* [W], that is, monotonous repetition of words, interjections, or parts of sentences, often with quite nonsensical construction—and this may occur either temporarily, only on certain occasions, or in certain phases of the illness. Thus a patient verbigerated for months on end the words: 'Anna mia mara Kochlunsky o Landleben'. It is simply a symptom, of activation, since this patient repeated this phrase over and over, and was not significantly disturbed in this way even by eating. However, at the same time, speech was restricted to predetermined motor tracts, since, when verbigeration ceased, she was not yet in a position to talk, despite clearly wanting to do so; in other words she had a motor aphasia. I speak here of a patient already known to you (p. 6), who has remained dumb for 5 years, and then, with great effort, had to learn to speak again. In other cases, a link of this sort between verbigeration and mutism may be seen. Incidentally, I should point out here that verbigeration can also occur in writing, obviously in those who are not totally motionless.

Parakinetic phenomena analogous to verbigeration are also to be seen when immobility ceases. These are the so-called *movement stereotypes* [W], that is, certain movements of the limbs that are repeated rhythmically in unchanging manner, and are therefore designated as 'pseudo-spontaneous movements' [Ed] of a certain uniform type. Once again, in these situations, the clinical connection with *absence* [Ed] of movements—the state of immobility—is clearly recognizable in many instances. We have become acquainted with examples of this in one of our cases, Miss M. You will have the chance to see other examples during clinical rounds. Thus one patient makes constant movements with her mouth, which she everts like a snout; another utters at fairly regular intervals a half-groaning, half-grunting sound, without any other Affective signs. You have met another patient who, while eating, aimlessly dips his spoon, time and again into the bowl, taking it out empty again. He behaves like someone who, deep in thought, does something quite mechanically. We saw another who made constant rocking movements of his trunk, yet another making only nodding movements of his head. One patient performs a more complex movement, in that he passes one hand through his hair, then describes a circle around his head and calmly returns to his former position. Occasionally, the evident aimlessness of such movements is concealed by the fact that an object is manipulated in the proper manner, such as when a patient lifts her bed covers again and again by one corner and smoothes them. Yet in these cases, the handling itself is clearly aimless. Moreover, more-or-less forcible movements of the entire body may occur, as when female patients frequently make coitus-like movements of the trunk. Even very complicated coordinated movements, which appear to be spontaneous, are proved to be pseudo-spontaneous by their connection with mutism and other akinetic symptoms, as well as by their rhythmic repetition. For instance, a patient continuously marches to a certain corner of the room, then returns, and then goes back, like a pendulum. They are therefore movements restricted in an unchanging manner to certain muscle groups, or to a definite coordinated movement. Similar movements, repeated rhythmically, can be grouped with other hyperkinetic symptoms, but never in such a circumscribed and localized manner.

Besides negativity and waxy flexibility, another disorder is encountered quite often, to be differentiated in relation to passive motility of limbs, trunk, or head. Patients seem strikingly willing to yield to passive movements; sometimes it even appears as if they actually *assist* [Ed] them. Any body position thus reached is then usually maintained. This symptom, in which any joint resistance is lacking, may be grouped with waxy flexibility as *Pseudo-Flexibilitas* [W]. Easy acceptance of these movements by patients is usually akin to actual flexibility. The freest interpretation of this symptom, which is usually found only in moderate levels of immobility, is that it is based on some sort of 'suggestion' [Ed] exerted on the patients. In some way, an examiner suggests to the patient the execution of a movement, towards which the patient is apathetic. It is easily understood that akinesia, the absence of spontaneous impulses on muscles, provides the most favourable basis for this. The *pseudoflexibilitas* [Ed] then often appears only when real waxy flexibility abates, and the patient's condition is seen to improve. It thereby shows itself as the mild degree of disturbance just mentioned. In keeping with our view that it is due to the effect of suggestion, at this stage of the illness it is sometimes possible, through verbal suggestion, to exert a favourable influence on other akinetic symptoms, such as mutism, food refusal, and lapses of personal hygiene. However, it is also only in such cases that suggestion as a method of treatment can be employed successfully. It is the general experience of all observers, including the most passionate devotees of hypnotism, that, for all other psychoses, one struggles in vain.

Maintenance of certain body positions is not found in exclusive combination with symptoms of waxy flexibility or pseudo-flexibilitas; it also occurs independently of these, in that patients of their own accord, apparently spontaneously, adopt certain positions and maintain them with abnormal persistence. Most often in this respect, we meet the remarkable manifestation that the head is held above the pillow with the neck in a flexed position, an uncomfortable one relieved usually only during sleep. Such a patient explained why she held her head in this position: She had the feeling that her head might otherwise fall backward, it being totally slack (see also: information from Patient M., p. 246). The next most commonly seen sign is adopting and maintaining a particular squatting position, often quite uncomfortable, for instance with legs crossed or trunk turned half to one side, or preservation of a position midway between sitting and reclining, while one arm is used as a support, etc. Totally abnormal positions are less common, and tend not to be maintained for long, for instance, when a female patient adopts the gynaecological knee-elbow position, or a male patient stands on his head, leaning against the wall. Any attempt to correct such fixed positions, is met with varied reactions. Some patients quietly accept what is indicated, but immediately turn round and resume their former position; others become resistant, and in some cases violent. The same goes for cases when it is desired to prevent pseudospontaneous movements or series of movements located in particular muscle groups.

Gentlemen! The present attempt to describe the main akinetic symptoms must include a number of apparently heterogeneous phenomena. In the endeavour to describe only what fits together, I have been guided exclusively by experiences in the clinic. However, you will have noticed how much it comes down to the greater or lesser extent of the akinetic symptoms. Some symptoms, such as waxy flexibility and muscle rigidity belong exclusively, or largely to severe levels of generalized immobility; others, which we find to be prominent only in partial akinesia, or in generalized akinesia of only moderate degree, prove to be symptoms indicating *susceptibility* [Ed]. In this group, we can include mutism, negativity of mouth, jaws, and neck, and also refusal of food. In akinesia of moderate severity, spread over the whole body, we can find generalized pseudoflexibilitas, circumscribed pseudospontaneous movement, and mutism which is exclusively reactive. It is common to the great majority of cases, and by the very nature of akinetic symptoms, no information can be obtained about inner processes and probable motives for patients' motor behaviour. Most often, one can ascertain, either during periods of remission or after the illness has passed, that alleged voices, commanding or vetoing in their content, had influenced such behaviour; However, I need discuss no further that these phonemes explain nothing, after my previous remarks on the significance of hallucinations, and particularly of phonemes. Rather, they themselves need an explanation; and it is easy to find in them the Affective state of motor disarray, which we can generally assume to be present for disorders of motor identification, described unmistakeably by a proportion of patients during or after their illness. The basis for this is just that a certain level of activity in the sensorium is retained.

Gentlemen! We thus come to the further question as to how far akinetic behaviour allows us to make conclusions on the *state of the sensorium* [W]. In this respect, we propose with certainty that the state of the sensorium shows clear dependence on the extent of akinetic symptoms, just as this might also be claimed for muscle rigidity. In states of severe generalized immobility, clouding of the sensorium is generally found, and this can go so far that it is impervious even to painful stimuli. Accordingly, any memory of time spent in this state either does not exist at all, or does so only in that dream-like hallucinations, or actual dreams may appear, in fragments, and are considered to be real. When the aetiology is hysterical, the state of the sensorium usually corresponds more to one of so-called 'ecstasy' [Ed], and remaining memories are endowed with feeling tone of supernatural events. In such patients, you also encounter fixed body positions, as are also found as expressions of enraptured ecstasy. Those cases which have led to the special clinical picture called *catalepsy* [W], are particularly well known. Ever since Kahlbaum introduced us to knowledge of motility psychoses, this alleged type of functional nervous disorder has increasingly been disappearing from textbooks. Without disputing that periods of an akinetic state may occur in hysteria, which are of shorter duration than elsewhere, and with specially favourable outcome, I should say explicitly that these cases *do* belong amongst akinetic motility psychoses. We find a contrast to these dream-like states in cases like that of Miss M. (p. 242), when there is no doubt about clarity of consciousness. All cases lying in between show a more or less clear sensorium, with either a lesser extent or a lower severity of akinesia. When the sensorium is significantly clouded, despite only moderate extent or severity of akinesia, features of delirium such as restlessness, or signs of occupational delirium are often simultaneously present. In comparison, the deepest levels of unconsciousness are to be found in the rare, extremely acute cases, in which the muscular rigidity is intermingled to a degree akin to epilepsy, seen occasionally also in epileptic seizures, but of longer duration, and leading to death in a few days.

Gentlemen! The state of severe generalized immobility has always been known to alienists; it was probably also called atonicity and considered the essential basis of a unique clinical picture: *Melancholia attonita* [W], or *Melancholia cum stupore* [W]. I feel no need to deny that this illness has anything to do with Affective melancholia in our sense; I recommend rather to drop this term and replace it with 'akinetic motility psychosis' [Ed]. That a whole series of other motor symptoms besides atonicity belong together clinically was proved by Kahlbaum [3] in his monograph on catatonia. He explained its relationship with melancholia, and emphasized the importance of the state of muscle rigidity amongst mentally ill people. In these respects, Kahlbaum must be acknowledged as the real founder of the theory of motility psychoses.

Gentlemen! It is proper that I take this opportunity to do justice to Kahlbaum's contributions. After Meynert [4], we are indebted to this great investigator and observer for the greatest advancements that clinical psychiatry has made in more recent times. You will readily grasp that I adopt the same view as Kahlbaum in validating the concept of catatonia, the more so as the importance of his work is acknowledged more and more, and a few gifted younger 'psychiatrists' have taken it up as well. Nevertheless, the value of Kahlbaum's work must be perceived essentially in the fact that he gathered a number of important stones for erection of his structure, while the structure itself is not durable. He has not escaped the fate of all authors who laboured on monographs in a designated domain, and has outlined much too broad a clinical picture, a step backward, in so far as the narrow concept of *Melancholia attonita* [W] or *cum stupore* [W] has fallen by the wayside. One can thus also account for the difficulty this clinical picture has met with in gaining general acceptance, as well as the still-lively opposition to it. Motility symptoms described above are not confined at all to my so-called 'motility psychoses' [Ed]; they are to be found amongst a great number of other, far more complex cases, and not merely those of acute origin. Only where they constitute the clinical picture, solely or in greater part, as in the above cases, are we justified in accepting a special *illness* [Ed] whose essential symptoms are motor in content. In particular, I would particularly emphasize that 'catatonic' [W]—or, in our sense, specific motor—symptoms, tend to appear in the majority of chronic progressive psychoses at some phase of the illness. We are thereby warned to confine our clinical picture of akinetic motility psychosis within the narrowest possible limits.

Gentlemen! Much as we may want to debate this, the practical clinical perspective is sufficient: It allows us to claim that it is impossible to recognize a single dimension according to its boundary; and that, in the background to akinetic motility psychosis more extensive disorientation may be present, which may temporarily conceal essential akinetic symptoms. Perhaps at some future time, we will acquire data which allows us to differentiate in this dimension between pure parakinetic motility psychosis and its combined forms; but at present, given the existing state of knowledge, we would be forced, artificially, to split apart those cases where there is an essential coherence with respect to akinetic symptoms. Involvement of the sensorium, present in the most pronounced cases, undeniably signifies that the disease process should be extended into the psychomotor realm. We are accustomed to contrasting symptoms arising as part of the sensorium, as a general illness, with focal symptoms of brain diseases; yet we must not forget that they, like the indirect focal symptoms which I differentiated, are based on summation of several deficits; and, like them, represent secondary effects of focal illness ('long-range effects' [Ed] of other authors). On the other hand, we must recognize that more drastic clouding of the sensorium constitutes definite disorientation in all three domains of consciousness, and so we see that the greater extent of the illness process cannot, by its very nature, be separated from its intensity. Corresponding with this, severe involvement of the sensorium is observed exclusively when there is greater severity of generalized immobility. There must therefore be other criteria by which we can try to differentiate within the clinical picture of akinetic motility psychosis; and we find these chiefly by studying the course of the illness. Accordingly, we want to include as akinetic motility psychoses those acute cases of illness which present, as a rapid development, that complex of akinetic and parakinetic symptoms described above, which are sustained in continuity throughout a longer duration of illness. That the further course can then be organized along entirely different lines, is understood just as easily as what we already know, that after an apoplectic attack with marked loss of consciousness, complete restitution can sometimes occur, while at other times a series of focal symptoms remain. As is generally known, such focal symptoms, occurring in the context of some major insult in this restricted sense, gives us the prospect of recovery, the significance of this fact doubtless lying in the fact that a focal symptom arising in this way is a secondary effect, often an indirect focal symptom; but, naturally the same apoplectic onset can also be direct, and therefore accompany incurable focal symptoms. Likewise, in akinetic motility psychoses, a proportion of such cases in which stupor and muscular rigidity occur, show themselves capable of recovery, our university professor being the most convincing example.

The start of an akinetic motility psychosis may be very sudden, almost apoplectiform. The above (p. 253), briefly mentioned, very acute cases, with a rapidly worsening course, appear to have had an apoplectiform onset. However, irrespective of these, a similar acute-onset sometimes occurs. For us, over the course of the year, it has happened repeatedly that such patients had been found on the street, or on the floor, in a strange house, motionless, and were brought into our clinic; and it was subsequently established that the patients had carried on their usual occupations right up until then. At other times, an initial stage of a few days was reported, where disarray was present, not exclusively of a motor type, with outbursts of anxiety and despair, dominating the picture. Our university professor is an example of this. A special class can probably be made up, characterized by an initial stage of 'delirium of relatedness' [Ed] lasting for weeks. The duration of the akinetic and parakinetic state usually amounts to a few weeks. Undoubtedly, the reciprocal relationship is thus that akinesia represents a more intense symptom; and so, parakinetic symptoms usually appear first when remission in the akinesia is seen. In rarer cases with severe, more extensive akinesia but relatively intact sensorium, parakinetic symptoms, such as verbigeration, stereotypical movements, altered gait, etc., are especially likely to appear, if, along with pronounced akinesia for initiative movements, reactive movements can still be elicited. Following the akinetic and parakinetic stages, in which we will find the peak of the disease curve, there is usually a paranoid stage, in which parakinetic symptoms are intermingled to greater or lesser extent. Only in this paranoid stage might it become apparent whether, and how far other disorders of identification, such as those in the psychomotor domain, are included in the clinical picture. Those like our professor belong amongst the most favourable cases, where the paranoid stage might be assumed to exist just as long as perfect insight into dreamlike events of the akinetic state had not yet been acquired. In most cases with a favourable course, as in this case, hypochondriacal symptoms stand out in particular as signs of more widespread somatopsychic disorientation during the paranoid stage.

Persistence of sporadic delusions, which correspond to dreamlike memories, indicates merely the suggestion of a paranoid state. Signs of mental weakness, like 'emotional incontinence' [Ed] and mild exhaustibility, are also mingled with other symptoms, in such favourably proceeding cases. At other times, the akinetic/parakinetic stage is soon followed by prominent dementia, which can still end in recovery, although usually after a quite long duration of 6 months to 1 year; or, at other times, this becomes the definitive outcome of the illness. Not uncommonly, the stage of dementia follows an intervening paranoid stage, and these cases seem largely to terminate in a permanent state of dementia. If the paranoic stage is very marked, that is, if it has expanded into formal systematization, remediation can still occur; and then an increasing level of insight into the illness, growing slowly but steadily, can be seen. Finally, in about 1 year, there may be complete recovery, without residual deficits. In such a favourable course, elementary symptoms of phonemes and delusions of relatedness soon disappear. In other cases, progressive systematization occurs, when religious, grandiose, and persecutory ideas arise—so-called 'prophetic delirium' [Ed]—which may build up from the most fully thought-out premises, evidence of great intellectual productivity. Significant memory deficits may accompany this paranoid stage, as well as the demented stage; these are related to the akinetic stage.

Gentlemen! If we ask ourselves why it is that the akinetic-parakinetic stage is followed at one time by a paranoid stage, at another by a demented stage, naturally only by reviewing a large number of cases can an answer be provided. It thus seems that the state of the sensorium during the akinetic phase is an important matter for consideration. The greater its involvement, and the more the state approximates to sleep or unconsciousness, the more likely is it that a stage of dementia will ensue, and this tends to follow especially in cases of so-called twilight states with attendant symptoms of accompanying delirium. If, on the other hand, the sensorium is only slightly involved, pronounced states of paranoia usually occur, although these can still be curable. Although this result is based on a statistical review of cases, it also confirms what we might already have expected. Delusion formation in the paranoid stage is based here, as in other cases, chiefly on explanatory delusions, and for their formation, a prerequisite is a certain intactness of the sensorium. Indeed, the case of Miss M., which I reported to you, might be an example of this, yet explanatory delusions with perfectly clear sensorium, failed to appear. Nevertheless, it is noted that this case is of relatively recent onset, and according to all precedents, explanatory delusions may be expected to occur later on. As for the outcome of our illness, I must state very clearly that an outcome of complete recovery is by no means rare, and I have seen this after both slight—or after more pronounced indications of paranoic stages, and also after a stage of dementia; while in Kraepelin's [5] textbook, dementia is described as the regular outcome for such cases. Here, as well as elsewhere, we come across little by way of thought, plus an ignorance of facts, which features are arguably unsuited to a textbook. Moreover, the tendency to recurrence, emphasized by Kraepelin, is in no way greater than in most other acute psychoses.

As for the *aetiology* [W], akinetic motility psychoses have a predilection to affect persons of young age, and of those, predominantly the female sex. It is not unrelated to menstruation. Relatively often, the *post partum* [W] state or other exhausting influences are to be found as the immediate precipitating factor. Emotional states have often preceded it, and hysteria, as mentioned above, has occurred in a proportion of cases. The percentage of cases that had earlier presented with a moderate grade of congenital imbecility or at least of retarded mental development is quite high.

Diagnosis [W] meets no difficulties for the akinetic state, if one adheres to the above description. Beyond our narrowly-defined clinical picture of acute akinetic motility psychosis, diagnosis is possible only when the previous history is known, when it can be established that akinetic symptoms have an independent significance, and are not accessories to another type of pre-existing illness. Therefore, a definite duration of continued akinesia is important for differential diagnosis between it and other motility psychoses, a point to which I return later. Only a remitting pattern of akinetic behaviour should be mentioned, which sometimes occurs, to be interrupted by abatement of symptoms for a few days. We have already discussed sporadic interruptions of immobility by apparently spontaneous acts, which are, in reality, reactions to hallucinations. I only touch on differential diagnosis in relation to melancholia here, owing to the still-prevailing confusion in nomenclature. Prominent cases of so-called *Melancholia attonita* [W] or *cum stupore* [W] all belong here. Only akinesia of dementia, with its intrapsychic hallmarks, and so-called depressive melancholia could be mistaken for our illness. However, pronounced reactive akinesia is never found; as in akinetic motility psychosis, the contrast between the lack of initiative and the well-retained reactivity to external stimulus is therefore always most noticeable. Furthermore, both in dementia, and in depressive melancholia, the specific motor symptoms of muscle rigidity, negativity, *Flexibilitas cerea* [W], and pseudoflexibility are absent.

Treatment [W] of akinetic motility psychosis has as its objectives a series of most important tasks, connected to very definite symptoms. Foremost amongst these is the struggle to overcome food refusal. Cases usually need artificial feeding, that is by means of a tube, for a long period. Much has been said for and against the effectiveness of this measure, and there are still some authors who abhor it, on account of associated dangers. Far from denying these dangers, I prefer to emphasize that even with careful manipulation and much practice in this manoeuvre it can occur that patients aspirate liquid food and suffocate in this manner. This happened to me once, and the tracheotomy, which was carried out immediately, did not avert a fatal outcome. However, this should serve only as a warning against forced feeding at all costs, but rather to stop at once when any violent strangling or coughing interferes with the flow of the feeding mixture, and particularly if there is any suggestion that the tube is located in the trachea. A mechanical difficulty is sometimes encountered, consisting of paralytic depression of the larynx, a condition which can also occasionally interfere greatly with introduction of the tube in acute bulbar paralysis. In other cases, this condition is not present, but spasm of the pharynx, with the larynx pressed against the pharyngeal wall posterior to it will produce the same hindrance. The oropharyngeal or intranasal tube then impinges on the upper border of the reclined epiglottis, and if this obstruction can be successfully bypassed, comes against the open glottis. If it is necessary to battle against such difficulties, it is advisable first to pour in a small quantity of some indifferent test fluid, such as clear water, through a funnel. In every case, wait until choking and coughing have stopped, at least partially. If this method fails, the attempt to feed should be given up this time and repeated later. Should it not succeed even then, although the indication for forced-feeding still exists, under some circumstances you will have to resort to use of light anaesthesia. Ether rather than chloroform is recommended, but narcosis should not be taken beyond the point where the swallowing reflex is abolished. At other times, it would be preferable to dispense entirely with introducing the tube, and to be satisfied if sometimes only small amounts of fluid are swallowed spontaneously; also, nutritional enemas should be tried. However, there are always certain exceptional cases where such difficulties are encountered, perhaps when you encounter a vigorous and energetic conscious resistance, or when there is dreamlike, impulsive resistance with total failure to grasp the situation, or when a patient is overwhelmed by hypochondriacal and anxious ideas. On the other hand, in the vast majority of cases, artificial feeding can be achieved without substantial resistance, and it would be an error not to employ it in these cases, because of the danger it presents in other cases. Often, patients quickly adjust to the procedure and even assist, or otherwise give recognizable signs of gratitude. The widely preferred material is a thick-walled *Nélaton* catheter with lateral openings. Feeding through the nose is by far more practical and usually also more easily achievable than by mouth. Most highly recommended as a nutritive fluid is a mixture of milk, sugar, and eggs, mixed according to Voit's recipe. Any medications or wine may conveniently be poured in after the feeding. Feeding is usually carried out twice every 24 h.

The need for feeding is based in part on the very severe nature of the illness. I mention the case of a young girl admitted to the clinic 8 days after acute onset of her disease and who died within 3 weeks, with an anomalous fever and rapid loss of strength. No difficulties were encountered in feeding, and took place quite regularly; but weight loss had nevertheless amounted to 18 pounds at time of death, almost 1 pound/day. Autopsy revealed no organic illness of any kind, but brain mass was abnormally low

(1,100 g). A similar loss of body weight, despite sufficient nourishment, is often seen in akinetic motility psychosis, and shows how seriously the whole clinical picture should be regarded.

Next in importance after taking care of nutrition, is attention to defaecation and voiding of urine. Quite commonly catheterization of the bladder is needed, at least from time to time. Moreover, by getting the patient out of bed and to the toilet at regular intervals, one aims to develop some sort of habit. If there is a very sluggish sensorium or as a consequence of other conditions, and voiding takes place in bed, care has to be taken over most scrupulous cleanliness. However, the risk of bedsores is so slight that I have never seen it in this illness.

Gentlemen! In my opinion the behaviour of the musculature is a special and rewarding objective for treatment, although I cannot claim extensive experience here, because conditions in the clinic do not favour this. However, if we consider the great value provided by the state of the muscles, in part for overall metabolism, in part for subjective well-being of patients, systematic treatment of the muscles should be attempted in all cases where it is allowed by external conditions. This treatment should consist of regular passive movements, massage and local electrical stimulation of muscles. I need not call any special attention to a proper care of the skin by ablutions and baths.

The *prognosis quolad vitam* [W] of the illness is always questionable, not only because of the dangers due to individual symptoms, such as refusal of food, but also from the whole character of the illness, as I already emphasized. What is more, the initial acute stage is particularly dangerous in many cases, in that physical disarray can promote suicide attempts. I have already quoted a case in which multiple attempts at suicide had been thwarted before the patient was admitted [6]. If a patient survives the akinetic stage, there is generally no longer a threat to life provided there are no special complications, of which I mention only those of stomatitis and scorbutic-like haemorrhages into the tissue. On the other hand, at this stage it becomes relevant to ask whether full restitution, or outcomes in dementia, or as a progressive chronic psychosis are to be expected. In many cases, prognosis in this respect may be judged from the curve of body weight. Rapid increase in body weight with corresponding improvement in mental symptoms allows one to conclude with fair certainty that there will be complete recovery. On the other hand, if a pronounced stage of dementia occurs, increase in body weight is of no guide to prognosis; even after a longer duration of the dementia—up to 6 months or more—patients can still come belatedly to recovery. A rapid rise in the body weight curve, at the same time that a prominent paranoid stage is developing, appears to be an unfavourable sign for the final outcome.

References

1. Goltz FL. Beiträge zur Lehre von den Functionen der Nervencentren des Frosches. Berlin: A Hirschwald; 1869.
2. Cramer A. Die Hallucinationen im Muskelsinn bei Geisteskranken und ihre klinische Bedeutung, ein Beitrag zur Kenntniss der Paranoia. Freiburg im Breisgau: P. Siebeck; 1889.
3. Kahlbaum KL. Die Katatonie oder das Spannungsirresein. Berlin: A Hirschwald; 1874.
4. Meynert T. Klinische Vorlesungen über Psychiatrie auf wissenschaftlichen Grundlagen für Studierende und Aerzte, Juristen und Psychologen. Vienna: Braumüller; 1890. p. 17.
5. Kraepelin E. Psychiatrie: Ein kurzes Lehrbuch für Studierende und Aerzte. 2, gänzlich umgearbeitete Auflage des Compendium. Leipzig: Abel; 1887.
6. Wernicke C. Krankenvorstellungen aus der psychiatrischen Klinik in Breslau. Breslau: Schletter; 1899. vol. 2, Case 2.

Lecture 35

35

- Akinetic phases of hyperkinetic motility psychosis
- Cyclic and complete motility psychosis
- Significance of the paranoid phase
- Excursion into intrapsychic akinesia
- Indicators of psychomotor akinesia
- Theoretical considerations for understanding motility psychoses

Lecture

Gentlemen!

To gain a firm standpoint, it was most opportune for us to see initially the two clinical pictures, of hyperkinetic and akinetic motility psychosis, conceived as narrowly as possible; and from these it would seem possible to penetrate the area in which we find by far the majority of cases defined specifically by motor symptoms, yet which in one way or another are more complicated than cases already considered.

Primarily we have to consider here the differences in course, and in the combinations between the opposing states of hyperkinesia and akinesia. We find such combinations represented by two main types. The *first* [Ed] type consists of a picture in which, either from its onset, or at some time during the course of a hyperkinetic motility psychosis—within hours or a few days at most—an akinetic motility psychosis occurs. In such cases, it is evident that, as the disease process becomes augmented, deficit symptoms appear in place of symptoms of activation. Likewise, in the clinical picture of agitated confusion, one can sometimes see such an increase from hyperkinetic to akinetic symptoms. In two cases of this kind, the acute onset of confused mania was made up of a 1- and a 2-day akinetic-parakinetic stage. The *second* [Ed] type of combination consists in mutual separation of the opposed states of hyperkinesia and akinesia, with each single phase producing pictures of hyperkinetic or akinetic motility psychosis, as described above. The main difference from the first type lies therefore in the more protracted continuous course of each phase. You see, gentlemen, that it is a parallel with the familiar circular psychosis, which in pure cases shows just such an alternation between mania and melancholia. In fact, just as in circular psychoses, frequent changes from akinetic to hyperkinetic phases may occur, even if not with the regularity of circular psychoses. These cases seem to stand out by their poor prognosis.

Much more frequently, however, the combination results in only a single cycle of this sort, in which case I avoid the term 'circular' [W] and speak of the special form of *cyclic motility psychosis* [W]. I have seen cases of this sort almost exclusively in young girls and women, and their aetiology seems to be predominantly menstrual and post-natal. The hyperkinetic stage always occurs first; and a distinct stage of exhaustion

R. Miller, K.J. Dennison (eds.), *An Outline of Psychiatry in Clinical Lectures*,
DOI 10.1007/978-3-319-18051-9_35

stupor is often inserted between it and the akinetic stage, or after the latter; the final outcome is either recovery, death or profound dementia. Mixed in with the hyperkinetic stage is often a stage of mania, whilst in the akinetic state, a state of melancholia is often added; in other words, at one time intrapsychic hyperfunction, at another, *loss* [Ed] of intrapsychic function. At the same time, patients are usually completely disorientated; and motor disarray is always very prominent. In these cases, one could speak of the substitution of one clinical picture for the other. More often, however, here also the akinetic symptom is always an expression of increased intensity. In such cases, of cyclic motility psychosis onset of the akinetic phase may appear earlier in some subdomains of motility than in others. In particular, it is observed that motor loquacity has already passed into mutism, while the motor impulse lasts a few days more, before it passes on in similar fashion to immobility. In unfavourable cases, the hyperkinetic stage often has an anxious hypochondriacal content, with corresponding phonemes [1].

Having just seen that such opposite states as motor hyperkinesia and akinesia can occur in combination, it will not be strange that we quite often encounter cases whose main feature is a mixture of akinetic, hyperkinetic, and parakinetic symptoms. These cases of mixed or, if you will, *complete motility psychosis* [W] therefore do not present particular phases belonging only to one category, but they occur in rapid alternation, at one time predominantly hyperkinesia, at another, akinesia or parakinesia, or—simultaneously—there may be akinetic, hyperkinetic or parakinetic symptoms, but in different muscle regions. Special mention must be made here of certain recurrent cases lasting only hours or days, associated with the most severe Affective states and total disorientation, followed by a stage of exhaustion and amnesia. Such cases occur occasionally as the so-called transitory psychoses; and I have found that, in cases where they recur at short intervals, the course is always unfavourable. The easy assumption that epilepsy is involved, has not been proven. The fact that in such cases of complete motility psychosis it is still possible to communicate with patients, reveals a difference with respect to disorientation. The sensorium is likewise only temporarily clouded or remains perfectly clear. It may be found in some cases that motility is almost exclusively affected, and such cases seem to be characterized by rapid development of explanatory delusions, therefore without unfavourable progression. It is from such patients that the best information about purely motor symptoms can be obtained after their recovery.

Gentlemen! Experiences in the clinic do not allow us to define any exclusively parakinetic form of motility psychoses. Where altered forms of movement dominate for a long time, or throughout an entire illness (as you saw in one case [2]), it transpires that phases of akinesia and hyperkinesia can be differentiated, so that the parakinesia, even when striking, does not exist independently. The concept of parakinesia is evidently only an abstraction, just as we might analyze paraesthesia arising in peripheral nerves in part as hyperaesthesia, in part as paraesthesia, without losing any essential part of the symptomatology.

Gentlemen! As we have seen above, it is in the nature of akinetic symptoms, that it is often totally impossible to decide how far they are intermingled with other identification disorders, and at other times this is possible only after the akinetic stage is over. So we must then take into account the possibility that the above clinical picture of akinetic motility psychosis, derived entirely empirically, is too broad, and still contains cases in which the motor symptom complex is merely grafted onto another syndrome, which is just as significant, and encompasses it. How justified this concept is, we see in some cases of 'complete motility psychosis' [Ed]. These reveal at the outset, apart from the ever-changing motor symptoms, images of 'fantastic menacing delirium' [Ed] with severe disorientation in all three areas of consciousness, and which always seem to have an unfavourable outcome. Very similarly, the fantastic menacing delirium in the paranoid stage of an akinetic motility psychosis is sometimes the only expression of disorientation, that was previously concealed by the akinetic stage.

These cases also have a largely unfavourable prognosis. At other times, the fantastic menacing delirium occurring within well-retained allopsychic orientation is to be seen in the same paranoid stage, combined only with hypochondriacal sensations, mainly intestinal in nature. These cases also follow a predominantly unfavourable course, so that we are to some extent justified in regarding the fantastic menacing delirium in motility psychoses as a generally unfavourable prognostic feature.

Gentlemen! To understand other more complicated cases of motility psychoses, it may help to discuss together all those symptoms based on disorders of identification within the psychomotor pathway *Zm*, as we always did hitherto in analogous cases. However, it has been proved necessary, above all, to clarify how intrapsychic akinesia is to be differentiated from psychomotor akinesia. A digression into *intrapsychic akinesia* [W] therefore cannot be avoided.

Gentlemen! Affective melancholia presented us with an example where symptoms derived from a hypothetical scheme, and these alone, make up a clinical picture which, in reality, is met very often. The situation is not so simple for that state of illness—a more severe grade of intrapsychic functional disorder—namely a deficiency of psychically induced movements, which is a striking form of akinesia in objective terms. The independent significance of such a condition, which provisionally, I would like to call *depressive melancholia* [W], has become more and more questionable over the years. To begin with, I want briefly to present the hallmarks of this condition, as derived from our schema. Patients of this type, of their own volition, stop speaking or doing anything; they therefore present symptoms of mutism and akinesia for initiative movements. Expressive movements are correspondingly fewer, the face less animated, while reactive movements are also involved, but less severely so. Insofar as reactive movements *are* [Ed] affected, this depends on the patient's intrapsychic capacity, certainly not on changes in activation of muscle groups. With complete failure of processes of association, the Affective response that is linked to subjective feelings of inadequacy likewise ceases, and in place of that overvalued idea, a *lack* [Ed] of thought prevails, perhaps even, at times, complete standstill of thinking. An anxious Affective state might be possible once we remember that failure of processes of association represent, in a certain sense, a threat to the body. On the other hand, specific motor symptoms such as flexibility, pseudo-flexibility, muscular rigidity and negativity are missing.

Patients fitting this picture are not rare. Affective melancholia may occasionally show some similarities, and I believe that in the past, I have observed transitions of one condition into the others, in which the picture of depressive melancholia corresponded to more severe grades of the illness, cases which always showed a much longer course than the vast majority of cases of Affective melancholia. In particular, a characteristic of these cases, it seems to me, is strangely intact reactivity in speech, a clearly difficult way of giving an answer, with just a soft flat voice, or with much effort—just when I have turned away from the patients. The same hesitancy, the same complication and retardation, apparently involving overcoming some sort of inhibition can, in such cases, also extend to all other reactive movements. I now think it likely that these transitions from Affective to depressive melancholia do sometimes actually occur, and so I can no longer maintain that depressive melancholia is significant as an independent illness. More detailed examination of such cases during the last few years has always revealed to me additional symptoms which are there to be found, but only when you know what you are looking for. Without having arrived at a conclusive judgment of this, I want briefly to share my experiences.

First [Ed], I have collected a series of statements, in part from the patients themselves, in part from their relatives, according to which a specific condition continued for hours, or occasionally days, at the time of onset of motility psychoses, corresponding most closely to what I have just described—the cessation of any kind of ideation. Sometimes a definite body position was maintained which, in itself was in no way abnormal or constrained. Information given later by patients indicated a complete stand-still of thoughts, as occurs normally in the state of the so-called bewilderment, but then only momentarily. A female patient of this kind was found in such a state on her admission, persistently immovable, her clothes pulled up, and in a foot bath ordered for her. The motor character of this disorder only became clear later on, because she had had mutism already for a long time and could not protrude her tongue, while all other reactive movements were carried out promptly. A *second* [Ed] series of cases consists not only of short-lasting conditions, such as those just described, but correspond to a separate clinical picture of longer duration, always lasting over a year, for which the name *pseudomelancholia* [W] might be appropriate. This 'pseudomelancholia' [Ed] usually forms the first stage of a compound psychosis, which in general has an unfavourable prognosis, although the possibility as an exception, of a favourable outcome always exists. This clinical picture has been spoken of before (p. 103). Cases in this class usually present with some signs of Affective melancholia, so that they might be identified as borderline cases between this and the above clinical picture, constructed on the basis of theory. However, sooner or later in their course, they produce further signs, in that delusions of relatedness join in, this being entirely foreign to melancholia. Cessation of melancholia—which may last for a year or more—then usually gives way to a further, worsening stage of persecutory delusion, and soon also of grandiosity.

The *third* [Ed] case, is the most important, which, on its own would justify establishing a separate clinical entity of depressive melancholia. I have often seen cases of illness, which by any criterion, present primarily with a pure type of intrapsychic akinesia, but which, later on, sometimes after 6 months, turn out to be cases of progressive paralysis. Paralytic symptoms, particularly ones arising from the projection pathways, first emerge here when supposed depressive melancholia is starting to improve and a favourable turn of events is anticipated. Far more often, however, we meet cases of depressive melancholia in which hallmarks of paralysis are there right from the outset, either through participation of the projection system, or by actual deficits. When combined with a mild degree of somnolence, a special subgroup among such cases seems to be defined, which, to judge by results of specific therapy, should be grouped among the luetic brain diseases. Of Heubner's cases [3], a few might belong here.

Gentlemen! As you see, in these cases, as in pseudomelancholia, we are dealing with a definite phase—usually the initial one—of a compound psychosis (see later). In the case of a combination of severe loss of intrapsychic function and hypochondriacal symptoms, it is different, and allows one to interpret the first of these, and the resulting akinesia representing as merely the sequel, induced psychologically, of a severe feeling of physical illness. These cases, which are in large part curable, present the same combination of symptoms throughout the entire illness, and thus form a uniform, albeit mixed, clinical picture. In contrast to hypochondriacal melancholia, mentioned earlier (p. 162), this is driven throughout by disorders of psychosensory identification of the patient's own body, except that, by its very nature, this exercises special influence over motility. The Affective reaction is psychosensory, and thus consists of hypochondriacal feelings of misery and attendant anxiety. At times of remission, or with a favourable response to a medication such as opium, you may hear from patients that they feel too ill to think, or speak or to do anything. In brief, the akinetic reaction is therefore psychologically motivated and not reflexly induced as in the previously mentioned (p. 132) cases. Aberrant sensations can have various locations, usually intestinal.

Gentlemen! I must make special mention of the frequent cases of acquired dementia whose chief characteristic is intrapsychic akinesia. Here I give only bare essentials to differentiate this from depressive melancholia. It may be claimed that the intrapsychic akinesia of acquired dementia is the same as that in depressive melancholia: A deficit in objectively visible movements depending on reduction in intrapsychic function is the indication of those symptoms of Affective melancholia which are felt only subjectively, the inability to take decisions, the coldness of psychic feelings, and the blunting of interests. Therefore, the motivation for voluntary movements is deficient; patients sit or lie around in an apathetic state, and do not present any trace of autopsychically-induced Affect. On the other hand, the obvious sluggishness of thought often means that psychic capability is overburdened, and then leads to expressions of discontent, and, of impoverishment of knowledge, judgments, and often even of ideas. That the latter 'symptoms of deficit' [W], however prominent they may be, do not of themselves bring about intrapsychic akinesia, will be evident to you from my remarks at the beginning of our clinical studies (p. 54).

From all these experiences, we can take the following to be characteristics of intrapsychic akinesia.

1. The disorder is always uniform and general, corresponding to our assumption of diffuse degradation of excitability extending over the entire organ of association. Distinction amongst different muscle groups is never seen. Most noticeably, speech reactions are impeded and retarded in exactly the same way as are all other reactions. Complete failure of speech reactions does not occur, or does so only when more complex psychic performance is required, and to that extent.
2. Initiative movements are in general affected more severely than are reactive ones. This is especially true for speech, which may cease entirely unless there is some external influence—'initiative mutism' [Ed]—although a response is always given to simple questions, albeit sometimes only very softly or tonelessly, with very slight lip movements, slowly and sometimes at the very last moment. As for expressive movements, they are indeed few, yet not absent; and when conveying Affects, such as the above-mentioned hypochondriacal feeling of misery, they occasionally appear as expressive movements. A part of this is the habit of looking at the questioner during oral conversation. In intrapsychic akinesia this special form of reaction is never lost.
3. It has already been adequately demonstrated that intrapsychic akinesia is not accompanied by previously mentioned, specific motor symptoms.

Gentlemen! Before I pass on to describing psychomotor akinesia in detail, I would like to mention a symptom which is encountered occasionally in cases of total motility psychosis, or in those of compound motility psychosis, the so-called *imperative speaking* [W]. Patients in question, during attacks which sometimes last only minutes, at other times up to an hour, may utter, with evident effort and every sign of anxiety, either single words—often quite disconnected—or a definite series of words, such as a series of numbers, or sometimes whole sentences, usually in a fairly loud monotonous raised voice, approximating the mechanical expressionless impression of recitation by a schoolboy. The content—where it is coherent—may be derived from the current situation. One patient of this type generally uttered punctuation aloud, which, in his opinion, belonged with the sentences that he was delivering, somewhat in the following manner: 'When I speak, comma, it strains me, fullstop. I cannot do otherwise, semi-colon'. These patients state that what they say, has been said to them or dictated, and they must repeat it. The compulsion which actually occurs is manifest unmistakably in the mechanical way they repeat; in the evident effort employed, which often radiates out to other areas of musculature; and also finally in patients' facial expressions, sometimes more involuntary, sometimes anxious and perplexed. As this continues, a patient may finally come to be bathed in perspiration, sinking back in total exhaustion, then needing a long rest to recover from the effort. According to patients' own testimonies, there is no doubt that they experience a compulsion to repeat voices they have heard.

In these cases, patients themselves state—and also demonstrate by their conduct—that they are subject to a compulsion; while at other times we may observe directly that their 'will to speak' [Ed] encounters certain resistance. An irradiation of the volitional impulse may be seen, especially in patients who succeed in breaking through psychomotor mutism, which far exceeds the muscle area whose activation is intended. For example, a patient closes his jaws convulsively, opens his eyes wide, wrinkles his forehead, dilates his nostrils, tenses his neck muscles, throws his head back, elevates his shoulders, presses his arms against his body, and then words are uttered in a wheezing, forceful manner.

In contrast, in the familiar pseudospontaneous speaking, which is (for example) the basis of the psychomotor loquacity, the feeling of compulsion is not evident either subjectively or objectively. This is the same difference as that between autochthonous ideas and obsessive ideas.

Gentlemen! A few further facts can be cited here, which serve to explain more fully the nature of the akinetic symptoms. As already indicated, it sometimes happens that generalized immobility takes the form of a flaccid paralysis, instead of its being combined with muscle tension. I have seen this for instance in attacks lasting several hours in the acute stage, a very severe complete motility psychosis, terminating within 6 months in a state of confusion. In these attacks, which were most closely similar to *states of syncope* [W], a patient acted as though she was totally lifeless; and when someone raised her limbs, they fell back in perfectly flaccid fashion, obeying nothing other than the law of gravity; pain sensations and reflexes seemed to be completely eradicated, even including those to the sensitive mucous membrane of the eye; pulse was accelerated but barely palpable; respiration seemed imperceptible. There was no cyanosis, but an unchanged sallow face. Artificial respiration was employed repeatedly for hours until, after repeated attacks, the harmlessness of the condition was revealed. Suddenly, that is after a certain duration of this condition, the patient was able to get up, and then began to dance about with theatrical gestures, and to sing songs of a pious nature; perhaps she was then in an ecstatic semi-rapturous state. I have seen similar states, once again with apparent respiratory arrest lasting several minutes, which pass rapidly into a state of hystero-epilepsy between two attacks, when there was a striking, complete unsteadiness of the head, just like a flaccid paralysis. Moreover, in these states we must not ignore that more things are taking place than just a paralysis of volition: Absence of 'will' [Ed] seems to exist temporarily in cases where patients—for example—suddenly let themselves fall to the ground from a sitting position, or occasionally cannot walk, and then let their legs hang lifeless while they are being carried. Both were observed at a somewhat later stage in the selfsame patients who had passed through conditions similar to syncope. Here, I do not want to neglect—at least to touch on—the so-called hysterical palsies. They have an intimate relationship with conditions just described, even though we should not deny their peculiar nature in any way.

The so-called *hypochondriacal palsies* [W] provide evidence that elimination of will can be manifest in localized muscle areas. These palsies are quite rare, and seem to occur almost exclusively in severe hypochondriacal psychosis. Of course they never amount to palsies of individual muscle and nerve areas, but of whole limbs, or at least of whole sections of limbs. However, these should not be grouped with Charcot's 'psychic palsies' [4] [Ed], which I regard as by-products of suggestion, so that they can easily take on any favoured form. If these are disregarded, the most frequent occurrence is hypochondriacal paraplegia [5], albeit with easy transition to hysterical paraplegia. In my own experience, I can report a case of hypochondriacal hemiplegia, which was right-sided, complicated by motor aphasia. It involved a hypochondriacal psychiatric patient, who soon stubbornly refused food, and who died several months later, death not being attributed to any complication. Careful brain autopsy was carried out, with essentially negative findings. The right-sided paralysis in this case presented peculiarities, differing at first glance from organically based hemiplegia, as shown most conspicuously by the awkward, stiff gait, the affected leg being dragged like a heavy weight. One might have considered this to be simulation, had this been excluded beyond all doubt, by the severe course of the mental illness. Unfortunately, I do not accurately recall the condition of this patient's arm; but I know that arm and shoulder appeared to be deliberately fixated, and that a very unusual picture resulted, which resembled a simulated palsy. In contrast, Charcot's psychic paralysis is usually a flaccid one. One might object that occurrence of hypochondriacal paralysis provides evidence of the possibility of psychic paralysis in Charcot's sense, and, as a possibility, this should not be challenged. However, in separating hypochondriacal and psychic palsies, the latter may occur in mentally healthy people, and one fundamental difference remains: that the latter is based on the abolition of the will in the context of a normal, albeit hidden motive; while for the former, there is the same anomaly of the will, but in consequence of an unhealthy motive. If adhere to this, treatment of psychic palsies is the same as that of simulated palsy.

Related to the so-called hypochondriacal palsies are cases of 'fixed contracture' [Ed], which sometimes—in rare instances—may remain as the residue of the same symptom present during the acute period of illness, but after its termination, while all other disturbances of motility have disappeared. According to the little experience I have had of this, extremities of the limbs seem to be affected preferentially, so that at one time contracture was confined to both hands, at another time to one hand with foot-drop of both feet, combined, in the first case, with moderate degree of dementia, and in the second case with a severe degree. According to the unusual way in which these contractures originated, it was impossible to decide if they were combined with real paralysis; but one can say, at least, that patients' ability for spontaneous work with the muscle areas affected was lost. Of course, these were not cases of progressive paralysis. I have no hesitation in regarding these cases as analogous to ones already familiar to you—of motor and partial sensory aphasia, whose deficits remained after a severe episode of motility psychosis; and I explain them by summation of individual deficits of the psychomotor pathway *Zm*.

With regard to interpretation of the akinetic symptoms, special consideration is needed for pseudo-flexibilitas, in which perfectly clear and alert consciousness is usually present. A patient's independent volition to do something other than whatever is forced on him by passive movement, seems to be absent here, and so one is tempted to trace the moderate generalized akinesia in these cases back to an absence of volition, that is to intrapsychic influences; and the fact that positions imposed on a patient are maintained also fits this interpretation. However, clearly we almost always see that such positions are maintained for a longer duration if one of us is present and busy with patients, than when the patients are left to their own devices. As already indicated above, we must regard this condition as being an effect of suggestion from manipulations performed by an examiner, that is, an involuntary influence derived from existing volitional processes. Cases of negativism, with full retention of activity in the sensorium, display just the opposite: We saw, for example, the following behaviour: A patient, who is perfectly conscious, sits in bed with his eyes open and evidently notices what is going on in the ward. He is requested to raise his right arm. When he does not comply, an attempt is made to make the movement passively; but this meets resistance, increasing in proportion to the strength used. When the patient becomes reluctant, we attempt to explain this difficulty in psychological terms as intentional resistance. Nevertheless, from the rest of the patient's behaviour, it is shown beyond doubt that he did not lack the good intention needed to carry out our request, and that otherwise he shows no tendency to oppose other requests of the physician. We then consider the fact that the patient often exerts very great strength in his resistance, out of all proportion to other volitional manifestations; and so that we get to the idea that volition *is* [Ed] present, which cannot be expressed because of internal resistance, and effort is exerted in the opposite direction, the patient then usually feeling that he is subject to a compulsion. In a similar manner, in attempting to part the patient's lips and separate the lower jaw from the upper jaw, the opposite result is produced: The lips become more tightly closed, masseters and temporal muscles spring into action, although it is soon apparent that the patient really intended to open his mouth; at one time, this cannot occur at all, at another, only with great effort. Sometimes we gather information after inquiring about motives for this behaviour, that voices forbad a patient from performing the movements. However, they are the same voices that subsequently prevented his making the movement spontaneously: Characteristic assertions include: 'They do not let me speak; now they strain and drag me'. I need not emphasize that these voices, with their vetoes and commands, do not explain the patient's strange reactions; in our sense, they are no more than the expression of physical disarray connected to the particular situation. I have already called your attention to the irradiation of the volitional impulse in such cases.

Without doubt the most remarkable and most specific reaction of patients to passive movements is the third form, that is, waxy flexibility. This manifestation, met with exclusively under psychotic conditions, might not at once arouse suspicions of its being based on an aberrant change in volitional action: It must evidently be regarded as a specific cortical reaction to passive movements, which appears in pure form only under certain pathological conditions. These conditions, however, are ones of severe immobility, for only then can it be observed. In other words, it occurs only when the 'will' [Ed] cannot be exercised in passive movement; hence, as part of this disorder, imparted positions persist in unquestioning manner. Once we reach this point of view, pseudo-flexibilitas as well as negativism seem to be just modifications of *Flexibilitas cerea*, [W] which occur when the possibility of *some* [Ed] volitional influence is retained. Attempts to make passive movements are perceived within the cortex. At one time, this might arouse the idea of a movement to be performed, and facilitates the corresponding volitional action; at another time, thought of the impracticability of the movement arises; that is, coupled with the idea of the movement to be performed, is also the 'inhibitory thought' of the required expenditure of effort, which, subjectively, often seems very great. The effect of the will is thus inverted into its opposite. From such an overestimate of the necessary expenditure of effort, the volitional impulse then radiates to wider areas of musculature, as observed under certain conditions (see above).

In patients who are otherwise immobile, a number of muscle contractions appear in the form of negativism, as soon as the attempt is made to change a patient's position, possibly having significance similar to that of a 'modified cortical reflex'. However, persisting contractions and those independent of passive movements are so invariably combined with states of unconsciousness or marked stupor, that one might be compelled to relate them to some form of volitional action. I confine myself to suggesting that there are sufficient clinical and experimental data to prove that central projection motor fields are the origin of tonic spasms and contractures.

Gentlemen! In the literature of our science you will come across the term 'abulia' [Ed] many times, used to designate states of immobility at different levels of severity. We are now in a position to show how inapt this term actually is. It would be justified only for the akinesia of initiative movements in melancholia and dementia, albeit even then an unnecessary term. Amongst motility psychoses, it is not an aberrance of the will, nor does it indicate the impossibility of having notions about objectives for actions; rather it is a disorder of identification between those notions about objectives and the central projection motor fields. Hence one can account for the possibility that localized contractions and palsies can remain even after states of acute psychosis have ended; hence also the possibility of hypochondriacal hemiplegia combined with motor aphasia. To assume a unilateral condition of the will would be nonsense, whereas, deficits in the function of—or actual interruption of the pathways available to—the will, for activation of the motor centres of one hemisphere, is conceivable and not without analogies. Only in this way can occurrence of the Affective state of motor disarray, and of numerous and strangely-coloured explanatory delusions, and many other symptoms, be explained. Under some conditions, one might observe directly that certain notions about objectives are initiated *by* [Ed] motor behaviour itself, for example, when a patient who is made to drop to his knees, raises his head and eyes upwards and puts his hands together as if in prayer; or a body position that is imposed accidentally reminds him of the situation of a fencer or an acrobat, and, at once, he executes those movements which help to complete the picture. Pseudo-spontaneous movements, as primary manifestations, which have been mentioned occasionally, often produce Affective reactions habitually combined with them, such as 'cheerfulness' [Ed] or 'attack' [Ed]. Likewise, emphasis has constantly been placed on the fact that all expressions of movement in hyperkinetic motility psychoses occur without cooperation of the will, to be regarded as primary signs of attendant trains of thought and Affective states. This is true even more when strictly localized pseudo-spontaneous movements are repeated rhythmically, and which occur in akinetic motility psychoses, and where contracture of affected muscles may precede paralysis.

Gentlemen! From such arguments, it seems that in motility psychoses, consciousness of personhood—in our sense, that 'grand complex of ideas' [Ed] which makes up the ego—is to a degree detached from motor mechanisms of the body, over which 'the ego' [Ed] has become used to exert control. As a witness, the 'ego' is confronted with motor processes, and also with the failure of this machine, and in turn, is initially affected by this. It is evident that only dissolution of associations, our hypothetical process of sejunction, can be the basis for this behaviour. Through this connection of events, special light is shed on that group of movements which are almost exclusively under the control of the integrated personality, namely expressions of speech. They are the ones most readily damaged, and provide the finest indicator of the motor character of a psychosis; and we obtain confirmation of this from experiences in the clinic. When you encounter a new patient who responds to your questions with striking silence, and thus makes examination difficult, do not omit, gentlemen, to move his limbs and arrange them in certain positions. You will often be surprised to find quite prominent symptoms of pseudo-flexibilitas and maintenance of imposed positions; and I have myself experienced that, as motility psychosis abates, a type of reflex muteness, that is, a failure to answer questions put by a physician—our reactive mutism—forms the last remaining motor symptom, while all the other reactions are prompt, this being seen so often that I have to consider it to be a regular feature. That it is 'reactive mutism' [Ed], and the fact that it emerges when confronting a physician, is immediately understood, if I remind you of the distinction favoured by a temperamental colleague, between a 'super-' [W] and a 'subconsciousness' [W]. Likewise, we will find it natural that under these circumstances the speech mechanism fails, especially for questions about this very this symptom. Even after lengthy persuasion, the only answer you may get is an understandable Affective outburst (In a 26-year-old Jewish merchant a speech impediment of this sort existed entirely alone. He consulted me in a peculiar manner by handing me a note of the following words: 'Almost always when I want to speak with deliberation, I am unable to utter a sound, despite the greatest effort. Involuntarily I speak very fluently, likewise in reading and singing. This condition has existed since school days, and becomes ever more manifest, so that at times I believed I might be dumb.').

Gentlemen! I remind you now of the account I gave you of consciousness of corporeality, at the start of these clinical discussions. Musculature must have a prominent place in this, and indeed we must presume some vague awareness of the state of our muscles, which constantly accompanies us in our waking state, to regulate posture and gait. We must thus ascribe to the curve of 'psychophysical movements' [Ed], the attribute of their being raised above the general level of body awareness to a moderate degree of excitement. If we remember this, we must also appreciate that expressions of movement in a patient, just like those in a healthy person, immediately presuppose a process of excitement, elaborated within our consciousness of corporeality. Abnormal expressions of movement, which have occupied us here, would find their simplest explanation by assuming that there was a disorder in consciousness of corporeality. We might then modify the definition of volition, which you would take to be present, in such a way that motor projection fields make up a part of bodily consciousness. The idea of 'expenditure of effort' [Ed], necessary for execution of any definite movement likewise belongs with bodily consciousness. Under certain conditions, an aberrant change in the framework of motor ideas, built one upon another, impacts on awareness of the whole body. This has the effect of increasing expenditure of effort, to an abnormally high level, as judged subjectively, for every simple movement, so that movements are avoided, and immobility is the result. Patients adopt abnormal body positions, and—once they are made to stand or walk—also adopt abnormal stance. This is explained in an equally simple manner as disturbed bodily consciousness, such that relationships between trunk and limbs are felt to be changed in certain parts of the vertebral column or in the normal complementary activation of muscle groups cooperating symmetrically in their relative positions, in their proper association. A patient who initially remained motionless and, when forced, tried to avoid locomotion, then discovers that his motor mechanism is in a state of confusion. Clearly, this process cannot be placed on a par with hallucinations, for there, aberrant and abnormally intense stimulation is the main feature, whereas in our case, loosening of firmly established associations suffices as an explanation. Similarly, maintenance of certain abnormal positions may reveal only subjective sensations of changed balance between motor impulse and its collateral and antagonistic [6] activation of definite muscle areas [7], which cooperate in normal positions. Automatically repeated movements, distinguished by their uniformity, are similar to autochthonous thoughts in the domain of personhood. They are autochthonous ideas in the area of corporeality, and are therefore uniform, because everything in this area of the consciousness is localized.

Rhythmic repetition in such cases can be based on existence of a local abnormal stimulus limited to certain uniform movements, which must grow to a certain intensity to produce the movement itself. At this point, some sort of discharge is effected, such that the incentive for movement is relieved until the same process reappears. It is very similar for the process of verbigeration; here too, local stimulation which leads to rhythmical repetition must stick to certain patterns of speech delivery. Imperative talking, that is compulsory repetition of hallucinated words, gives us an example where the starting point for such aberrant stimulatory processes in motor areas can also lie within central sensory areas, if aberrant stimuli there encroach on bodily consciousness. For primary auditory hallucinations, hearing is indeed to be regarded as a stimulation process that arouses not only acoustic patterns, but also related organ sensation; and, beyond the intensity of the original stimulus, it is only the presence of a well-worn pathway, which has always served for repetition, that explains irradiation to the motor speech area. In this way, in the same cases, this aspect of consciousness of corporeality, namely the motor speech area, turns out to be inaccessible to the patient's will, or harder to access than normal. An analogue to this reaction of the motor area in bodily consciousness of stimuli streaming into it from central sensory regions, is to be found in the following observation. Such a patient is found sitting in bed holding his right hand in a position as though he were holding something in it, although nothing is to be seen. Specifically, the thumb is pressed against the first two fingers and the ends of the fingers pressed together. This is the same patient who is teased and enticed by voices. I now request him to raise his left arm, which he does readily; I then request this of the right arm, but without success. Repeating the request leads to the same result. I now try to place his right arm in another position and at once meet growing resistance, and then vigorous signs of unwillingness on the part of the patient. Careful examination of the fingers shows that the patient has a tiny bit of cloth between his fingers, that came from his woollen duvet. After this has been taken away, he makes all required movements with his right hand, just as he had done before with his left hand. While such examples reveal an abnormally strong influence of intercortical pathways, other observations, in which garbled words are sometimes uttered by the same type of patient, indicate that the influence of these pathways—which are always normally used in speaking—can meet similar difficulties in the effect of will on speech movements; without this, it is impossible for speech movements to be uttered suddenly in paraphasic form. This instance can likewise be generalized. Consider for example that in walking and standing our movements must be constantly regulated by centripetal stimuli, then here, too, one must acknowledge the influence of intercortical pathways on movement ideas required for standing and walking. The same inhibition, which is responsible for immobility of the patient, transfers to such intercortical pathways, and then seems very well suited, just as in the speech area, to produce the paraphasia (*sit venia verbo*).

References

1. Wernicke C. Krankenvorstellungen aus der psychiatrischen Klinik in Breslau. Breslau: Schletter; 1899. vol. 1, Cases 6, 15, and 21 are examples of cyclic motility psychosis.
2. Wernicke C. Krankenvorstellungen aus der psychiatrischen Klinik in Breslau. Breslau: Schletter; 1899. vol. 1 (Cases 15 is an example of cyclic motility psychosis.)
3. Heubner JBO. Die luetische Erkrankung der Hirnarterien: nebst allgemeinen Erörterungen zur normalen und pathologischen Histologie der Arterien sowie zur Hirncirculation, eine Monographie. Leipzig: FCW Vogel; 1874.
4. Charcot JM. Oeuvres complètes: Leçons sur les maladies due système nerveux. Progr Méd. 1890; 3:299–359.
5. Wernicke C. Krankenvorstellungen aus der psychiatrischen Klinik in Breslau. Breslau: Schletter; 1899. vol. 3 Case 23 is an example of hypochondriacal paraplegia.
6. Boulogne GBA. Physiologie des mouvements démontrée à l'aide de l'expérimentation électrique et de l'observation clinique, et applicable à l'étude des paralysies et des déformations. Paris: Baillière; 1867.
7. Hering HE, Sherrington CS. Über Hemmung der Contraction willkürlicher Muskeln bei elektrischer Reizung der Grosshirnrinde. Pflug Arch Ges Physiol. 1897;68(5):221–8.

Lecture 36

36

- Simple or basic forms of acute psychoses
- Mixed and compound psychoses
- Examples

Lecture

Gentlemen!

You will recall how strongly I have always emphasized that our clinical knowledge of the psychoses is still very incomplete. You must also bear in mind that the cases I present exemplify most of the more frequent types of illness; yet, taken together they do not constitute the majority of the main types. In other words, the more complicated and therefore less familiar cases predominate in number. The principle that has guided me in this selection is well known, and readily understood, namely to serve teaching purposes. Thus, you had to be shown simple cases, composed of a few elementary symptoms, where we could gain as full an understanding as possible. For us, they form the foundation of a theory of illness, to which we must refer continually in order to understand more complex cases. In this sense we could designate types of illness considered so far as fundamental forms of psychosis. It is not my intention now to attempt to describe just those cases which extend beyond the simpler situations: However, I cannot neglect a few brief comments on the perspective you will have to use in evaluating those cases which predominate in practice. Obviously, we should not attempt to force them artificially into some kind of schema, even if it be one like ours, which has been tried and tested. Nevertheless, our scheme does so much to help analyze presenting symptoms in these complex cases.

Firstly, I remind you that, between any two familiar forms of acute psychosis, we have already found many transitional cases. These are amongst the simplest examples of those more complicated *mixed psychoses*, [W] as we shall call them. Thus borderline cases of anxiety psychosis and Affective melancholia, which I briefly outlined earlier (p. 149), are familiar to you. Because of their high frequency, they deserve to be emphasized. Less common are cases of delirious anxiety psychosis, briefly mentioned earlier (p. 147), fairly pure cases of acute autopsychosis whose content was one of anxious belittlement, in which essentially only the course and contribution from the projection system are borrowed from *Delirium tremens* [W]. The clinical picture of agitated melancholia, which I likewise characterized for you as an anxiety psychosis (p. 148), is perhaps amenable to a uniform explanation, if we assume that the frequent occurrence of ideas of anxiety leads to loquacity and flight of ideas. In any case, coincidence of these two manic symptoms with anxiety psychosis is quite exceptional. Moreover, agitated melancholia corresponds to one of the more frequent illness types. These cited examples

R. Miller, K.J. Dennison (eds.), *An Outline of Psychiatry in Clinical Lectures*,
DOI 10.1007/978-3-319-18051-9_36

represent mixed forms, which wholly or partly include autopsychic disorientation, so that they always remain within the larger illness group of autopsychoses.

As a transitional case between autopsychoses and somatopsychoses, we have become acquainted with the example of hypochondriacal melancholia (p. 162). In Affective melancholia, the 'overvalued idea' [Ed] is a feature taking its content from bodily consciousness, and whose derivation from a hysterical sensation is usually unmistakable. In depressive melancholia, the somatopsychic element predominates by far, whenever it is derived from severe hypochondriacal mental illness (p. 262). In both cases, we can assume that other sets of symptoms have a conditional relationship, but in opposite directions. Thus, in hypochondriacal melancholia, the hypochondriacal element appears as a consequence, while in depressive melancholia, it becomes the origin of the autopsychosis. In hypochondriacal mental illnesses, we regularly encounter similar mutual conditionality based on the fact that the symptom of anxiety, which is seldom absent, can have as a consequence, corresponding autopsychic ideas of anxiety, which lead to autopsychic disorientation in the form of belittlement. Thus we conclude that somatopsychoses occur only rarely in pure form, but usually fit the concept of 'autosomatopsychoses' [Ed], and thus really belong among the mixed psychoses. You will find that in my presentation of the somatopsychoses I always took this into consideration. In contrast, I deliberately said nothing about another combination, which is seen no less often. It consists of that form of disorientation which often occurs quite acutely, and which we can designate as 'hypochondriacal delusional state of persecution' [Ed]. Moreover, there exists internal connection between somatopsychic symptoms, and (in this case), allopsychic symptoms, due partly to simple explanatory delusions, and in part to the elementary symptom of somatopsychic delusions of relatedness, which, at the time, we categorized as new-formed associations. In acute psychoses, the latter connection evidently predominates, and often does so, either just initially, or entirely, even in cases which lack autopsychic disorientation via belittlement. We include such cases amongst acute allosomatopsychoses, a well-defined hybrid between allopsychoses and somatopsychoses. In other cases, this combination develops on the same basis, while anxiety soon reaches a very high level, with disorientation in all three areas of consciousness, and characteristic content which is fantastic, and at the same time a hypochondriacal, menacing delusional state. This is often a very acute clinical picture of total sensory psychosis, usually associated with a huge numbers of hallucinations, fear of being touched and blind defensiveness. In the autopsychic area, it often comes down not only to ideas of belittlement, but also to the opposite picture of grandiosity; and the disorientation often has a tendency to gravitate in the latter direction, while belittling ideas, in the guise of phonemes, are strongly rejected, and the Affective state of disarray prevails in this respect. The helpless compulsion towards movement described above (p. 232) is peculiar to all these cases. As a result of the disorientation, the most diverse acts of disarray may occur: among them, running about blindly; breaking windows; attacks on people round about; and self-harm in most diverse ways, according to the location of hypochondriacal sensations; finally, we should explicitly mention the refusal of all food. Differentiation of the clinical picture described here, is mainly made in the motor domain, in that we can include only cases in which actual motility symptoms are entirely absent. The clinical picture of acute total sensory psychosis, with content of fantastic hypochondriacal menacing delusions, occurs quite often as very brief attacks, lasting only a few hours or days, based either on intoxication or degenerative processes. Chronic alcoholism is particularly involved in the case of intoxication; in the case of degenerative states, those with hysterical and epileptic disposition make up the majority of the so-called *transitory psychoses.* [W] Prior head injuries predispose to this. For longer states of this sort, I am unaware of any deeper aetiological relationship. I need not mention that this is always a life-threatening situation. If maintained, a more-or-less severe state of exhaustion, with memory deficit, tends to follow, which may merge into convalescence. A paranoid stage is not observed. With respect to the course of acute fantastic hypochondriacal menacing delusional states, their development up to their peak may be reached within a few quarter-hours in cases of transitory psychosis; in other cases it develops over a period of a few weeks, from an initial hypochondriacal stage, in which delusions of relatedness with hallucinations in all the senses occur, as well as explanatory delusions of most diverse kinds. Even for these cases however, as the severe state endures for longer periods, a predominantly sensory character and evident worsening course tends to develop, mainly with motor symptoms and of various hyperkinetic, parakinetic, and akinetic types, which can lead, at this stage, to profound exhaustion and death. I have seen many such cases, mainly amongst those with a severe hereditary predisposition; they deserve to be called *acute progressive sensory psychosis* [W]. One case of this kind, involving a 40-year-old kyphoscoliotic labourer with hereditary loading, not addicted to alcohol, ran through this course within 2 months, during which the patient lost 24 lb in body weight despite extensive feeding during the last week. Moreover, the majority of cases of transitory psychosis tend to be accompanied by more specific motility symptoms.

Gentlemen! The picture outlined above of acute fantastic hypochondriacal menacing delusional states is amongst the most severe Affective states we know. When it has lasted somewhat longer, often even after a few days, the general finding is that it leads to a degree of damage of such severity as is found elsewhere only in the most severe general physical illnesses. Shrunken features; general muscular tremor; hoarse, rasping voice; dry, scaly coating on the lips, tongue and teeth. Quite often, and probably then as a *sequela*, signs of incipient blood decomposition or severe trophic disorders foretell impending demise. Disorders of nutrition can also find a basis in pathological anatomy, for example as inflammatory foci in the anterior horns of the spinal cord, with multiple gangrenous areas in skin (autopsy carried out by Cohnheim). It is mainly such cases, which other authors have called *Delirium acutum* [W]. However, we cannot acknowledge this as a special sort of illness, but recognize only the readily comprehensible consequences of a particular clinical picture, with acute features, rapidly taking a severe toll on available energy. Such extremely severe cases are fortunately quite rare, although a proportion of them also present with additional symptoms from the projection system, so that they are claimed as cases of the so-called 'galloping paralysis' [Ed]. Moreover, you would be wrong if you thought that total sensory psychosis always had characteristic contents of fantastic hypochondriacal menacing delusions. That is by no means true, as it shows up mainly as mixed cases, with only moderate levels of Affect, and with delusional ideas whose content covers various types of partial disorientation, differing greatly amongst individuals. For example, somatopsychic disorientation may be limited to delusions of pregnancy, autopsychic disorientation to accompanying ideas of having sinned, and allopsychic disorientation restricted only to certain time periods and certain relationships, so that the prevailing situation can still be recognized correctly. Phonemes and explanatory delusions then form accessory parts of the clinical picture [1]. At other times, partial disorders of orientation are found in isolation, at least in their not being mixed simultaneously with significant motility phenomena, which usually endow the explanatory delusions with a definite magical aura in their content. You will find several examples of this type, characterized, I should say, by a relatively rapid favourable course, described as mixed acute sensorimotor psychoses, among the patient demonstrations from my clinic [2].

Mixed forms, lying between motility psychoses and more-or-less extended sensory psychoses, are familiar to you, in part from descriptions I have already given. So I remind you of facts highlighted in discussing confused mania, that hyperkinetic motility psychosis may be associated with allopsychic disorientation, for which combination I reserve a special place. These cases have the same menstrual basis, and the same tendency to periodic recurrence as hyperkinetic motility psychoses, and deserve the name 'hyperkinetic allopsychoses' [Ed]. Less often we encounter the combination of hyperkinetic motility psychosis, or agitated confusion with more severe hypochondriacal symptoms, yet I have had a few cases of this kind, in which hyperkinetic symptoms were replaced by (and seemed partially to be grafted onto) a hypochondriacal stage lasting only a few days, with tendency to severe self-harm. Hypochondriacal symptoms in these cases represent a brief stage at the very peak. Affiliation of motility symptoms with changed body awareness is thus illustrated again. At other times, acute hyperkinetic motility psychoses are associated from the start with total disorientation, which we learn from the adverse behaviour at the time of the aroused state, and later from information given by the patients. Very recently, we saw an example of this kind [3]. I already mentioned that the more-or-less prominent picture of a hyperkinetic motility psychosis may later be added to a state of total sensory psychosis; and that this may be the basis of the severe course taken by certain cases of acute progressive psychosis. You will remember in this eventuality, that it is not usually a hyperkinetic motility psychosis whose progressive course unfolds, but a complete motility psychosis.

For akinetic motility psychoses, from the outset we should abandon the idea of considering only pure cases; the fact that we usually have to deal with mixed cases is therefore quite well known to you. Nonetheless, I want to emphasize explicitly that a definite combination, specifically that with hypochondriacal symptoms, makes up an almost normal picture; again this indicates that motility psychoses should be included with the broader concept of somatopsychoses. On the other hand, in many cases, the fact that complete allopsychic orientation is retained, has been established with reasonable certainty. In one such case, there was complete somatopsychic orientation, yet complicated by fantastic delusions of belittlement, and in general by a picture of Affective melancholia. Irrespective of the latter, we deal here with cases whose course is unfavourable, whereas other cases, with total disorientation in the sensory area, recover completely, even though this may be years later in some cases. There seems to be no compelling case for drawing an analogy between the differentiation amongst these cases and the quite circumscribed nature of direct focal symptoms in brain diseases. I have already emphasized sufficiently the fact that cases of akinetic motility psychosis associated with total sensory disorientation and fantastic menacing delusions require special interpretation, and generally have an unfavourable prognosis.

Gentlemen! Cyclic motility psychoses have given us the opportunity to become familiar with forms which mix mania and melancholia in two opposed phases of illness. Quite apart from motility psychoses, such combinations, and resulting cases of mixed psychosis, are not rarities; and we can understand that disorientation of any sort, not itself an effect of mania or melancholia, is often enough associated with diffuse augmentation or reduction of excitability in association pathways. Most often, we are dealing with very different cases of illness, which are still unknown. On the other hand, certain combinations of a more familiar kind are also occasionally encountered. Thus I mentioned previously (p. 240) certain cases of manic allopsychosis; and, to complete what I said earlier, would add that in cases of hyperkinetic motility psychosis orientation to the outside world seems to be damaged directly, if patients are at the same time manic, or have presented with a prominent, purely manic picture as the early stage of their illness.

The combination of allopsychotic symptoms with mania is important practically, and deserves special mention. The clinical picture of *choleric mania* [W], found quite often as an independent illness, consists essentially of a combination of mania with ideas of anxiety and corresponding phonemes, but without any necessary allopsychic disorientation. Usually however, allopsychic delusions of relatedness and hypermetamorphosis are present. Complaints of anxiety itself are made, and fear of being approached, and terror are also sometimes observed. A very typical case of this kind occurred at intervals of exactly 4 weeks, and lasted 14 days, without menstrual aetiology being possible, since it was in an

18-year-old youth at the stage of puberty, who was strikingly backward physically, and with a strong hereditary taint. Choleric mania generally seems, as in this case, to have a favourable outcome. Choleric mania in paralytics, which is not uncommon, usually makes up no more than one phase of the illness.

Through confused mania, I have come into contact from time to time with a further combination, not of mania, but of consecutive asthenic confusion with allopsychic disorientation; and likewise I have emphasized that the same combination is also to be observed in primary, asthenic confusion (pp. 241, 242). It remains to be decided whether a causative connection exists between demonstrable weakness of association and allopsychical disorientation. Occurrence of asthenic autoallopsychosis in young girls, mentioned in this connection, certainly supports this.

The intermingling of Affective melancholia with these other psychoses is much less familiar than their combination with mania; and then I need do no more than mention the combination. I refer to previously mentioned (p. 274) co-occurrence of melancholia with akinetic motility psychosis, or with the akinetic phase of a cyclic motility psychosis.

Gentlemen! Besides mixed psychoses, with which we have just been dealing, we can differentiate *compound psychoses* [W]. These are distinguished by the fact that in them, illness proceeds in distinct stages or phases, independent of one another. I make a general comment on the importance of the independence or individuality of these phases. In most acute psychoses, we must acknowledge an initial stage which, as we have seen, owes its hallmark to the specific Affective state of disarray. Disarray can rise to the level of anxiety and despair; or anxiety can itself be regarded as a special somatopsychic form of disarray. We cannot regard this initial stage as an independent manifestation, because the prevalent Affect is merely a reaction to the same elementary symptoms that lead to disorientation, and which determines the special features of a definite simple psychosis. As you will remember, this initial stage provided the first reason to envisage the course of every psychosis as occurring in stages; the first stage should accordingly be a melancholic one, in the sense used by older authors. Had the acute psychosis gone beyond its peak and developed to a special paranoic stage before actual recovery, we would not be able to perceive it as an independent stage, in the sense just suggested. For us, this stage is nothing more than the more-or-less pure picture of disorientation, after abatement of those acute symptoms which led to the disorientation. Where, instead, it goes on to a paranoic or, after that, a demented stage, the same reflection is just as true, because it also represents a *sequela* [Ed] like the paranoic stage. Moreover, the final outcome in an incurable state, that is either chronic mental disorder or dementia, cannot, for us, be a real stage in this sense.

You see, gentlemen, that in this way we can exclude from the concept of compound psychoses most psychoses that we know about, be they simple or mixed. Only in one respect might we remain in doubt, namely over whether the sequence of contrasting states such as mania and melancholia is to be interpreted as a set of independent stages. Here too the possibility is raised that increased excitability, which is the basis of one stage, only prepares for—or induces—the reduced excitability in the other stage, just as we see in the peripheral nervous system: These two stages often follow each other. As you know, Meynert [4] actually advocated such a causal connection, and explained it through vasomotor influences. The same principle could be extended to consecutive phases of hyperkinesia and akinesia. However, I would like to make use of this notion only in so far as I acknowledge that the convalescence from mania (p. 209) preceding melancholia, and likewise the reverse relationship, as such *sequelae*. In either case we should bear in mind the circular mental illness and the cyclic motility psychosis as special cases of composite psychoses. If we adopt this viewpoint, it gives support to the idea that composite psychoses are encountered far more rarely than simple or mixed psychoses, as Ziehen already correctly recognized.

Cases of *composite motility psychoses* [W] arouse our special interest, because it is clearly these which led Kahlbaum [5] to formulate his clinical picture of catatonia. By 'composite motility psychosis' [Ed], we understand quite generally all those acute psychoses which occur in different stages, if one of these fits a picture of motility psychosis. The most common event is the transition, mentioned several times already, from an anxiety psychosis to a motility psychosis, and indeed we can then speak of a composite motility psychosis, even if the first stage—the anxiety psychosis—has a much longer duration, months at least, so that it cannot be interpreted simply as an initial stage. Very often, the anxiety psychosis develops into an akinetic–parakinetic motility psychosis [6], and then often with a particular coloration signifying that the Affect of anxiety remains, either always intermingled with, or at least occasionally breaking through the akinesia. The later course of such cases seems usually to be unfavourable. More rarely, in cases with especially severe Affective symptoms, development to a hyper-parakinetic motility psychosis takes place. The first stage has thus a content of fantastic belittlement and menacing delusions, with the usual fluctuations appearing to be improvements in the anxiety psychosis. Motor symptoms are more uniform than in hyperkinetic motility psychoses; parakinesia predominates, mainly as expressions of anxiety, for example, as rhythmical yelling. Instead of the anxiety psychosis shifting directly into motility psychosis, an increase of the anxiety psychosis is often seen, initially to total sensory psychosis with content of fantastic menacing delusions, and then, with further worsening, to the picture of a motility psychosis, a course which, like the above-mentioned clinical picture, corresponds to an acute progressive psychosis. Instead of a *total* [Ed] sensory psychosis, it is also often transformed into a state where the only impairment of awareness of the outside world involves frightening hallucinations, without orientation being directly affected. In all such cases, motility psychosis appears at the peak of a worsening and rather extended trajectory of the illness.

Now, if we acknowledge that the most common form of acute progressive psychoses is an anxiety psychosis, escalating to a motility psychosis, other forms also often occur, where the peak takes the form of a motility psychosis, while, at onset of the illness, some other psychosis prevails. This is particularly common in the case of acute hallucinosis—quite similar to anxiety psychosis—with which we have already become acquainted, as a particularly progressive form, which can lead to complete motility psychosis. Moreover, the special form of circumscribed autopsychosis mediated by overvalued ideas, may take a similar progressive course. An especially instructive case of this kind involved a 41-year-old night watchman, admitted in December, 1895, who presented initially only with the overvalued idea that a cultured young lady was in love with him, and had led him to recognize this by her conduct towards him (an autopsychic delusion of reference). His detention led to the explanatory idea that a rival wanted to take his place. After just 2 months, I presented this patient in an entirely changed state, since he now believed that he was being widely persecuted, his body destroyed by poison, and imagined himself to be seriously ill and weak, believing that he was a count, and had been abducted in childhood by robbers; and he became threatening and, at the same time, violent. Occasionally, at this stage, hyperkinetic and parakinetic symptoms were mixed in. Here, therefore an illness which was entirely circumscribed, followed a basically progressive course, right to the point where motility symptoms occurred. The only striking feature of this initial, and otherwise quite pure stage of circumscribed autopsychosis, was that it was associated with numerous, peculiar phonemes—peculiar in that they consisted exclusively of terms of endearment on the part of that young lady, so that the patient had coined the technical expression 'language of the heart' [W]. For aetiology, sexual abstinence undoubtedly played a part, since he had lived apart from his wife for 2 years, and had had too little sleep in the last year; there was no alcohol abuse. The illness of a 30-year-old maidservant began in the form of an acute allopsychosis with allopsychical disorientation, which lasted several months. She then gradually became completely motionless and, for about 18 months, presented a picture of akinetic motility psychosis. After gradual abatement of the akinesia and finally, also the disappearance of the mutism, she now appears to have entered convalescence without signs of deficit. The case of a 28-year-old tailoress ran in three separate stages: She appeared melancholic for 9 months then, with rapid increase in symptoms, remained disorientated with respect to the outside world and body awareness for a further 3 months, and finally presented a symptom complex of akinetic motility psychosis. I was able to present her to you about 6 months after the beginning of the third stage, when she was totally demented, with contractures of both hands, a fixed position of trunk and head reminiscent of Meynert's celebrated optic thalamus case; walking and standing in the *Pes equinus* [W] position or on the outer edges of the feet. Rapid transition of the first into the second stage was characterized by emergence of incoherent delusions of persecution and grandiosity.

The gradual transformation of one clinical picture into the other, and the evident progression which occurs as the range of symptoms extends, results in the separation of special stages in such cases seeming somewhat artificial; the opposite view is held only by those observers who see the patients only rarely, with long intervening intervals.

The situation is quite different in a number of other cases. Thus, some time ago, I showed you a patient presenting a picture of akinetic motility psychosis with marked stupor, who, allegedly, was acutely ill. Certain indications in the case history led us to suspect that we were dealing with a paralytic illness, and, in fact I could show you the same patient not long afterwards, free from motility symptoms, but in a state of that fantastic grandiosity, which we recognize as a specific paralytic form of expansive autopsychosis (p. 219). Here, one condition had replaced the other. Mania also commonly includes a stage of composite motility psychosis. This can follow an akinetic motility psychosis, either immediately or after an intermediate stage of apparent dementia, usually not quite pure, but with admixed hypermetamorphosis or agitated confusion with sensory mediation (pp. 235, 236). In this combination, the manic stage appears to be a favourable omen, leading to recovery, either directly or after a further stage of exhaustive stupor. Mania proved to have the same favourable significance, in a case where it appeared as the third stage, after a stage of agitated motor confusion, and a second one of residual hallucinosis. Severe phthisis came in as a complicating factor, which prevented significant increase in body weight. With regard to aetiology, this female patient, a 32-year-old straw hat seamstress, aside from significant hereditary influence, presented with overwork, trouble, and worry, haemorrhage from an external injury, and finally, an attack of influenza. I would briefly like to mention the combination of complete motility psychosis, defined purely by motor symptoms, with severe hypochondriacal psychosis developing after the motility psychosis had totally abated, leading us to the definite expectation of imminent recovery. In one case, a further separate, apparently unfavourable stage of delusion-formation, based on sensory symptoms, led to a single attack of cyclic motility psychosis of puerperal aetiology. One case must arouse our special interest, in which a 16-day stage of ordered mania was followed by an apparently lucid interval of 2 days, preceded by an akinetic motility psychosis, which continued for 4 months; and even in its full picture, never reached the level where the patient's personal hygiene lapsed, and which was then followed, in turn, by a paranoid stage and finally by dementia. Notably, the manic picture of the first stage, at times of greatest excitement, had a mixture merely hinting at a motility disorder, in that the patient sometimes persistently adopted domineering postures, and thereby presented a rather rigid manner of expression. This 20-year-old patient had some hereditary loading, and a mentally ill brother.

In addition, the picture of choleric mania, which is itself already a mixture, may occur as a stage in a composite psychosis. This was so, in a case of hereditary, degenerative aetiology in a 15-year-old boy, leading to a second stage of hyperkinetic motility psychosis, followed by a further stage of severe exhaustion-stupor; the patient, who had repeatedly had brief attacks of psychosis, was initially perfectly well. Recurrent attacks of choleric mania, lasting only a few hours at irregular intervals of 1–4 days, whose interim periods were sometimes approximately normal, were sometimes largely replaced by states of anxiety with terrifying hallucinations. This led to the second stage of a composite psychosis lasting 6 months, starting with anxiety psychosis lasting about 1 month. Residual *sequelae* involved severe confusion with autopsychic and allopsychic disorientation corresponding to previous hallucinations and a moderately irritable mood. This 52-year-old female patient presented no prospect of further recovery, and was transferred to a secure unit. For further examples of compound psychoses, I still return, on occasion to the aetiological grouping of psychoses, and I would like to emphasize here only one point, that progressive paralysis, when it proceeds as a composite psychosis, often also produces a stage of choleric mania, and especially at the time of acute onset of the illness.

References

1. Wernicke C. Krankenvorstellungen aus der psychiatrischen Klinik in Breslau, vol. 3. Breslau: Schletter; 1899. Case 9.
2. Wernicke C. Krankenvorstellungen, vol. 1, Case 28 and vol. 2, 1899. Case 2.
3. Wernicke C. Krankenvorstellungen, vol. 3, 1899. Case 20.
4. Meynert T. Der Bau der Grosshirnsrinde und seine örtlichen Verschiedenheiten, nebst einem pathologisch-anatomischen Corollarium. Leipzig: Engelman; 1887.
5. Kahlbaum KL. Die Katatonie oder das Spannungsirresein. Berlin: A Hirschwald; 1874.
6. Wernicke C. Krankenvorstellungen, vol. 2 Case 21, vol. 3 Case 18 are examples of this.

Lecture 37

37

- Progressive paralysis, an aetiological group of diseases
- Prodromal symptoms
- Spinal and cortical symptoms
- Various forms of paralytic psychoses
- Course as a compound psychosis
- Paralytic dementia
- Remissions and paralytic attacks
- Atypical paralysis
- Worsening paralysis
- Diagnosis
- Treatment
- Anatomical findings

Lecture

Gentlemen!

We have often met Progressive paralysis in the course of these discussions, and in such different forms that you will have already reached a conclusion as to the importance of this group of illnesses. However, the main theoretical significance of the group is far greater: For, alone among all the psychoses, cases in this group show almost constant anatomical findings, and in addition, as we also know, the constancy of this finding corresponds with constancy of certain symptoms common to almost all cases; while, beyond that, very different localization of the disease process is also to be found, but with corresponding differences in symptomatology. Thus, it gives us an example of a brain disease in which anatomical findings and symptoms correspond with one another. Of course, up to now this principle has applied only to symptoms arising in the projection system, and to the symptom of disintegration, namely dementia. However, by analogy it is permissible to conclude that what applies here, applies also to an equally large diversity of clinical psychiatric pictures, if one were in a position to locate these clinical pictures symptomatologically. Thus, progressive paralysis offers us a way into a general anatomical foundation for the psychoses. You see, gentlemen, that from this point of view, we again need to hold to the view that progressive paralysis represents no more than an aetiological recapitulation of psychoses, which otherwise differ widely from one other.

Paralytic aetiology shows itself to be related most closely to toxic effects, with the sole difference that it is a toxic effect to be seen as arising repeatedly anew within the organism. The progressive deleterious character of the disease can be explained in no other way. This necessary concept can be explained by analogy with the spinal disease *Tabes dorsalis* [W] and an assumed 'metasyphilitic toxin' [Ed], in contrast to the syphilitic aetiology. Despite this, you still cannot avoid accepting bacterial action as the basis for this peculiar behaviour. But I want to comment here that sporadic exceptions to this deleterious progression are to be seen. Over the years,

R. Miller, K.J. Dennison (eds.), *An Outline of Psychiatry in Clinical Lectures*,
DOI 10.1007/978-3-319-18051-9_37

however, amongst thousands of cases of severe paralytic psychosis with a clear syphilitic basis, a few cases have recovered completely, and not relapsed. As you can see from these comments, I perceive paralysis to be the epitome of syphilis-related psychoses, a viewpoint finding increased general recognition, and which appears justified by experiences in our Clinic. It would already be clear to you from my periodic utterances that a certain psychosis cannot be said to have an *exclusive* [Ed] causal relationship to syphilis. You can never recognize anything more than the *preference* [Ed] of a particular aetiology for a particular form of illness.

With this restriction, you must consider as specific to paralytic psychosis, the fantastic grandiosity, that is the earlier-mentioned (p. 219) *expansive* [W] form of *autopsychosis* [W], seen almost exclusively in the context of syphilis. But I have already alluded (p. 220), though not often, to the occurrence of Kahlbaum's [1] so-called *Progressiva divergens* [W], which probably was not syphilitic—and I presented to you the case of an 86-year-old woman with the same fantastic grandiose delusions—which certainly was not. The fantastic grandiosity, like other yet-to-be mentioned, and more distinct psychoses, often forms the first stage of a composite psychosis [2] usually lasting only weeks or months.

The *prodromal symptoms* [W] of progressive paralysis, usually accompanied by feelings of severe illness, are well known. They consist of headaches, insomnia, and irritable mood, and can precede outbreak of acute psychosis by 1–2 years. However, quite often, headaches are denied. In this prodromal stage, often indistinguishable from severe neurasthenia, you often also hear complaints of forgetfulness and failing ability to perform, although these symptoms cannot be verified objectively. However, early on in some cases, and in this prodromal stage, symptoms derived from the projection system may be prominent. To recapitulate briefly, they usually consist just of a suggestion of facial palsy or tongue deviation; the so-called 'paralytic speech impediment' [Ed]; and a tremor of the *voice, tongue, and lips*. The *paralytic speech disorder* [W] ranges between two opposites, which we can describe as 'stumbling over syllables' [Ed], and blurring of speech—if you prefer to avoid the anatomical terms of cortical and bulbar speech disorder. To assess stumbling over syllables, you can use test words to be repeated, like 'civilization' [Ed], 'army reorganization' [Ed], 'extraterritoriality' [Ed], etc. The voice becomes tremulous, up to the point of aegophony. If these symptoms, which are decisive indicators of palsy, are missing during the prodromal stage, diagnosis may still be possible, as soon as you can detect characteristic spinal symptoms. These *spinal symptoms* [3] [W] sometimes precede all other paralytic phenomena, and are therefore the most valuable diagnostic tools. Here, they indicate no more than signs of the so-called 'column disease' [Ed] of the spinal cord, symptoms derived partly from dorsal columns, partly from lateral columns. From the former, one must expect rigidity of the pupillary reflex. Without doubt, little value can be placed pupillary inequality. I particularly draw your attention to certain characteristic signs of combined columnar disease, although there are two types that are equally valid: Respectively, they are increased passive mobility of the legs with simultaneous increase of tendon reflexes; and reduction of passive mobility, producing prominent rigidity, together with reduction or even a total absence of tendon reflexes. Through prolonged observation, we see one of these patterns being replaced by the other; for example, return of a lost knee jerk! As regards their diagnostic value, it is important to note that in neurasthenia there may be an increase in tendon reflexes, but never a reduction.

As for the immediate precipitant of the illness, undoubtedly strenuous mental activity has often preceded it. However, we would be giving a false impression if we took into account only the 'quantum' [Ed] of work; we often see men with unceasing and strenuous mental activity who reach their later years full of vigour. Indeed, I would like to suggest that strenuous mental work is even beneficial to health. What is harmful by itself is to work under emotional pressure. Whoever finds himself forced to work beyond his individual strength, under tight time pressure, taking on responsibilities beyond his capacity, must struggle with excitement, grief, and sorrow which can easily lead to impairment in purely. Undoubtedly all-pervading careerism encourages such damage. From this fact, and similarly from the increased prevalence of syphilitic infection, we can explain the significant predominance of the male sex, particularly amongst educated classes. The age of maximum risk is between 30 and 50 years, especially 35–45.

Alongside expansive autopsychosis we find paralytic mania; in this respect I refer again to my earlier remarks (p. 219). Usually, the picture of mania is coloured by simultaneous presence of fantastic grandiosity. At other times, it is not so pure, in that hypermetamorphosis or hyperkinetic symptoms accompany the mania. Nevertheless, cases of almost pure mania of paralytic aetiology undoubtedly occur [4]; and after running its course, only very rarely is there complete recovery, although there is often very good remission over a prolonged duration. At other times, the mania subsides, but is transformed into a more restrained state of simple fantastic grandiosity.

Affective melancholia may also have a paralytic aetiology, even if it is not usually entirely pure but rather an admixture with either mild delusions of relatedness, or symptoms of anxiety psychosis, or both, these being foreign to pure melancholia. It is widely known that melancholia occurring in the age range 35–45 years raises suspicions of paralysis.

Depressive melancholia of paralytic origin has already been mentioned. Here, too, delusions of relatedness are frequent additions, so that the differential diagnosis of pseudomelancholia comes into question.

Amongst paralytic allopsychoses, I stress the importance of *paralytic delirium* [W]. In contrast to previously mentioned forms of paralytic psychosis, which occur preferentially in initial stages of the illness, the delirious condition can appear in any phase of the illness, often quite suddenly and unexpectedly. In most cases, it is therefore not difficult to make a correct diagnosis. Incidentally, the clinical picture can be the same in all detail as that of *Delirium tremens*, as already emphasized (p. 174). However, this is nevertheless rare. Mostly, one is struck by the dominance of the twilight state, and the impossibility of patients being awakened from this state. The most obvious outward feature is clouding of the sensorium, so that one can speak of a *paralytic stupor* [W]. Delirious features that add a peculiar colour are often no more than adjuncts derived from the projection system through muscle or vocal tremor, and muscle rigidity. Instead of restless movement, akinetic behaviour prevails.

Of other allopsychoses, I must mention one case in which the purest picture of presbyophrenia showed up in its delirious form for several days. Its nature was then clarified as a case of paralysis, when a paralytic attack occurred, with subsequent specific paralytic symptoms derived from the projection systems. Instructive as the case is for relations between concepts, I introduce it only as a rare occurrence. Of the hallucinatory allopsychoses, I remember an equally rare case involving a prostitute, who was in the clinic for 2 years as 'chronic hallucinosis' [Ed] to be presented as such every semester. You will remember that, at her last presentation, to my surprise, symptoms derived from the projection system became noticeable, which shed light for us on the paralytic aetiology, a diagnosis which was confirmed during the subsequent course. Moreover, with regard to acute hallucinosis there are cases with paralytic aetiology whose true significance becomes apparent only after the paranoid stage has ended, through striking deficits, loss of retentiveness in memory, and paralytic speech disorders. However, exclusion of alcoholic pseudoparalysis (see later) is often difficult, and can be achieved only through a detailed knowledge of the case history. Here, I want to mention that the belief about the rarity of hallucinations in paralysis, which is still widely held, is quite wrong. In our clinic, we have had many acute paralytic psychoses in which hallucinations were represented as strongly or even more so, than in corresponding cases of different aetiology.

When discussing anxiety psychoses, I have already stressed (p. 149), that they often have a paralytic aetiology. In particular, hypochondriacal anxiety psychosis raises suspicions of paralysis, as indeed does the large class of somatopsychoses which provides some of the most severe cases of paralysis. I already mentioned examples, amongst which bouts of most severe somatopsychic disarray and disorientation occurred, one of which led later to a purely demented form of paralysis (p. 163). However I must also include here an earlier-mentioned case (p. 74) of severe hypochondria that I cited as an example of residual hallucinosis, with a favourable outcome after acute psychosis. Already, in this first illness there was a suspicion of paralysis, since a history of syphilis was known. After 5 years of perfect health, a relapse occurred, this time taking the form of expansive autopsychosis whose deleterious course led to death within a year. A case with the most rapid course deserves mention here. Initially there was a simple intestinal somatopsychosis for some weeks gaining no fantastic significance, and it was treated as a genuine intestinal disorder. However, this was followed by a phase of hypochondriacal symptoms, which were quite fantastic in character: The patient described schemes that were running through his brain, in which an entire factory operation, with all manner of manipulations was going on; and soon it developed into the most severe threatening hypochondriacal delusion. Amongst other things, the patient had been tormented over the last few weeks by a tiger lying on him and tearing away at his liver. The entire course of illness in this 38-year-old man lasted 4 months. It had been preceded 10 years earlier by syphilis and had been treated several times. When total sensory psychosis occurred, as already mentioned (p. 273), acute worsening psychoses occurred, presenting in paralytic form, as a so-called 'galloping' [Ed] form of paralysis. Moreover, in such cases, at the very beginning or in the subsequent course, symptoms of threatening hypochondriacal delusions become clear. During cases mentioned, Affective states that are downright fearful made themselves manifest, but sometimes, according to the severity, with content of different coloration; and in other cases, which fortunately are more frequent, just the opposite is seen. The most severe hypochondriacal presentations show themselves with hardly any Affective component, such as having no head, no heart, no lungs, no stomach, or being completely hollow, 'only a tube' [W], as one educated patient put it so starkly. This phenomenon stands on its own, in no way dependent on the dementia, which may show up at about the same time. You will find a typical case of this sort in the patient presentations from my Clinic [5]. However, for weeks, in an earlier acute stage of his illness, the same patient presented the picture of most severe somatopsychic disarray, admittedly not as agitation, but only as almost total inaccessibility and helplessness, while only occasionally were there isolated expressions and actions pointing to total loss of bodily orientation.

With regard to motility psychoses of the paralytic variety, I have already often mentioned the hyperkinetic variety. Usually their manic features, fantastic grandiosity, and hypermetamorphosis are mixed together, this clinical picture developing mainly at a later stage of the illness, over several weeks. If worsening sensory psychosis reaches maximum severity, then hyperkinetic symptoms often join in with the paralytic aetiology [6]. A relatively frequent event, I should emphasize here, is the isolated *loquacity* [W] of *paralyzed patients* [W], a loquacity linked to flight of ideas, yet without any specific hyperkinetic shading, and also without actual mania. This peculiar isolated loquacity in otherwise apparently circumspect behaviour is limited almost completely to paralytics, the only exceptions known to me being the mildest cases of circular mental illness. Isolated hyperkinetic-parakinetic symptoms such as verbigeration, and stereotyped movements are met with very often in paralytics at later stages. You will remember that I have often used paralytics to demonstrate just such symptoms. Even in their relationship with aphasia and paralysis, these cases are sometimes very instructive. A type of *Echolalia* [W] may be touched on briefly here. It is occasionally seen in paralytic patients at the same time as severe motor disarray, producing such a rapid 'reflex' [Ed] reaction that it is uttered simultaneously, rather than being repeated later. You will find an example of this in patient presentations [7] from my

Clinic. Incidentally, elsewhere one usually finds responses in echolalia limited to a one- to two-syllable echo, sometimes in patients who are already quite demented, and in expressionless paralytics. The following conversation would be relatively typical:

'Are you big?'
'Big.'
'Are you small?'
'Small.'
'Are you a husband?'
'Husband.'
'Are you a wife?'
'Wife.' etc.

Akinetic motility psychosis in progressive paralysis is encountered relatively rarely in pure form, given that widespread muscle rigidity of paralysis originates specifically in the spinal cord. Hints of it are not so rare in later stages. However, in some cases that I know, prominent akinetic motility psychosis appeared as the first acute stage of the paralysis, followed by a second stage of agitated sensory confusion, and then a third stage of paralytic dementia with paralytic seizures. Every so often, you meet clinical pictures exhibiting a peculiar mixture of a paralytic delirium with akinetic motility psychosis. Moreover, akinetic-parakinetic conditions that obtain special coloration through predominance of motor disorientation and disarray should be mentioned [8].

Finally, I do not want to omit mention of certain twilight conditions, with clouding of the sensorium, which occur after paralytic attacks just as they do after epileptic attacks; usually they have certain focal symptoms, for example, combined with signs of sensory aphasia, and they tend to regress after lasting several days.

If we survey the whole picture of progressive paralysis, in so far as it can be regarded as a genuine psychosis, then in most cases, it is virtually the very model of a composite psychosis, passing successively through all different stages. Each stage may be a pure, simple psychosis; yet usually the clinical picture includes strange components, amongst which common falsifications of memory should not be forgotten. One of the more frequent possible combinations is one in which a stage of fantastic grandiosity is followed by one of mania, with allopsychic disorientation, and finally a stage of marked hypochondriac symptoms. However, just as often, a course is observed which is widely regarded as specific: cases of simple psychosis, distinguished from other simple psychoses only because of their rapid transition to dementia, and an admixture of above-mentioned symptoms derived from the projection system. Alternatively, it amounts to a colourful mixture of ever-changing symptoms, and thus to a complex clinical picture related only remotely to each simple psychosis.

The regular outcome in dementia here supports the view—highlighted at this time particularly by C. Westphal [9]—that paralysis almost always allows one to detect early signs of dementia. This is true even for cases developing just as simple psychoses, in which, by the nature of their entire clinical picture, more detailed analysis is often impossible in this regard. Nonetheless, the easiest symptom to establish here is reduced attentiveness, albeit not absolutely attributable to dementia. Even this loses its significance when there is a very severe Affective reaction. On the other hand, there are cases where no trace of deficit or loss of attentiveness can be found, like the examples of paralytic mania already cited. Fantastic grandiosity in such cases does presuppose a definite deficit in judgment, since the reality of things is apparently ignored; however, herein we find a contradiction that is no greater than the known fact (and in my opinion also wrongly evaluated as a symptom of deficit)—the failure that all mentally ill people show, to criticize the veracity of their hallucinations. Incidentally, you can find an example of paralytic mania *without* [Ed] fantastic grandiosity in my *Krankenvorstellungen* [10].

In a substantial proportion of cases, progressive paralysis follows a course, not as one or several periods of psychosis, but as a more regular progressive dementia—sometimes more regular, sometimes more intermittent—a continuous form that has led to it being designated *Dementia paralytica* [W]. I come back to this course when

I deal with acquired dementia. In all such cases, either prominent spinal symptoms or paralytic attacks with subsequent focal symptoms, can be found, occurring at the same time. Loss of mental acquisitions comes about here without the circuitous route of some other psychoses, just as does the gradual increase of direct focal symptoms in organic mental illness; it begins with autopsychic deficit, and ends in physical disorientation.

Included in the latter course, the most uniform and continuous trajectory is manifest as a curve, rising slowly in its extent, and actually belonging amongst the chronic psychoses. Whenever actual psychoses appear during the course, the illness always shows an acute character, at least temporarily, and Meynert [11] explicitly classed it with the acute psychoses.

Gentlemen! This description is still not enough to capture the multifaceted picture of progressive paralysis. It lacks some of the variations in intensity of the disease process that become established in most cases of longer duration and, may represent stages in the more-or-less uniform progression of the illness. These variations show up in opposite ways as remaining aspects of the illness: as the so-called remissions, and as acute exacerbations—the so-called paralytic attacks. *Remissions* [W] are often immediate outcomes of acute paralytic psychoses, most often with paralytic grandiosity, or specific paralytic autopsychosis as already mentioned, or of paralytic mania. One can usually differentiate remissions as being good or bad, by indications of insight into symptoms of illness in acute psychosis. If insight into the illness does not appear, while just the acute symptoms of illness disappear or abate, remission usually lasts only for weeks or months. However, in exceptional cases, even this incomplete remission (in an anatomical sense), as judged by the criterion of insight can lead to definitive recovery. This was so in a case known to me for 13 years, in which lack of insight in the early years was shown through repeated complaints, sometimes quite extreme, about our clinic. Good remissions are characterized not only by insight into the illness but also sometimes by almost complete disappearance of deficit symptoms. Quite often such a remission progresses to provisional cure, that is, one lasting more than a year and a day.

The *paralytic attacks* [W], as Lissauer [12] (see later: p. 290) first noted so incisively, undoubtedly signify an increase in acute features of a disease process, already known to be present. I come back later to discussing the anatomical findings, but note here that current monographs deal with progressive paralysis in a wholly inadequate way on this one point, relapsing in a questionable way into antiquated ways of thinking. I restrict myself to the most essential clinical data: Paralytic attacks are sometimes simple fainting episodes, or even just attacks of vertigo, while at other times they may be longer-lasting states of syncope, sometimes apoplectiform, sometimes epileptiform seizures. At the beginning of the illness, simple fainting or attacks of vertigo are to be seen, almost always followed by a short-lived speech impairment and faciolingual paresis. After a duration of hours or days, such symptoms tend to dissipate. The speech disorder can differ greatly in severity, but can amount to motor aphasia for a short time. Apoplectiform seizures can be very similar to apoplectic attacks of organic brain diseases; they usually leave behind hemiplegia or hemiplegic symptoms in a wider sense, such as hemianopia, sensory or motor aphasia, unilateral paralysis of the trunk, tactile anaesthesia of one hand, etc., generally matching the usual picture of fresh hemiplegia. Epileptiform attacks are sometimes *actual* [Ed] epileptic seizures, resembling exactly those of epileptic neurosis; however, they show a remarkable propensity for recurrence, and meet criteria for *Status epilepticus* [W]. More often the pattern of the attack corresponds more closely, or entirely, to that of the so-called cortical epilepsy, in that initially, without loss of consciousness, a specific muscle area such as the faciolingual region is affected, the onslaught then spreading further with the familiar regularity. In addition, these bouts of cortical epilepsy tend to leave focal symptoms in their wake, including, quite remarkably, even those of a sensory nature, such as sensory aphasia or hemianopia, and often also combined sensory symptoms right up to the level of asymbolia. Such focal symptoms tend to disappear rapidly, often within a few hours; but once seizures of this type have appeared, they tend to recur in just the same form. Accompanying focal symptoms then tend to last longer and longer, and finally to remain as permanent features. It is from such cases that Lissauer [12] derived his fundamental views on paralytic seizures. That bouts with bulbar and spinal character can occur in progressive paralysis was first shown by Cl. Neisser [13] in a commendable work. Severe paralytic seizures are also associated with a significant rise of body temperature.

If we start by disregarding focal symptoms arising in the wake of the paralytic seizures, then each case is clinically important as a portent of detectable emergence of dementia. Following a paralytic attack, but especially after each series of such attacks, there is a stage of stupor, whose regression follows slowly, step by step to a degree of dementia more severe than seen before. With regard to the frequency of paralytic seizures, there is hardly a single case where they are not at least hinted at. About half of all attacks are quite prominent, while a lasting residue of distinct focal symptoms is seen in only a fraction of cases. After bed-rest as treatment was generally introduced, paralytic attacks in our clinic became relatively rare. One encounters exceptional cases where apoplectiform or epileptiform seizures with subsequent focal symptoms dominate the clinical picture, so much that they must be attributed to organic brain diseases, according to clinical criteria. Such *atypical cases* [W] of paralysis have likewise been studied in greater detail by Lissauer [14], and their anatomical findings established.

In the *course* [W] of paralytic psychoses, the clinical form taken by each illness has some influence, as I repeatedly indicated. Moreover, the duration of individual cases, right up to the lethal outcome, differs widely and can range from a few weeks—galloping forms—to more than 10 years. On average, a large proportion become patients for a period of about 1¼ years from the time of entry into institutional treatment.

Gentlemen! *Diagnosis* [W] of progressive paralysis is easy in most cases, since the combination of a distinct psychosis with the above-mentioned symptoms deriving from the projection system is quite characteristic, especially if the latter show up in near-complete form, and at the same time, dementia is already prominent. If cortical or spinal symptoms are rare, the following points should be considered: Chance occurrence should always be considered when a spinal disease coincides just with a psychosis, for example, when a person with *Tabes* [W] or spastic spinal paralysis or a chronic myelitic focus suffers acute psychosis with no internal connection between the two illnesses. In such a chance concurrence (which, in my experience, is extremely rare), the case history will then indicate that an independent spinal cord disease existed long before. More frequently, actual paralytic psychosis is combined with pronounced paralysis arising in the spinal cord, and simple paralytic dementia is most likely to develop. These cases have been well distinguished as a *worsening form* [W] of paralysis, or have been assigned the name *Taboparalysis* [W]. Meynert ascribed to them a particularly rapid course, evidently having in mind only cases of actual paralytic psychoses, not those of simple paralytic dementia. If there is no historical evidence of long pre-existing spinal cord disease, then, detection of the so-called dorsal column or lateral column symptoms, or more definitely, a combination of both with the near-universal symptom of reflex rigidity of the pupil in paralytic disease of the spinal columns, the diagnosis of a paralytic psychosis can be made safely. A mere difference in pupil size, shown by the existing light reaction has long been known to have no diagnostic value. It should be noted that certain symptoms of *Tabes*, such as gait disturbance, or the Romberg sign can be completely concealed by the increased sense of personal agency in paralytic mania. Similarly, it should be considered that psychosis could coincide with cortical symptoms just by chance. In this respect, it is particularly important to recognize that each earlier phase of motor aphasia, though outlasted successfully, and otherwise well-compensated, can leave behind prominent, long-term, stumbling over syllables. It has already been emphasized repeatedly that certain paralytic psychoses meet diagnostic criteria through their specific clinical form.

The main difficulty in diagnosis is not psychoses of other aetiology, but organic brain diseases. An especially difficult case here is that mentioned earlier, of atypical paralysis designated by Lissauer as 'abnormally localized' [W]. Such cases are definitely not to be diagnosed as deriving from foci of organic brain disease, especially when you consider their great rarity, compared to the relatively common occurrence of cortical epilepsy in tumours of the cortical mantle. Apart from such cases, the main task is differential diagnosis from cerebral syphilis, and probably as much from gumma, as from syphilitic endarteritis, or from the frequent combination of both. The main criterion here is maintained insight into the illness, which is found for cerebral syphilis. If there is even *any* [Ed] underestimation of existing focal symptoms, one is led to suspect paralysis. The speech disorder is not such a useful criterion, for the reason given above; rather more useful is the very characteristic disorder of handwriting, arising from a combination of irregular tremor and paragraphia. If focal symptoms have developed slowly with no previous apoplectiform or epileptiform seizures, this favours neurosyphilis rather than paralysis. By its very nature, the clinical picture of paralysis can develop later out of that of cerebral syphilis; and corresponding to this, transitions between the two illnesses occur quite often. You will find an instructive example of this in my patient presentations [10]. You will readily grasp that this question is of utmost importance, since in paralysis we have an illness that is no longer influenced by specific treatment, whereas cerebral syphilis requires most energetic anti-syphilitic treatment, but is then curable.

Diagnosis of a paralytic attack claims an independent significance. Gentlemen! You are so often called to deal with a so-called 'stroke' [Ed] that your first question must be whether you are dealing with a possible paralytic attack. If you find that the attack is not simple apoplexy but also includes increase in temperature and epileptiform symptoms, then paralysis becomes more probable. As always, a careful case history is the only way to find out whether familiar prodromes of paralysis had preceded the attack, or whether a dizzy spell with transient speech disorder had occurred earlier, or that signs of mental disorder had been noted. If you learn of any earlier-striking dementia dating from a particular point in time, and if you are dealing with the most common age of paralysis between 35 and 45 years, then the probability is very high. Usually the behaviour of the pupils can be used diagnostically, because pupillary rigidity is one of the most common spinal symptoms of paralysis [3]. Other spinal symptoms are unlikely to be useful, since the apoplectic attack can lead either to a flaccidity or—admittedly more rarely—to some degree of limb rigidity. However, it should be noted that the very hemiplegia of a paralytic attack can be identified because, very early on—that is after 1–2 days—it may be associated with reduced passive mobility. The timing depends on return of spontaneous movement, which is always to be expected very soon after the paralytic attack. Moreover, the hemiplegia of a paralytic attack has no special features; at most it could be emphasized that in a paralytic attack conjugate deviation of the eyes, and sometimes of the head as well, to the opposite side is more common than in attacks of the so-called organic brain diseases. The hemiplegia of the paralytic attack is usually quite short in duration, sometimes only a few hours, but more often a few days. It usually tends to regress completely, as does existing motor aphasia or other focal symptoms. Therefore, you can understand the great importance of having a proper diagnosis, to predict the near future. Of course prognosis for the distant future in a paralytic attack is much more gloomy. On the other hand, if you are faced with an apoplectic or an epileptic attack, or *Status epilepticus* [W], then the differential diagnosis is to be made in comparison with genuine or symptomatic epilepsy or the so-called eclampsia where, in any case, the medical history—and where necessary a urine test—will provide evidence. Blood sampling is absolutely contraindicated in a paralytic seizure.

Gentlemen! In terms of *treatment* [W] of paralysis, certain tasks fall to the medical practitioner. I confine myself just to general measures, mainly in the field of prophylaxis. If you know that your patient has previously survived syphilis, and you find the prodromal symptoms I have described, or other symptoms of the so-called cerebral neurasthenia, or if there is perhaps a marked predisposition to disorders of the nervous system, or to psychosis, you must not shy away from the most drastic measures to counter the impending danger. However, anti-syphilitic treatment is indicated only when existing syphilis can be detected, be it in the brain, or in other organs; and then it is to be carried out with the utmost caution, so that any weakening of the constitution, especially a decrease in body mass, is avoided. The first condition for initiation of such treatment must therefore be that the patient curtails his occupation, and soon finds himself in the role of patient. Any measures applied while the patient pursues his occupation are often quite unhelpful. The most expedient is any invasive treatment combined with long-term bed-rest and over-feeding. If there are no traces of florid syphilis, antisyphilitic treatment is contraindicated. However, potassium iodide administered in small doses (from ½ to 1 g per day) over a long period, appears to work favourably. Nevertheless, the main thing is to enhance nutrition and correct those noxious influences that we have come to recognize as immediate causes of paralytic psychoses. Should occupational activities bring such damaging effects with them, the patient should not shy away from interrupting them for a half to a full year and, when this is ineffective, should not flinch from giving them up altogether. An investigation of spinal or cortical symptoms of paralysis will usually provide the criteria you need, to decide about such interventions.

If you no longer have any doubt, and paralysis is established to be present, it is your job to bring it to an end as quickly as possible, since any delay results all too frequently in material and social ruin of the whole family. If you are in any doubt over whether and when to bring the patient into a mental institution, it is always safest to decide in favour of this. Admittedly, in many cases, a specialist will postpone the date of containment for a long time.

Anatomical findings [W] in progressive paralysis are best described by dividing them into macroscopic and microscopic. The *macroscopic findings are* [W] prominent only after the illness has run a prolonged course, since it represents mainly the end result of a florid anatomical process, just as cirrhosis forms the outcome of liver disease. The outcome is atrophy of the cerebral cortex, most obviously in its documented loss of weight. This loss is not spread evenly across all parts of the cortical mantle, but, averaging across brains, the greatest shortfall occurs in the frontal lobe—although it should be noted that the frontal lobe in Meynert's [11] sense also included the anterior central gyrus. However, this average conceals the fact that isolated cases preferentially involve temporal, parietal, or occipital lobes; or, for these three lobes, or when there is mainly a bilateral illness with the same localization, 'abnormal localization' [W] does occur, as the atypical cases of Lissauer prove. I have assembled the following values from Meynert's table, which has never been surpassed by more recent authors in the care taken in weighing, and in the number of cases. In a substantial proportion of cases, weight loss also involves the brain stem. The cerebellum seems always to be least affected, so that from it, one has figures for comparison with values for other regions.

Taking brain-weight of manics to be approximately normal, their averages (in grams) were:

	Total weight	Cerebral cortex	Brainstem	Cerebellum
39 males	1,376	1,082	148	146
53 females	1,221	957	131	133

Paralytics, on the other hand, gave averages of:

	Total weight	Cerebral cortex	Brainstem	Cerebellum
145 males	1,215	933	135	146
29 females	1,068	819	119	130

The parts of the cerebral cortex had the following proportions amongst manics:

	Total weight	Frontal lobe	Temporal lobe	Occipital lobe
Among men	1,376	450	251	380
Among women	1,221	404	213	339

Amongst paralytics, on the other hand the proportions were:

	Total weight	Frontal lobe	Temporal lobe	Occipital lobe
Among men	1,215	380	216	337
Among women	1,068	323	202	294

Apart from loss of weight, atrophy is expressed by visible change on the brain surface and in the ventricles. On the brain surface there is more or less extensive loss of cortical substance, distributed in a very irregular way. Often the entire cerebral cortex, and at other times large sections of it, show reduction in the cortical grey substance of up to half or a third of the normal width; occasionally you even find scattered locations where cortical substance is missing entirely. The medullary strips of the gyri and the common underlying white matter are likewise revealed as significantly narrowed. Corresponding with this atrophy of the cerebral cortical substance, there is usually an increase in free cranial fluid, as *Hydrocephalus externus* [W].

The reaction of the pia mater shows two contrasts. Most obvious by far, you find that the pia is relatively soft, although often cloudy, the latter again especially over the frontal lobes, and thus the pia adheres so firmly to the brain surface that it appears to have fused with it. In any case, if you try to separate the pia, shreds of brain tissue remain adhering to it, often to a great extent, but often also only on the crests of the gyri [Ed], and there remains an ulcerated cortical surface, which soon turns reddish on exposure to the air. This so-called *decortication* [W] was formerly taken to be evidence of widespread inflammation of the brain surface—'periencephalitis' [W] or 'meningoencephalitis' [W]. People have usually distanced themselves from this view, since microscopic examination does not confirm the interpretation. From experiences in our clinic, this is almost always a sign of maceration, which takes a little time to form. If one has the opportunity to perform an autopsy soon—or only a few hours—after death, it is almost always possible, with caution, to avoid the decortication. Only a small proportion of cases prove to be exceptional, where examination of thin slices reveals real adhesion of the pia to the brain surface. It is known that the same phenomenon of decortication occurs in other conditions favourable for maceration, especially when cortical tissue is pressed against the tightly stretched translucent pia by *Hydrocephalus internus* [W], in meningitis or by a brain tumour, and the convolutions are flattened outwards and against one another. In contrast to these main cases of decortication, one often also encounters the opposite reaction, of a markedly thickened pia, richly saturated with fluid and usually also hard to tear. In these cases the pia tends to be very easily removed from the brain surface without any loss of substance.

The gyri differ in their prominence, with many depressions and pleats, corresponding to the grade of atrophy; their texture is apparently thickened. In all old cases, you also find expansion of ventricles and *Hydrocephalus internus* [W], a sign of general atrophy. Ventricular walls are very often abnormally firm, presenting the so-called *Ependymitis granulosus* [W] found especially at certain preferred sites, and this can even extend to the fourth ventricle. I hasten to add that despite this finding on the ventricular surface, hydrocephalus is no more than a result of diffuse atrophy, arising to fill the vacuum. We also find such consequences in the roof of the skull and in the dura mater. In the roof of the skull diffuse thickening is often present with no other structural deviation. Sometimes, however, there is a more-or-less widespread loss of diploë, and a type of eburnation. This finding might be interpreted independently as syphilitic bone disease. Frequently changes of the so-called *Pachymeningitis haemorrhagica* [W] are to be found on the dura mater, usually by chance, and undiagnosable in life. These consist in part of isolated blood stains, and their organized remnants, and in part as recent signs of major bleeding next to multiple membranous formations left as residues from previous haemorrhagic episodes. Only rarely does the extent of the bleeding reach as far as the base of the skull; usually it is mainly the convexity that is affected and one hemisphere can also appear flattened by such a pool of blood. However, it is most likely that atrophy of brain substance and the vacuum so created first precipitates these bleeds. As regards symptoms of haemorrhagic pachymeningitis, I have already noted that, in my own view, even cases in late stages of paralysis with very prominent anatomical changes are usually undiagnosable. Only in the case of unilateral papilloedema, which has often been observed when the bleed extends right into the sheath of an optic nerve (according to Fürstner [15]), will diagnosis sometimes be possible.

In some cases, especially in the atypical form of paralysis mentioned above, a gross anatomical finding of marked atrophy of the optic thalamus on one or on both sides can be seen in addition to the above findings. The white *Stratum zonale* [W] of the thalamus may thus appear grey over large stretches, the appearance being altered so much that for example the pulvinar protrudes like a sharpened ledge; and the texture becomes spongy. Lissauer's work grew from such findings.

All the above changes can easily be regarded as *sequelae* of the underlying process of tissue destruction as revealed in *microscopic findings* [W], whereas earlier, following Virchow's [16] doctrine of inflammation, the belief was always that there was a primary process of inflammation in the supporting vascular tissues, and in the neuroglia. For true insight into the real process we should thank Exner [17], for his discovery of the abundance of myelin in the cerebral cortex, and Tuczek [18], for his work based on this. Perfection of Weigert's [19] method of staining myelin sheaths, and the work of Lissauer have provided us with the most significant advances in our knowledge. (Preparatory work for a comprehensive publication is included in part in the posthumous draft of a habilitation thesis. A revision of this manuscript, often understandable only to the most well-informed, is one of the next tasks for the workers in my clinic. It will emerge from this, just how far Lissauer was ahead of all his co-workers in his penetrating knowledge of the paralytic process. His only publications on this are given below: [12, 14])

In what follows, I restrict myself just to the quintessential, and most important microscopic findings, stressing that I have secure knowledge of modern neuroscience teaching and how it is applied to disorders of peripheral nerves and spinal sections in degenerative neuritis. Primary disintegration and necrosis of neural elements, analogous to degenerative neuritis in the peripheral nervous system, is, from the onset, and throughout the course, the essential process determining all symptoms of paralysis. Earlier changes in supporting vascular tissues and in fibres of glia-like cells, which have been taken as signs of primary inflammation, are secondary or reactive to changes resulting from the primary necrosis of neural structures. They are thus consequences and outcomes of the illness, a *quasi-scar* [W] formation, replacing healthy tissue, not the actual disease. The disease is generally progressive and pernicious, so that I had earlier [20] drawn a parallel between it and progressive muscular atrophy. We can explain this by the presence of a constantly-unfolding toxic effect which has the specific effect of causing degeneration of the neural elements of the central nervous system, mostly in the cerebral cortex. Necrotic decay is detectable first in axons, but they are to be regarded as the main targets of toxicity only because they are dependent on nerve cell bodies for their nutrition. Corresponding to this, the first success was to detect degeneration of nerve fibres; and indeed we have known since Tuczek that axons are usually lost initially in the most superficial cortical lamina that which Meynert [21] identified as the first, purely grey lamina. Later, the network of fine fibres in supraradial and intraradial layers is affected, and finally the radii themselves. At first, cell bodies seem to be quite unchanged. However, in later stages, one concludes [20] that there is significant cell loss in all layers of the cortex, so that the cell layers become uniformly narrowed. In addition, I have always found cortical sites where the number of ganglion cells is visibly reduced, and the microscopic appearance of the cortex is changed in such a way that, instead of the normal, regular, and delicate delineation, a disorganized jumble of fibres, cells, and glial components is found.

Now it is known from the work of Nissl and his successors [22], that ganglion cells of the cortex, in every case of paralysis, also suffer severe changes. (Nissl's methylene blue stain is equivalent in its importance for pathology of the ganglion cells as is Weigert's myelin sheath stain. The reader will find information about the method in refs. [23] and [19]; see also [23, 24].) However, credit for first finding cell shrinkage of the entirety of the cortical layers undoubtedly goes to Lissauer. This researcher succeeded in proving, in cases of atypical 'abnormally localized' [W] paralysis, a laminar degeneration in those cortical regions in the parietal and occipital lobes which were identified as the point of onset of the focal symptoms. Cell loss in these cases did not extend continuously over the cortex, but came in irregularly-distributed patches, and involved mainly layers of densely arranged, small pyramids, arranged in rows, and increasing in size inwards, in other words, Meynert's second and third layers. Macroscopically this can be identified on the hardened brain as a bright stripe running parallel with the cortex, in the middle of the grey cortical substance, darkly stained by chromium solution. These cases also enabled Lissauer to show that secondary degeneration of myelinated fibres from these locations could be traced through the otherwise intact medullary white matter to other locations, and especially downwards into the corona radiata and internal capsule; and that generally changes of the white matter in paralysis are consistently based on secondary degeneration. Clinically, Lissauer's atypical cases were distinguished, in that mainly only focal symptoms of the parietal and occipital lobe were present, namely loss of tactile sensation and hemianopia, and that these had developed in connection with paralytic attacks in the manner indicated above. 'The paralytic attacks then appear as a sudden violent surge of the paralytic process in certain cortical territories.' That the changes in the white matter were largely to be regarded as systematic, was already highlighted by Tuczek, who emphasized especially that the degeneration he demonstrated in six cases, in the shortest association bundle lying just deep to the cortex—Meynert's *Fibrae propriae* [W]—always involved sites where myelin degeneration of the cortex was also prominent.

In Lissauer's cases, thalamic tissue also showed itself to be abnormal, providing evidence that secondary degeneration occurs in subcortical ganglia whose importance von Monakow has rightly emphasised. Moreover, this degeneration leads to disappearance of axons and cells, so that only coarse spongy tissue remains, within which the regular, delicate markings of thalamic tissue are completely missing. According to the type of focal symptom, different regions of the thalamus showed themselves to be changed in this manner, confirming Monakow's [25] theory of the thalamic nuclei. The anterior region of the thalamus and the lateral geniculate body appeared to be unaffected by secondary degeneration in cases mentioned, while the medial geniculate body behaved as the other nuclei of the thalamus, with secondary degeneration and sensory aphasia as a result of the paralytic disease of the temporal lobe.

Lissauer's findings show that the paralytic process can differ greatly in intensity and extent, so that, at certain locations, it can progress to actual paralytic focal disease in the cortex and that this progression becomes manifest in the form of paralytic seizures. The white matter pathology consistently shows the hallmarks of secondary degeneration. (This sentence from Lissauer finds striking confirmation in the work of Starlinger [26]). Thus some fundamental empirical facts have been gained, that are no less important than Tuczek's work.

Regarding the localization of the paralytic process, the following should be noted. In all his cases, Tuczek found the frontal lobe to be involved, and had come to the view that fibre loss generally progressed in an antero-posterior direction, and would go no further than the region of the central gyri. However, in contrast, Zacher [27] had already found that the parietal, occipital, and temporal lobes were also abnormal, sometimes more so than the frontal lobes, and that Tuczek's statement that fibre loss always started in tangential fibres of the outermost cortical layer, only later to involve the deeper layers, had no general validity. Lissauer's findings also suggest that the paralytic process has a very irregular, patchy distribution, by no means beginning exclusively in the outermost cortical layer. Common to virtually all cases, however, is a remarkable fibre loss in the insula, Broca's gyrus [28], and the lower extent of the central gyrus, corresponding to clinically detected speech disorder, and paresis of the faciolingual area in almost all cases. Such mainly focal localization, as in the other atypical cases, is however very rare.

Moreover, it is noted that the paralytic process is not limited to the cerebral cortex: Beyond the thalamus, other subcortical regions can also be affected. Thus, A. Meyer [29] demonstrated loss of myelinated fibres in the cerebellar cortex; and H. Schütz [30] showed that the myelin of the periaqueductal grey matter and motor cranial nerve nuclei had been attacked. Perhaps the diversity of paralytic seizures is connected with this.

Since Weigert has taught us about normal distribution of glial cells in the brain, we are also in a position to evaluate also the localization of glial cell proliferation. Amongst other things, Meyer's finding in the cerebellum is confirmed in Weigert's [31] great work. Proliferations of glia arise everywhere where neural parenchyma have degenerated; therefore, the location of this indicates localized loss of nerve cells. At a particular stage in such proliferation, we have observed the occurrence *en masse*, of giant astrocytes; and indeed they correspond to the more recent stage, seen temporarily soon after loss of neuronal tissue. Later, for the most part, they disappear again, but a proliferation of fibrous glia remains permanently. In some cases, however, such a glial reaction fails to occur; and all that remains are regions with a wide-meshed net of normal glial fibres forming rarefied stripes or patches.

Recently Binswanger in his careful monograph [32] obtained similar results with regard to the primary parenchymatous nature of the disease. We learn from him about occurrence of inflammatory changes and, where it applies, disintegration of adhesions of the pia to the cerebral cortex. 'Destruction of cortical tissue, with its consequences, leads to greater accumulation of pathologically-altered lymph fluid in the extravascular lymphatic system. It drains mainly into areas formed by glial sheaths and areas for collection on the brain surface. Here the accumulated lymph fluid of dying tissue changes by coagulation and hyaline necrosis, but it also evokes hyperplastic processes in the adjacent pia and its vessels. In consequence of the latter, partial adhesions of the brain surface to the pia mater occur, with scleropathy of large sections of the epicerebral space, relocation of the confluences of extra- and intravascular lymph spaces.' It is readily apparent that in this way the outermost cortical layers can easily succumb to a maceration process after death. Moreover, it seems to me that Binswanger overestimated the influence of these processes on the course of the disease, and he is particularly mistaken in their application to paralytic seizures.

Gentlemen! If you ask me what final result is to be drawn from these cortical findings for the theory of illness, it is briefly as follows: The paralytic process almost always leads to rapid loss of neural elements of the cerebral cortex, which is significant, but subject to great local variation in its extent. According to Meynert [11] loss of weight within a year amounted to about 100 g. Corresponding to this is the dementia that accompanies the course of the illness in most cases from the outset. This dementia is therefore dependent on the extent, not the localization of the paralytic process, and is thus to be regarded clinically in its entirety. Preferred localities for early attacks, as described above, correspond on the other hand to the most frequent cortical symptoms derived from the projection system. With this concept there need be no surprise that Zacher also found extensive loss of fibres in the cerebral cortex among senile, alcoholic, and epileptic demented patients, and that this has been confirmed many times since. Here too, breakdown of the clinical phenomena coincides with anatomical findings.

As for the changes in the spinal cord, they are certainly based in part on secondary degeneration, for example when, in late stage of the illness, general helplessness occurs, with muscle rigidity and increase in tendon reflexes. On the other hand, the above information on premature recurrence of spinal symptoms in paralysis reveals that severe illness of the spinal cord often takes place independently. The connection with the paralytic process in the brain is evidently the production of the same active toxin. We also know from the *Tabes dorsalis* [W] that it, like paralysis, is a *sequela* of syphilis. That at one time only the spinal cord is affected, while at other times, the brain is involved exclusively or predominantly in a form of paralysis, and that *Tabes* [W] sometimes persists as such, while at other times after existing for many years, can still lead to paralysis, must be considered as depending on the respective predisposition of different individuals and particularly on the functional harmfulness of the process.

References

1. Kahlbaum KL. Die Gruppierung der psychischen Krankheiten und die Eintheilung der Seelenstörungen. Danzig: AW Kafemann; 1863.
2. Wernicke C. Krankenvorstellungen aus der psychiatrischen Klinik in Breslau, vol. 3. Breslau: Schletter; 1900. Case 14 is a good example of this fantastic grandiosity.
3. Gaupp RE. Über die spinalen Symptome der progressiven Paralyse, Psychiatr Abhandl, vol. 9. Breslau: Schletter; 1898.
4. Wernicke C. Krankenvorstellungen, vol. 3, Case 30 a case of paralytic mania, is relatively pure. 1900.
5. Wernicke C. Krankenvorstellungen, vol. 3, Case 26. 1900.
6. Wernicke C. Krankenvorstellungen, vol. 2, Case 8 is a good example of paralytic hyperkinetic motility psychosis. 1899.
7. Wernicke C. Krankenvorstellungen, vol. 2 Supplement, Case 18. 1899.
8. Wernicke C. Krankenvorstellungen, vol. 2, Case 18 is an example. 1899.
9. Westphal CFO. Über einige durch mechanische Einwirkung auf Sehnen und Muskeln hervorgebrachte Bewegungs-Erscheinungen. Arch Psychiatr Nervenkr. 1875;5:792–802.
10. Wernicke C. Krankenvorstellungen, vol. 3, Case 30. 1900.
11. Meynert T. Klinische Vorlesungen über Psychiatrie auf wissenschaftlichen Grundlagen für Studierende und Aerzte, Juristen und Psychologen. Vienna: Braumüller; 1890.
12. Lissauer H. Sehhügelveranderungen bei progressive Paralyse. Dtsch Med Wochenschr. 1890;16:561–4.
13. Neisser C. Die paralytischen Anfälle. Klinischer Vortrag. Stuttgart: F. Enke; 1894.
14. Lissauer H. Klinisches und Anatomisches über die Herdsymptome bei Paralyse. Vortr Ver ostdtsch Irrenärzte am 2.3.1891. Zbl Nervenheilk Psychiat. 1891;2:295–7.
15. Fürstner C. Weitere Mitteilungen über den Einfluß einseitiger Bulbuszerstörung auf die Entwicklung der Hirnsphären. Arch f Psychiatr. 1882;12:612.
16. Virchow R. Die Rolle der Gefässe und des Parenchyms in der Entzündung. Virchows Arch. 1897;9(3):281.
17. Exner S. Über das Sehen von Bewegung und die Theorie des zusammengesetzten Auges. Sitzungsber Wiener Akad Wiss. 1876;72(3):156–90.
18. Tuczek F. Beiträge zur pathologischen Anatomie und zur Pathologie der Dementia paralytica. Berlin: L Schumacher; 1884.
19. Weigert C. Die Markscheidenfärbung von Fibrin. Ergeb Anat Entwickl Gesch. 1897;6:3–25.
20. Wernicke C. Lehrbuch der Gehirnkrankheiten, für Aerzte und Studierende. Kassel: Fischer; 1881. p. 539.
21. Meynert T. Der Bau der Grosshirnsrinde und seine örtlichen Verschiedenheiten, nebst einem pathologisch-anatomischen Corollarium. Leipzig: Engelman; 1887.
22. Nissl F. Mitteilungen zur pathologischen Anatomie der Dementia paralytica. Arch Psychiatr. 1896;28: 987–92.
23. Nissl F. Über eine neue Untersuchungsmethode des Centralorgans zur Feststellung der Localisation der Nervenzellen. Neur Centralbl. 1894;13:507–8.
24. Alzheimer A. Beiträge zur pathologischen Anatomie der Hirnrinde und zur anatomischen Grundlage einiger Psychosen. Mschr Psychiat Neurol. 1897;2:90.
25. von Monakow C. Gehirnpathologie. Wien: A Holder; 1897.
26. Starlinger J. Zur Marchi-Behandlung; ein Apparat zur Zerlegung in dünne, vollkommen plnparallele Scheiben. Z Wiss Mikrosk Mikrosk Tech. 1899;16:179–83.
27. Zacher. Über das Verhalten der markhaltigen Nervenfasern in der Hirnrinde bei der progressive Paralyse. Arch Pychiatr Neurol 1884;18:p. 60, p. 348.
28. Broca PP. Nouvelle observation d'aphémie produite par une lésion de la moitié postérieure des deuxième et troisième circonvolutions frontales gauches. Bull Soc Anat. 1861;36:398–407.
29. Meyer A. Ueber Faserschwund in der Kleinhirnrinde. Arch Psychiat Nervenkr. 1890;21(1):197.
30. Schütz H. Anatomische Untersuchungen über den Faserverlauf im centralen Höhlengrau und den Nervenfaserschwund in demselben bei der progressiven Paralyse der Irren. Arch Psychiat Nervenkr. 1891;2:525.
31. Weigert C. Beiträge zur Kenntnis der normalen menschlichen Neuroglia. Frankfurt: Diesterweg; 1895.
32. Binswanger O. Die pathologische Histologie der Grosshirnrinden-Erkrankung bei der allgemeinen progressiven Paralyse mit besonderer Berücksichtigung der acuten und Frühformen. Jena: G Fischer; 1893. p. 169.

Lecture 38

38

- Notes on the aetiology of acute psychoses
- Aetiological groupings of the psychoses
- Alcoholic psychosis
- Alcoholic jealousy mania
- Alcoholic stupor
- Pseudoparalysis
- Cocainism
- Polyneuritic psychoses through lead poisoning and arsenic poisoning, in tuberculosis and syphilis
- Hereditary psychoses
- Epileptic psychoses
- Perseveration

Lecture

Gentlemen!

Progressive paralysis deserved a detailed discussion; but I repeatedly made reference to the aetiology of acute psychoses. My lecture today is a summary, with some expansion of my earlier comments.

Every specialist is forced to some general notions: Very often we find some debilitating event being specified as a proximate cause or occasion for outbreak of acute psychoses, that is, some influence that significantly reduces the nutritional status and general wellbeing in a short space of time. Blood loss, or repeated blood losses through *Menstruatio nimia* [W] pregnancy, the puerperium, and lactation usually act as disease-inducing factors in this way, but the same can be said for untimely or excessive low-fat or vegetarian diets, prolonged gastritis, continued grief and sorrow interfering with sleep and nutrition, and finally, acute illnesses. Amongst the latter, endemic influenza should be highlighted, because, it meets at once the prerequisite of producing rapid reduction in body weight. Monographs on various acute illnesses as causes of psychosis teach you that it would be quite wrong to propose a regular relationship between this type of illness and the clinical forms of subsequent acute psychosis. Nevertheless, if, by way of example you speak, hear, or read of 'exhaustion psychoses' [Ed] as a specific clinical entity, this is the same misunderstanding to which I have already repeatedly drawn attention. Even more can one say, with some justification, that in the sense just discussed, by far the majority of acute psychoses are 'exhaustion psychoses' [Ed].

Of course, a certain degree of inanition due to such illnesses or other injurious influences is usually no more than a trigger. What is also needed is a pre-existing disposition, before mental illness occurs. This predisposition may be either congenital or acquired. You will long have known the major role that innate predisposition or (according to Griesinger [1]) heredity plays in mentally ill people, and in the so-called functional nervous disorders. Evident degeneration, which can be followed in many families, is based on this. I want

R. Miller, K.J. Dennison (eds.), *An Outline of Psychiatry in Clinical Lectures*,
DOI 10.1007/978-3-319-18051-9_38

to make just one point here, that I still do not find sufficiently emphasized: that a strong hereditary predisposition may be present without its ever leading to acute or a chronic psychosis. However, in all cases where it is present, a doctor must bear in mind the need for his patients to avoid, as far as possible, aforementioned adverse triggers. Nonetheless, hereditary disposition does not in itself enable diagnosis of a mental illness to be made. I should not forget to mention here that I find phthisis to be specified surprisingly often among the forerunners of acute psychoses; yet it is a well-known fact that this does not generally worsen the prognosis of the fundamental hereditary predisposition, this depending, as usual on the clinical form the psychosis takes.

The acquired predisposition to mental illness is based usually on adverse influences that are also expressed as organic changes in the brain. These include *Hydrocephalus internus* [W], even if this has reached the stage of recovery, as we often see; but we also see it even where no conspicuous alteration of the head has been left behind, but only partial adhesions or diverticular formation within the cerebral ventricles, a finding rightly emphasized by Meynert [2] in particular. Survivors of childhood meningitis, and any head trauma that has definitely been accompanied by concussion, also imply acquired predisposition. I should comment that recovery from meningitis, and also from tuberculars, should be recognized more readily than has been generally accepted. Childhood cramps, for whatever reason, although successfully outlasted, must likewise be regarded as noxious influences predisposing to mental illness. The impact of epileptic seizures, especially if they are clustered, is, in itself, not only a consequence but at the same time, also a cause of gross anatomical changes in the brain that cannot always be totally repaired. Similarly, the relationship between acute psychoses and severe infectious diseases such as typhus or malaria, survived from earlier times, must be taken into account. We assume that during the course of these ailments, anatomical changes can become enduring features in the brain. Finally, I mention as one of the most common precursors of acquired predisposition, certain toxic effects, foremost amongst which is prolonged alcohol abuse.

I have repeatedly drawn attention to the fact that times of normal physical change, such as puberty, menopause, and finally senescence, are particularly likely to predispose to onset of psychoses, based on the great importance that bodily changes have for consciousness. This widespread general predisposition will certainly have an effect, as it does normally and even when acquired disposition already exists through previously mentioned organic changes.

After such general preliminary remarks, we can proceed to study the influence which certain aetiological events might have on the nature and course of mental illnesses to which they lead. It is best to start from familiar territory: We have come to know *Delirium tremens* [W] as an acute psychosis [W] that is specifically alcoholic [W], a form of delirious allopsychosis almost always due to chronic alcoholism. However, I have already pointed out certain exceptions that, at least, deserve our attention.

I remind you that we have learned about the chronic and protracted *Delirium tremens*; but I have occasionally mentioned an even more acute alcoholic psychosis: It is commonly referred to as pathological intoxication [W], and we know that it usually takes the form of a very acute allopsychosis with allopsychic disorientation and dream-like hallucinations. The content of this altered state seems always to be fantastically threatening, and corresponding to this is an extreme Affective state which accompanies pathological intoxication, which is different from *Delirium tremens*. This condition lasts no more than a few hours, so that we can regard it as an example of a transient psychosis. It is followed by deep sleep, usually with complete amnesia. I have already mentioned that very similar transient psychoses can occur after a single bout of alcoholic intoxication or even without one, whenever there is a strong predisposition to mental illness.

I dealt with acute hallucinosis in greater detail earlier. However, I may have presented the prognosis of the initial illness in such cases too favourably, because recently I have repeatedly encountered a state of chronic hallucinosis, continuing after acute hallucinosis in alcoholics. On the other hand, it has long been known that the clinical picture of chronic hallucinosis (pp. 102, 103) that I mentioned earlier, whose content is a state of physical persecutory delusions, is often found among alcoholics.

Polyneuritic psychosis, which we have also discussed already, is often mainly alcoholic in origin. This illness, which is usually curable, can, under some circumstances, progress to a clinical picture of visual agnosia and asymbolia. You will recall such a case from my patient presentations [3].

So far, whenever we have had to deal with various forms of allopsychoses, autopsychosis also comes our way, this, of course, being not exactly alcoholic in origin. I mean here the 'second state' [W] also called *Semmelwochen* [W]. It is even likely that the same condition always occurs among the so-called 'degenerates' [Ed]; but there is the added possibility of the condition being self-inflicted through alcoholism in some cases.

The importance of a circumscribed autopsychosis based on an overvalued idea probably includes the so-called delusional jealousy of drinkers [W]; at least, this is a feature of several pure cases of this type. The overvalued idea on one occasion was based on a husband having been repeatedly rejected in his claims for marital intercourse, by his slightly-older wife, already richly endowed with children. In a second case, the underlying Affective experience could not be definitely proven, but was presumed to be a similar situation, and delusional jealousy was thus actually identified, because the subsequent delusion of reference was directed so specifically to that single issue, that the entire clinical picture could be understood only as a circumscribed autopsychosis based on this overvalued idea. Although these cases are chronic in character, they also belong amongst the acute psychoses on account of their more acute stage of origin.

Much more often, perhaps even most often of all—if you also include abortive cases—are anxiety psychoses in drunks. In my patient presentations you will find a few such cases, amongst them a very instructive case of abortive anxiety psychosis [4].

Alcoholic stupor [W] deserves brief mention. Here, clouding of the sensorium, and somnolence, comparable only to that found in tumour patients, can exist for several weeks or even months, making the clinical picture so similar to that of organic brain diseases that, for my part, I do not doubt that it has an organic basis in hydrocephalus internus [W]. Moreover, the gait disturbance that such patients show as soon as they can leave their beds, can be compared only with that of senile hydrocephalus internus [W]. Correspondingly, the pulse can be fairly slow. General muscle stiffness, with great increase in mechanical excitability of muscles, is common both in these cases and in senile hydrocephalus internus [W]. Papilloedema tends to be absent in both cases, but, as a residue after surviving alcoholic stupor, I have seen atrophy of the optic nerves with significant visual impairment. Generally the disease is curable, sometimes most definitively so, if permanent abstinence can be achieved. In other cases, stupor can turn into a state of deficit to which traits of asymbolia may be added, although to widely varying degrees.

Cases of the so-called pseudoparalysis [W] claim a special place amongst alcoholic psychoses. They are seen especially after long-continued, very severe excess of alcohol intake. The paralytic character of the resulting acute psychoses is expressed as disturbances of speech—by now familiar—and of the cranial nerves, just as in delirium tremens, and probably is again organically based. Beyond this, signs of disease of the spinal cord, differences in pupil size, and pupillary rigidity may be present, as they are in genuine paralysis. The acute psychosis usually has added delirious features at least initially. Later the picture corresponds mostly to acute hallucinosis but with added independent states of anxiety, temporary allopsychic disorientation, and traits of dementia. Moreover, a paranoid stage does not develop. A highly fluctuating clinical picture can exist for years and yet finally reach a state of recovery. At other times, at least a moderate degree of deficit remains, which need not progress further, given abstinence. I note explicitly here that the recovery relates only to the psychosis and the specific paralytic concomitants of speech disorder, tongue tremor etc.; the actual spinal symptoms tend not to recover. Fainting spells, which occur in the course of the illness can make diagnosis of true paralysis even more complicated.

One often encounters psychoses [W] related through combined morphine and cocaine abuse [W], although I have yet to see real psychoses caused exclusively by morphine abuse. Sudden occurrence of physical persecution delusions, with rapid systematization and, strange tactile and combined hallucinations of the skin, so that the patient sees and feels 'fungus' [Ed], or mould [Ed], or hair-like structures growing out of their skin, which seem fairly specific to such cases.

Closest to the alcoholic psychosis are isolated cases that in all probability can be attributed to lead or arsenic poisoning. In connection with the former, I have in mind the example of a 30-year-old typesetter whose clinical picture consisted mainly of sensory confusion, continuous pressured speech, generally incoherent flight of ideas, with very prominent hypermetamorphosis, but no significant addition of any Affective reactions. After an illness lasting about 10 months, he started to become demented, and was failing physically. Death occurred a year later, after general muscle tremor had occurred, with temporary states of excitation including a content of hypochondriacal fantastic threatening delusions. Polyneuritic symptoms were not present in his extremities. For chronic arsenic poisoning, I should probably go back to the case of a 50-year-old maker of artificial flowers, who had had much to do with arsenic green for 30 years. She suffered headaches for many years, and finally also dizziness, and suddenly became ill with symptoms of anxiety psychosis and hallucinations. Soon however, pseudospontaneous movements of the mouth also developed, with rapid increase of all symptoms (confused pressured speech, grandiose ideas, verbigeration, transitional parakinetic movements, spatial fixation of her eyes, yet orientated temporally). She then showed a sudden physical decline, despite adequate food intake, and died within 18 days. Autopsy revealed a brain weight of 1,250 g, moderate *Hydrops ventriculorum* [W]. The illness closely preceding this was a cystitis that lasted several weeks. With remission of the motor restlessness, rigidity of her legs, and ankle clonus could be demonstrated; a few days before death, paresis of the left facial nerve, of peripheral origin, appeared. I have come across similar cases of mixed sensorimotor psychosis, whose course proved severe, and suddenly fatal, which seemed to have no basis in the clinical symptoms; *inter alia* [W] there was a typical anxiety psychosis which became fatal within 7 weeks; and at autopsy, despite signs of developing phthisis, no other explanation for the rapid decline could be found. Conversely, I remember a patient in the last stage of long-standing pulmonary tuberculosis who, in his last 14 days presented one of the purest pictures of akinetic–parakinetic motility psychosis. In all such cases, one could not dismiss out of hand the suspicion that the acute psychosis is a polyneuritic one with unusual clinical symptoms.

Regarding the polyneuritic psychosis [W]—which belongs here because it owes its name to it—I refer you to my earlier lecture. In the literature, you almost always find it called 'Korsakoff's psychosis' [Ed], terminology also recently accepted by Jolly [5]; and it was in fact Korsakoff [6] who first directed attention to certain typical features of the clinical picture seen amongst those suffering from polyneuritis. However, you will find the cases described by Korsakoff in this group to be far more complex than the picture I have painted, which was condensed as tightly as possible. For this reason, even now, I consider the name 'polyneuritic psychosis' [Ed] to be more accurate, while far from wishing to disparage Korsakoff's merits. The main objection, which could be levelled against my preferred name, gives him special credit, in my esteem. As I wanted to suggest through previously mentioned cases, the polyneuritic basis for psychoses applies, in a broader sense, to degeneration of neural elements in the brain, similar to polyneuritis, assumed to have an anatomical basis in psychosis, but probably extending far beyond the narrow concept of the so-called polyneuritic psychosis. Since we have also made corresponding findings in paralysis, the above facts confirm only the long-established fact that degenerative neuritis develops most often in the context of syphilis, chronic alcoholism, and tuberculosis. Beyond this, as already mentioned, the high incidence of tuberculosis as a forerunner in individuals with acute psychoses of the most varied types, gives one pause.

One can only speak in most general terms of hereditary psychoses [W], since a hereditary predisposition in the broader sense is very frequent among acute psychoses: In my estimate it is present in about half of all cases. The percentage might be even more marked, if you include not only chronic psychoses, but also the frequent cases on the borderline between psychoses and mentally healthy persons. I have already mentioned this point (p. 104) when referring to Magnan's [7] work. In the latter category, those suffering from obsessions are special cases, but so also are healthy individuals. Obsessional psychoses tend to have a severe hereditary loading; but it is again highly instructive that I could present to you a very pure case of obsessional psychosis [8] in which it was certain that only senile involution of the brain was implicated as an aetiological component, heredity being totally excluded. As with obsessional neurosis, hypochondriacal neurosis also finds its main members amongst those with hereditary loading. You will recall that, amongst hypochondriacal psychoses which I reported to you, some particularly severe cases occurred similarly in persons with severe loading. Such individuals are particularly predisposed to febrile delirium, which is regarded as a special form of symptomatic psychosis. Again, amongst more marginal cases, are otherwise healthy people, prone to unhealthy impulses. Frequently, the effect of suggestion plays a role here, such as the almost-endemic suicidal impulse that prevails in some families. No less common in the same 'degenerate' [W] families is kleptomania [Ed] at the time of menstruation, sexual perversions, etc. Transitory psychoses, including pathological intoxication, show unambiguous predilection to affect individuals with a hereditary burden. Finally, I mention once more 'moral autopsychosis' [Ed] (pp. 193, 194), and a particular form of primary dementia, which sets in at the time of onset of puberty, particularly among children with a heavy hereditary loading. With regard to mania, Affective melancholia, and circular mental illness, I refer you to my earlier comments on their aetiology.

It cannot be denied that amongst psychoses related to heredity, extremely severe cases sometimes occur. Nevertheless, these are outweighed by far by milder cases, and notably by the so-called borderline ones, which suggest a more bourgeois existence than do severe acute psychoses. On the whole, I would impress upon you, that a genetic trait certainly can increase the tendency to mental illness; but, except for a few special cases, these have a no more severe psychosis, but rather a milder course, when it erupts. Of course, one must also acknowledge an increased tendency to its recurrence.

Epilepsy [W] plays a very important aetiological role in psychoses. In general, the so-called twilight state can be recognized as a specifically epileptic psychosis, but with limits on its aetiological relationships, that we have already met. As a main feature of the twilight state, we know of clouding of the sensorium, with total allopsychic disorientation. This disorientation in the epileptic twilight state not uncommonly grows to the point of asymbolia, when an easily understandable failure of will—a real abulia—may also be present. At other times, dreamlike actions are carried out, especially ones of a severe violent nature, apparently under the influence of dreamlike hallucinations. When such twilight states are seen, lay people are always surprised by the disturbed, and weird actions of the sick person, produced by allopsychic disorientation. These states are usually quite short-lived, lasting half an hour, up to several hours, and seldom more than a day. Their behaviour in epileptic seizures is different. Predominantly these states make their appearance post-epileptically, but sometimes pre-epileptically or as part of an epileptic attack. Mostly, there is no later recollection; however, except for one—albeit cursory—reminder, we find that the violence was perpetrated as defence against a threatening situation. While minor actions are quite common in this twilight state, the epileptic tantrum [W] in its most typical form is only the blindest thrashing, screaming, and drooling as a defensive Affective reaction, enhanced to maximum extent. These attacks of a 'frenetic' [Ed] twilight state, which can be compared only to the behaviour of a cornered animal, last only for minutes, or at most half an hour, and are followed by total amnesia. In contrast to this, prolonged twilight states are sometimes seen, which can even last for weeks, with harmless delirious urges to keep moving. Such patients, like those with delirium tremens, can focus their attention momentarily, but cannot hold it as long as in a delirious patient; yet, on the contrary, their retentiveness is surprisingly well preserved. At other times—but rarely, or so it seems—exactly as in those with genuine delirium, the twilight state only becomes obvious when a patient is left to himself; otherwise, he may seem quite bright and attentive. Moreover, in these cases, well-retained retentiveness is quite striking, and should be regarded as a feature of delirium specific to epileptic bouts. You will remember a case [9] in which retroactive amnesia existed at the same time, and then differential diagnosis from polyneuritic psychosis could be made, due to the well-retained retentiveness.

Where the twilight state dominates more strongly, the symptom of perseveration [W] (Neisser [10])—persistence with previously used expressions, well known from organic brain disease, notably aphasia—often becomes very prominent. This symptom is best illustrated by a conversation that you yourselves witnessed, in a recent clinical demonstration.

'What is your name?'
'Martha Glockner.'
'How old are you?'
'Martha Glockner.'
'Where are we?'
'Martha Glockner.'
'How old are you?'
'22 years.'
'Where are we?'
'22 years.'
'What is your profession?'
'22 years.'
'Who am I?'
'Cousin Georg.'
'Who is this gentleman?'
'Cousin Georg.'
'Who is the other gentleman?'
'Cousin Georg.'

The patient in this conversation, a 22-year-old woman, with an epileptic father, had herself suffered epilepsy from childhood, and had survived severe *Status epilepticus* [W] 3 days earlier. You will not have forgotten her strange movements, which I described to you at the time as the languidness of a dandy, but with the greatest exaggeration. Even these movements had a tendency to be repeated, for example when she attempted to embrace me as her supposed cousin. The patient looked weak and frail, stumbled visibly from her weakness, and in the ward lacked any initiative, even to the point of keeping herself clean. She showed such striking resistance to change of position, and maintained such persistently uncomfortable positions, that we were led, involuntarily to compare her with Goltz's [11] decapitated frog. We could attract the attention of this patient only with difficulty, and allopsychically, she was totally disorientated, not actually dazed, but appearing 'mentally empty' [Ed]. For that reason her retentiveness could not be tested. Only the simplest instructions or questions were understood; she failed everything else, and tired very rapidly. As you may remember, I attempted to differentiate such symptoms of exhaustion from other symptoms of the twilight state, as temporary consequences of the Status epilepticus [W]. However, there is no denying that the residual state of fatigue which often remains after epileptic seizures and which is referred to as post-epileptic stupor [W], shows smooth transitions to any kind of actual twilight state.

The same female patient, who I have just introduced as an example of a post-epileptic twilight state, 6 months previously had become an exception, on account of a post-epileptic psychosis; but at the time, it was a totally different situation, namely a hypochondriacal psychosis, whose main symptom was a supposed unilateral paralysis, on the left side. It was not a genuine paralysis, and weakness was evident only for the first 3 days. Facialis muscle and tongue remained unaffected; passive movement and reflexes were normal; but sensibility was markedly involved. Eight days later, the patient could be discharged as recovered. This report will call to mind a case, again post-epileptic, of hypochondriacal paraplegia of short duration, with flaccid paralysis of both legs. The particular mode of origin of the paralysis, through disturbance of psychomotor identification could be demonstrated in an instructive way in this case [12]; but it was a rare occurrence.

Far more often, one sees severe sensory psychoses with extensive disorientation, with content mainly of fantastic hypochondriacal threatening delusions, almost always mixed in with grandiose ideas, and hyperkinetic and characteristic parakinetic motility psychoses, usually post-epileptic and with a duration not exceeding one or a few weeks. Thus, I remember an epileptic who, during his psychosis, practised the most dangerous acrobatic tricks while mute, and apparently allopsychically disorientated. The complexity of these movements distinguished these cases as real psychoses; but we also see, and far more often, that restlessness of jactation accompanies deep unconsciousness of post-epileptic stupor, sometimes lasting for hours or days.

You have already come to know, (p. 134), a typical example of the fearful hallucinatory states seen amongst epileptics. One could summarize these states, by their essential characteristics, as cases of the most acute hallucinosis. They last for half an hour, or a few hours; they are related to the 'frenetic' [Ed] twilight states, but are distinguished from them by their allopsychic orientation. I have yet to see cases of epileptic melancholia. In contrast, manic states are seen in rare cases, albeit not quite pure ones, since they are combined with isolated hyperkinetic symptoms. You have yourselves occasionally seen an example of this [13].

Whether the so-called 'second state' [Ed] occurs in actual epileptics or is rather more specifically hysterical in nature, I would regard as not clearly resolved, despite the case that I personally experienced, mentioned earlier (p. 191). French authors emphasize that such states are distinguished from others in the same series, through a certain stereotyped character of behaviour, with precise recurrence of the same actions, as was the case in the example already mentioned. However, exactly this uniformity of attacks seems also to apply in the so-called second state. Moreover, we observed exactly the opposite: namely a rather 'polymorphic' [Ed] behaviour for the various seizures in the same individuals.

If we look elsewhere for characteristic features of psychoses related to epilepsy, a rapid sequence, usually leading to a recovery, is common to almost all cases. However, there are almost always recurrences. Cases of epilepsy complicated by psychoses tend finally, and often quite soon, to lead to dementia. Moreover, such epileptic psychoses involve mainly, but by no means solely, the so-called twilight states. However, the sensorium can be completely clear, and allopsychic orientation totally intact. If the psychosis does not exist in a twilight state, it tends to show Affective coloration, with sudden flaring of angry outbursts being particularly common. There is often actual muscle twitching, or exaggerated, expansive, violent, and purposeless movements that occasionally fall outside the clinical picture typical of motility psychoses. We seem to see in these phenomena, suggestions of increasing motor excitability being due to adverse consequences of repeated epileptic seizures. It is known, that in many epileptics, hints of focal symptoms are also to be found, which become especially pronounced after severely-adverse impacts, and after a series of seizures. The same is also sometimes reflected in the epileptic psychoses, particularly with hints of paraphasia. Furthermore, persistence—or perseveration—both in sensory and motor relationships, can be regarded as a common peculiarity of many cases of epileptic psychoses.

References

1. Griesinger W. Herr Ringseis und die naturhistorische Schule. Arch Physiol Heilk. 1842;1:43–66.
2. Meynert T. Der Bau der Grosshirnsrinde und seine örtlichen Verschiedenheiten, nebst einem pathologisch-anatomischen Corollarium. Leipzig: Engelman; 1887.
3. Wernicke C. Krankenvorstellungen aus der psychiatrischen Klinik in Breslau, vol. 2. Breslau: Schletter; 1899. Case 9.
4. Wernicke C. Krankenvorstellungen, vol. 1, 1899. Case 12.
5. Jolly F. Über die psychiatrischen Stoerung bei Polyneuritis. Charité Ann Berlin. 1897;22:580–612.
6. Korsakoff SS. Über eine besondere Form psychischer Störung kombiniert mit multipler Neuritis. Arch Psychiatr Nervenkr. 1890;21:669–704.
7. Magnan V. Psychiatrische Vorlesungen. Vol. 1. Über das 'Delire chronique a evolution systematique', Paranoia chronica mit systematischer Entwickelung oder Paranoia completa. Leipzig: Georg Thieme; 1891.
8. Wernicke C. Krankenvorstellungen, vol. 2, 1899. Case 17.
9. Wernicke C. Krankenvorstellungen, vol. 2, 1899. Case 7.
10. Neisser A. Krankenvorstellung (Fall von 'Asymbolie'). Allg Z Psychiatr. 1895;51:1016–21.
11. Goltz FL. Beiträge zur Lehre von den Functionen der Nervencentren des Frosches. Berlin: A Hirschwald; 1869.
12. Wernicke C. Krankenvorstellungen, vol. 3, 1900. Case 23.
13. Wernicke C. Krankenvorstellungen, vol. 2, 1899. Case 24.

Lecture 39

39

- Continuation of aetiological grouping of the psychoses
- Hysterical absences
- Hysterical delirium
- Pubertal psychoses or hebephrenic psychoses
- Kahlbaum's Heboid
- Senile psychoses
- Menopausal psychoses
- Menstrual psychoses
- Puerperal psychoses.
- General and special aetiology
- Inanition delirium
- Symptomatic psychoses

Lecture

Hysterical psychoses are related to epileptic psychoses in many respects, for example in their tendency to so-called twilight states. Some variety is often seen in this, especially among hystero-epileptics in connection with seizures, which French authors defined as a unique stage—the hystero-epileptic attack. However, it is not so much the 'pre-syncope' [Ed] of the sensorium, as the total allopsychic disorientation—usually of only short duration—that forms the main feature of these conditions. Patients behave as if they are in a fantastically altered situation, intensely Affect-laden. In particular, any misfortune that has befallen them—loss of relatives etc—plays a role. This so-called emotional stage of hystero-epileptic seizures thus falls within the area of delirious allopsychoses.

The so-called hysterical delirium corresponds even more closely to this concept—it being an acute psychosis that occurs independently, with an urge to move induced by sensory factors, and with total allopsychic disorientation, but with no definite prevailing Affective state. Due to their multiple sensory distractions, spontaneous expressions of these patients are also highly incoherent, reflecting their hypermetamorphosis. Only occasionally and momentarily can patients' attention be fixed sufficiently to obtain answers from them. Tactile hallucinations and phonemes, localized with abnormal precision, play a major role. Addition of asymbolia is likely, as indicated by the patient's behaviour towards food intake and bodily care. General muscle tremor, occurrence of the so-called lateral column symptoms [1], and physical decline can accompany the psychic symptoms, and lead to death within a few weeks. Moreover, mainly hypochondriacal symptoms may be seen during hysterical delirium. In like manner, in a severe case, after 6 weeks, the sensory agitation made way for a typical picture of agitated motor confusion, namely a hyperkinetic motility psychosis with manic features. This reversal appeared to be attributed to recovery of strength and general condition as a result of continued artificial feeding. An equally rapid reversal led to full restitution

R. Miller, K.J. Dennison (eds.), *An Outline of Psychiatry in Clinical Lectures*,
DOI 10.1007/978-3-319-18051-9_39

with insight into the illness; but a recurrence happened 18 months later. I am not aware of the outcome.

I have already mentioned (p. 253) the so-called *catalepsy of hysterics* [W], that is, a relatively short-duration akinetic motility psychosis. The sensorium usually becomes deeply insensitive, and often, to judge from the rapturous facial expression, is filled with ecstatic, religious dream experiences. A residual condition of weakness, without a paranoid stage, passes rapidly into healing. However, it also happens that such ecstatic states recur, and merge into a clinical picture of continued total immobility. I saw such a case end in death: These cases are serious psychoses. Often enough cases of illness are seen that have not so much the pattern of acute psychoses, but rather, represent transitional cases, or mixed ones between hysterical degeneration or impoverished personality, and isolated psychotic symptoms. In psychiatric wards in big cities, such as in our Clinic, prostitutes make up a very large proportion of these very troublesome cases of illness, because of their lax discipline. However, illnesses arising in quite civilized situations raise similar doubts: Is it misbehaviour and moral deficit, or illness? Tests on their spiritual *endowment* [W] and memory retention often show the former to be strikingly restricted, the latter to be significantly reduced. However, these are not necessarily lasting deficits. Treatment of such cases is extremely difficult, with a chance of success only if one always starts by assuming that a patient's behaviour is conditional on some pathology. Quite recently, cases have been described by Ganser [2], in which patients with apparently clear sensorium, and quite sound mind, answered questions put to them in such an inaccurate and twisted manner that one had to assume an intent to deceive, the more so since some of them were prisoners. However, detection of the so-called hysterical stigmata led the author, justifiably we believe, to assume that a so-called twilight state exists in such cases. This is supported by the fact that previously-described, undoubtedly hysterical patients, often present the same symptom of deliberately meaningless answers. The only objection is to the name 'twilight state' [W] for such cases, for reasons mentioned earlier: The sensorium is not impaired, although existing mental material is restricted in its extent. There is a 'narrowing' [Ed] of consciousness, suggesting being hypnotized in a waking state. Thus, one sees in otherwise hysterical patients, quite atypical cases of psychoses, such as a delusion of persecution directed against only one person, where the sensory presence of this person is hallucinated, while allopsychic orientation is retained. I have already said what is necessary on the specific hysterical 'second state' [W].

Independent of hystero-epileptic seizures, I have often seen short-duration hysterical psychoses lasting a half to several hours, especially in children and school students during adolescence, recurring quite irregularly, often after demonstrable emotions of any kind. They have to be subsumed under 'transitory psychoses' [Ed]. Such seizures usually consist of anxious misunderstanding of situations, similar to the popular image of *Pavor nocturnus* [W] of children. In milder cases, they represent a type of abortive anxiety psychosis, that is, not so much a misunderstanding of the situation and people, but a vivid display of anxiety, sometimes in the guise of phonemes, with seemingly impulsive dragging, clinging to family, or blind lashing-out, ripping, rummaging, etc. These hysterical psychoses, which are rapidly cured with appropriate treatment, but likewise gradually subsiding without it, are usually precipitated by emotions, and by any kind of debilitating eventuality, such as mental strain, too little sleep, etc. They are usually accompanied by a precursor stage, with headaches, palpitations, and fainting spells. Almost always in these cases, phrenic nerve insufficiency can be demonstrated as the basis for the fear. Twilight states lasting several days sometimes occur in young people in connection with major emotions, with total allopsychic disorientation almost to the point of asymbolia, blended with episodes of parakinetic symptoms. Thus—incidentally—I presented to you a 15-year-old apprentice baker, who had too little sleep for a long time; short-duration 'absences' [Ed] in preceding weeks, mostly at night, with subsequent amnesia; and he became acutely ill after an act of embezzlement he had committed came to light.

Far more common in our area of interest than hysterical psychoses, are hysterical neuroses. I mention only obsessional neuroses and anxiety neuroses. Exceptionally however, these can lead to corresponding genuine psychoses.

Gentlemen! You will assume from this description, that hysterical psychoses are frequently diagnosable from the clinical picture that they present. However, the main means of *diagnosis* [W] is always that hysterical symptoms can be detected before onset of the acute illness. In this respect it is important to know that the main source of hysteria among young girls is increased mental work beyond their individual capability. Only rarely will you encounter girls who take their Bachelor of Teaching exam without having become hysterical. In many cases, detection of the so-called hysterical stigmata at the time of the acute illness is possible, thereby confirming the diagnosis.

As for the *prognosis* [W] of hysterical psychoses, for a long time it had been decided that this was not so reliable as it is for the epileptic psychoses, which usually recover rapidly. However, one is often surprised by recovery in cases that seemed clinically unfavourable. Hysterical delirium almost always seems to recover; in other words, there need be no fear of residual chronic mental disorder. Hystero-epilepsy, in cases complicated by psychosis, just like epilepsy in such cases, appears, in the end to lead to dementia. Hystero-epilepsy by itself does not have this outcome, whereas known epileptics, with frequent seizures, always become demented. The prognosis of acute psychoses is generally favourable; however, the danger of recurrence is great if there is no recovery from the basic hysteria.

The psychoses of puberty, or *hebephrenic psychoses* [W] have already been mentioned a number of times. You will remember, gentlemen, that I have earlier referred to the term hebephrenia, and have acknowledged the particular type of illness described by Kahlbaum and Hecker [3]. However, from experiences in our clinic, I have become increasingly dissatisfied with this viewpoint, and can now deal only with hebephrenic aetiology, which *is* [Ed] of great importance. Rather than 'hebephrenia' [Ed], I am inclined to accept Kahlbaum's 'heboidophrenia' [Ed] or, for short, 'heboid' [Ed], as a specific psychosis of puberty. This clinical picture is defined far more sharply, as one in which 'Affectuosity' [Ed] (generally uniquely related to puberty but accentuated here) plays such an important role, and which seems to occur only in the context of puberty. Of course, I must then assume that certain symptoms that are consistently present have not been adequately observed by Kahlbaum. I mean mainly experiences of anxiety, outward signs of anxiety, and hypochondriacal sensations. Otherwise, I refer you to Kahlbaum's descriptions of relevant cases; they are relatively rare, so that I have encountered only a few such.

Much more common, and again specifically hebephrenic, are cases mentioned earlier, in which the clinical picture of the so-called primary lunacy is accompanied by a rapid progression to dementia. Such cases of illness, examples of chronic psychoses, earn the name *hebephrenic expansive autopsychosis* [W]. However, the clinical picture in some of these cases does not remain the same, but shifts, sometimes after 3–6 months, to a state of atonity, which, for its part, gives way only to most profound dementia.

Next most common might be motility psychoses of any kind, but particularly akinetic motility psychosis, which find their next occasion for occurrence at time of puberty. The familiar tendency for akinetic motility psychosis to be transformed into dementia might be based in part on this aetiological relationship, as is their tendency to recur, falsely attributed to this particular form of illness. Yet I also know of cases of akinetic motility psychosis occurring during puberty that were followed by such a complete recovery that it has not disturbed the life-transition of the young men involved; nor had any recurrence occurred. Thus the unfavourable prediction that Kräpelin [4] makes for such cases, does not always apply to those during puberty.

Furthermore, hypochondriacal anxiety psychosis, the particular form of somatopsychosis closely related to simple anxiety psychosis, undoubtedly occurs preferentially during puberty. Nonetheless, in a proportion of cases, the clinical picture becomes continuous and prominent only after a long period, when up to a year has passed with no more than isolated attacks of anxiety lasting no more than an hour, and an unhappy mood; and by then a correspondingly reduced capacity has emerged. In one case of this sort, which finally recovered, the patient falsely interpreted perceived pollution and erections, combined with olfactory hallucinations—a stench of death referred to his genitals—and attacks of increasing anxiety as the principal element of the clinical picture, which slowly faded. Definitive recovery ensued only after some years. In the meantime, reduced retentiveness and rapid fatigue when challenged by mental demands became disturbingly noticeable even to the patients themselves. However, the mental *status quo ante* [Ed] was never regained. Such a mild course corresponds perhaps to an 'abortive' [Ed] case of hebephrenic psychosis. In any case, far more often, cases are to be found which could be described as slowly worsening somatopsychoses, in which a hypochondriacal psychosis emerges, in a sense 'slipping in' [Ed] unnoticed. It is often bodily discomfort of undetermined or changeable localization, but sometimes leading to an outcome of complete inactivity. An acute episode leads to total sensory psychosis with a content of fantastic hypochondriacal threatening delusions, pointing to a more florid disease process, often developing only years later. The residual deficit state then presents with features of Kahlbaum's hebephrenic weak-mindedness, which is sometimes very striking.

Finally, I mention the extremely acute psychosis already touched on (p. 244), that I have seen repeatedly in young girls. This seems not to be a chance occurrence, but supports a hebephrenic aetiology for their illness. I already stressed that they can still recover without deficit.

To validate my position on hebephrenia, I limit myself to the following remarks, which as you know, are by no means exhaustive. On the whole, we must recognize that hebephrenic psychoses in most cases show some characteristic traits. They are not to be found in the specific childhood form, in which, the resulting feeble-mindedness in silly and foolish beings, would seem only natural: Rather than a predilection to a certain clinical picture which, in its tendency to recur, is by no means limited to puberty, there is a prevailing tendency to an unfavourable outcome, or, if there is a favourable outcome, at least a temporary occurrence of actual deficit symptoms; and in the event of a chronic course, for worsening with each episode, so that the most acute clinical pictures occur in between. Finally, in cases with the most-acute onset—but sometimes also in chronically developed cases—it is stressed that they proceed as composite psychoses, that is, by producing totally different clinical pictures at different periods. So much is this so, that, in one case, with profound—almost animal—dementia, over many years, I have seen hyperkinetic motility psychosis occurring; and since this occurred during continuous stay in the institution, there were no harmful external influences. Consequently, you had the opportunity of seeing a case that I presented to you in one semester as Affective melancholia; and in the following semester as a picture of hyperkinetic motility psychosis; and finally as the pure deficit condition of severe feeble-mindedness [5]. It was in the context of this case that I drew your attention to what is frequently seen in cases of hebephrenia: This is the relatively 'busy' [Ed] face that gives no indication of inner emptiness. This is particularly surprising when it is compared with the smooth and stupid face of most paralytics, even in early stages of this illness.

Little is known about the influence of senescence or *senile involution* [W] of the brain on the form and course of psychoses; yet here also we can group psychoses according to their aetiology, namely presbyophrenia, as already described. You will recall that this clinical picture, in its essential features, matches another psychosis, of polyneuritic aetiology. However, differences can be pointed out in some peripheral features. Thus allopsychic disorientation of presbyophrenia seems to change in degree over time; at least I have often seen this. With polyneuritic psychosis this feature tends not to change, nor do delirious states of presbyophrenia. Sometimes they occur only at night, and there are borderline cases in which such nocturnal deliria, plus actual deficit symptoms account for the whole clinical picture. I have already emphasized that the notion of senile dementia does not include presbyophrenia. Here too, the attentive facial expression and prompt reaction to stimuli are evident, quite apart from the curability of acute-onset delirious cases, which you already know about.

Moreover, senility seems to produce very different clinical pictures. Cases of Affective melancholia are fairly common, although borderlines cases predominate, which are familiar to you and belong more in the area of anxiety psychoses. Apart from senility, the prognosis of such cases, as you will remember, is generally favourable, except that the risk of recurrence is greater than usual. We were able to define senility as the sole aetiology in one case of obsessional psychosis [6], and one of circumscribed autopsychosis due to overvalued ideas [7]. We have met examples of acute anxiety psychoses that showed a special course, deviating from usual, in that a very physical and 'altruistic' [Ed] persecutory delusion was created, which quickly became associated with total allopsychic disorientation. We then came to suspect that we should attribute the course in such cases to a definite senile aetiology. It now appears that, right from the start, chronically progressing cases of 'chronic hallucinosis' as we named it (even without development of the delusion systems of physical persecution), can often lead to the same outcome of allopsychic disorientation in old people. A 78-year-old woman I have in mind, misjudged everything within a context of imprisonment, yet showed intelligent, level-headed, and active behaviour. Furthermore, a case of akinetic motility psychosis presented, in the paranoid stage with surprising allopsychic disorientation. This case is remarkable in that the psychosis, despite advanced age, proceeded to full recovery within 2 years. It was only the signs of senile amnesia, which remained for the duration, that prevented real insight into the illness, because of memory deficit for the period of acute psychosis.

As far as the specific aetiology of senile psychoses is concerned, a stroke is often found to be the immediate origin of the psychosis, even in cases where hemiplegic symptoms have regressed completely. This is especially true for cases of presbyophrenia; but it is sometimes also true for other types of illness. I would particularly like to mention a case of hemiplegia in an elderly woman, in whom the psychosis had the content of a uniquely coloured hypochondriacal delusion of persecution. Specifically she believed the persecutor to be a man who lay beside her in bed, and had taken possession of the paralyzed half of her body.

The influence of the *menopause* [W] on development of psychoses is well-known. We can probably point to a closer connection with a special clinical form of acute psychosis, specifically of anxiety psychosis, and instances of anxiety neurosis, which also prove troublesome at the time of menopause in otherwise normal women; and find ways to understand it in various vasomotor disturbances. At other times the illness develops chronically, with slowly, creeping delusions of relatedness; or a subacute outbreak is seen, with episodic relapses indicating exacerbations. Menopausal psychoses tend mainly to progress unfavourably; yet even here, the form of psychosis is likely to be influential, since a case [8] was presented to you in convalescence, on the borderline between Affective melancholia and anxiety psychosis. In addition, I can recall cases of complete menopausal motility psychosis that had a favourable outcome.

Menstrual psychoses [W] have been discussed several times already. We have encountered hyperkinetic motility psychosis, confused mania (or agitated confusion, related to it by its close connection with menstruation) as specific forms of menstrual psychosis. I remind you of the fact that the two clinical pictures have close connections with each other; indeed they can replace each other, and they usually tend to recur in sequential attacks at about 4-weekly intervals. However, sporadic cases are also seen that likewise occur within a four-weekly period, and, at their best, progress to complete recovery without a paranoid intermediate stage. The moment of the outbreak, which is always very acute, is most often premenstrual; sometimes it coincides in time with the period, or the end of it. If, instead of this recurrent course, there is continued or longer-lasting psychosis, a paranoid stage remains, usually at the same time as a residual hallucinosis; but this can also lead to recovery. Outcome in dementia is to be feared only if menstrual hyperkinetic motility psychosis or confused mania at the same time is understood as a hebephrenic psychosis.

The next most frequent risk related to menstruation—likewise usually with a periodic or recurrent course—is any kind of mixed form of mania. Pure mania with a menstrual basis is relatively rare. Of the mixed forms, a special introduction is needed to manic allopsychosis and manic hyperkinetic allopsychosis: These are clinical pictures that would correspond to the type of confused mania or agitated confusion, but with added allopsychic disorientation. Wrathful mania should be mentioned here—the mixture of anxiety psychosis and manic symptoms that I have occasionally described already. Since agitated melancholia represents a mixed psychosis with some components of mania and some of anxiety psychosis, it is perhaps necessary to interpret the concept of wrathful mania in somewhat greater detail. Wrathful mania preserves the general character of mania; in agitated melancholia by contrast, despite the compulsion to speak, and the flight of ideas, we cannot forget that it is an anxiety psychosis. Thus, in wrathful mania we find the sophisticated, imperious, brutal, sometimes even obscene behaviour of manic patients, and usually also prominent grandiose ideas and, at least temporarily, abnormal euphoria. The differential diagnosis should therefore focus mainly on the mania, but of course, it is usually very easy in this respect. Pressured speech and flight of ideas are frequently distracted and interrupted by hallucinated expressions of anxiety, by delusions of relatedness, and sometimes by fear of approach, while hypermetamorphosis also claims attention. All these are symptoms that are foreign to pure mania. I have already stated that wrathful mania often shows up as a recurrent type, and not only when the aetiology is menstrual. Akinetic motility psychoses and anxiety psychoses closely linked with menstruation occur relatively rarely, but are still recognizable.

On the likelihood of recovery from menstrual psychoses, the general view puts them in a worse light than they deserve. In particular, it is probably the periodic cases and experiences coming from earlier times, when treatment was less careful, that gave rise to this unfavourable judgment. In my experience, most cases, even after multiple recurrences, tend finally to heal, but of course, treatment needs great care. As is generally known, when there is a severe hereditary load, recurrent mania is often seen at the time of puberty, or the first appearance of menstruation. Such cases, which, as I have repeatedly stressed, unjustly bear the name of 'periodic mania' [Ed], may in part have been confused with menstrual psychoses.

Gentlemen! Amongst *puerperal psychoses* [W], puerperal mania is best known to you all. However, you have learned that hyperkinetic motility psychosis, that, up to now could not be clearly separated from mania, represents the most common form of puerperal psychosis. Quite remarkably, puerperal cases of hyperkinetic motility psychosis tend to show multiple recurrences, at about four-weekly intervals, and these are the more favourable cases. Equally common is when the first attack of puerperal hyperkinetic motility psychosis shows only the beginning of a cyclic pattern. Finally, if the regular pattern is curtailed, a complete motility psychosis appears; and such cases are always judged to be very serious, especially if they go beyond a single cycle. Less common than these cases, but still seen quite often are the pre-existing akinetic motility psychoses. Pure mania is relatively rare, but such cases are distinct by their rapid, favourable course. Moreover there are some—mainly severe—clinical pictures of psychoses related to the puerperium, especially when, apart from the puerperium, other harmful circumstances are present, such as excessive lactation, febrile illness, or painful mastitis, that have reduced the levels of energy. In such circumstances the most severe hypochondriacal psychoses may occur, with allopsychic disorientation. Experienced experts are unable to agree on whether such puerperal psychoses have a favourable outlook with regard to their curability.

Gentlemen! This overview allows you to see the benefits that an aetiological approach offers for knowledge and understanding of the psychoses. However, throughout this, it will have confirmed for you the maxim that, so often, I sought to instill, that aetiological considerations offer a benefit only if we separate them sharply from clinical definition of the various psychoses, making no claims to artificial construction, or to clinical forms defined exclusively by aetiology.

Perhaps, at this point, a classification of 'aetiological moments', according to their importance [Ed] is to be recommended. Every reason then suggests that we should always separate the 'general aetiology' [Ed] and the 'special aetiology' [Ed] (in the sense of an immediate trigger). Sometimes, one or the other type of physiological effect is unaccounted for; but often, both are detectable, or the same adverse consequence can be attributed just as well to general as to special aetiology.

I have already mentioned that I cannot recognize 'exhaustion psychoses' [Ed] as a special group, because any [Ed] variety of 'exhausting moment' [Ed] can be seen as the immediate cause of illness in the vast majority of acute psychoses. In contrast, a delirious state can be recognized in states of inanition. We are thus getting near to the notion of *symptomatic psychoses* [W] that is, those psychoses which, in their appearance and course, show unmistakable dependence on other physical illnesses. Each febrile delirium would, in this sense be interpreted as a symptomatic psychosis; but it would probably be better to contrast this with actual psychoses, as psychotic states. To all these delirious states, apart from familiar symptoms of hallucinations (in particular dream-like hallucinations), occasional ideas of anxiety, and a restlessness more-or-less reminiscent of jactation, an allopsychic disorientation appears always to be distinctive, at least temporarily.

Moreover symptomatic psychosis might still require a more precise study according to the criteria that you have met here in my clinic. According to my few experiences, symptomatic anxiety psychoses which come to our notice—dyspneic states being most common—tend to be regarded as anxiety neurosis, as long as such obvious disease processes are absent. They occur in the wake of diseases of heart, kidney, and lung, at all levels of severity, even down to simple cases of anxiety. Moreover, almost all clinical forms might occasionally appear symptomatically. Thus, for example, I have observed symptomatic Affective melancholia in perityphlitis, and a 3-day hyperkinetic motility psychosis with febrile illness, caused by pus formation in the mastoid antrum. However, mostly it is acute infectious diseases that predisposed to symptomatic psychoses, and most commonly with a picture of anxiety-coloured, delirious twilight states. Symptoms of muscle tremor and speech disorder caused by severe physical illness can then give rise to confusion, with delirious states of progressive paralysis. The *prognosis* [W] of symptomatic psychoses depends exclusively on the course of the underlying disease, whose prospects of course can only be unfavourably influenced.

References

1. Bonhoeffer KFOH. "Seitenstrangerscheinungen" bei akuten Psychosen. Psychiat Nervenpath Abh. 1896;2.
2. Ganser SJM. Über einen eigenartigen hysterischen Dämmerzustand. Arch psychiatr Nervenkr. 1898;30: 633–40.
3. Hecker E, Kahlbaum KL. Hebephrenia: A contribution to clinical psychiatry. Arch Pathol Anat Clin Med. 1871;52:349–429.
4. Kraepelin E. Über psychische Functionsstörungen. Allg Ztschr Psychiatr. 1890;46:522–4.
5. Wernicke C. Krankenvorstellungen aus der psychiatrischen Klinik in Breslau. Breslau: Schletter. vol.2, Case 16.
6. Wernicke C. Krankenvorstellungen vol.2, Case 27.
7. Wernicke C. Krankenvorstellungen vol.1, Case 23.
8. Wernicke C. Krankenvorstellungen vol.3, Case 22.

Lecture 40

40

- Course of disease
- Body-mass curve
- Intensive and extensive disease curve
- Accumulating and substituting course
- Outcome in death, mental invalidity, or paranoid states
- Material confusion
- Dementia or idiocy and imbecility
- Congenital and acquired dementia
- Principal signs of acquired dementia
- Causes of the same
- Paralytic dementia, post-apoplectic, epileptic, alcoholic, hebephrenic dementia

Lecture

Gentlemen!

The factual material that I have presented to you so far allows us to put forward a few general observations about the course of the psychoses and their outcomes. We moved on from there to differentiate chronic and acute psychoses. However, closer examination of these differences of the course over time soon showed that acute clinical pictures are occasionally to be found in chronic cases, somewhere along their time line. This situation is to be explained by the fact that acute episodes interrupt the chronic course, but also by addition of symptoms that in themselves, or in their practical consequences, bring with them severe Affective states. We should always stipulate that a continuous course, uninterrupted by symptom-free periods, is a criterion to recognize a psychosis as chronic. We should not expect to include the so-called periodic psychoses amongst the chronic psychoses, since, in reality, they are recurrent or relapsing psychoses, even though recurrences follow so closely on one another that in practice there is no significant difference. In general, chronic psychoses have a worsening course, that is, they lead to ever-increasing disorientation. This is particularly true when acute psychoses are separated from actual chronic psychoses, and cases of chronic mental disorder remain as I did earlier. In contrast to such cases of chronic psychoses, we can also define—as we would in general medical parlance—an improving course, provided the condition does not remain stable and unchanging, which is rarely the case. The improving course is then synonymous with gradual recovery of orientation, without it ever being fully achieved.

We must subdivide acute psychoses according to their time course into peracute, acute, and subacute psychoses. This distinction is of practical importance; however, we would only apply it when we deal with a clinical picture of acute coloration, which has developed slowly over time, to distinguish it from chronic psychosis. Thus, for example, paralytic psychoses usually develop subacutely. The differentiation of a peracute illness onset is less useful in practice, but finds its

R. Miller, K.J. Dennison (eds.), *An Outline of Psychiatry in Clinical Lectures*,
DOI 10.1007/978-3-319-18051-9_40

use in the so-called transitory psychoses. If you want to include here all cases where a severe clinical picture emerges within 24 h, then a significant percentage of all acute psychoses would be excluded. Of course prodromal symptoms, which are purely physical in nature, such as insomnia, lassitude of limbs, headache, indisposition, etc., must be omitted. Included amongst the rarities, are cases such as the previously mentioned (p. 186) Miss v. F. in whom an acute psychosis existed in full force from one particular instant—her awakening from sleep—but then continued on an improving course. We might properly consider such cases as apoplectiform, and thereby rare cases would automatically come to mind of polyneuritis, within which the same clinical picture intrudes. Moreover, these very acute-onset cases remain for some time at the peak level of illness, before their intensity diminishes. Of course, their outcome can also be death or dementia.

The great number of acute psychoses, in which onset of illness occurs within the bounds set by the above-mentioned borderline cases, nevertheless correspond to a trajectory of disease that proceeds relatively slowly, compared with physical illnesses. Such psychoses thus find closer analogies amongst certain chronic illnesses, such as *Phthisis pulmonum.* [W] Correspondingly, most acute psychoses, notably all subacute ones, initially show a worsening course. An example of this is given by acute hallucinosis, which well illustrates the preceding sentences. The clinical picture, apparently rises rapidly to full disease intensity in accord with its Affective coloration, and shows a rising course of physical symptoms, and soon also altruistic delusions of persecution are added in to an increasing extent over succeeding weeks. Thus, in the paranoid stage, a definite peak of allopsychic disorientation is achieved, while at the same time symptoms that led to this are starting to subside. The latter enables orientation to return—a subsequent improving course. Repeated bouts of this kind may often result in an attack whose outcome is unfavourable. This is due to the fact that elementary symptoms, rather than subsiding, continue and even increase, so that the aftermath of the Affective outburst depends solely on habituation, and accommodation to external conditions. This course therefore is continuously worsening, leading to ever-more-remote alienation from reality. One could characterize such a course—because of its fateful significance—as a progressive course of acute psychoses. You will remember that I often spoke of acute progressive psychoses in this sense. If there is an improving course following the peak stage of the acute psychosis, then evidently we are dealing with three distinguishable stages: an incremental stage, the peak, and a decremental stage, as has long been known in all acute physical illnesses.

However, the course just described is still continuous. There are, however, not only continuous courses but also remitting and intermittent ones. In effect, we should call the course intermittent if there are one or more lucid intervals. In this sense, one could therefore refer to many cases of mania and confused mania as having intermittent courses. However, in practice, intermissions of the shortest duration are best ignored. We should then identify an intermittent or recurrent course only in cases in which a series of individual attacks succeeded one another, as is the case in hyperkinetic forms of menstrual psychosis. The intermissions here must be included in the actual duration of illness, especially since they are often beset with states of physical and sometimes mental fatigue. There is no question that such intermissions do not merit the term 'intermission' [Ed] in its strict sense, if they do not lead to full insight into the illness. Such cases would therefore be examples of a remitting course. Sometimes, chronically worsening psychoses show an intermittent start. For example, two distinct instances of a delirious state formed the precursor to primary major and consecutive delusions of persecution in a 35-year-old man who was not a drinker. In such cases, insight into illness gained in the first intermission was lost in subsequent ones. Here the course is remitting or, probably more accurately, rising in a staggered fashion. The remitting course often both rises and falls in a staggered way. Most anxiety psychoses are examples of such a remitting course, in which anxiety, and the autopsychic disorientation based upon it, usually exist in a persistent fashion, but are increased in attacks that lead to allopsychic disarray and corresponding ideas of allopsychic anxiety, in the guise of phonemes. This fluctuating—perhaps 'remitting' [Ed] would be better—course of anxiety psychoses has been mentioned repeatedly.

Gentlemen! In remarks just made, you will recognize the effort made to express the course of psychoses in part in the form of a curve. It would be a great step forward if we could obtain a rapid overview of such illnesses, which often stretch out over years, by producing a true disease curve, as an immediate focus for our attention. However, we must not hide from the difficulties in the way of such an undertaking. What criteria could guide construction of such a curve, if we want to avoid being quite arbitrary? Surely it would have to make exclusive use of tangible objective data. We find such data for example in body mass, and from my comments about the remarkable influence of mental illness on nutrition and metabolism (p. 100), you will not be particularly surprised if I tell you that the closest method of constructing such a curve is to use data on body mass as the ordinate. In fact, in a large number of cases, a curve constructed in this manner seems, at first glance, to match the disease curve surprisingly well—surprisingly, in so far as all emerging clinical variations in the course seemed to reflect inverse variations of the *bodyweight curve* [W]. Moreover, in acute episodes of chronic psychoses, this behaviour often comes strongly to the fore. Furthermore, it is often seen in recurrent courses of acute psychoses, for example in hyperkinetic motility psychosis or wrathful mania, that the bodyweight curve rises in a staggered way in intervals between attacks, while, at the same time, clinical forms of these attacks become milder, until the continual increase indicates definite recovery. However, deviations from this behaviour *are* [Ed] observed, even when not explained by inter-current illnesses or accidental complications, although frequent occurrence of such complications often hinders evaluation of bodyweight curves to measure a disease trajectory. A glance at chronic psychoses also teaches us that often enough the patient's general condition is in no way mapped out in his suffering. Certainly therefore, we can acknowledge the practical value of the bodyweight curve as a mirror image of the disease curve for most cases of acute psychoses; but we should also not overestimate it and, above all, should admit *a priori* [W] that its scientific value is provisional and doubtful.

Moreover, theoretical considerations point us in other directions. In psychoses, as everywhere, we must obviously differentiate between intensity and extent of the disease process. Accordingly, a special curve must be constructed for intensity and extent for each case. What we have to understand by extent, is not hard to specify: It is the number of elementary symptoms which can be specifically identified in the resulting changes in content of consciousness; or, in other words, the scope and degree of disorientation. We know of psychoses whose extent is consistent throughout their course, and in which disorientation varies only in degree but not in extent. Thus Affective melancholia and pure mania persist as the same symptom complexes throughout their entire course. Accompanying disorientation (in other words belittlement of self, even to the point of delusion), or the hubris of grandiose delusions, remain limited not only to the area of personhood, but also to an unchanging and specific line of thought. There are essential variations in the degree of orientation here, and these depend in distinctive ways on the intensity of Affect. The name we give—autopsychic anxiety ideas (we might also call them 'misfortune ideas', undermining ideas of happiness) [Ed]—shows their derivation from an Affective state. As a result, a *curve of intensity* [W] suffices in such cases, to represent the course of the illness completely. In contrast to such cases, we see gradual summation of elementary symptoms, and substantive changes in psychoses proceeding in a purely chronic manner. Here a curve just of *extent* [W] will reproduce completely the progression of the disease. We could also express this relationship by setting in one type the curve of extent, in the second that of the intensity lying parallel to the abscissa.

Gentlemen! From the overview that I gave you at the conclusion of the clinical presentations, you will have seen that cases that I differentiated as the so-called 'basic forms' [Ed] or 'simple psychoses' [Ed], present mainly the same complex of symptoms throughout their entire course. For all such cases, the intensity curve is of predominant importance. However, this applies only in a broad sense; to be specific, there are many variations in extent. I mention only cases of intestinal somatopsychosis that increase rapidly to almost total disorientation over the entire body. For the vast majority of acute psychoses it would therefore be essential to plot both curves. Take the above-mentioned example of acute hallucinosis: There the course is summarized from two curves of totally different shape, following the overall impression given earlier. The acute onset of illness corresponds evidently to its greatest intensity, while the desperate decision of suicide can be viewed just as an external index of this. During hospitalization, and probably as a result of it, intensity tends to diminish significantly; and it shows occasional elevation, related to external causes such as a change in circumstances. Finally, the Affective reaction is progressively lost, and the intensity curve approaches the x-axis quite rapidly. The summary representation of the disease process given above could not take such a pattern into account; it appears to correspond to a one-sided consideration of the curve of extent of disease, whose shape tends generally to be a reciprocal of the intensity curve, that is, the worsening form progresses and only later, more or less rapidly does it approach the abscissa. From this example we also see what yardstick we need to represent the intensity of the illness. The Affective reaction is the exclusive consideration for this purpose: Its variations in degree give a good general discrimination. Whatever fear, unhappiness, despair, or bewilderment present is forced on each observer without further thought. I must point out only that a deeper sense of our curve of intensity curve requires that all levels of these different Affective reactions are to be conceived as expressions of the one basic Affect for all acute psychoses, namely disarray. I even believe that the abnormal euphoria of manics is due in part to disarray, but surely in other manic states, such as manic allopsychoses, the evident joy, and inclination to laugh, can often be attributed to the patients' finding the supposedly changed situation funny. However, I would specifically like to emphasize that those Affective states which cannot be attributed to disarray must remain unused in constructing the intensity curve. I would prefer deliberately to omit more specific information about the shape of the two curves, and their relationship to each other in the various psychoses that you have studied in greater detail, because this part of our clinical task is still very much under development. I limit myself to suggesting that the curve of body weight depends predominantly on the curve of intensity, and prognosis of individual cases seems related to the relationship of the two curves to each other.

Gentlemen! I have yet to mention a peculiarity in the curve of extent that is essential to characterizing all those psychoses in which it is of primary importance: We have seen above that the majority of acute psychoses initially take a worsening course. For the curve of extent, this usually amounts to summation of symptoms of illness, so that we can speak of an *accumulating course* [W] of the disease. You will remember my description of composite psychoses. Consider these now in relation to their curves of intensity and extent: The purest type of composite psychosis is seen when the succession of clinical pictures has come about not through an accumulation of symptoms, but through some manner of mutual separation of different symptom complexes. Apart from a cumulative course, we must therefore differentiate a *substituting course* [W], and see that the latter relates only to the curve of extent. The difficulty to which I already drew attention in the context of composite psychoses, was that a later phase of the illness can simply be regarded as augmentation of an earlier phase. This appears in a special light, given this consideration. Perhaps it would even be correct to restrict the concept of composite psychoses solely to cases characterized by substitutional behaviour in the curve of extent. One could perhaps use different colours on the curve, to indicate the significant diversity of symptoms in these cases.

Gentlemen! I come now to a brief summary overview of the *outcomes of psychoses* [W] and take the opportunity to draw attention to a point that I have never found emphasized sufficiently. Psychoses, if not conceived too narrowly, are so common that at least two per thousand of the population are undergoing treatment in asylums, these belonging to the most hazardous and truly life-threatening illnesses. Even the statistics of large asylums, provided that they are not exclusively secure units for chronic cases, reveal mortality of about 10 %. If we add the myriad of suicides carried out outside institutions by psychiatric patients who were not hospitalized at the time, we get a mortality figure approaching that of the most difficult surgical procedures. Outcome in death is intrinsic to all acute mental illnesses, a fact which, *a priori* [W] must remain as part of one's reckoning. This outcome is sometimes brought about by incidents arising from the unpredictability of the sick, such as self-harm, but at other times as a result of the illness process itself, as I have repeatedly stressed, along with many examples. Fever is sometimes present in such cases, but one can often find—even at autopsy—no explanation other than the disease process in the brain itself. Between these two extremes lie a large number of cases of illness in which death is to be explained as a result of insufficient nutrition, lack of sleep, and continued restlessness—that is through inanition and resultant wasting away. Finally, wound complications, and internal illnesses should be mentioned.

The exact opposite outcome—in complete recovery—is encountered only in acute or subacute psychoses. Fortunately it is far more common than is known in lay circles, averaging at least 30 %. Nearest to this is 'cure with deficit'. Such disabled people do indeed recover, without evident gross deficits, but are not sufficiently resilient to survive, at liberty and independently, without help from others. Every adversity they encounter puts them in danger of relapse; and hallucinations in particular, usually in the context of delusions of relatedness, occur easily in such Affective states. The result is that such patients, after repeated attempts at discharge, finally remain permanently in the institutions, where they find necessary protection and care, and also an opportunity for useful activity.

The outcome for paranoid states was dealt with in detail earlier. I want to emphasize once more (p. 66) that it is expedient to differentiate two groups: residual mental disorder which is simply chronic, and chronic psychoses which develop further. The former fall mainly into two different forms. In one, we find, after the acute psychosis has subsided, that certain elementary symptoms persist, either permanently or temporarily and hinder recovery of insight into the illness. These are mainly phonemes and delusions of relatedness. We referred earlier to such cases as residual hallucinosis. In contrast, other cases show a straightforward picture—the end-result of any acute psychosis: Falsification of contents of consciousness, naturally without any insight into the illness, but often also with no acute elementary symptoms. We can call this outcome 'forgery of consciousness' [Ed] or 'confusion of substance' [Ed]. The expression 'confusion' is appropriate to this state, in which we often find well-preserved formal logic: Any more extensive forgery of content of consciousness must evoke the actual *appearance* [Ed] of confusion. The requirement for intellectual material to 'conform' [Ed], which is necessary for mutual understanding between people, falls away here, and therefore patients, despite accurate and logical thought processes, become incomprehensible to us. Of course, linguistic expressions of such patients often acquire a different sense, and in particular may make use of a number of technical expressions invented solely for their own use, and this must further reinforce the appearance of confusion. In the expression 'voices' [W], you already know of such widespread technical expressions. There are still many such phrases used similarly by mentally ill people in remarkably similar ways. Thus many make use of the expression 'mirror language' [W] to denote that their own thoughts, in some manner inexplicable to them—rather through 'reflection' [Ed]—have become known to others. I took the following small sample from a document:

> 'Illness due to withdrawal of My physical regulation and of My armour in the civil registry. The collection of lost power-watches that my Holy Father gave me, clothing outfit-power watch, jewel

> watch, wardrobe watch, sickness watch, health maintenance-power watch etc. is in full intercourse. Because my civil status did not allow me to visit the present ruling imperial house, I have been ordered into the asylum for the insane in order to await the end of the collection of my powers and the full physical armour. Majesty Elisabeth Margaretha, according to my educator's time reckoning born 15th. February, 1868.'

The important outcome in dementia, that is, idiocy or feeble-mindedness, must be discussed in somewhat greater detail, since the same symptomatology often occurs as a primary independent illness.

Gentlemen! We can distinguish *congenital* [W] and *acquired* dementia. [W] Only the latter, which also forms the outcome of many mental illnesses, should concern us in detail here. Regarding the former, I limit myself to referring you to presentations by Emminghaus [1] and Meynert [2]. In the latter, you will find descriptions of the main types of deformity of the skull. Dementia acquired in early childhood should be grouped alongside congenital idiocy, because it also hinders further development of the brain. According to Emminghaus (with whom we concur), in congenital or early-acquired idiocy, three levels can be distinguished, depending on its severity, based on the level of mental development reached: For the level remaining from earliest childhood: *idiocy* [W]; for that remaining from later childhood: *semi-idiocy* [W]; and when there is no more than an inability to reach full mental maturity from puberty onward: *imbecility* [W]. Separating these three from one another is of course quite artificial, and in many borderline cases cannot be achieved; but otherwise, it is easily applied in practice.

Gentlemen! Let us now move on to examine *acquired dementia* [W]. Of course we still need more extensive and detailed investigation of how we are to understand idiocy or feeble-mindedness. Certainly, it is a 'failure' [Ed] phenomenon, a state of deficit, and one might be tempted to apply an exclusively quantitative scale, equating idiocy with loss of intellectual *endowment* [W] or contents of consciousness of any kind. However, you will soon be concerned that normal mental *endowment* [W] differs greatly, as I myself have already stressed at the beginning of these lectures (p. 54). You might then still suppose that we had adequate criteria to claim a reduction of mental *endowment* [W] only if this had previously been demonstrated to be significant. We might thus also have found an essential difference between innate and acquired dementia. However, this criterion is subject to definite qualifications, because, without doubt, much of the mental *endowment* [W] is normally lost, as is easily determined, if you challenge an elderly physician, lawyer, or mathematician with a test of word form in ancient Greek. Loss of positive knowledge can therefore be seen as abnormal only if it has been acquired quite recently, or has been refreshed repeatedly since its acquisition, or has found its use. Whether a certain area of knowledge is retained or has been lost can perhaps provide a usable scale for the so-called memory deficits. In any case, loss of most common knowledge, assumed to correspond to the level of education, can be a valuable criterion of acquired idiocy.

We should not regard this as crucial, for there are states where severe deficits of this kind can exist, yet patients have full insight into the fact, and thus retain sound judgment. If such patients take account of their failures, and at the same time are circumspect and capable of holding their attention, we will rightly be cautious before labeling them as 'stupid' [W]. Special weight has therefore always been placed on a person's ability to make judgments; and reduced ability to do this, was intended to establish the main finding—of idiocy. In fact, we must recognize that this criterion, in so far as it includes a quantitative element (as we shall soon see, p. 318), in measuring the performance of the organ of association, appears particularly suitable for use in disorders of mental activity—because each judgment is based on this. However, a source of error must be taken into account here: This relates to judgments a patient demonstrates towards their own delusional ideas, or indeed to all elementary psychotic symptoms. You scarcely require that a patient distrusts the evidence of his senses and should therefore recognize a hallucination as being not real, just in so far as it conflicts with other experiences. Similarly, one *might* [Ed] require an open judgment to be made about a delusional idea, however absurd it may be in factual terms; yet whoever does this—and you can find such a view very widespread—disregards the truest essence of all mental illnesses, which consists of the very fact that opposing ideas *can* occur, *can* co-exist side-by-side. Of course this does not happen without an Affective reaction, even the Affect of disarray (except for a very slow insidious approach of opposites as occurs in entirely chronic psychoses). Attempt to balance such opposites made within normal consciousness is the basis of systematization, already familiar to us. Earlier, we learned of the existence of several quite different—and normally mutually exclusive—groups of ideas lying side-by-side in the same organ of consciousness, leading to the erosion of personhood, these being outcomes of an earlier pre-existing psychosis. I have often drawn attention to the fact that in highly acute cases of illness, such as most acute attacks of hallucinosis in epileptics (p. 135), analogous juxtapositions of contrasting ideas can be seen. Even Meynert's intellect, penetrating more deeply into this phenomenon than any other, did not quite assimilate this fact. When for example he characterized delusional ideas of paralytics simply as 'idiotic' [Ed] and finds this idiocy itself to be founded on a lack of association, he undoubtedly goes too far: 'When the paralytic declares himself to be a rich man, a king, he shows himself different from the paranoid, who almost always raises only claims; but the former explains his delusion as facts. The delusional personality must harbour certain attributes: Something must have *preceded* [Ed] production of the delusion, which he would at least have had to interpret. That the lack of any attributes of a rich man, or a king, is not noticed by him, amounts to a lack of association.' These are Meynert's words [2]. As you know, however, this deficit in association is a quite general aspect of any delusional idea, based on the most fundamental process of all mental illnesses, namely sejunction. Where the delusional idea comes from is therefore of relatively little importance. Just as in such a typical example of 'paranoia' [W], so also the primary grandiosity resulting from primordial delirium is inexplicable to patients themselves, and is therefore regarded no less as a fact, provided confabulation has not yet gained a firm footing. For us, this example is nothing more than a clear *a priori* [W] symptom of failure—that is autopsychic disorientation—which, within a prevailing feeling of happiness, takes on a content of grandiosity. Such disorientation can only be based on dissolution of associations, our postulated process of sejunction. If, instead of primordial deliria, it is a question of grandiosity arising through autochthonous ideas, as in the cases of A. and Sch. mentioned earlier (p. 194 *seq.*), then the mechanism of its formation is known in only a slightly better way, but, as before, it is due to sejunction. In such cases, there is no real failure of intelligence. Moreover, the lack of judgment shown by patients prone to fixed ideas, for instance when they produce whining complaints derived from their overvalued idea, is not to be interpreted otherwise; and the viewpoint of Hitzig [3], who sees it as a lack of intelligence and a degree of feeble-mindedness is quite wrong. By the same token, one could interpret allopsychic ideas of anxiety in acute cases, that always have contents at odds with reality, but yet with well-preserved allopsychic orientation—meant in the strict sense—ideas which victoriously assert themselves, as evidence of idiocy. Delusions in the somatopsychic area can be of a most far-fetched character without ever permitting one to conclude that there is a lack of judgment, a fact that you will understand most easily from their particular mode of origin. From these observations, we are entitled to specify a special form of paralytic, expansive autopsychosis, without concluding that idiocy is present. Where, as in most cases, idiocy *is* [Ed] nevertheless present, it can often be viewed as a completely independent feature. However, sometimes it happens, and you yourselves have seen a patient of this sort, that fantastic grandiosity is associated with well-preserved mental *endowment* [W], and even with good memory retentiveness. You will remember that, at the same time, this patient [4] gave evidence of striking insight into his illness, but also gave an apt expression of his feelings of happiness, by remarking that 'one could probably put up with such an illness' [Ed]. These grandiose ideas, despite their fantastic coloration, are therefore nothing more than a companion piece to the equally fantastic ideas of anxiety; they are notions of happiness.

From these arguments we can conclude that deficits of judgment amongst mental patients do allow one to identify idiocy or feeblemindedness (the lower grade of idiocy), but only to the extent that they relate to matters outside their own delusions or any other existing psychotic elements. However, given this proviso, erroneous judgments can probably be used; for example, when patients are incapable of judging the behaviour of other mental patients correctly as abnormal, when set alongside otherwise appropriate behaviour. Also, in planning for the future, a clear inability to make judgments is often revealed, such as when an accountant can no longer solve a simple arithmetic problem, yet thinks he can return to his former position. However, the best test of a person's capacity for judgment is found in his actions, as we shall soon see.

In congenital idiocy we see numerous examples, that sometimes a person is still able to lead an active and useful life, but in simplified conditions. In the rural locations, you come across high-grade feeble-minded individuals everywhere, who can carry out specific monotonous work quite satisfactorily, provided they do not need to adjust to any change of conditions. However, if unforeseen circumstances happen just once, their lack of judgment is revealed by inappropriate actions, often in situations that any child would be able to assess accurately. For example, such a feeble-minded man had, for a long time, been involved on his own, with the job of collecting wood, hewn and sawn up in the forest, putting it on a wagon, and driving it into the yard. One day a large stone was lying on the road, and he ran into it. Instead of moving the stone aside, he repeatedly drove his team into it and beat the animals half to death. Likewise, for persons with acquired idiocy and feeble-mindedness, we can make particular use of actions that are performed under modified conditions, to rate their capacity for judgment.

In many cases, feeble-mindedness reveals itself through an even more accessible, crude feature, namely a reduction in the number of concepts. I do not mean to identify this symptom simply with lack of judgment, for which a certain complexity of the tasks is still required. Essentially, it is a lack of discrimination between related terms. Applying this criterion to more complicated, abstract terms, it can be used to detect even subtle deficits, which might otherwise easily escape notice. Such tasks include the differences between 'civilization', 'education', and 'culture' [Ed]; 'nation', 'people', and 'state' [Ed]; between 'religion', 'faith', and 'belief' [Ed], etc. In addition, what we call 'skill' [Ed] and 'tact' [Ed] but especially, choices of an apt expression, are based on such finer distinctions; and thus a crooked, inaccurate, or quirky expression can represent the most striking symptom of feeble-mindedness [5]. By chance, this has led to a particular type of wit, as in productions of that eternal third-year grammar student 'Karlchen Mießnick' [W], and the equally famous 'Wippchen' [W] war correspondent of the *Berliner Wespen* [W]. However, much coarser distinctions may also become impossible for these impaired people, for example, between 'Prussia' and 'Germany' [Ed], between 'Parliament', the 'House of Representatives', and 'Mansions' [Ed], between mountain and mountain range, between lake and pond, between outside wall and inside wall, between door and gate, between husband, son and brother, between wife, daughter, sister, and girl, between ox and calf, steer and cow, and so on. The loss of concepts can go so far that the sense even of simpler questions, such as the season, the skies, religion, is no longer understood, despite behaviour still remaining attentive.

While lack of discrimination between various concepts reveals a quantitative loss of what we have called contents of consciousness, the pattern of conscious activity in the end gives rise to the most fundamental symptom of acquired idiocy—failure of unsolicited movements deriving from intrapsychic activity, the necessary condition for inactivity. In depressive melancholia we already came to know two phenomena: Patients stop talking, and they stop doing anything, as objective features of intra-psychic akinesia. For any significant degree of acquired idiocy, exactly the same phenomenon is entirely to be expected, although, according to opinion, it is essentially cases where idiocy has been acquired somewhat more acutely, where we see this similarity to the familiar disease state of depressive melancholia. In such cases of more acute coloration it is also quite natural for it to be impossible to make a differential diagnosis between this and depressive melancholia—which is in itself curable, and certainly still a viable clinical picture; or between it and primary dementia. Under certain circumstances, reduced retentiveness can also be a partial manifestation of idiocy or feeble-mindedness; but we have also seen that this symptom is often seen in acute psychoses, in circumstances where there is no question of idiocy. The situation is similar for attentiveness, except that this is affected much more frequently and in the most varied ways, particularly in relation to concomitant stimuli; and indeed, the most severe cases of idiocy will also be characterized by the fact that attention can be activated or captured only with difficulty, if at all.

As regards the *causes* [W] of acquired idiocy or feeble-mindedness, this is by no means exclusively a result of mental illnesses. There are numerous other causes, which I should address very briefly, so that such important facts are not completely unknown to you. Idiocy following head injury is probably organically based. We should probably assume such a link, especially in cases where symptoms of concussion appear after the injury, since we now know that concussion is accompanied by a local change in the arachnoid fluid, with multiple vascular lesions. Trauma produced in this way can be so extensive that it leads to degeneration of neural elements of the cortex over large stretches. In other cases, the intermediate link of *Hydrocephalus internus* [W] may play a role, but because we know so little of this rare disease, it seems much more likely that a proportion of such cases can be traced back to head injury. Given the prominence of degenerative conditions in individuals, the possibility should be taken into account that even milder head trauma, unaccompanied by concussion, nonetheless can initiate degenerative processes in neural elements, which then progress independently. Of organic brain diseases, multiple sclerosis in cases with widespread sclerosis of white matter is an exquisite example of primary, slowly worsening dementia. Such cases are not infrequently diagnosed from the accretion of paraplegic symptoms, ocular palsies, optic atrophy, or even other well-known features of the sclerotic process. Cerebral syphilis sometimes leads to clinical pictures that are almost indistinguishable from those of multiple sclerosis, but perhaps with rather more acute coloration, and with its admixture of stuporous symptoms. In an adult, following meningitis I have seen a high level of residual idiocy, along with profound suppression of vegetative functions. The resulting marasmic state led to death 2 years later. During puberty, a relatively rapidly developing dementia is sometimes seen, which can reach severe levels, without its being accompanied by other significant psychotic symptoms. At other times, such a primary degenerative dementia of puberty develops, accompanied by harmless delusions of relatedness, especially autopsychic delusions of reference, and after previous bouts of severe headache. Outside puberty, I have seen on a few occasions, cases of continuous, subacutely developing primary dementia that recovered; but I would now consider it more appropriate to consider these as examples of depressive melancholia, which two would in any case be difficult to differentiate clinically. We will soon discuss in greater detail, senile dementia, epileptic dementia, post-apoplectic dementia, and alcoholic dementia. Paralytic dementia, separate from idiocy after mental illnesses, will be given special consideration as well. Moreover, it should be stressed that there are particular clinical forms of psychosis, which, if not progressing to recovery, tend to result in idiocy. In this respect, motility psychoses of any kind, especially akinetic motility psychosis, are not very different from paralytic psychoses.

Gentlemen! If we now focus on feeble-mindedness or idiocy, highlighting those characteristics that differ depending on the different aetiologies, we find only a few relatively reliable points of reference. *Paralytic dementia* stands out because of its practical importance, since diagnosis of this common disease, upon which depend far-reaching implications, depends on detecting dementia. It cannot be denied that most cases of acute paralysis are associated with early dementia—either exclusively, or in company with other acute patterns of disease; and this is prominent from the start, and then gradually increases. Paralytic dementia can now be distinguished particularly by the fact that in most cases, right from the outset a change of personality itself is also included. We find this *character alteration* [W] interpreted by Meynert [2] with his usual mastery. The complex, interlocking mental coordination which represents personality, falls apart in chronological order, the reverse of their formation, according to Meynert's presentation, so that an ever-simpler, less composite, primary, childlike personality remains, which in turn becomes individualized sensory activation of dominant impulses for behaviour. This character change is based on aggravation of association through loss of brain elements. Healthy intelligence includes in its thought processes both synergistic and antagonistic impulses, like the coordination of movement through synergistic and antagonistic muscles; but it also has an effect on the most complicated area for coordination, since it constructs personality; and in moments of brain activity across the whole life-span, while it is defining each of those moments, it also assimilates all those previous experiences. In paralytics, from early stages, impulses for action can no longer perform in accord with that unknowable coordination; and we understand that the character change represents a smooth transition from the forewarning stage. The change in personality so described, for paralytic patients, therefore has an origin very different from that described earlier, for manic patients. It is based on *deficiency* [Ed] in mental activity and consequently on increased predictability based on immediate stimuli, whereas in the latter case, there is an *excess* [Ed] of mental activity, but a levelling of ideas. The changed personality of paralytic patients is revealed by their words and actions; and dementia is revealed by both. An example will best illustrate this: A prison inspector who has so far conducted himself impeccably, institutes a capricious rule, in place of the earlier orderliness; makes indecent proposals to his female convicts; fraternizes with his subordinates; allows himself to be bribed by suppliers; spends his time on duty largely in taverns, etc. At his usual dining table he brags about the advantages of his position, the many women available to him, the incidental revenue that he achieves through his corruption. If he has to face questions, he probably says that only stupid people would do otherwise. Taken to task by his superiors, he has a euphemism for everything; denies everything; or construes his behaviour as having given the wrong impression; judges as false or spiteful persons who are hostile towards him, so that those not completely aware of detailed conditions can find almost nothing abnormal in his speech. The owner of a renowned millinery shop made romantic overtures in a most unabashed manner, which was also most offensive manner to well-liked customers, while he served them. Another made so bold, on an open street, to begin an abbreviated overture to love by exposing his penis. Nonsensical purchases and acquisitions of patients fit in here. Thus an official, of very moderate means, bought an upright piano, a harmonium, and a barrel organ, all in 1 day. Quite correctly, Meynert remarked that a patient with advanced paralysis still has the motivation for all such senseless actions. One undresses himself to nakedness, and makes the excuse that children were also walking around naked. The fact that he is not a child does not perturb him. Another declares himself to be God, yet humbly kisses the doctor's hand because the trappings of superhuman existence never enter his mind. However, even in early cases of paralysis, exactly the same nonsensical actions occur; to him the motives of the moment are sufficient. Although senseless, demented actions are characteristic of paralytic patients; the change in personality that we take from them is only one of the conclusions we can draw: This is actually a failure phenomenon, a failure of associations, the exclusion of links to time and place. I emphasize this, because, in your expert activities, you will often have to deal with criminality of paralytic patients. A judge will not easily recognize that a changed personality is abnormal; but if there is evidence of idiocy, namely dementia revealed by actions—he will readily concede the point.

Nonsensical actions can also occur at times when no impairment has appeared in a patient's prudent outward behaviour and formal attitude. At other times, manic behaviour appears, as a part of paralytic mania, along with myriad drives to action, and also the levelling of ideas. However, actions resulting from this alone, such as wandering around, travel, making plans, and undertakings of the most diverse kinds, have a different mode of origin and therefore intrinsically have less direct bearing on the simplification, characteristic of dementia.

A second equally important characteristic of paralytic dementia, in many cases, is inaction and silence, which, *a priori* [W] is quite striking. It is initially noticed that patients at home tend to become silent and stop doing things, yet at first continue professional duties in the usual way. For example, an official remains at home 1 day; probably he also answers reproaches of his family by explaining that he is dispensable, yet makes no apology for his absence. If you talk to him about this, all you get is euphemisms, perhaps a promise to get back to the office; but actually he remains at home, passive and indifferent. In such cases, the incentive for conversation often encourages the patient's thought processes and answers to become appropriate and correct; nor need there be any sign of speech impediment. It is therefore often difficult for investigators to understand failures of action, which are very characteristic, and to judge them accurately. However, in such cases, on closer examination, one will almost always find other indications of the diagnosis of paralytic dementia. Experience shows that patients eat unusually large meals, in a greedy manner; tests of memory retention show this to be reduced; side-by-side terms, such as Prussia and Germany cannot be distinguished. These matters are equally important when prominent spinal symptoms are found.

Paralytic dementia finds a further early objective indicator in the smooth and inert, and at times decidedly idiotic facial expression that is sometimes seen. This facial expression is all the more remarkable in that it can be associated with a certain emotional lability, slight irritability, or sudden flaring to boisterous merriment on minor occasions.

It is particularly important to distinguish paralytic dementia from *post-apoplectic dementia* [W]. It is known that most cases of apoplexy have outcomes where there is no significant deficit in intelligence. For some cases however, this rule does not apply, and we see obvious idiocy. We can explain this behaviour as major atrophy in the affected hemisphere, by an ancillary finding made by Hitzig, that after specific ablation in the brain there is often atrophy of an entire hemisphere. In my experience post-apoplectic dementia has only one specific sign, that it offers most severe emotional lability, aptly termed in English 'emotional incontinence' [Ed].

Epileptic idiocy [W] usually has likewise certain characteristic features. These consist immediately of irritability and intolerance unique to most epileptics, in their tendency to display brute force and occasional fits of rage. In addition there may be an obviously ostentatious, quite superficial piety among epileptic patients with idiocy that one might take to be no more than a purely chance encounter. Finally, there is often—but not always—a surprisingly intact retentiveness in memory, apart from just after an attack. The loss of concepts is often striking, revealed as a twisted, clumsy manner of expression. Not uncommonly this clumsiness in selecting words reaches the level of isolated paraphasic infelicities. You will find a good example of these peculiar manners of expression in my *Krankenvorstellungen* [6] [W].

Alcoholic dementia [W] is indicated particularly by blunted intiative and brutality, which is often very pronounced when any deficit in mental *endowment* [W] is limited in extent. Later, however, it always includes a significant deficit in the most common knowledge. Obviously, signs of chronic alcoholism are always present.

Hebephrenic dementia is the most general indicator of an immature stage of development, corresponding to the age of puberty. Hence we see childishness and foolishness in behaviour of such patients, highlighted particularly by Kahlbaum and Hecker. In the near future, I would like to use the idea of 'mental laziness' [Ed] as to some extent specific for hebephrenic dementia. It is often expressed in quite characteristic ways. Patients answer questions randomly just as it suits them, no matter whether or not they then contradict themselves. Questions that were previously answered with 'yes' [Ed] are soon to be answered with 'no' [Ed]; or the answer consists of a most non-specific style of talking. Gradually during the course of examining a patient an unmistakable unwillingness or discontent becomes clear, linked to overburdening of mental effort. From leading questions, one probably also learns that thinking itself is a strain on a patient: An unwilling 'turning away' [Ed], or the expression 'Leave me alone!' [Ed] Under some circumstances, an actual outbreak of anger, signals the end of the interview. It is hard to arouse the attention of such patients, and particularly difficult for purposes of making an examination. Memory retention is often surprisingly good, if judged by memory for particular events. Moreover, one may be surprised by such patients, in that they occasionally reveal fragments of knowledge, for example speeches or other learned and memorized material, which one seeks in vain during a systematic examination. Their facial expression remains one of hebephrenic idiocy, even at times more-or-less distorted—yet mostly very lively—as one might anticipate, from the level of idiocy. You will find a very obvious case of hebephrenic idiocy after chronic psychosis under my *Krankenvorstellungen* [7] [W]. The indicator of a twisted, oblique, and inappropriate manner of expression is very pronounced in many cases, which is easily understood, given the chronological age of patients; but in my experience, in hebephrenia, it is not at an age-characteristic level, nor is the appearance of inertia of thinking described above.

Age-related dementia [W] leads mainly to general mental dullness, an egotistical narrowing of interests, which can go as far as the most unwholesome greed and obvious unkindness to family, sometimes rising even to moral aberrations. The main indicator is, however, the almost total loss of retentiveness and corresponding loss of memory for the immediate past. In contrast with this, the memory of the distant past can be well retained. Every now and then, a tendency to confabulate, and delirious behaviour at night can intervene. For age dementia, physical complications are quite common: senile tremor, weakness of sphincters, an unhelpful, wide-legged, tripping gait, and a bowed body posture. None of these complications has a close relationship with senile atrophy of the brain, any more than do pseudo-apoplectic attacks, yet to be mentioned. These are probably based on hydrocephalic effusions, and may be simple faints, sometimes longer-lasting somnolent or comatose conditions, and they differ from apoplectic attacks by the absence of unilateral symptom profiles. Moreover, patients usually survive such attacks, even though one of them will finally lead to death; and, while recovering from them, weakness and disability of the legs, usually coupled with bladder weakness, is the most surprising symptom. Moreover, such attacks can also be seen without any degree of age-related dementia having existed previously or subsequently.

Senile brain atrophy or senile involution of the brain is mapped as an anatomical substrate for age-related dementia. That a preceding apoplectic attack can give a premature impetus to the same changes in the brain, and to corresponding clinical findings has already been mentioned above.

References

1. Emminghaus H. Die psychischen Störungen des Kindesalters. In: Gerhardt CJAC, editor. Gerhardt's Handbuch der Kinderkrankheiten. Tübingen: Laupp. 1887;8.
2. Meynert Th. Klinische Vorlesungen über Psychiatrie auf wissenschaftlichen Grundlagen für Studirende und Aerzte, Juristen und Psychologen. Vienna: Braumüller; 1890. p. 274–297; 221–222.
3. Hitzig E. Über den Querulantenwahnsinn, seine nosologische Stellung und seine forensische Bedeutung. Leipzig: FCW Vogel; 1895.
4. Wernicke C. Krankenvorstellungen aus der psychiatrischen Klinik in Breslau. Breslau: Schletter. vol.3, Case 25.
5. Wernicke C. Ein Fall von Schwachsinn leichteren Grades. Mschr Psychiatr Neurol. 1897;1:398–409.
6. Wernicke C. Krankenvorstellungen vol.2, Case 24.
7. Wernicke C. Krankenvorstellungen vol.2, Case 28.

Lecture 41

41

- Dissimulation and simulation of mental disturbance
- Functions of institutional treatment
- Final remarks on the prospect of a pathological–anatomical rationale of the psychoses

Lecture

Gentlemen!

These lectures can hardly be intended to introduce you to the practical medical specialist training course for the asylums. Whoever wants to dedicate himself totally to our specialty is of course expecting to spend a considerable part of his life in mental institutions, and among mentally ill people, a task that in some respects you can imagine is not sufficiently challenging, but also not sufficiently gratifying and interesting. However, each of you will, at some time, be in a position of deciding on the placement of a patient in a mental hospital, or having to issue a certificate that health has been regained, and it is therefore imperative to give you some orientation on practical issues, including the specific tasks of the asylum, and the simulation and dissimulation of mental illnesses.

Let us not underestimate the fact that a major source of evidence in psychiatry is language, in other words, the messages that patients themselves provide about the content of their consciousness. Clearly, it is only in this way that you can learn anything more complex about the thought processes of a patient. A prerequisite for this is either the goodwill a patient shows towards communication, or in illnesses such as mania, when there is an intrinsic desire to communicate. If such prerequisites do not apply, it can happen that patients remain intentionally silent for weeks, months, even years, or speak only on exceptional occasions. Amongst the best proven ways of bringing such patients to speak, is a clinical presentation, although of course you should be prepared for all manner of surprises and, under some circumstances, even quite dramatic turns to the conversation. This *deliberate silence* [W] naturally has nothing in common with mytacism, the incapacity to speak. Usually, it involves negative, suspicious, and embittered patients, overcome by ideas of persecution and grandiosity—those paranoid states which have already been mentioned. On the other hand, it may happen that the silence is deliberately restricted to those points that a physician needs to know, in order to assess the mental illness; that is, the patient dissimulates his delusions. Most frequently such *dissimulation* [W] occurs in patients who have long survived in a calm state, after having previously come through an acute period of illness. Having now regained the discretion that is necessary to monitor their statements, they are inspired by a lively ambition to rid themselves of restrictions to their freedom, that is, life within a mental institution. They therefore strive, with

R. Miller, K.J. Dennison (eds.), *An Outline of Psychiatry in Clinical Lectures*,
DOI 10.1007/978-3-319-18051-9_41

greater or lesser success, to deny their delusions, once they have found out what ideas a physician might regard as abnormal; this having been learned in any favourable circumstance, such as their presence during examination of similar cases. However, in such patients, it is always possible, by asking appropriate questions, to determine the truth. For this purpose, the method consists of provoking the patient's judgment about his symptoms, as previously observed, and thereby determining that actual insight into his illness—the main criterion of health—is still missing. If the patient's silence persists in a stubborn manner, on points that matter, then you cannot consider him healthy. Sometimes, it turns out that the patient cannot give the information you need, because, as part of his illness, a memory deficit exists; and then, naturally it is not required that the patient admits them. Generally, patients seldom deny their delusions; and even where it seems appropriate to them to do so, they do it only reluctantly, and are easily driven to adjust the boundary where expediency might prevail rather their delusion. Compared with such frequent cases, it may happen, albeit rarely, that a patient with early-stages of a chronic worsening psychosis dissimulates his delusions, at a time when he is himself still unclear how far the intrusive ideas and alleged observations correspond to reality. He declares this or that strange expression he had used, to be a joke or a misunderstanding, or he attempts to give it a more harmless character. In the end, he probably becomes indignant, and denies the questioner the right to meddle in his affairs. In such cases, reliable information from the family or other persons close to the patient is essential in order to justify crucial decisions that the patient be detained against his will, for observation in an institution. Such information could be about comments and actions that have raised suspicions of mental illness. A case like this is before me at present, where my encouragement led to the patient being admitted voluntarily into the institution, where however, his trust was lost on the very next day, when I had to refuse his discharge; from then on, he refused to give any further information. After that, he existed only for his discharge, and finally sought to force this through, by refusing food. Under the circumstances, I was extremely embarrassed to use force, but it was unavoidable, and it was therefore, against vigorous resistance, that artificial feeding was enforced several times, at which point, he decided to give up his resistance. After several weeks had elapsed the family then decided, much against my advice, to remove the patient from hospital treatment. Apparently they were right, for there was no further recurrence of the delusions he had expressed previously, and he resumed his earlier work in a business. Even though it appears that, with a history like that, the doctor got it wrong, yet this very case is the most irrefutable evidence that in all similar cases no greater benefit can be rendered to the patient than his being forcibly transferred to the mental institution. To be specific, when, in such cases, recovery is possible—relatively so, as it appears in this case—it is brought about firstly by the fact that the morbid ideas were overcome by his own forceful protests; and there is no more powerful protest against delusions that are not completely fixed, than to realize that they inevitably lead to his being detained, against his will in an asylum for the insane. Thus the patient had to thank his undeniable improvement, perhaps even his healing, had this been achieved meanwhile, mainly to the fact of his transfer to the mental institution. (I must now correct these lines, written about 10 years ago. The patient's mytacism resumed after a year, and later he became incurable.)

After such experiences, we must pose the question: To what extent should everything that is said by a patient claim the value of an objective symptom? Rather, are not utterances of patients completely dependent on their volition? Under some circumstances, could not a healthy person imitate the speech of a mentally ill person; or, apart from this case, could not a patient intentionally say things other than what he is actually thinking? Our standpoint here is briefly as follows: Language may indeed be influenced very much by volition; yet it still remains a function of consciousness, that is, of that brain activity which we have to examine. This function may not always be so simple, so that the willingness of a patient cannot easily be assumed to comply appropriately with questions addressed to him. Nevertheless, with proper conduct of the physician, and as soon as the patient's trust is won, only seldom do we find that a mental patient's words are at odds with what is in his heart, and intended to mislead the doctor. Where a patient is prone to violent Affective responses, then the self-control that would be necessary for this approach is already ruled out. Usually, the rest of the patient's behaviour enables a reliable judgment to be made about whether or not he comes to meet the doctor willingly. In some cases however, the particular decision on whether, and to what extent, a mental patient is simulating, can be made only with great difficulty. Two aspects should then not be ignored in the assessment. Firstly, there are mentally ill people who confront their nonsensical intrusive thoughts *en masse* [Ed] with their own quasi-criticism, so that, for example, they even laugh about the nonsense that they produce in given moments. These patients usually belong with those otherwise characterized as motility psychoses. The content of the delusions is often religious, characterized simultaneously by both fantastic coloration and repetitiveness. The repetitiveness often rises to the point of verbigeration. The rest of these patients' behaviour dispels any doubts over whether they had been serious about their delusions, even after achieving success in getting them to confess that they had just been talking nonsense. Of course they then tend to reinforce what they said: It just came to them; they could not explain it themselves. This phenomenon has a certain similarity with the compulsive speaking we encountered in the same class of patients. The second case is more difficult, where usually even external circumstances raise the suspicion of simulation. This usually involves prisoners, in whom there are suspicions about whether it was true mental illness, or simulation; and they have therefore been sent to the mental institution for observation. Experience teaches that most of these individuals *are* [Ed] actually mentally ill, even when they are apparently simulating. Pure simulation without existing mental illness or feeble-mindedness is rare in itself, so that even the most experienced alienist sees only isolated cases. If you consider that a mental patient usually experiences the inconvenience of imprisonment with all the embarrassment of someone who is mentally healthy, and therefore takes advantage of feelings of mental illness coming over him, that fact seems like putting a gift into his hands. At least the prospect of being transferred to a mental asylum holds no terrors for him, and therefore has no power to motivate his self-control. If this is so, a few days of indulgent, confidence-inspiring treatment in a mental hospital usually suffices to allow the clinical picture to emerge in purer form, and for arbitrary excesses to disappear. Of course, there often remains a disconcerting clinical picture, such as one that does to fit any form of illness, or crude violence, or all manner of shameless acts, coprophagia, etc. However, such modifications become understandable to us, in that, in such cases we are dealing with morally depraved and neglected people, coming mainly from families where they were forced to become criminals. In other cases, it turns out that, although mental illness is simulated, it is nevertheless based on either congenital or acquired feeble-mindedness, often complicated by epileptic seizures. Nothing is as hopeless as wanting to turn around malingerers of such kind by coercive measures such as starvation, etc. Leaving aside these two possibilities, the number of remaining true malingerers, as said above, is very small.

Gentlemen! During the course of these lectures I have emphasized countless times that in terms of the *treatment of mentally ill people* [W], your main task consists of timely transfer of the patient to a mental institution, forcibly if necessary. Now, there are experienced alienists who adopt the view that, by properly setting up a private residence, the same can be achieved as in institutional treatment. We must realize immediately, when discussing the purposes of institutional treatment, that this is not entirely true.

Institutional treatment [W] has the following tasks to resolve:

1. *Monitoring of the patient* [W]. This includes restriction of personal freedom, not to be separated from institutional treatment. Only a mental institution, with its internal services specially organized for this purpose, its seclusion and various measures to make escape of the patient more difficult, can, at the same time, grant the patient individually beneficial

measures of personal freedom. Where walls and fences are missing, as in the so-called 'free institutions' [Ed], watchful staff ensure that patients will not go beyond the terrain of the institution. Of course, escapes from the institution can never be completely avoided; at least those in penal servitude and similar places, with refined cunning, and bent only on escape, will always find ways and means to gain their freedom; but here the main obstacle standing in their way is not sentries with loaded weapons, as tends to be the case elsewhere: With regard to precautions taken to prevent escape, a mental hospital should in no way be reminiscent of a prison or penitentiary. Prevention of escape is certainly not the main purpose, or one of the main purposes of the institution; generally one might even claim that escape of a mental patient is a harmless event. Nevertheless, a well-established institution will make escape so difficult, that at least among those patients where it matters, one can be completely reassured. Foremost amongst such cases are those at risk of suicide, but next, the not-so-rare cases of delusional patients whose sharp focus is hostility against specific people. A good institution also provides the best guarantee against any form of self-harm.

2. Constant *medical observation* [W]. In no other type of patient is it so important that any change in state should be detected immediately by the doctor, and necessary measures put in place. Where a patient has otherwise lost all orientation, he often shares his confidence with a physician, because the latter may bring the greatest understanding to information so imparted. In these cases, responses of an expert physician cannot be replaced by any other, at least by well-meaning relatives who have often been affected in the first place by changed feelings and beliefs of the patient. In good institutions, doctors are together with the patients for a greater part of the day; in any institution a physician is immediately accessible when a need arises, a situation that occurs quite often, be it due to the seriousness of the clinical picture, or to incidents caused by unpredictable actions of mentally ill patients. Even diet makes many mental patients in need of constant medical attention.
3. *Maintenance of social instinct* [W]. Due to changes in content of their consciousness and the varying degrees of disorientation and scope thereby imprinted, many patients are almost totally deprived of means of communication with the outside world, and especially with people from their own environment. They are then either continuously resistant, or totally passive and, in any case, in a helpless position, in need of intervention by other people. Here the deep-rooted herd instinct that patients often still retain, comes to the aid of medical services, where other means of communication have been applied in vain. The example given by other patients in the same room, who likewise get up, wash, and dress themselves, eat unaided or let themselves be fed etc., also has its effect, by regular monotonous repetition, in such cases. Participation in walks, in collaborative games, devotions, singing practice, etc., produces an educative effect in a similar way.
4. The possibility of total *isolation* [W]. In some situations, it is desirable to keep patients totally isolated for hours, days, or weeks without the room or their clothing providing any means for self-harm. This requires specially equipped rooms without any—or with only fixed—furniture, with solid smooth walls, the same for the floor, and with solid, ideally opaque windows. Similarly the bed and the patient's clothing can be made from firm material. We call rooms made up in this fashion 'calming rooms' [Ed]; the institution provides them, and, even if they are seldom used, and assigned only for specific indications, they belong among the most useful and salutary installations of the institution. Citing the special indications for this would go beyond the scope of this lecture. Moreover in good institutions—and this is particularly stressed—isolation of patients is always instituted only by special order of the physician, and undertaken under his supervision.

5. Appropriate application of means of *coercion* [W] as may become necessary. Use of force is required if the patient threatens to harm himself, has already done so, or does not want to leave wound dressings on, and so on. The most protective process under these circumstances is a straitjacket with long sleeves that are closed in front, and taper down into a type of belt. In an emergency, securing the patient's arms to the sides of the bed, or application of the so-called force belt across the patient's torso may be required in addition, so that the patient is prevented from changing his position too much in the bed. Only a mental institution offers the appropriate paraphernalia for this purpose—or it should at least always have them available. Furthermore, only a mental institution enables continuous supervision of such coercive measures by medical staff.

Gentlemen! We have reached the end of our reflections. And it could be that the large series of new facts with which you have become familiar, and the so-very diverse cases of illness that I have presented to you, have misled you into believing that you have thoroughly learned about existing mental illnesses. I must regretfully disagree, and make clear to you that we have not gone beyond the first basic concepts of psychiatry in these meetings. You will have plenty of opportunity to convince yourself of this, when you face the bewildering variety of cases in practice. I can only take credit for having sorted out certain of the simplest cases from the rich material of my clinic, and thus having gradually prepared you to approach more complex cases with some understanding. I need not emphasize that this difficulty applies mainly to acute cases. By my naturally very-subjective estimate, those acute cases that I have discussed here may make up only about half of all cases. You can get a clearer idea of the richness of clinical material that is to be mastered, from the three volumes of clinical cases, totalling over a hundred, which I have published, from my clinic [1]. Overwhelmingly, these were selected for teaching purposes, so that simpler cases predominated. You might get the clearest idea of the richness of our clinical material if I tell you that I still encounter cases—indeed not so rarely—that are so markedly different in symptomatology and course from anything seen before, that I have to classify them as 'new' [Ed] and 'never seen before' [Ed]. Every older alienist says the same, as I have discovered through many enquiries. Hence, there is great difficulty in getting an overview of the great body of clinical material, and keeping it in mind. The difficulty of filtering out only the basic facts that can be taken from the material is even greater; and finally, we have the most serious task of selecting the most common, or the most important, types of illness for any attempt at an objective and true-to-life representation.

Certain errors are associated with my task, which are inextricably linked, to which I should not avoid drawing attention. My presentation is based on approximately 5,000 carefully kept medical records that have been prepared over the course of 15 years, under my direction and supervision. Unceasing study of these case histories, their monitoring by continuous observation, the comparison of similar cases with one another, in addition to special study of individual symptoms in these patients, required such an expenditure of time that it was impossible for me also to evaluate studies of other authors in the literature to the extent that would have been necessary for my purposes. The individual cases gave me the advantage that they were very fully examined for my purposes, especially since, through my photographs, which form an integral part of our medical records, I usually managed to call to mind the entire personality. You will therefore find many things not mentioned, thought to be important by discerning professional colleagues, as well as everything that was superfluous to my immediate purpose. In the naive viewpoint of Griesinger [2], who relied almost exclusively on material from other institutions in his textbook—material not even observed by him—in which you will probably find the more culpable errors of an opposite type. I cannot therefore lay claim to completeness. Thus I deliberately did not touch on issues of practical importance in judicial psychiatry, an omission not based on a lack of personal experience. If you require further guidance in this area, I refer you to excellent guidelines on judicial psychiatry by A. Cramer [3]. Moreover, for the difficult area of idiocy and imbecility you will find extensive instruction in Emminghaus' book [4], already-mentioned; and for the area of sexual pathology, not a tasteful read for everyone, the book by von Krafft-Ebing [5].

Despite these shortcomings, I believe that I have generally pointed you in the right direction, and opened up for you some understanding of psychoses. I also believe that I have gained a firmer foundation, upon which further work can be built. There can be no doubt about the goals that hover over us. In addition to broader expansion in teaching of clinical pathology, our immediate task is to substantiate the pathological anatomy of the psychoses. Just 20 years ago, you had to prepare yourself to be ridiculed by clinical representatives of our profession, if you claimed this goal to be in any way achievable in the future. This exclusively critical—and sceptically barren—viewpoint can expand with no danger to itself. In a few concluding remarks, I want to try to show how very much closer we are now to achieving that objective.

I proposed that, for the vast majority of acute and chronic psychoses, anatomical findings are still pending. Alleged findings, listed in most textbooks, such as opacity and thickening of the pia mater; increase or decrease in blood supply to the brain; oedematous infiltration of the brain; increase in ventricular fluid, and so on, cannot be used in any way, since they belong among the most common findings in the widest variety of physical diseases; and are caused very often by the type of agonal process, position of the corpse, and other random influences, and by complicating physical illnesses. It would only obscure the facts, if you wanted to give any value to such findings, for mental illnesses from which patients survive. For most psychoses, their basis in pathological anatomy stands just as it did for cases of degenerative polyneuritis about 30 years ago. The breakthrough in recognizing these cases came by detection of microscopic alterations in most cross-sections of peripheral nerve, and results in a striking and systematic preference for motor nerves. You should be familiar with the fact that we are now inclined to view degeneration of these most distal ends of the motor nerves always as the result of disease of those nerve cells, related to motor nerves by means of the axonal processes and fibres of the ventral roots. We have long been accustomed to consider ganglion cells of the anterior horn as nutritive centres of the ventral root fibres. Disease of the ganglion cell itself can thus remain inaccessible, and concealed from our current methods of investigation. It must now be apparent to every unprejudiced person that the one group of psychoses for which a constant anatomical finding is available, namely progressive paralysis, initially produces a similar finding—that is fibre degeneration which apparently does not affect ganglion cells. I refer to my earlier presentation in this regard. As Lissauer [6] has shown, this loss of fibres is now been proved to be a systematic loss, corresponding to secondary degeneration; and Lissauer also succeeded in demonstrating the source of this secondary degeneration in the destruction of entire cell layers, in certain cases. Where he succeeded with the laborious method of tracking the granular cells, we now see brilliantly confirmed in Starlinger's [7] work, using the improved Marchi method. A glance at the table accompanying this work is sufficient to bring out the systematic nature of all these degenerations. Likewise, thanks to the improved method of Nissl [8], pathology in ganglion cells is now established with certainty in every case of paralysis. As you know, paralytic psychoses usually present with a certain added component of idiocy, right from the beginning. It is probably no coincidence that in this very group of psychoses, in which there are such coarse deficit symptoms, that a constant anatomical change—fibre degeneration in the cortex—has been demonstrated first. On the other hand, it has been shown that psychoses in other aetiological groups—senile, alcoholic, and epileptic—show the same changes in the cerebral cortex in the form of axonal damage and loss, once they have led to deficit symptoms, just as in paralytic psychoses (p. 292). Widespread fibre loss in the cerebral cortex is therefore not peculiar to the paralytic process, since the cellular pathology, substantiated in the case of paralysis, according to Nissl's authoritative account, represents a form of pathology not specific to paralysis. One should therefore be prepared for the finding that, as a result of alcoholic, senile, and epileptic aetiology, analogous pathology of the ganglion cells will be present in the cerebral cortex. Where it does not reach the level of a deficit symptom, as in all curable acute psychoses with an alcoholic, senile, or epileptic basis, we might expect to see cellular pathology without actual degeneration of fibres, that is, a curable process within the ganglion cell. This is one line of thought for which an anatomical basis can be expected in the not too distant future, applying to a large number of acute psychoses.

Other facts leading to the same conclusion are purely clinical. Already, the one fact that we have come to know is that a particular form of psychosis, accompanied by polyneuritic changes of the peripheral nervous system, can be assessed for some internal relationship between polyneuritic disease and that which plays out in the brain, and produces psychosis. In its symptomatology, this polyneuritic psychosis is identical with the specifically senile psychosis, presbyophrenia. For the latter therefore, we can expect the same change in the brain, especially when we consider that the symptom of severe memory deficit is common to both diseases. That presbyophrenia is not accompanied by polyneuritic palsies, may lead us not far astray here, since polyneuritic psychoses often have to be diagnosed—on the basis of the clinical picture—without polyneuritic changes being found in the peripheral nervous system. A truly remarkable case of this kind later revealed itself to be undoubtedly paralytic. When the clinical picture of polyneuritic psychosis is seen, along with fibre loss in the cerebral cortex—but without the anticipated 'polyneuritic' [Ed] changes, that is, degenerative neuritis—then it must be interpreted as an independent illness of the brain, occurring without disease of the peripheral nervous system. Conversely, there is some possibility that other clinical pictures of disease can arise from the same basis as the polyneuritic pathogenesis. I remember that possibility, when I mentioned a case of agitated confusion after lead poisoning, and in a case of unusually pure akinetic motility psychosis in the last weeks before death from long-lasting pulmonary tuberculosis; and further, in various forms of alcoholic psychosis and the frequent occurrence of tuberculosis, as mental illnesses worsen. If we consider that the paralytic process in the cerebral cortex also carries the imprint of degenerative neuritis, at least in its usual outcome of fibre loss, then we are forced to accept the consequence that, for a large proportion of acute psychoses, we may find the same as in degenerative neuritis of the peripheral nervous system, that they should be attributed to the toxic effects of alcohol, of syphilis, and of tuberculosis, impacting on ganglion cells.

Gentlemen! I have repeatedly pointed out that paralytic psychoses, in their symptomatology, not only differ greatly one from another, but often represent precisely the same diseases as psychoses with other aetiologies. These cases may even lack the accompanying early signs of dementia, as I have stated, especially for paralytic mania. Since we cannot doubt that there are general reasons for paralysis mediated by a tangible pathological process, we must also ascribe to the most diverse paralytic psychoses a characteristic anatomical finding. It would be most strange if the same mental illnesses of different aetiology should not likewise yield anatomical changes in the same localities, although perhaps of a different type, in consequence of a different toxic effect.

Gentlemen! I have repeatedly emphasized that mental illnesses should be regarded as serious and life-threatening, compared to other life-threatening internal diseases. Often they are accompanied by fever, without any complications being found to explain the fact. At other times, for no apparent reason, they lead to a rapid decrease in body weight and death, without any disease process being detected in other vital organs. In such cases, should not the brain itself be the starting point of the observed clinical symptoms, and also the site of the illness, and that these should be detectable, at least microscopically? This expectation has, in fact, been confirmed in a series of acute psychoses leading to death, in which the brain has been examined. I mention in particular, cases by Cramer [9] after insolation; cases likewise by Cramer, of the so-called delirium [10]; and, finally, a very recent work by Alzheimer [11, 12]. In all such cases extensive illness can be demonstrated either by Weigert's method for staining myelin, or using the Nissl method with methylene-blue for staining ganglion cells, be it of fibres, or cortical ganglion cells, so that the generality of this finding in most cases of very severe psychoses is not to be sidestepped. Determining the nature of this cellular pathology is still essentially a task for the future. For the time being, it suffices our clinical needs that we can distinguish relatively benign and reversible forms of disease from destructive forms. Paralytic cellular pathology belongs amongst the latter. Moreover, an important result of Alzheimer's work seems to me to be that in certain diseases of ganglion cells, the glial cells are also affected very early; but in others, this is not the case. The latter seem to represent relatively benign, milder forms of the pathology of ganglion cells. Correspondingly, in paralysis we tend to encounter, almost without exception, glial cell proliferation; yet other non-paralytic psychoses of severe form, such as acute motility psychoses with rapid outcome in dementia, belong amongst the severe forms with disease of the ganglion cells, connected with some stimulatory effect exerted on glial cells.

Do the few cases I have in mind allow us to conclude that *all* [Ed] acute psychoses, as well as the less severe cases, would reveal similar anatomical findings, were they to reach autopsy? Admittedly they might not be tangible, but yet visible microscopically. In my opinion this question cannot be supported. We must concede that 'functional psychosis' is a broad area, even if the currently prevailing tendency to extend this area without limits is resisted. We are forced to adopt this assumption about purely 'functional psychoses' [Ed] because, amongst other reasons, cases of pure mania and Affective melancholia that appear combined in circular psychosis in such a way that they can switch from one phase to the opposite, within a few hours. Coarser anatomical changes are likely to be ruled out completely by such behaviour. Even for cases of pure mania, which completely match the manic phase of circular psychosis, this conclusion is already true, because we generally encounter conditions of increased excitability of the nervous system without major anatomical changes. In contrast, for independent cases of Affective melancholia, which we traced back to general reduction in excitability in the organ of association, the possibility of more severe damage by analogy with the peripheral nervous system is admitted for some exceptional cases, and corresponds fully with the experience that Affective melancholia, in exceptional cases, is incurable, and leads finally to dementia. I have deliberately avoided discussing hitherto the mechanisms of the functional disturbance that bring about opposing states of intrapsychic hyperfunction and loss of function. However, I must mention here, Meynert's [13] quite plausible hypothesis, according to which, in the case of neurosis in a subcortical vascular centre—probably involving the medulla oblongata—which leads to the opposite states of diffuse hyperaemia and anaemia of the organ of association. Permanent anaemia could, under some circumstances, lead to real damage to neural elements, which indeed seems quite understandable to us. Here I remind you of the contrast, in Meynert's ingenious approach, between functional hyperaemia due to 'nutritive attraction' [Ed] of tissue elements, which allows very fine localization, and the diffuse hyperaemia, which shuns any localization. Just as with mania and melancholia, one will have to assign to the 'functional psychoses' those acute and chronic psychoses arising and persisting exclusively in the context of increased, yet not abnormality of, function. What I have called the 'fixed ideas' [Ed], with all their subsequent *sequelae* [W], belong here. Only where phenomena occur in the further course, independent from these sources, such as in cases of acute progressive psychosis, which begin as circumscribed autopsychosis, might one also expect anatomical findings.

This raises a further question: Could an anatomical finding also be provided in cases of completely cured, acute psychosis? This would provide an occasion to evaluate autopsy findings scientifically in those cases of illness that, after recovery, die later as a result of inter-current illness. Of course, only empirical knowledge can reveal this. Meanwhile, *a priori* [W] it is likely that the organ of consciousness itself can sustain a degree of loss of nervous elements without any remaining deficit being detectable. We had intended to demonstrate the site of the most severe pathological process, even after recovery from illness, using Weigert's [14] method for staining glial cells. However, where it is really a case of 'healing with deficit' [Ed], for example in the case of severe motility psychosis, which I mentioned at the start of these lectures, and where partial motor and sensory aphasia remains, then we would almost certainly expect a positive result in such a momentous method of study.

You see, gentlemen, difficult as the tasks are that await us, it would be foolish to deny that, given the present state of our knowledge, they can be undertaken with a definite chance of success. Of course we should always remember that even a significant anatomical finding is meaningless if it cannot be brought into close relationship with definite clinical data. I might expect the same anatomical finding only in cases that are perfectly matched clinically. Hence preliminary work is needed, in which you have participated in these lectures.

There is no shortage of pessimists who declare that my comments, as expressed previously, on the prospect of an anatomical–pathological basis for the psychoses is quite redundant, and, wherever possible, seek to tone down hopes nourished thereby. However, since the views I have expressed, acquired, as they were, on the basis of 25 years experience, might also be declared to be 'uncritical' [Ed], I therefore had a very special reason to dwell on them with some force. You have learned in this way that the anatomical findings brought forward so far, varied as the cases were, always revealed to us the same anatomical change, namely degenerative processes in ganglion cells and myelinated fibres of the cortex. For overall pathology of the psychoses, this circumstance, that we may confidently generalize, is of utmost important. If it is universally the same degenerative processes of neural parenchyma, there remain only two standards for scientific classification of psychoses: These must be taken either from the different localization of the anatomical process, or from the diversity of their aetiology. I intentionally avoided detail about the difficult field of classification in these lectures, and must refer you to a lecture [15] held elsewhere if you want to know more about it. However, in conclusion, I want to draw your attention to one point, and that is that these, my last comments, should serve to remind you of the need for those theoretical considerations which occupied us in the first half of our clinical studies, but, for you, perhaps often quite difficult to understand.

References

1. Wernicke C. Krankenvorstellungen aus der psychiatrischen Klinik in Breslau. Vols. 1–3. Breslau: Schlettersche Buchhandlung; (1899–1900).
2. Griesinger W. Die Pathologie und Therapie der psychischen Krankheiten für Ärzte und Studierende. 3rd ed. F Wreden: Braunschweig; 1871.
3. Cramer JBA. Gerichtliche Psychiatrie. Ein Leitfaden für Mediziner und Juristen. 2nd ed. Jena: Gustav Fischer; 1900.
4. Emminghaus H. Über Kinder und Unmündige, Schwachsinn und Blödsinn in forensischer Hinsicht. In: Maschka J, editor. Handbuch der gerichtlichen Medizin, vol. 4. Tübingen: H. Laupp'schen Buchhandlung; 1882.
5. von Krafft-Ebing R. Psychopathia sexualis. 9th ed. Stuttgart: Ferdinand Enke; 1895.
6. Lissauer H. Klinisches und Anatomisches über die Herdsymptome bei Paralyse. Vortr Ver ostdtsch Irrenärzte am 2.3.1891. Ref. in: Zbl Nervenheilk Psychiat 1891;2:295–7.
7. Starlinger J. Zur Marchi-Behandlung; ein Apparat zur Zerlegung in dünne, vollkommen plnparallele Scheiben. Zeitschrift für wissenschaftliche Mikroskopie und für mikroskopische Technik. 1899;16:179–83.
8. Nissl F. Mitteilungen zur pathologischen Anatomie der Dementia paralytica. Arch Psychiatr. 1896;28:987–92.
9. Cramer JBA. Faserschwund nach Insolation. Zentralbl f allg Pathol. 1890;1:185.
10. Cramer JBA. Pathologisch-anatomischer Befund in einem akuten Falle der Paranoiagruppe. Arch f Psychiatr. 1890;29(1):1–24.
11. Alzheimer A. Das Delirium acutum. Monatsschr f Neurol u Psych. 1897;2:64.

12. Alzheimer A. Beiträge zur pathologischen Anatomie der Hirnrinde und zur anatomischen Grundlage einiger Psychosen. Monatsschr f Neurol u Psych. 1897;2:90.
13. Meynert T. Psychiatrie: Klinik der Erkrankung des Vorderhirns begründet auf dessen Bau, Leistungen und Ernährung. Vienna: Braumüller; 1884. p. 230.
14. Weigert C. Beiträge zur Kenntnis der menschlichen Neuroglia. Frankfurt: Moritz Sierterweg. Aus d Abhandl d Senkenberg naturforsch Ges. 1895; 63–209.
15. Wernicke C. Über die Klassifikation der Psychosen. Nach einem in der medizinischen Section der vaterländischen Gesellschaft zu Breslau gehaltenen Vortrag. Breslau: Schletter. 1899.

Editorial Commentary

I. Lecture-by-Lecture Synopses

Synopsis of L1: This, the very first lecture, is one of eight comprising the first main section of *Grundriss*, outlining Wernicke's overall understanding of normal human brain processes in relation to subjective awareness. However, he starts with his basic *credo,* that mental illnesses are brain diseases. He expresses the view that psychiatry, compared to other specialties, is backward in its development (although he suggests later that he has something better to offer). The rest 'sets the scene' in relation to clinical concepts, clinical practice, and neuroscience of the day.

Synopsis of L2: In this lecture, the point of departure and the topic he understood best is the cerebral representation of language—but this is merely a device to move into other territory. He moves quickly at the start of the lecture to clarify the notion of the 'supposed' Conceptualization Centre mentioned in L1. Although he was a pioneer for the notion of cerebral localization of function, by the time *Grundriss* was written he had moved beyond simple localization. Soon other issues arise, raising several philosophical questions. Much of the emphasis is that all symptoms in psychiatry can be reduced ultimately to a patient's movements, which are all a physician sees directly. This strongly materialist tone was common in Germany, after Griesinger, a leading 'Somatiker' of an earlier generation. Towards the end of the lecture, he provides his classification of symptoms in a three-by-three table: The columns are: 'Psychosensory', 'Psychomotor', and 'Intrapsychic'; the rows are: 'loss of', 'excessive', or 'aberrant' excitability (e.g. 'anaesthesia', 'hyperaesthesia', and 'paraesthesia' in the Psychosensory column). This classification gains prominence in the clinical lectures.

Synopsis of L3: The main topic of this lecture is Memory Images (*Erinnerungsbilder*) sometimes rendered here as 'remembered images'. Much of the lecture is devoted to separating perceptual/sensory images from 'memory images'. In modern terms this is the distinction between sensation and perception. The former implies 'awareness' arising directly from sensory input, the latter has added implications of a degree of interpretation or analysis of that input, to be given lasting representation in memory.

Synopsis of L4: The main topic of this lecture is the way in which remembered images, acquired separately, come together to create a coordinated picture of the external world. In describing how remembered images of objects are assimilated to become representations of concepts, Wernicke sees an exact analogy with formation of memory images from sensations, represented in the primary visual areas by linking various active 'perceptual elements' (primary visual cortical cells).

R. Miller, K.J. Dennison (eds.), *An Outline of Psychiatry in Clinical Lectures*,
DOI 10.1007/978-3-319-18051-9

Synopsis of L5: This lecture focuses on how the brain represents our body (using interchangeably 'physicality' and 'corporeality'). A conceptual distinction is made between sensory *content* and *tone* of sensation, a near-synonym for the latter being 'organ sensation', a term whose meaning is discussed in section XVI: 'Terminology'). 'Corporeality' includes what we now call visceral sensation, notably that from the large intestine.

Synopsis of L6: The main topic of this lecture is representation of movement. Amongst evidence referred to is that obtained by electrical stimulation of muscles: This procedure, well known at the time, was pioneered earlier in the century by Duchenne de Boulogne, who used it to study actions of individual muscles and muscle groups. Later, Wernicke discusses how full perceptual awareness depends on combining passive sensory awareness with exploratory movements. The latter notion builds on ideas first mentioned in L3, on elaboration of tactile perception by combining immediate sensation with exploration (especially manual exploration), an idea now well understood by somatosensory physiologists. Wernicke draws exact parallels here between tactile and visual perception/exploration.

Synopsis of L7: The subject matter of this lecture is how our brains construct for each of us an image of ourselves as a (somewhat) unified person. In English, the word 'personality' refers to the unique quality or 'essence' of each person. Another word—'personhood'—is used in legal discourse, signifying 'status as a legal person'. In this lecture, and later, 'personality' will be used as just defined, while 'personhood' is used in a more generic, abstract sense, referring to our sense of 'being (to a degree) a unified person', whatever the detail of each individual's personal quality. Sometimes the phrase 'personalized consciousness' seems to capture Wernicke's meaning better than a literal translation. The word 'individual' refers to a single human, without implying that he/she approximates to any sort of unified entity. A central notion, to be developed in later clinical lectures, is that memories from which each individual constructs his sense of personhood consist of three components. These are the sense of one's own body (corporeality), one's sense of the outer environment, and personal memories or beliefs acquired in one's own life experiences. An additional topic introduced here is not so much the 'contents' of consciousness (upon which earlier lectures focused) but the 'processes' by which such contents are laid down, and are subsequently manipulated and retrieved. Wernicke knew the importance of this topic, although current understanding in the nascent discipline of neuropsychology was quite limited.

Synopsis of L8: Much of this lecture is psychological theory, about psychological *processes,* rather than content, such as might have been found in writings of his American contemporary, William James. This includes the phenomena of attentiveness, and of 'narrowness of consciousness' (i.e. selectiveness of attention), the process by which memory is acquired, and the role played by Affective states. Much of the lecture consists of shrewd reflections based on introspection, which was easier before psychology became 'objective' when behaviourism came centre-stage. The lecture also brings to the fore the scientific tradition in which Wernicke is best placed—not so much that of most biomedicine of his day, but that of natural philosophy (which became physics). This conclusion can be reached not only from his use of analogies from physics for processes envisaged to occur in the brain. More important are methodological features such as his balance between experiment and theory, typical of natural philosophy (but seldom found in biomedicine); his freedom in postulating hidden variables which could not be directly demonstrated (as were many concepts in the history of physics); and notably his close reasoning from fundamental principles, based on sensory and motor processes. This allowed them to be traced back to the core language of the natural sciences.

Synopsis of L9: Lectures 9–17 make up the second main section of *Grundriss,* dealing with chronic states of 'paranoia', and dealing mainly with long-stay patients in his institution. One such patient is described in vivid detail. In this first lecture dealing with clinical matters, Wernicke outlines basic concepts. First he distinguishes '*real* mental illness' from 'mental disturbance': In lectures so far, when 'illness' has been mentioned, the German word was *Geisteskrankheit.* Here he uses *Geistesstörungen*. Wernicke also enunciates a principle, that one should start one's analysis with the simplest situations, before moving to more complex ones. He points out (as he often does in later lectures) the similarity between normal mental processes and mental processes he sees in his patients, an emphasis no doubt intended to dispel as far as possible the idea that patients were somehow 'alien' to the rest of humanity. It is already clear here that psychiatric symptoms are to be the major focus of *Grundriss.*

Synopsis of L10: This lecture is a succession of case presentations, continuing those in L9, and referred to in later lectures. It gives insight into medical practice and institutional life in the asylums of the day, Wernicke's clinical style, his approach to symptoms, as well as initial ideas about his approach to classification.

Synopsis of L11: The focus here is on separating chronic cases from residual ones where the disease process has apparently run its course, and patients have recovered, without their gaining insight into their illness. Wernicke outlines his classification, based on which of the three components of memory is falsified—a patient's sense of corporeality (somatopsychic), of the outer world (allopsychic), and life experiences from which personhood is built (autopsychic component). Falsification in each of these is seen as secondary, a normal attempt to explain other experiences, whose abnormality *is* primary. Two such primary areas are identified: 'autochthonous ideas' (not 'created by usual processes of association'), and hallucinations.

Synopsis of L12: The first half of this lecture attempts to define what for Wernicke is a key concept, which he calls 'sejunction', purportedly a neuropathological process occurring at the level of nerve cells by which associative links are broken, and through which primary abnormal symptoms are to be explained. As in L11, he accounts for delusions not mainly as an abnormality in the process of interpreting experience, but rather as a more-or-less rational attempt to explain other subjective experiences, which he sees as primary abnormalities. His concepts appear to be imprecise or over-inclusive. This is perhaps inevitable when there are major gaps in background knowledge, and when the most useful way to define concepts is unclear. Sejunction is the obvious example here, making this one of the more contentious of his lectures. This lays him open to a sceptic's charge of 'neuromythology', especially when components drawn from his analogies are used subsequently as premises for further steps in supposed scientific reasoning. Much of the second half of the lecture is vividly descriptive, but also attempts to systematize, even to explain.

Synopsis of L13: The first part of this lecture is about hallucinations (identified as 'sensory deceptions'), recognized then, as today, as most often of the verbal auditory variety ('phonemes' in his terminology). These are taken as primary abnormalities, a consequence at the symptom level of the hypothetical 'sejunction' process at the neuronal level. Later parts of the lecture deal with explanatory delusions, envisaged to arise by quasi-rational processes, as patients' accounts of primary abnormalities they experience.

Synopsis of L14: The preceding lecture examined explanatory delusions occurring *immediately* to account for unusual primary experiences. *This* lecture explores delusions distorting *earlier* events, held in memory, as 'retrospective delusional explanation' and 'falsehoods of memory', to match current abnormal experiences.

Synopsis of L15: Wernicke's idea that each patient's symptomatology arises from a single 'elementary symptom' was mentioned in L14. Such symptoms, by virtue of a range of internal interactions, lead secondarily to other symptoms. The concept of an 'elementary symptom' is part of the title of L15, yet is not well explained. A review by Krahl and Schifferdecker, (1998) [1] suggests that he developed the idea in relation to 'anxiety psychosis' and 'hallucinosis', to which can be added 'autochthonous ideas', plus 'overvalued ideas' dealt with in this lecture.

Synopsis of L16: This lecture is important for both clinical science, and hospital administration, and Wernicke sketches out systems of classification to cover both. Much of the chapter attempts to decipher what might be the core pathological processes, by excluding other disturbances, seen as normal, albeit working to resolve tension set up by primary abnormalities, especially sejunction.

Synopsis of L17: A major part of this lecture is devoted to Wernicke's views on classification of mental disorders. He also introduces the term 'chronic hallucinosis'. Towards the end, an interesting section delves into recent history of psychiatry, as he saw it. In opening his first lecture, he already expressed his scepticism about contemporary categorization of mental disorders. Here his critique is expanded, more sharply, and in greater detail. He appears to reject most categories currently in use, favouring something simpler. Following a statement in his first lecture, he prefers to take as a starting point symptoms and the processes by which they arise, rather than supposed disease entities. Terms are introduced referring back to an earlier analogy, where intensity and extent of symptoms over time are plotted graphically. These are *aszendierend* (ascending) and *deszendierend* (descending), but henceforth, for clarity (since these words have other senses), we use the terms 'worsening' and 'improving', unless they clearly refer to anatomical relationships (such as in the gut), or refer directly to the original graphical analogy.

Synopsis of L18: The remaining lectures in *Grundriss* (more than half the series) cover acute syndromes of mental illness and defect states, as seen in Wernicke's practice. In this lecture he introduces the topic of acute mental illness, a topic he has already declared as more complex than that of chronic disorders. He also explores a topic touched on in L17, the separation between acute and chronic disorders. Later parts expand on the theme of delusions constructed to explain more primary abnormalities, and he suggests additional ways in which this may occur.

Synopsis of L19: The first two-thirds of this lecture give details of the phenomenology of hallucinations in major sensory modalities, and when modalities are combined. Later, he discusses the theory of hallucinations, starting with the history of attempts to provide such theory. Curiously, that presented here is different from, and based on assumptions different from those relating hallucinations to sejunction (in L13).

Synopsis of L20: This lecture continues discussion of the theory of hallucinations, and in passing, expands on issues discussed earlier on underlying neuroscience, notably the cohesiveness of acquired organization across widely separated cortical regions. Wernicke goes on to discuss other symptoms, including motor disorders of speech, hyperaesthesia, and what he calls 'hypermetamorphosis', 'an organically produced compulsion to take note of sense impressions, and to fixate attention on them'. This is presented as occurring mainly in neurological conditions, this being a precursor to subsequent lectures, where such symptoms arise in the context of mental disorders.

Synopsis of L21: This lecture deals with overriding features of any psychotic state, namely disorientation, and 'disarray'. The latter is an Affective state or reaction, and presents problems in translation, (section VIII(g) 'Wernicke's Distinctive Clinical Concepts in Psychiatry', *Affective Impact of Mental Illnesses*). These concepts divide according to the three-way split of contents of consciousness discussed earlier (allopsychic, somatopsychic, and autopsychic), to which, for the first time, a fourth subdivision—motor abnormality—is added.

Synopsis of L22: This lecture starts by enlarging on the concept of an overvalued idea, first discussed in L15, and leads to discussion of illusions. As already discussed for hallucinations, illusions originate as bias or distortion of perception resulting from a prevailing Affective state.

Illusions and hallucinations thus become hard to separate, but generally, the former are triggered mainly by concurrent events and their Affective impact, the latter arising more in the context of underlying illness.

Synopsis of L23: In this lecture, the style changes. It deals with identified disorders—'anxiety psychoses', including 'hypochondriacal anxiety psychosis'—and for the first time gives direct advice to students about treatment. The immediate symptom clusters, other than anxiety, are recognizably psychotic in modern terms, but may rapidly worsen to produce quasi-neurological symptoms, sensory abnormalities or akinesia, perhaps equating to classic conversion symptoms.

Synopsis of L24: This lecture, using Wernicke's terms, deals with 'hypochondriacal psychosis' and 'somatopsychosis'. The interest for today's reader is how concepts of mental disorder which today are considered separate, were then brought into relation with each other. They include somatisation, eating disorders, and a case of probable shell-shock from the Franco-Prussian war. Often these arise in conjunction with abnormal sensations arising from the intestines. A modern slant is given, attributing these to genuine abnormality of sensations from the body, perhaps exaggerated and distorted by patient's inaccurate lay knowledge about their internal organs.

Synopsis of L25: The focus of this lecture is 'Acute Hallucinosis', regarded by Wernicke as 'one of the best-defined forms of acute psychosis'. Usually this is the result of chronic excesses of drinking, probably mainly of hard liquor (cognac is mentioned), rather than beer or wine. The syndrome occurs rarely in other circumstances. Apart from description of symptoms, detail is provided on common patterns of recovery, aetiology, and danger of relapse.

Synopsis of L26: This lecture focuses on a specific diagnosis, *Delirium tremens*, starting with a case presentation, followed by discussion of symptoms, aetiology, diagnosis, differential diagnosis, treatment, and post-mortem findings. The clinical description is vivid, and raises important scientific questions about the nature of the abnormal mental state in such patients.

Synopsis of L27: This lecture follows from the previous one, amplifying the description of *Delirium tremens*, but moving on to 'polyneuritic psychosis' (otherwise known as Korsakoff's psychosis), common in people who have seriously abused alcohol. We now know this to result from nutritional inadequacy leading to thiamine deficiency, affecting both peripheral and central nervous systems. Wernicke did not know this, but hints that two pathologies may exist which cannot yet be adequately separated. Later parts deal with 'presbyophrenia', a mental disorder of the elderly.

Synopsis of L28: This long and complex lecture deals with disorders of personal identity ('acute autopsychosis' for Wernicke). The lecture does mention hysteria, but goes into most detail in describing a patient with a 'second state'. This had recently been described in France, but the emphasis here is different, with little stress on psychic trauma, and more on other ways in which such states might arise, including forms of epilepsy, or episodic binge drinking. Towards the end, discussion shifts to forensic topics, as 'acquired moral insanity', a term on which he is rather sceptical, and which he uses in a more restricted sense than some of his colleagues.

Synopsis of L29: Here Wernicke continues his account of 'acute autopsychosis', starting with two cases dominated by limited delusional ideas which distort personal identity, accompanied by prominent vasomotor symptoms, with acute onset and good prognosis. He gives them a provisional term '*acute expansive autopsychosis mediated by autochthonous ideas*'. He draws a parallel between disorders arising at the time when autochthonous ideas *appear*, and those arising on *disappearance* of thoughts. Later, he deals with obsessive neuroses and psychoses, commenting on differences between neurosis and psychosis. Finally he deals with the symptom of 'audible thoughts' ('thought echo').

Synopsis of L30: This important lecture starts by presenting two contrasting cases, one of severe melancholia (a variety of what is now called 'depression'), the other of florid mania. It continues with a fascinating account, with cogent reasoning to suggest that melancholia is primarily a disorder of 'will' (inability to resolve competing claims for action, leading to failure in taking decisions). Only when a person grasps their incapacity in daily activities, does it become a secondary disorder of lowered mood, along with symptoms such as 'delusions of belittlement'. The importance of accurately diagnosing the disorder is stressed, as well as the risk of suicide, and the good response to treatment in hospital (if it can be arranged).

Synopsis of L31: This complements L30, with an analysis of processes occurring in mania. Fundamentally mania is seen as 'pathological facilitation of acts of association' and, with it, an overall increase in activity levels in the cortex. It includes 'levelling of ideas' (as the level of activation of every idea is pushed to a similar 'ceiling'), course of illness, mania in progressive paralysis, combinations of mania and melancholia, and chronic forms of mania.

Synopsis of L32: This lecture starts with presentations of cases which Wernicke calls 'hyperkinetic motility psychosis', occurring either in the puerperium, or in relation to menstruation. Symptomatology is then extended from motor manifestations to speech pathology, and to compulsive choreatic movements; and there is discussion of what might today be called either akathisia or restless legs syndrome, and other syndromes driven by unusual sensations.

Synopsis of L33: This continues from L31, dealing with situations when 'intrapsychic hyperfunction', described in L31, escalates further. He thus deals with more severe grades of mania ('confused mania' and 'agitated confusion'), leading to discussion of 'amentia', a term originating with William Cullen and used by Meynert, but which Wernicke believes to be too broad to be helpful.

Synopsis of L34: This lecture, one of Wernicke's longest, complements L32, and deals with what he calls 'akinetic motility psychosis'. Early parts deal with symptoms such as 'waxy flexibility', muscle rigidity and catalepsy, and also with abnormal (that is *para*kinetic) movements. Much of the lecture, while dealing with psychiatric symptoms, reveals a world-class neurologist at work.

Synopsis of L35: This continues analysis of motility disorders, by exploring syndromes combining hyper- and a-kinetic symptoms (that is, compound psychoses). It also considers akinesia based on disorder of intrapsychic processes (including what Wernicke refers to as 'depressive melancholia'), and that based on psychsensory processes. It ends by considering the theory of motility psychoses (which started with Wernicke, and was retained in the Wernicke–Kleist–Leonhard tradition).

Synopsis of L36: This lecture is the first in which Wernicke starts 'winding up' the series of 41 lectures. As an overview, he discusses more complicated syndromes, in which different acute psychotic syndromes might be combined either simultaneously ('mixed psychoses'), or as separate phases ('compound psychoses'). Four components in such combinations are ones he defined earlier: allopsychosis, somatopsychosis, autopsychosis and motility psychosis. In turn combinations dealt with are: auto-somato-psychoses; allo-somato-psychoses; motility-allo-psychoses; motility-somato-psychoses; motility-allo-psychoses; and lastly, auto-allo-psychoses.

Synopsis of L37: This lecture, another long one, deals with the disorder mentioned many times earlier in passing, Progressive Paralysis. While he recognizes that it has some relation to syphilis, perhaps caused by a transmissible agent (not necessarily the same as that for syphilis), he is ambivalent about the relation between the two. This is understandable, since in 1900, when the lecture was written, the spirochete had not been discovered, nor had the Wasserman test to identify it been developed. Given this, Progressive Paralysis was of central importance to Wernicke, because its clinical manifestations overlapped with other forms of psychosis, and yet could be linked to identifiable neuropathological change, which could be correlated with specific clinical syndromes. It was thus an important basis upon which he could conceive a neuropathological basis for a wider range of psychotic syndromes.

Synopsis of L38: This lecture, spanning all earlier ones, is about aetiology of mental illnesses. Aetiology had already been discussed in the context of Progressive Paralysis (L37), with neuropathological evidence. Here, there is no neuropathology, the focus being on pathological processes inferred from symptoms, and 'proximate causes', that is the circumstance in which particular syndromes most often arise. Topics include psychoses linked to alcoholism, cocaine (then as now), poisoning by heavy metals (lead, arsenic compounds), infection diseases (tuberculosis, syphilis), the hereditary basis for mental illness, and links between epilepsy and psychosis.

Synopsis of L39: This lecture continues the aetiological grouping of psychoses, covering a variety of topics, especially disorders occurring at transitional periods of life. Topics dealt with include hysterical absences, psychoses of adolescence and puberty (including hebephrenia), senile psychoses, menopausal and menstrual psychoses, and puerperal psychoses. In addition, following recent new concepts in general medicine, he considers the separation of general and special aetiology (the latter originating in specific body systems or organs). This leads him to consider delirium due to inanition, and psychoses arising during other bodily disorders.

Synopsis of L40: This lecture discusses how the overall course of mental disorders might be represented and reported, including measures of intensity and symptomatic extent across time. The second half deals with dementia, a topic mentioned frequently in earlier lectures, and now in more detail. Wernicke considers this under heading both 'congenital' and 'acquired' dementia, and discusses terms for grades of dementia, ways of assessing it, and dementia occurring in several clinical contexts.

Synopsis of L41: Wernicke's final lecture covers a number of general topics, dissimulation (disguise) of mental illness, the opposite—simulation (or exaggeration) of it in healthy persons, and the proper role of mental institutions (and, in his view, the inadequacy of alternatives). His final section deals with his hopes for the future, especially the possibility of basing understanding of mental disorders on a secure pathological anatomy. Although Progressive Paralysis is an important pointer, he is clear that most 'functional psychoses' are unlikely to reveal any anatomical findings, were cases to come to autopsy. He nevertheless expresses in a closing section his optimism, in the face of numerous nay-sayers, for a future when there is a secure scientific basis for the subject of his major life's work. A century later, his hopes are still to be realized.

II. Unnamed Acknowledgment

In Wernicke's *Foreword* to the 1894 edition, he mentions an 'advocate of theoretical natural science' who provided 'stimulation and guidance', and may have been a critical supporter, without whose encouragement this work would never have seen the light of day. Who was this? It cannot be discovered from Wernicke's correspondence, since most of it is lost. Was he a neuroscientist, neurologist or psychiatrist of the time? The most likely such candidate would then be Theodor Meynert, his own mentor, whose portrait hung on the wall of his consulting room (see L26); but Meynert died in 1892, 2 years before the 1894 edition. Moreover, Wernicke gives thanks to the un-named person 'for his stimulation and guidance over the hours and days of a chance encounter'—hardly the acknowledgment he would give to his own, recently deceased mentor. Was it Gustav Fritsch (1838–1927), 10 years Wernicke's senior, Professor of Physiology at Berlin University, and who, with Edouard Hitzig, first showed, by electrical stimulation, the orderly layout of motor representation in the cerebral cortex? Was it Paul Flechsig, foremost German neuroanatomist of the day, also influenced by Meynert, and director of the Clinical

Institute of Psychiatry and Neurology at Leipzig (an easy journey from Breslau)? In his first Lecture, while praising such predecessors, notably Meynart, Wernicke sees significant weaknesses in their approach to scientific psychiatry, and he had little time for some of them (for instance Hitzig). This suggests that he intended to attempt something better. In several places in *Grundriss,* Wernicke makes it clear that he attempts to supersede Meynert's teachings.

It is noteworthy that he identified this unnamed person as 'an advocate of theoretical natural science', possibly hinting at a theoretical physicist. In the German-speaking world before Einstein, the foremost theoretical physicist was Ernst Mach (1838–1916), who, between 1867 and 1895 held a chair in physics at the Charles University, Prague, an easy journey from Breslau. Mach is best known for his philosophical and theoretical work. The main way in which this might have fulfilled his role of chair of *Experimental* Physics, was that his philosophy was that of a thorough-going empiricist. Theodor Ziehen, who together with Wernicke, founded *Monatschrift für Psychiatrie und Neurologie,* and was much cited by Wernicke in *Grundriss*, was himself much influenced by Mach [2], and is likely to have met Mach. That it was indeed Mach who inspired Wernicke is made plausible by several other facts: Mach himself made contributions to both sensory physiology and philosophy of science (both of which pervade *Grundriss*, especially in early lectures). Mach himself gained his inspiration in both areas from Gustav Fechner (1801–1887), who spent most of his life in Leipzig, and was also a major influence on Wernicke. The three of them worked in neighbouring university cities. Uniquely, Mach as a natural philosopher did not take variables such as mass and force as primary concepts, as did Isaac Newton. They were derivations, not ones related directly to empirical facts. Rather, his primary concept was 'sensation' ([3], p. 82). Corresponding to this, Wernicke never took disease concepts as the primary facts to be explained, these inevitably being indirect derivations and therefore of questionable validity, to which symptoms would then be secondary. Rather he took the *symptoms* he found in his patients as the primary facts. As discussed later, Wernicke's whole approach, and especially his emphasis on scientific reasoning, appears to be that of a natural philosopher, not that of a typical biomedical scientist. In the first eight lectures, many topics are referred to which correspond exactly to those with which Mach dealt. In his obituary Ziehen describes *Grundriss* as having being written 'almost as if a science of psychiatry did not yet exist' [4]. Of course it did exist, and had done so for a century; but Wernicke was independent of it. The final sentence of L41 reads as follows: 'I want to draw your attention to one point, and that is that these, my last comments, should serve to remind you of the need for those theoretical considerations which occupied us in the first half of our clinical studies, but, for you, perhaps often quite difficult to understand.' Clearly, in his first eight lectures, Wernicke was informed by insights right outside the field of study of his very able students, which he knew they might struggle to comprehend, and yet which he took to be of critical importance. In conclusion, we believe that it was Ernst Mach to whom this anonymous acknowledgment refers; but we have been unable to find any direct evidence of that 'chance encounter'.

In preparing the index for our translation (based on a translation of Wernicke's own index, plus items referring to this Editorial Commentary) we gained another insight into this matter. We realized that items which Wernicke chose to index were based on fairly orthodox concepts, while his most distinctive theoretical ideas, such as sejunction were under-represented. We conclude that, in indexing, he was playing to orthodox medical expectations of the time. However, careful reading of his text leaves us in no doubt that he thought the first eight lectures, and his more distinctive theoretical concepts were a crucial foundation for his clinical ideas; and also that they were likely to be beyond his audience, despite their being advanced students. Perhaps he was reticent, shy, possibly even a little embarrassed about his theoretical contributions. This is relevant to the 1894 foreword, and the acknowledgment to the anonymous person—who we think was Ernst Mach. Wernicke probably realized that the person to whom he addressed 'these apologetic intentions' really *was* a supreme scientific theoretician. In any case there is an enigma about why he did not name this person: The suggestion just made is not the only one possible.

III. The Medical Scene at Breslau in Wernicke's Day; Typical Psychiatric Practice

Breslau, located on the river Oder, was, at the time of Wernicke's first edition of *Grundriss,* a leading centre for medical research in the German empire, with many now-famous names working there; and a large proportion of contemporary clinical and scientific researchers, to whom he refers, were working there, or had done so. It was an exciting time in medical research. Recent discoveries included the transmissible agents responsible for tuberculosis, tetanus and diphtheria (and the toxins produced by the latter two agents). The neurone theory was coming to be generally accepted; and, building on advances in the German chemical industry, new stains were available which led to exciting new work in neurohistology and neuropathology. However, for most disorders, whether in general medicine or psychiatry, the best treatment that could be achieved was excellent nursing care and symptomatic relief. In L39 (p. 307), Wernicke writes, on psychoses occurring in the context of other bodily disorders: 'The prognosis of symptomatic psychoses depends exclusively on the course of the underlying disease, whose prospects, of course, can only be influenced unfavourably'. He thus accepts that, for most diseases, there was no effective treatment, although good general care favoured natural healing.

Through most of the nineteenth century, Paris had been the leading centre for medical research, but by Wernicke's day, Vienna and several German centres were worthy rivals, as French- and German-speaking worlds competed on several fronts. International conventions for defining diagnoses had not yet appeared, so there were no cross-national statistics on prevalence or incidence of diseases, and precious few national statistics. In L30 (pp. 210) Wernicke makes impressionistic comments on the high prevalence of melancholia; but only once (L40, p. 313) does he give any quantitative data on incidence of particular conditions, when he cites statistics on mortality related to mental illnesses *in asylums,* probably the nearest anyone could get to accurate statistics at the time. In 1893, at a congress of the International Statistical Institute, a French physician, Jacques Bertillon, made a distinction, for purposes of epidemiology, between general diseases and those localized to a particular organ or anatomical site (the *Bertillon Classification of Causes of Death*). The first conference to revise the International Classification of Causes of Death took place in 1900, from which, eventually the International Classification of Diseases (ICD) emerged as an administrator's instrument. The distinction made by Bertillon probably led Wernicke to write (L1, p. 4): 'Let us recall the division of brain diseases into focal disease processes and general diseases; mental illnesses will certainly not be subsumed under the former, but possibly under the latter.'

By the time that Wernicke was revising the text for the 1906 edition of *Grundriss*, he was working in Halle, and the prestige of the Breslau medical centre had declined. In its heyday, bacteriology and dermatology had been prominent specialties there. Sexually transmitted diseases, especially syphilis, were major topics for research. Of interest here, what was probably the first effective statute law on medical ethics was passed in Prussia in 1900, following a research scandal in the dermatology department in Breslau, deriving from research on syphilis. At the time, evidence on fundamental aetiology for brain disorders was very limited (except for correlations between lesion location and symptoms), a shortcoming reflected throughout *Grundriss.* However, perhaps because of the paucity of techniques available, those that *were* used, were employed with great care and in meticulous detail. In psychiatry, the one method that *was* available was documenting and analyzing psychiatric symptoms. *Grundriss* describes this in greater detail than one might find anywhere today.

The institution where Wernicke practised included many patients with what are now recognized as neurological conditions, as we read in his clinical descriptions. Moreover, many inmates of asylums suffered from the ravages of tertiary syphilis; and some of the phenomenology described by Wernicke (for instance in L20) is the result of this disease, rather than what we now recognize as mental disorder. Various syndromes, notably 'general paralysis of the insane' (GPI: German—*Paralyse der Irren*), now known to be syphilitic, would have been common in the asylum populations. In 1903, the causative agent was discovered, but the diagnostic test for the spirochete was not yet available, so the diversity of syndromes it caused was not yet clarified. Tuberculous meningitis, mentioned in L38 (p. 294), is now rare in developed countries, but is the commonest form of chronic CNS infection in developing countries, and probably was so in Wernicke's day.

Alcohol abuse was also a major issue for psychiatric practice. We now know that many of the psychiatric *sequelae* of excess drinking are not due directly to alcohol, but to poor nutrition, and deficiency of thiamine (vitamin B1). In L27 (p. 179) Wernicke refers to 'alcoholic degeneration' in the context of *Delirium tremens*. That state is, in itself, a withdrawal syndrome not linked with neuronal loss, but may become linked, when combined with chronic alcoholism, and thiamine deficiency. Later in the same lecture (p. 180), he mentions the poor general health and cachexia of such patients, an expected precursor of impaired memory, now known as a sequel of thiamine deficiency. Later in L27 (p. 182) he writes 'restoration of function' after a period in hospital.

Throughout the clinical lectures, Wernicke refers to links between mental disorders and a wide variety of problems in general medicine; and clearly he was competent both as a general physician and as a surgeon. In the lecture on progressive paralysis (L37, p. 286) he mentions gumma, a non-cancerous granuloma in tertiary syphilis which may appear in various organs (liver, brain, heart, etc.), and endarteritis, another pathology of tertiary syphilis starting with inflammation of arterial adventitia. In L38 (p. 294) he refers to 'childhood cramps', painful muscle spasms which may be provoked by exercise and various metabolic or hormonal changes, not viewed today as having adverse long-term *sequelae*. In his day, cramps may have been a 'proxy' for some more serious problem, related perhaps to poverty, poor nutrition, or some other aspect of life's hardships. In his discussion of extended regimes of tube feeding of akinetic patients (L34, p. 258) he is well aware of the danger of 'scorbutic', that is 'scurvy-like' lesions. The fact that scurvy could be cured by various dietary supplements such as citrus fruits had long been known. That the anti-scorbutic factor was 'hexuronic acid' ('Vitamin C'), was not proven until 1932. Wernicke clearly retained his skill in surgery, for instance when he writes L34 (p. 249) of a patient with a syndrome of rigidity in jaw muscles: 'I decided on "re-positioning" under chloroform anaesthesia, and fixed his jaw in a half-open position'.

Public attitudes to psychiatry appear to have been a mix very similar to those found today. In L9 we hear Wernicke, echoed by other enlightened practitioners, expressing concern about the poor grasp by the general populace of the realities of mental disorder, along with calls for public education. There are hints of difficult public relationships, where he refers to 'the familiar reformatory idea of those philanthropists'. In L17 (p. 101) he advises his students thus: 'I cannot emphasize strongly enough, that you have the right to declare a person mentally ill only when you can produce evidence of this by establishing definite psychotic symptoms; only then will you be spared the embarrassment of your opinion being exposed to justified attacks by lay people'. Then, as now, it seems, psychiatrists were targets of public suspicion, for which attitudes Wernicke had some sympathy. Concern over custodial practices in mental hospitals in German principalities went back to the early nineteenth century. By the 1890s this led to the first genuine anti-psychiatry movement, and, by the turn of the century, to calls for tighter legal control [5]. Some diagnoses, especially the so-called 'moral insanity' linked to the 'second state' (dual personality), were contentious then, just as today. In L28 (p. 193), he writes: 'You know that this is about cases of illness, which lawyers, unfortunately supported by clashing opinions, have been particularly reluctant to recognize, which, in our own view, has diverted attention from much of both the factual reality of these pathological conditions and their theoretical basis'. In L41 (pp. 322, 323) he asks '… could not a healthy person imitate the speech of a mentally ill person?' This, of course, has been carried out in an approximate way in recent times, to draw attention to the sometimes arbitrary compulsory detention in asylums. There is no suggestion of such activism in Wernicke's day. In any case, despite early 'anti-psychiatry' rhetoric, public views, as might be expected, were diverse and not always charitable. In L30 (p. 210), when arguing for hospital admission in cases of melancholia, we read '… the general view is that only the insane belong in institutions'. On public perception of links between mental disorder and violence, the issue was not schizophrenia (a term not yet coined) but epilepsy (which carried similar associations in the popular mind). In L38 (p. 298) he writes: 'Mostly, there is no later recollection [of acts committed during twilight states of epilepsy]; however, except for one—albeit cursory—reminder, we find that violence was perpetrated as defence against a threatening situation'. He hints here at unnecessary stigmatizing attitudes at the time towards epilepsy, just as people with schizophrenia or bipolar disorder are targeted today, yet are more likely to be victims than perpetrators of violence.

In L9, it is made clear that there *were* legal criteria controlling how and when patients might be admitted compulsorily to a mental hospital. L41 (p. 321), addressing his class, he states: 'Each of you will, at some time, be in a position of deciding on the placement of a patient in a mental hospital, or having to issue a certificate that health has been regained'. The laws were broadly the same across Germany, but with variations in different Länder [6]. There are clues to the lack of rigour (as understood today) in mental health law, and, just as today, in criteria for committal. In L15 (pp. 92, 93) a story is told about a master carpenter and his overvalued idea. Members of the public could initiate proceedings against people suspected of being mentally ill, which could lead to the latter being detained in an institution. There is no evidence of processes for legal scrutiny, or appeal against medical authority. However, in L41 (p. 322), Wernicke writes: 'After several weeks had elapsed the family then decided, much against my advice, to remove the patient from hospital treatment': Clearly legal provisions did not give doctors unassailable powers to detain patients. Medical and judicial authorities were probably not sharply separated, as was the case in other jurisdictions at the time and for some time to come.

In some respects, legal provisions and outreach of psychiatric services were far advanced. In L24 (p. 158), and again in L25 (p. 170) it is clear that patients could admit themselves voluntarily, a provision not possible in Britain until the 1930 Mental Treatment Act. A comment in L25 (p. 169) suggests that community follow-up was undertaken in the mental health system where Wernicke worked. In some places, then as today, the possibility of managing short-lived periods of serious mental illness at home, with intensive support, was given consideration (L25, p. 170). In L34 (p. 247) we read: 'Patient feels that he is very severely ill, and asks for reports': This should not be taken to imply that patients had the right to access their medical reports, a possibility in psychiatry which is rare even today.

Decisions about whether (and on what criteria) to discharge patients were of central importance, no doubt with financial issues in the background, but also taking notice of a patient's current mental state. In relation to the latter, we read comments such as (L10) '… the patient's behaviour is in no way normal but … requires so much patience and forbearance … that she can exist only in the special confines of an institution' (p. 60), or 'After recovery from actual mental illness, they prove themselves incapable of living anywhere else than in an institution, on account of their social incompatibility, their demanding and predominantly egotistical behaviour requiring constant supervision' (p. 61). Of course, then as now, such criteria might apply to many people who never had any mental illness, nor spent time in an institution. Overall the quality of care was as good as could be expected. In L40 (p. 313) we read 'Such patients, after repeated attempts at discharge, finally remain permanently in the institutions, where they find necessary protection and care, and also an opportunity for useful activity'. In administrative terms, it seems that patients fell into three categories: 'Recovered' (*geheilt*), 'Residual' (*geheilt mit Defekt*), and 'Unrecovered' (*ungeheilt*), a system of classification which probably applied across Germany [6].

In several places in *Grundriss,* Wernicke emphasizes that the best place to treat and care for patients with mental disorders *is* in institutions specially designed for this. In L30 he recommends this in the case of melancholia, because of the high suicide risk; and later (p. 209), urges that discharge should not be too early: 'After the illness has ended, a phase of mild manic exaltation is seen quite regularly, lasting only a few days or weeks; and it is always ill-advised to discharge the patient before this'. In L37 (p. 287) he makes a similar recommendation for progressive paralysis: 'If you are in any doubt over whether and when to bring the patient into a mental institution, it is always safest to decide in favour of this': Such general advice might not be given nowadays, in public hospitals at least, simply for financial reasons. One wonders what the financial tensions might have been for Wernicke.

In Breslau itself, there appears to have been a well developed public health system. In L32 (p. 229) reference is made to a 'female patient, previously healthy, had been in the public hospital', presumably a public *general* hospital. It was, after all, in Bismarck's Germany that a version of what we now call the 'welfare state' was first adopted. On alternatives to institutional care Wernicke writes (L41, p. 324): 'there are experienced alienists who adopt the view that by properly setting up a private residence, the same can be achieved as in institutional treatment. We must realize immediately, when discussing the purposes of institutional treatment, that this is not entirely true'. Ideas circulating then were the same as today, facing all the same dilemmas. In L24 (p. 158), reference is made to an establishment called a *Pflegeanstalt.* Such places, for mentally or physically disabled persons were half way between an asylum and what in Britain, from early nineteenth century, was called a 'nursing home'. In Britain and the USA, these were places for care of the elderly, under less austere and unsavoury conditions than obtained in the almshouses of the time in the USA, or the workhouses in Britain. In Germany, care of elderly or disabled persons or recuperating patients had long been undertaken by nurses linked to religious orders, although in 1869 Rudolf Virchow had recommended that nursing be secularized. By the turn of the century, a large variety of *Pflegeanstalten* existed, some secular (e.g. under the Red Cross), some religious [7]. Wernicke implies that such an environment might sometimes be more conducive to recovery than the institution where he worked. They were not free from compulsion, since, in L28 (p. 186) we read: 'During the unusually hot summer of 1886 she was detained for 2 months in a charitable institution.' In the Third Reich, they often became centres for euthanasia.

Communities outside the institution might accept or reject a patient after discharge, leading Wernicke to comment (L16; p. 99) 'Unfortunately, however, it is often inevitable that patients return to a life with no structure of regular activity nor any ordered social engagement, conditions that are harmful both through the lack of normal interests, and also even by predisposing them to emergence of depressive Affects. Their main interest may then remain focused on experiences of injustice; an Affect-laden state of mind sets in, and further delusion-formation is inevitable'. These lines ring true over 120 years. Issues of discharge planning, and the social milieu in which a patient might find him- or herself after discharge, applied then as much as now.

The harsh realities of care in institutions also seem to be similar then as they often are today. Ward staff are referred to not as nurses (*Krankenschwester*), but as 'warders' (*Wärter,* or *Wärterin*), although they were probably mainly skilled professionals (and in L34, [p. 250] Wernicke refers to the warder's notes recording rigid postures adopted by patients). Given the great vulnerability of patients, they are always likely to be subject to demeaning behaviour and attitudes (or worse) not only from the general public, but also sometimes from staff in the institutions, and, as we read in L9, these can lead to bitter complaints from patients. In L18 (p. 115) we read of violence within the ward: 'On inquiry we learned that he was not suffering headaches but experienced very unpleasant sensations in his head, which he described as dull and dragging—they were a result of mistreatment by the warders'. Then as now, it may be hard to avoid physical coercion in restraining agitated patients; although nowadays, there may be guidelines on suitable strategies to minimize this, training in ways to do it safely, and routines for reporting difficult incidents. Although Wernicke is well aware of similarities between normal mental processes and those in his patients, in L9, he confidently regards complaints of patients or former patients as 'false readings of reality'. Recovery of insight is more likely for the time of admission than for the fact of remaining in the institution. He describes the mental content of many patients as an amalgam of delusional and healthy material.

Some of Wernicke's descriptions reveal what might now be identified as signs of institutionalization, rather than intrinsic features of any illness. In L41 (p. 325) he writes: 'There are still many such phrases used similarly by mentally ill people in a remarkably similar ways'; and In L29 (p. 199), we read of patients' words, 'often heard in mental institutions, that thoughts were "drawn out of" them'. The specific experience described here would now be called 'thought withdrawal', pathological not so much for the experience itself but for the delusional interpretation imposed on it. However, Wernicke implies that interpretation of 'jargon' used by patients requires experience of the 'local scene'. In other words, linguistic use by patients to describe their experiences is developed collectively as much as individually in a long-stay ward, as in any other community. Other signs of institutionalization include descriptions such as (L10, p. 60) 'She regards her fellow-patients as men of the cloth, usually high-ranking clerics who are here in part for repentance'. Beliefs shared amongst patients in a long-stay ward are probably often not symptoms of active illness, nor (in the above case) of religious sentiment, but social constructions by disturbed people confined within a very strange environment, one where 'anything goes' conceptually, however absurd, as part of the 'organizational culture' in the ward. Likewise, complaints from patients may be driven by knowledge of—or resistance to—the abnormal situation of institutional life. We also read (L10, p. 59) '... she is persistently submissive by nature; she rises at each salutation and bows, doing this to every fellow-patient, even to a very feeble-minded female paralytic patient'. Such ritualized behaviour speaks of institutionalization.

Families of patients are mentioned a few times. In L22 (p. 140) there are two mentions of families. Again in L30 (p. 203), we read: '... takes no notice of visits by her relatives'. Clearly visiting was possible, perhaps into the main section of a ward, although, in L23 (p. 151), there is a reference to a 'visitor's room', suggesting that, as in many psychiatric wards today, visitors do not see the main part of the ward. In the recent memory of RM, this may be obstructed in psychiatric facilities, or visitors are shown only into a special 'quarantined' visitors' room; and even in general medicine, when charters for patient rights have been enacted in various jurisdictions, visiting rights are not necessarily included (for instance in the European Charter of Patients Rights of 2002) [8], the NHS Patients' Rights, 2013 [9]). However, in 2011 in the USA, legislation was passed about visitation rights [10]. How that applies to psychiatric institutions is not clear, but is likely to be more restrictive than in general medicine.

IV. Wernicke's Personal Style in Psychiatric Practice, Teaching, Writing, and in Scholarly Disputes

From the outset in L1 Wernicke shows that he is aware that psychiatry, perhaps because of its intrinsic complexity, was backward, compared with other specialties. At the very end, in a closing section of L41, he assures his students that attitudes to the discipline from other physicians, had improved over the preceding 20 years. He advises (L1) that a teacher in psychiatry 'should proceed as in sister disciplines of medicine'. Clearly he wanted to adopt standards and methods of general medicine, as did his contemporary Kraepelin, but in a very different way. In L1 he also accepts that there may be different types of mental disease, but as we shall see, his approach to classification was quite different from that of Kraepelin.

A critical aspect of the style of practice of any psychiatrist is whether, to what extent, and how, reunification of personhood can be achieved after it is fragmented by mental disorders. This is a core issue, more for psychiatry if practised well than for any other medical discipline. In L7 (p. 39) we read the following: 'After a person has recovered from a mental illness, it is required that we ensure that he has achieved insight into the abnormality of the state he has experienced; for the sum must necessarily be inaccurate if it contains false elements'. These words reveal what a fine clinician he must have been, in his hope that his patients recover full health, and in defining his own role in helping each patient to regain their sense of 'personal wholeness' to whatever extent this was possible. Nowadays, lack of such a holistic approach is the sharpest criticism made of many of today's psychiatric practitioners by service user groups. We get another clue his compassionate concern in L18 (p. 113). Unlike many chronic patients presented in earlier lectures, whose surname is given, here a patient is referred to just by an initial, because he is of some standing in the local community, and likely to remain so after discharge (which is to occur soon). He thus wanted to avoid his publication—which gives much detail about the patient—making life more difficult for him after discharge. Likewise, in L27 (p. 180), he uses initials only, to hide not only the identity, but also the former place of residence of a patient who is to be discharged; and in L30 (p. 203), for the same reason, an initial is given for the place in which one of his patients worked as a nurse.

We cannot miss Wernicke's careful and realistic assessment of what might be possible for each patient. In days when effective treatments were few, assessment of prognosis loomed larger than today. So, in L10 (p. 59) we read 'Frau Reisewitz, whose illness developed gradually over the last 5 years, from barely noticeable beginnings, and is expected to develop further'; in L16 (p. 97) '… cases where active illness is fully extinguished …': Clearly this bore implications for 'prognosis'. The prognostic indicators he used are discussed later. Footnotes in *Grundriss* were often added retrospectively, about the eventual outcome for patients he has presented and discussed.

A distinctive aspect of Wernicke's approach appears to be that he did not distance himself unnecessarily from his patients. Although he refers to doctors working in mental institutions as *Irrenärzten* (literally 'mad doctors')—never 'alienists'—he often drew parallels between normal psychological processes and those underlying symptom formation in his patients. We see this initially in L9, where the emphasis is no doubt intended to dispel for his students any idea that his patients were somehow 'alien' to the rest of humanity The emphasis is most striking when discussing delusions, seen mainly as plausible—even rational—attempts to explain more primary abnormalities of experience: In L13 (p. 82) he addresses his audience thus: 'Should anyone experience a feeling of deliberate rudeness when a greeting is omitted etc., then this also is an echo of a delusional interpretation'. He skilfully points out similarities, where they can be found, between the psychology he sees in his patients, and those in his audience. In L8 (p. 45) he speaks of 'herd consciousness' as a social phenomenon, in such a way as to make clear that this also applies to himself, accepting that he is not only a clinician and observant scientist, but also an object of study. Subject and object, clinician and patient, appear not sharply separated. In discussing the role of language in L8, he writes (p. 45): '… the main way to acquire a particular order to one's perceptions is through articulated speech'; but later, he steps back from his 'real self'—an articulate, supremely rational clinician-scientist—to defend himself against charges of over emphasizing language in defining human nature.

Wernicke knew how, as a skilled clinician, he could use those faculties of a patient still assumed to be normal, along with events occurring incidentally, or engineered by him, as a vehicle to correct delusional explanations. So, in L24 (p. 158) we read: 'this patient, was discharged from the nursing home after 6 weeks, allegedly completely recovered, probably as a result of the powerful impression that transfer there must have had on her.' He also knew how, on occasion, he could use the vividness of a clinical presentation for therapeutic purposes beyond any of the session's didactic aims; that is, to exert on a patient an impact more powerful, albeit subtle, than is possible in normal clinical encounters. He writes (L15; p. 94): 'Clinical presentation of such cases has proved useful to me several times, as is the process of 'internalization' itself, that is, a conscious ability to recognize mental illness, and to constantly accept paternal guidance: These are powerful and salutary corrective experiences.' Again in L41 (p. 321) he writes of mute patients: 'Amongst the best proven ways of bringing such patients to speak, is a clinical presentation'.

It is also clear that he does not hide from his own mistakes. In L34 (p. 257), he writes: 'This happened to me once, and the tracheotomy which was carried out immediately could not avert a fatal outcome.' Again in L41 (p. 322) after describing how a patient's family insisted on the patient being discharged, against his wishes, he writes: 'Apparently they were right, for there was no further recurrence of the delusions he had expressed previously, and he resumed his earlier work in a business'.

The one area where Wernicke seems to have a less subtle approach is with young patients. There are no descriptions of children in *Grundriss;* and in L39 (p. 304), when describing hebephrenic traits in adolescents, he writes: 'They are not to be found in the specific childhood form, in which, the resulting feeble-mindedness in silly and foolish beings, would seem only natural'. This comment, like ones in L40, betray him, uncharacteristically, as one with little sympathy for childhood or adolescence, almost as one with little knowledge of psychological issues faced by young persons.

Wernicke's teaching style is revealed from time to time. There was clearly a plan to cover the subject of psychiatry comprehensively (with a 'course curriculum' referred to in L24, p. 162). In L32 (p. 226) he refers to details presented in a 'past semester', so, probably the lectures were given across a whole year over two semesters. In the clinical lectures, he sometimes develops his arguments by referring to cases described by other psychiatrists or neurologists of the day in Germany or France (never Britain). Often however, patients were present—even several in succession—for at least some of the lecture, or sometimes, it appears, in sessions prior to the lecture (L24, p. 153). There are occasional hints (from comments such as 'To our great surprise, a turn-around occurred from yesterday' [L32, p. 223], and 'Chance has favoured us, in that I can present another patient' [L32, p. 225]) that choice of patients each day was sometimes quite opportunistic. In these clinical sessions he presumably demonstrated to the class his manner of interviewing each patient. Detail of such dialogue is seldom recorded, but in later lectures, verbatim dialogue is sometimes reported, showing his interviewing style, including his modelling for his students how to ask about suicide (L30, p. 202). In this situation, he states at one stage: 'As you see, his appearance is quite appropriate to the situation', (L9, 56). Clearly, Wernicke has his patient in the lecture theatre, seeing no incongruity about such candid public description of the patient's characteristics to the assembled audience. There might be more constraints in today's world! However, at times his comments leave it unclear whether they are the patient's view or his own. This ambiguity may sometimes have been necessary, when a patient about whom he is speaking is in the lecture theatre; and usually it does not matter.

As a lecturer, he knew how to engage his audience, often with personal anecdotes, or references to typical life experiences which all could share. Nonetheless, the lectures are dense with ideas, arguments and evidence, suggesting that, as delivered, they were each followed by extensive discussion, otherwise his students would have been left behind. In L28 (p. 193), he more-or-less invites discussion: 'This might be the place for me to respond to an objection that you could easily make'. Indications that this took place can also be found in the fact that some cross-references to earlier lectures refer to material, or patients not actually present in the text of *Grundriss.* For instance in L18, where patient K. is first introduced, there is no mention of his making a suicide attempt, but this detail *is* mentioned in L21, when referring back to this lecture. In L22 (p. 139) he revisits the notion of an 'overvalued idea' first introduced in L15; yet specific points mentioned in L22 are not mentioned in L15. In addition, sometimes two lectures (e.g. L9 and L10, L19 and L20) appear so closely connected as to suggest that they were given close together in time, even on the same day. Sometimes we are left to infer the occasions when patients, who are referred to, have been met in other situations, without knowing when or where this occurred. Later lectures often cite in-house reports (*Krankenvorstellungen aus der psychiatrischen Klinik in Breslau*).

His audience appears to have consisted of very advanced students. They were quite familiar with routine neurological problems, since, in L37 (p. 286) he writes: 'You are so often called to deal with a so-called "stroke" that your first question must be whether you are dealing with a possible paralytic attack'. In introducing L41, he begins: 'These lectures can hardly be intended to introduce you to the practical medical specialist training course for the asylums. Whoever wants to dedicate himself totally to our specialty is of course expecting to spend a considerable part of his life in mental institutions, and among mentally ill people, a task that in some respects you can imagine is not sufficiently challenging, but also not sufficiently gratifying and interesting … it is therefore imperative to give you some orientation on practical issues, including the specific tasks of the asylum, and the simulation and dissimulation of mental illnesses'. Clearly members of his audience are likely to become researchers; but here, he descends to mundane matters, likely also to be important in their subsequent careers. That his lectures were, in large part, research seminars is clear at the start of L21, when he acknowledges that the patient he is about to discuss is a 'very complex, and as yet little known form of illness'. He conveys that the lectures were research presentations more-or-less explicitly, when he writes (L41, p. 329): 'Hence preliminary work is needed, in which you have participated in these lectures'. There may, however, have been other courses, especially for future administrators of asylums.

Details are available on several members of Wernicke's class who went on to distinguish themselves. Many of the following names produced works cited in *Grundriss. Hugo Liepmann* (1863–1925), editor of the 1906 edition of *Grundriss*, was himself a noted psychiatrist and neurologist, who had worked closely with Wernicke from 1895 to 1899. He was noted for studies of cerebral localization of function, the first to describe several neurological syndromes, later becoming director of the *Herzberge* asylum in Berlin. *Ernst Storch* was Wernicke's loyal assistant, one of his first co-workers. He was appointed privat-dozent in Psychiatry at Breslau in 1902, and had previously been first-assistant in the psychiatric clinic there. In 1901, he published *Psychologische Untersuchungen über die Funktionen der Hirnrinde, zugleich eine Vorstudie zur Lehre von der Afasie* [11], recently republished. Biographical detail on Storch is obscure. *Karl Bonhöffer* (1868–1948) was a psychiatrist who worked briefly in Heidelberg (1903–1904), but moved to Breslau, where, under Wernicke, integration of neurology with psychiatry was possible. He gave detailed descriptions of *Delirium tremens* (L26, p. 175), and may have challenged Kraepelin's view that categorical disorders were to be defined by symptom clusters [12]. After Wernicke's death he defined the conceptual separation of endogenous from exogenous psychoses. His son, Dietrich Bonhöffer was the celebrated theologian who, from within Germany, resisted the Nazi regime, and was, imprisoned and executed in the last days of World War II. *Karl Heilbronner* (1869–1914) worked at Wernicke's clinic from 1894 to 1898, and between 1897 and 1903 headed an observation ward for mentally ill prisoners there. *Karl Kleist* (1879–1960) continued Wernicke's approach to description of symptoms, originated the terms 'unipolar' and 'bipolar' for Affective disorders, made detailed studies of many head-injury cases from World War I, and is known today as continuing what became the Wernicke–Kleist–Leonhard tradition. *Kurt Goldstein* (1878–1965) became an advocate of anti-localizationist neurology. When Hitler came to power, being Jewish, he was imprisoned for a short time in Berlin, then expelled from Germany, going first to Amsterdam, then to the USA, where he founded Gestalt therapy. *Heinrich Sachs* (1863–1928) was an early researcher on amyotrophic lateral sclerosis. After working with Wernicke at Breslau, he became head of the division of neurology and neurosurgery in the Jewish hospital there. *Otfrid Foerster* (1873–1941) studied under Babinski in Paris, returned to Breslau to become a pioneer neurosurgeon, and spending much time later in Russia. His most famous patient was Vladimir Ilyich Lenin, and it was Foerster who recommended that Oskar Vogt examine the latter's brain, after his death from stroke. *Edmund Forster* (1878–1933) was one of Wernicke's later students. During World War I, as a military physician, one of his patients was Adolf Hitler, who was treated and hypnotized by him after a gas attack, and whom he described as a 'psychopath with hysterical symptoms'. He committed suicide in 1933 under persecution; *Ludwig Mann* (1866–1936) studied with Wernicke and became professor at St Georg-Krankenhaus, Breslau. In 1896, he published *Klinische und anatomische Beiträge zur Lehre von der spinalen hemiplegia* [13]. *Robert Eugen Gaupp* (1870–1953) was an assistant to Wernicke at Breslau, and afterwards worked with Emil Kraepelin at Heidelberg and Munich, later to become a professor of psychiatry at Tübingen (1908–1938). He studied the relationship between psychosis and personality, advocated for 'pastoral psychology', and after World War II, headed the department of health and welfare in Stuttgart. In 1935, after passage by decree of the 'Nuremberg Laws' ('for protection of German Blood and Honour'), he came to the defence of a fellow physician, whose situation became precarious in a local society, on account of his Jewish wife. *Heinrich Lissauer* (1861–1891) was a neurologist and neuropathologist at the psychiatric institute in Breslau. Despite his early death, his name is associated with several significant advances, making studies on the pathology of Progressive paralysis, having a tract in the spinal cord is named after him, and the first to describe visual agnosia. Clearly Wernicke thought highly of him; *Paul Schroeder* (1873–1941) worked with Wernicke in Breslau, with Kraepelin and later with Nissl in Heidelberg, and with Bonhöffer in Berlin, to become professor of Psychiatry at the University of Griefswald in 1913. In 1937, he became first president of the International Society of Pediatric Psychiatry, but retired the following year.

In the first clinical lecture (L9) Wernicke enunciates the maxim that one should start one's analysis with the simplest situations, before moving to more complex ones. In consequence, he chose to deal first (L9–L17) with stabilized mental abnormalities seen long after acute stages of disturbance have subsided, before going on to acute states. His maxim may be sound; and given the realities of practice in his day, was no doubt applied correctly. Better this than trainees (then, and perhaps still today) being 'thrown in at the deep end', making it hard for them to reconstruct all the steps between normality and severe dysfunction. In psychiatry, the implied alien status of inmates could then only be reinforced. Whether this was true or not for Wernicke, it is likely that patients most commonly encountered in his institution were those whose acute disturbance had subsided to a stable state, however abnormal. However, in a number of areas of medical education, there is tension between what is best from a didactic point of view, and what is possible practically. For instance, one of us (RM) has argued [14] that, in teaching gross anatomy, spatial relationships in body cavities are grasped more easily by starting with, 'empty' cavities, and then adding organs one by one; which is exactly the opposite of what is normally possible in a dissecting room course. The way in which Wernicke's maxim might be applied could likewise be questioned in today's world: Mental states in chronic stabilized cases may *appear* simple, but to understand them fully depends on understanding processes leading to this 'end state', which are by no means simple. By L17 Wernicke reaches just this conclusion. In today's psychiatry, where most patients recover from acute psychosis, the best place to start education for trainee specialists may be open discussion with people who are distant from acute episodes, but whose memory for, and insight into those episodes is good enough to help such trainees grasp the unfolding processes. Indeed, in L18, Wernicke makes use of exactly such an insightful patient, who has reached near-complete recovery.

In addition, in L17, the last dealing with chronic conditions, he writes as follows (p. 105): '... after many years of work I had to decide to reverse my strategy, and to start working from the ground upwards, placing acute mental illnesses, which are still the main source of paranoid conditions, as the precursor of the latter [chronic conditions]': This sentence is important. In L9–L17, Wernicke deals with chronic conditions, paying little attention to their relation to acute ones. Here, however, he feels the need to reverse the emphasis; and later lectures fill out details of the shift in strategy. We comment here, that, in the sequence of 41 lectures we both had the clear impression that *Grundriss* is not so much a completely pre-planned presentation of Wernicke's ideas, but rather a progression of his developing ideas. In particular, in the transition from chronic to acute disorders, we felt that later clinical lectures were almost superseding earlier ones (although at times in the later lectures his consistency in use of terms defined earlier became looser, perhaps because he was writing in haste).

At various points in *Grundriss,* we get glimpses of Wernicke's methods of clinical examination. Basic assessment of sensory and reflex motor capability probably differed little from today. For auditory acuity, a test familiar today is described (L24, p. 158): 'On admission she understood speech whispered at 3–3½m.' ...'Over the first 2 months there was a clear decrease in her auditory acuity. This was noticeable even at ordinary conversational levels; for whispered speech, auditory acuity decreased to 30 cm on the left and 20 cm on the right.'...'we discovered particularly poor bone conduction; against the skull or mastoid process the clock was not heard at all.' In testing the pupillary light reflex we read (L24; p. 159): 'His pupils were fairly narrow, equidistant, and widened only a little, when his eyes were shaded.' In L34 (p. 397) we read 'Reflex excitability of cutaneous capillaries is normal'. Presumably this refers to the axon reflex, producing the reddening of the skin when scratched, a clinical test which, we believe, is not routine today. In L8, we read of Wernicke's simple clinical test to assess 'short-term memory', subsequently referred to as 'retention of memory'. Much as today, this involved testing recall of 'a three-digit number, a foreign-sounding word which she should have retained after interposing a short question' (L27, p. 180). In L30 (p. 203), we read of long-term memory tested separately for recall and recognition. Attentiveness was apparently tested separately for each of the three domains of experience (L27, p. 285). For speech articulation Wernicke had his special probe words (*Zivilisation, Armeereorganisation, Guiglelminetti, Exterritorialität* ['civilization', 'army reorganization', 'Guiglelminetti', 'extraterritoriality']). His test of cognitive capacity was to ask a patient to recognize, count, and make a tally of a number of coins. At various points he uses the phrase 'closed train of thought', attributed to Meynert. In L20 (p. 130), it becomes clear that this phrase describes a method of testing higher cognitive functions, where he writes of 'absent-mindedness, that is, the intractable nature of thought processes, and inability to follow a closed train of thought.'

Wernicke's written style is hard to separate from his style of reasoning, discussed later; and we are ill-equipped to assess it in comparison with that of contemporary German researchers. Overall, *Grundriss* is closely reasoned, with small phrases in early lectures being developed later, in a meticulous way, and special terms used with great efforts at consistency. However, there are many superfluous words, academic niceties, unnecessary qualifying words, double negatives, and tautologies. Perhaps this reflects how he delivered the lectures. Sometimes there are colourful idioms. For instance, in L13 (p. 83) a young man, embittered against his father, had the intention of 'setting him straight', without murdering him (*ihm etwas Ordentliches zu versetzen*); in L28 (p. 193), he writes: 'However, this assertion does not hold a candle' (*Diese Behauptung hält aber vor den Tatsächen nicht Stich*); in L35 (p. 290), he uses the phrase '*über jahr und Tag'*, familiar in English as 'for a year and a day'; and in L24 (p. 162) he uses the metaphorical term 'burnt out', which has been used in many ways. In medicine it might refer to the end-stage of an epidemic, or of an incurable disease such as leprosy (in Graham Greene's novel *A burnt out case*), or to the end-stage of chronic schizophrenia. In the nineteenth century, it led to mythology about 'spontaneous human combustion', a case of which is described in Charles Dickens' *Bleak House*; and today is revitalized as 'workplace burn-out'.

A few points need clarifying, where he is over-concise. For instance, in L31 (p. 219) where he writes '… the disorder is mainly one of form' he implies (we presume) but does not say 'rather than of content'; or, in L39 (p. 303) we read 'the familiar tendency for akinetic motility psychosis to be transformed into dementia might be based in part on this aetiological relationship', probably referring to (but not mentioning) Kahlbaum's concept that transitional periods of life make aetiological contributions to some mental disorders. Sometimes, the line of reasoning becomes hard to grasp when describing the 'second state' (L28). For instance, in L13 (p. 82), we read: 'Therefore, it follows from this that, as abnormal excesses of activation continue, phonemes, which tend to appear only intermittently in such cases, require a special amplification of activation before they come to a standstill.' We could not come to a conclusion of what was meant here. In L17, (p. 106) we read what seems to be a *non sequitur:* 'So, the great mystery remains for Griesinger: how such regularity of content can arise—the occurrence of ideas of grandiosity and persecution, in which "perhaps among ten patients, only five throughout the whole duration of the disease, form the main content of the delirium."' In L24 (p. 162) we read 'Muscle pains often underlie a very severe feeling of illness, as proven by occasional examples of rapid onset, resolved by relief of muscle pain.' We inferred the meaning here in respect of a single word we added, 'resolved'. What was actually written was: *Muskelschmerzen liegen Häufig einem sehr schweren Krankheitsgefühl zugrunde wie vereinzelte Beispiele rascher Herstellung durch Beseitigung der Muskelschmerzen beweisen.* In L28 he writes (p. 188): 'the sensorium is apparently well-preserved; on the other hand, to some extent, there is a break in continuity in consciousness of personhood, such that two personalities, very different from each other, override each other'; yet later (p. 191), again on the 'second state' he writes: 'Interrupted continuity in consciousness of personality is totally lacking here, and appears only temporarily during the recovery period.' Probably he was pointing to a contrast found amongst 'second state' patients, but gives little sign that he is actually making a contrast. In L33 (p. 241), what he writes seems to be repetitious: 'If … we must acknowledge confused mania as an independent clinical picture, and find its essential sign as an increase of the intrapsychic hyperfunction to the point of incoherent flight of ideas, we cannot consider it accidental, that such conditions tend to occur especially after severe attacks of confused mania or agitated confusion'. Occasionally sentences seem incorrectly phrased, as in L19 (p. 119), where the German reads: '*erfolgt das Abklingen der Phoneme in der Weise, daß die Kranken nicht mehr deutlich sprechen, sondern nur ein Flüstern hören*'. We translate this literally as: 'the phonemes fade out in such a way that patients no longer speak clearly but hear only a whisper.' Surely what he meant was 'the phonemes fade out in such a way that patients no longer hear clear speech but only a whisper.'

There are also some signs of Wernicke's haste in preparing *Grundriss.* In L6 (p. 34), his usual greeting to the class 'Mein Herren!' is abbreviated to 'M.H.'; and in L39, the greeting is omitted. In the later lectures, some clinical descriptions are synoptic, even to the extent of not being fully formed sentences; and his index included a few index items, but no corresponding page numbers.

Probably this reflected the pressured existence which he had to maintain, making perfection of written style a minor concern; and also a note-format may have been habitual amongst busy clinicians, then, as now. In L32 (p. 228) much of the last paragraph is in note form, but we expand it, to form full sentences. On p. 230 we render such a fragmentary section as accurately as possible in translation. Presumably he is reporting straight from Dr Kemmler's notes. In Wernicke's index, it seemed that some items did not refer to the page he had assigned for them.

Ambiguity about whether views expressed during clinical demonstrations were the patients' views or his own has already been mentioned. Usually it does not matter; but a 100 years later a little clarification may be needed. In L29 (p. 199), we read: 'At times she showed a feeling of anxiety, which severely disturbed her sleep because of her thoughts'; and in L35 (p. 246) he writes: 'Stress and many sleeping drugs were given as the cause of the illness': Of course, sleeplessness, while no doubt accompanied by vigorous thoughts, probably has its own causes, at the level of brain biology, rather than in the realm of thought content, or 'stress'. In L34 (p. 246), our translation reads: 'When she closes her eyes, she sees bright colours. She must be watched, when she closes her eyes'. Here there is a sharp juxtaposition of a clinician's identification of a symptom (based on a patient's report), and the patients self-referential statement.

Wernicke clearly kept abreast of contemporary developments in other centres: He was well aware of developments in Vienna, where he had studied, as well as other German-speaking centres, including Prague, mentioning Arnold Pick, who he met in 1875 when they had both worked under Westphal in Berlin [15]. There appears to have been on-going dialogue with Freud (section VIII,(s) 'Wernicke's Distinctive Clinical Concepts in Psychiatry'—*Wernicke's Links to the Emerging Dynamic Tradition in Psychiatry*). His awareness of developments in Paris include several mentions of Charcot, and L7 mentions a 'recent case' described by him. Since Charcot died in August 1893, this was unchanged from the 1894 edition. Other references to French researchers of the time include Magnan (L17) as well as a Esquirol, a pioneer of an earlier generation (L19). It is not clear that he knew of the work of Pierre Janet, who, although working at *Hôpital de la Salpêtrière* in Paris during the period when *Grundriss* was written, was not so well known, and was at this time no longer focusing on hysteria [16]. Some of Wernicke's ideas, notably the division between positive and negative symptoms, and on hierarchical organization in the brain were similar to those of his English contemporary, the neuropsychiatrist, John Hughlings Jackson (L2; L11, p. 66; etc.). Both were fluent practitioners in areas where psychiatry and neurology intersect. There is no evidence of direct influence of Jackson, and none of the sources he cites were in the English language. A few are in French; one assumes that Wernicke could not read English papers.

Academic disputes are normal amongst researchers, and not always gentlemanly. Wernicke's style in controversy seems to have been quite generous, sometimes with touches of gentle humour. In L17 (note), after giving his views on his French rival, Dr Magnan, he adds: 'I am delighted to be able to state that in my critical opinion of Magnan's teaching I have encountered heat. But furthermore, I believe that in the fundamental ideas that he expresses in his important book on the delusion of querulousness, despite all the polemic directed against me, I perceive that I detect a pleasing agreement.' He also writes 'Works of an eminent French psychiatrist, Magnan, have drawn us, even here in Germany, in his direction, in the back-and-forth swirl of public opinion': The hint at enduring hostility between Germany and France can be understood, given that Wernicke had been a surgeon during the Franco-Prussian war. His generosity of spirit, does not prevent his making wry jokes over national difference. In L4 (p. 22), he writes: 'Not everyone is a Shakespeare, but you will be surprised when we soon pass to the other extreme (among civilized nations!): the vocabulary of an English seaman does not exceed a few hundred'. (The exclamation mark is Wernicke's.) In L30 (p. 207), he writes: 'The consequence of self-knowledge of this is a state of pathological indifference and inner emptiness, whose prototype is the blasé attitude, the renowned 'spleen' of the

English.' Metaphorical use of the word 'spleen' has shifted over time—for Shakespeare, it was 'irritable'; in eighteenth and nineteenth century England, 'hypochondriacal' or 'hysterical', or 'in bad humour'; and today, 'prone to outbursts of anger'. It is not quite clear what Wernicke thought to be typical English traits, but he seems not to be paying any compliments!

In L17 Wernicke has sharply critical words directed against the concept of *Paranoia chronica simplex.* This refers to one of four types of paranoia proposed by Theodor Ziehen [17], then about 30 years old, but who is not named. Wernicke's target may have been more senior, perhaps Otto Binswanger at Jena, under whom Ziehen was working at the time. In L33 (p. 236) there is milder criticism on a matter of terminology. Ziehen later became professor in Halle in 1903, 1 year before being replaced by Wernicke. From 1897, they jointly edited *Monatsschrift für Psychiatrie und Neurologie,* and Ziehen published an eloquent and generous obituary therein at the time of Wernicke's death. Even with those who took opposed positions on basic philosophy, he is generous. Heinrich Neumann preceded Wernicke as director of the institution in Breslau (with Wernicke as his assistant) until the latter's death, and was one of the last *Psychiker* psychiatrists, and opponent of Griesinger [18]. Despite their having opposed philosophies for mental disorder, Wernicke has no hesitation in citing and commending his work, in preference to his own mentor, Meynert (L19, p. 124). The gentlemanly approach to rival research *personalities* shifts to a sharper tone, when dealing with *issues*, especially in L17, those of classification. Following his cautioning trainees against over-hasty diagnosis of mental illness without firm evidence of symptoms (beginning 'I cannot emphasize strongly enough …') he continues (pp. 101–102): 'The "general impression" sometimes relied on even by better-known representatives of our profession, when they fail to elicit definite psychotic symptoms, is no better than everyday parlance and must elicit the deepest suspicion, when used as the basis of diagnosis of a paranoid state. It deserves to be rejected most strongly when, in cases of this kind, the claim is made that we are dealing with a well-known, and relatively simple disease state which is given the accurate name of *Paranoia chronica simplex.* Then it is easy to arouse the impression of intentional deception, for both judges and lay people, thereby harming the reputation of the entire alienist profession.'

The anonymous acknowledgment in the Foreword of Wernicke's 1894 edition is sometimes taken to refer to Theodor Meynert, his former mentor. It is thus interesting to see how Meynert is cited. (See [19] for a recent appraisal of Meynert's scientific work.) Certainly Meynert is the most cited of all researchers in *Grundriss.* In L1 to L8, he is mentioned with non-specific praise. So, in L1 we read 'Work of men like Griesinger, H. Neumann, Kahlbaum, Meynert, Emminghaus and many others, has not been in vain'; 'Psychiatry today enjoys more general recognition, and this would have been welcomed as progress by a thinker like Meynert in his time.' In L2 (note), the reader is referred to the collection of Meynert's 'popular scientific treatises'. Sometimes he is cited as having established what by Wernicke's time had become basic facts about the nervous system: 'We learned from Meynert that voluntary muscles and sense organs are linked with the cerebral cortex by conducting pathways that extend, in physiological continuity, through the brain, the spinal cord, and the peripheral nervous system. Meynert named the aggregate of these pathways, where the 'law of isolated conduction' predominates, the *projection system*' (L1). Meynert's conceptualization of faculties remaining after transection at the level of the cerebral peduncle is mentioned in L5, and his classification of movements, into 'defence' and 'attack' is cited several times. Sometimes his analogies are cited. (Meynert, polymath that he was, included poetry amongst his talents, so naturally thought in terms of vivid metaphors [20]) The 'enclosed pipe system' (L4) as an analogy for the entirety of associative processes is Meynert's, as is the analogy between human and mollusc (L5). Occasionally Meynert's hypotheses are mentioned, for instance, in L5 (p. 29), that intestinal sensation might be represented in 'the ganglia of the striatum', or that the thalamus was a central station for all sensory pathways

(L19, p. 123). A few distinctive phrases and concepts originate with Meynert. For instance Meynert used the metaphorical phrase 'a train of thought', which goes back centuries, into psychiatric vocabulary, describing his own thought processes (L19, p. 123). It was conceived to have a clear physical basis in the cerebral cortex. In L31 (p. 215) Wernicke writes: 'In my introduction, I developed the idea that a strictly terminated train of thought is the result of practice and training, that is, of functional acquisition' (see also L33, p. 236: 'closed thought'). These lines probably refer to Meynert's 'enclosed pipe' metaphor.

The most distinctive concept Wernicke attributes to Meynert is 'primary Ego' (*das 'Ich'*), dependent especially on the sense of corporeality (L5, L17). In the first few lectures on chronic conditions, the only mention of Meynert is to this concept (L17). In later lectures he is more ambivalent and nuanced in appreciation of Meynert, certainly not seeing him as an irrefutable authority. In L30 (p. 213) we read: 'Even in the clinical lectures of Meynert, to whom we owe so much, you will find this clinical picture [melancholia] defined far too broadly'. In L33 Wernicke mentions Meynert several times, showing how his own associationism grew from similar, though less well-formulated views of Meynert. According to Meynert (L33, p. 236), there was a direct link between local cerebral blood flow and associative activity in the brain. The more the cerebral arteries narrowed and restricted blood supply, the less associative activity could occur in regions supplied [21]. According to him, active brain tissue attracted higher blood flow to supply nutritional needs—an uncanny forerunner of principles on which functional imaging is based today—as in the following quotation: 'If we accept Fechner's theory, that the cortical images and their connections may be stimulated to one of two variable degrees of intensity, and that in any particular mental act those images which are actively utilized stand above the threshold of consciousness while others remain below the level of consciousness, then accepting this theory, we may interpret it to mean that elements bearing processes standing above this level exhibit a greater nutritive attraction than those elements which are not then called into play' [22]. This highly metaphorical—and partly vitalistic—account by Meynert of the formation of associations is an analogy with 'attraction', possibly magnetic, or of 'animal magnetism' (whose popularity was still remembered). It applied at both cellular ('molecular') and mass levels to account for strengthening of connections between co-active cortical sites. Wernicke's version was more precise, and in the fullness of time, became a testable hypothesis.

In L33 Wernicke's expresses his sincere, but nuanced appreciation of his former mentor as follows (L33, p. 240): 'I have repeatedly indicated how important I consider Meynert's clinical lectures to be; in my opinion, they have provided the foundation for better understanding of the symptomatology of acute mental illnesses. However, it must be expressly stated that Meynert also succumbed to the general fate of other authors, who have laboured hard on their monographs in certain provinces, in our discipline … Nevertheless, the chapter on amentia is of lasting value for all time, and indicates the greatest advance psychiatry has made clinically since Kahlbaum's work on catatonia, since it contains the first real theory of mental illnesses and especially of acute psychoses, founded on hypotheses derived entirely from the condition of the affected organ'. In L36, he is mentioned again in relation to the hypothesis about local blood flow, which Wernicke hardly believes, and his 'celebrated optic thalamus case'. In L37, an issue of classification of progressive paralysis (acute vs. chronic) is mentioned where Wernicke does not quite agree with Meynert. He also mentions Meynert's system for cortical lamination, and—with high praise—his data on brain weight in various conditions. In L38 he compliments Meynert on his findings about hydrocephalus internus. L40, on dementia, he is sometimes critical, sometimes full of praise, and in L41, Meynert's hyperaemia notion is mentioned again. Overall, from this survey of Wernicke's citations of Meynert, it is hard to believe that it was the latter to whom the anonymous acknowledgment was made, given the terms in which it was expressed.

What about Emil Kraepelin, his real rival? In L34 (p. 256), dealing with akinetic motility psychoses Wernicke writes: '… in Kraepelin's textbook, dementia is described as the regular outcome for such cases. Here, as well as elsewhere, we come across little by way of thought, plus an ignorance of facts, which features are arguably unsuited to a textbook. Moreover, the tendency to recurrence, emphasized by Kraepelin, is in no way greater than in most other acute psychoses'. It was probably the textbook to which he refers (L28, p. 192) with the words: 'as I constantly regret, it is impossible for me to recommend to you one of the best-known textbooks of psychiatry for your private studies'. Here for the only time, Wernicke 'takes off his kid gloves' in opposing a rival. This is the most specific and potent personal attack on any of his colleagues or rivals to be found in *Grundriss*.

There is one other striking sentence (L31, p. 221): 'When attacks of recurrent mania finally outweigh in duration the lucid intervals, they do not turn into a chronic mania, at least not in the strict meaning of the term, *that I alone can defend*'. (Emphasis added here.) Clearly, Wernicke knew that in some of his views, he *was* a lone voice.

V. Contemporary Knowledge in Neuroscience; Contemporary Practice in General Medicine and Psychiatry in Wernicke's Day

Wernicke's *Grundriss* contains much detailed description in the clinical lectures, but, throughout, he attempts to explain what he saw, on the basis of neuroscience of the day. To understand the strengths and weaknesses of his attempts, it is important to understand what he knew, and, just as important, what he did not know about structure and function of nerve cells, nervous tissue, functional organization of the brain, and the state of clinical knowledge at the time. In this section, common knowledge, and prevalent misunderstandings are described. Wernicke's own contributions come later.

Basic neuroscience: In1894 Wernicke would have known of the neurone theory, for which Santiago Ramón y Cajal and Camille Golgi were jointly awarded the Nobel Prize in 1906. Their conclusion, that nervous tissue consists of discrete cells, not a syncytium, was developed between 1887 (when Cajal learned Golgi's staining method) and 1894 (when Cajal gave the Croonian lecture, focusing on cortical pyramidal cells). Other staining methods in neurohistology were that of Nissl (mentioned in L41, p. 323) which stains neuronal cell bodies (the 'Nissl' granules in their cytoplasm) but not axons or dendrites, and that of Weigert to stain myelin deep blue, with degenerating portions yellow, and another of his methods to stain neuroglial cells. The distinction between neurones and glial cells was well understood in Wernicke's day, as well as some of the subtypes of glial cells, since, in L37 (p. 291) he writes: 'We have observed the occurrence *en masse*, of giant astrocytes; and indeed they correspond to the more recent stage, seen temporarily soon after loss of neuronal tissue'. In L4 (p. 24) 'fusiform' (spindle-shaped) cells in the visual cortex are mentioned. This probably refers to a classification of cell types by von Kölliker [23], long before the Golgi method was in use. Wernicke suggests that their existence 'contradicts our intuition to accept nerve fibres that cannot prove their origin from any nerve cell', implying that aspects of Cajal's neurone doctrine were not yet fully resolved.

In L16 (note) we also read '… we see only *remnants* of pathological change in the organ of association: That is, growth of glia. Of epoch-making importance in this regard is the work of C. Weigert [24] … We would hope that a pathological anatomy of psychoses may be built from this.' The role of glial cells in neuropathology, especially the proliferation of some types of glia, was not proven until the 1920s. However, it was shown by the Romanian, Georges Marinesco (1863–1938) that non-neuronal cells acted as phagocytes, removing remnants of injured or dying cells [25]. This was published in 1900, but may have been known earlier; and Wernicke may have been alluding to this.

With regard to signals carried by nerve cells, there was *some* crucial knowledge, but many gaps. In L1 the *law of isolated conduction* (initially proposed for the peripheral nervous system, but implicitly applying to the central nervous system) is mentioned. This states that signals remain isolated in each axon, despite transmission over long distances [26]. This extended Johannes Peter Müller's *Law of Specific Energies*, which stated that the function and subjective impact of activity in a nerve pathway depends on what it is connected to, rather than what initiated the activity (be it a sensory stimulus, applied electrical or chemical stimulus, or whatever). Conduction velocity in peripheral nerves had been measured in 1850 by Helmholz, but nothing was known of conduction time in central axons. In L5 (p. 26), in developing a 'thought experiment' Wernicke writes 'Sensations would, as before, reach consciousness, but with a slight delay caused by the longer pathway.' He was thus aware of conduction time in axons as a significant variable, but could not use this in explanatory reasoning. Nothing was known of the physical basis of axonal conduction. The all-or-none law was known to hold for cardiac contraction from work of Bowditch at Harvard Medical School in 1871, but that it applied to axonal conduction was accepted only in 1909, from results of Keith Lucas [27]. This indicates that signal transmission in axons is independent of the energetics for generating signals. Wernicke's ignorance of this was part of the context which enabled him to develop the imaginative (but incorrect) sejunction hypothesis. Chemical transmission was a completely unknown principle.

Basic neuroanatomy of the brain had advanced in decades before *Grundriss.* In L1 a term used by Wernicke (after Meynert) was *the projection system,* a metaphor derived from optics. We read of 'the fact of physiological continuity, if not anatomical continuity' in such pathways. This refers to cytological findings of Cajal. Knowledge about cranial nerves went back a long way, but there were still uncertainties, even over their exact number, and details such as the exact innervation of the tongue for touch and taste. At the time of writing much was known about ciliary nerves (long and short)—the visceral innervation of the eye itself (as opposed to the retina)—most of which knowledge went back to the eighteenth century [28]. L6 touches on the possibility that there is position sense in the eyeball, transmitted via the ciliary nerves.

The laminar layout of the cerebral cortex was first described by Bailarger, with more detailed description provided by Meynert; but terminology was not settled. References to cortical laminae include: 'the cortical layer (or layers) immediately adjacent to white matter would represent consciousness of corporeality'. ('*Die schichtenweise Übereinanderlagerund der Ganglienzellen der Hirnrinde begünstigt eine solche Annahme wonach die der Markleiste nächste Schicht (bzw die nächsten Schichten) das Bewusstsein der Körperlichkeit repräsentieren würden*)' (L5, p. 30). We also read 'the most superficial cortical lamina, that which Meynert identified as the first, purely grey lamina' (L37, p. 290), presumably lamina II, in modern terminology.

The French edition of Cajal's *Histologie du Système Nerveux de L'Homme et des Vertébrés* was published in 1909–1911, and was already known in its Spanish version in 1905 (*Textura del sistema nervioso del hombre y de los vertebrados*, vol. 1, published in Madrid in 1899; complete in 1904). These works do not use the modern 6-layer terminology. Later in L37 (p. 290) we read 'Cell loss in these cases did not extend continuously over the cortex, but came in irregularly distributed patches, and involved mainly layers of densely arranged, small pyramids, arranged in rows, and increasing in size inwards, in other words, Meynert's second and third layer': This refers to laminae now known to be major origins of cortico-cortical axons (although some descending axons were identified). This point is relevant to Wernicke's view of the cortex as the 'organ of association', and of mental disorder involving disruption in such connections.

In 1905, it was unclear whether taste and smell had their own cortical projection area (L5, p. 26). Wernicke occasionally refers to the basal ganglia (although terms he uses leave doubt about which structures he means). Karl Friedrich Burdach (1776–1847) provided the first account of the anatomy of the basal ganglia [29]. Nothing was known of their function, but there were many ideas, including Meynert's (L5, p. 29), that the 'corpus striatum' (*Ganglien des Streifen*) represented intestinal sensation. It is unlikely that uncertain whether this refers either to 'the striatum' (part of the basal ganglia) or to the 'nucleus basalis of Meynert'. Meynert was also the first to suggest that Parkinson's disease might arise due to abnormality there [30]. In the 1880s, Hermann Nothnagel (1841–1905) named the striatum *nodus cursorius,* implying a role in locomotion. Motor functions of the basal ganglia became known early in twentieth century, and wider aspects of their function were revealed later.

Wernicke refers to several issues about central nervous function. In L3, in analyzing the difference between perceptual and memory images he mentions visual after-images as a model of the former. His statement that after-images arise in retinal ganglion cells is incorrect: Classical after-images, such as seeing an orange spot after staring at a blue light, or a black (sometimes white) spot after staring at white light is due to saturation of pigments in photoreceptors [31]. In L5 (p. 29) he assumes that the ability to locate the source of a sound reflects processes in the inner ear ('organ of Corti'), but we now know this to depend on comparison in the brainstem of timing of sounds from the two ears.

Important principles of functional organization were well known. The concept of reflex action was important for both neuroscientists and clinicians, but the emphasis was different from today: Supposedly automatic reflex action was easily extended to include psychic processes, for instance by Russian physiologists Ivan Sechenov, and I.P.Pavlov, and in Austria, by a young Sigmund Freud. This was easier then than now, because it was less clear that reflex action was independent of conscious awareness (with support from the philosophy of psycho-physical parallelism). In psychiatry, Kahlbaum [32] formalized this with terms such as 'centripetal', 'intracentral', and 'centrifugal' for the stages of 'psychic functions' [33]. In L34 (p. 236) Wernicke refers to 'reflex excitability of cutaneous capillaries': This probably refers to the cutaneous 'flare response' or 'axon flare reflex', responding to sharp mechanical stimuli such as scratching. That it was an involved local axonal conduction, but no central transmission or integration was known since 1889, as described by Sokovnin and Rozhansky, and apparently discovered as early as 1873 [34].

Early in his career Wernicke made major contributions to the concept of cerebral localization of function. Orderly representation of sensory surfaces and motor control in the cerebral cortex (somatotopy, retinotopy', etc) was well understood, although in a simpler way than today. Larger principles of organization linked basic neuroscience to clinical topics. In L5 (p. 27), writing on protective reflexes, he compares humans to lower vertebrates: 'Where a large cerebral hemisphere is present, as in mammals, and more so in humans, we see similar mechanisms of movement transferred to central projection fields of the cerebral cortex (as shown experimentally by Munk for eye movements)' This is similar to ideas of Hughlings Jackson (1835–1911), and before him, of Herbert Spencer, who, in 1855 had published 'The Principles of Psychology' [35]. Their view, based on evolutionary doctrine, was that the central nervous system has a hierarchy of levels, reflex activity being the lowest. Related ideas were promoted by Meynert [22], for whom mental illness arose due to conflict between cerebral cortex and sub-cortical regions (a view still widely held today).

Bacteriology and Infectious Disease: Advances in bacteriology in years immediately prior to publication of *Grundriss* provided a new model of disease. Researchers in psychiatry saw a potential cause for disorders in their own field. 'Phthisis' is mentioned several times in *Grundriss*, a term implying no more than a 'wasting disease' (as did 'consumption'), qualified, in English, as 'pulmonary phthisis'. The name tuberculosis was given by Schoenlein (1793–1864), based on characteristic lesions—tubercles—seen in the lungs *post mortem*. The term 'phthisis' was used well into the twentieth century, and was used by Wernicke (pp. 294, 296), but sometimes he used the German term *Lungenschwindsucht*. Discovery by Robert Koch of the corresponding micro-organism, *Mycobacterium tuberculosis*, dated from 1882.

Knowledge of the symptoms of tetanus after wounds went back to antiquity. That it was caused by a bacterial toxin was proven in 1884 by Arthur Nicolaier (1862–1942). The bacterium responsible (*Clostridium tetani*), its transmissibility, and its role in producing symptoms of tetanus were discovered in the 1890s; and by 1897, an antitoxin had been produced, giving immunity. In L34 (p. 296) catatonic rigidity is compared to tetanus. The diphtheria toxin was discovered in 1890 by Emil Adolf von Behring (first Nobel laureate for physiology and medicine) working in Marburg [36]. The idea that bacterial toxins could cause mental illnesses appears often in writings of Wernicke and Kraepelin. Discovery of the spirochete in 1903, in experiments on monkeys by Metchnikoff and Roux, and the development of the Wassermann test in 1906 clarified the fact that syphilitic disease could take many forms. Prior to this, diagnosis had been based solely on clinical evidence, as in most of psychiatry to this day. Epidemics of 'dengue fever', mentioned in L28 (p. 190) were long known to occur in tropical and subtropical regions. Its transmission by mosquitoes was known from 1906, and its viral aetiology from 1907.

Neurology: There are several references to advances in neurology in *Grundriss*. Wernicke mentions 'degenerative neuritis'. In L1 he refers to the fact, already known, that peripheral neuropathies can lead to differential loss of sensory vs. motor function, or of specific types of somatic sensation. Many manifestations of syphilis were well-known to neurologists; but at the time of revising *Grundriss*, it was not clear that GPI was syphilitic; it was seen as a mental rather than a neurological disorder (in so far as the two were distinguished) [37]. Several clinical tests were devised in the context of syphilis: In one, the Romberg test (L37, p. 229), a standing patient is asked to close his or her eyes. Loss of balance indicates that the contribution of proprioception to balance is compromised. The test was devised as early as 1840 by the Berlin-based neurologist Moritz Heinrich Romberg (1795–1873), to diagnose *Tabes dorsalis* (L36, p. 280), an aspect of neurosyphilis in which axons in the dorsal columns of spinal cord are lost, leading to differential loss of discriminative somatic sensation. *Tabes* had been named as early as 1836 and given a full description by Duchenne in 1858. It was shown to be late-stage syphilis in 1885 by Jean Alfred Fournier (1832–1914), who suggested that GPI ('Progressive Paralysis' in Wernicke's terms) was syphilitic in origin. However, when Wernicke was writing, this appears not to have been fully accepted [38]. Another test involved pupillary reflexes and Wernicke refers (L37, p. 280), to 'rigidity' of pupillary reflexes, termed 'Argyll Robertson pupil' in the English-speaking world [39]: The accommodation reflex was intact, while the light reflex was lost. Argyll Robertson, a Scottish-trained physician studied in Prague and Berlin, and identified the syndrome in 1863, calling it 'spinal miosis'. In fact, none of the pupillary reflexes (light reflex, accommodation reflex, and papillary dilatation) involve spinal pathways. Wernicke's qualifying phrase—'the *so-called* column disease'—suggests he was referring to a named syndrome, rather than to symptoms arising strictly in the spinal cord. Only later was it found to be an early sign of general CNS involvement in neurosyphilis. It is now rare in the developed world.

A major issue, mentioned throughout *Grundriss*, was what was called 'Progressive Paralysis' ('of the Insane': [40]). (Today 'Progressive Paralysis' has a different meaning, referring to several clearly defined neurological conditions.) Mainly, progressive paralysis is another manifestation of neurosyphilis. In 1894 Wernicke was unlikely to have known that it was part of a sexually transmitted disease, caused by an identifiable micro-organism. When revising the 1906 edition he *could* have known of the 1903 finding, but detailed discussion of Progressive Paralysis occurs in one of the last lectures (L37), so any revision he may have intended was forestalled by his death. There is however no hint of the finding in earlier lectures. Indeed, in L17 (p. 103) he separates syphilis from Progressive Paralysis, referring to '… disease of the posterior columns [attacked] by alcoholism and syphilis and, finally, the most famous type, of progressive paralysis …'. In L36 (p. 280) he draws a contrast between *Tabes* and syphilis and in L37 (p. 286) discusses the differential diagnosis between Progressive Paralysis and syphilis. However, he seems to have suspected *some* relationship, since this lecture, focusing on paralytic disorders, makes reference to syphilis, and sometimes implies sexual transmission. Likewise, in L35 (p. 262) he writes 'When a mild degree of somnolence is mixed in, a special subgroup among such cases [of paralysis] seems to be defined, which, to judge by the results of specific therapy, should be grouped among the luetic brain diseases' ('Luetic': venereal—sexually transmitted). He also mentions that paralytic attacks were sometimes accompanied by fever (although that might have been due to another infection impacting on the CNS, or simply to the mental disorder itself—as mentioned in L41). In L36 (p. 280) he applies the word 'bacterial' to syphilis, implying perhaps that symptoms were caused by a bacterial toxin. Despite his not understanding the origin of Progressive Paralysis from syphilitic infection, he clearly recognized that it was a chronic, progressive illness, with many mental symptoms (L36, p. 285). He may have suspected it to have a bacterial in origin, involving a different agent, but could not have known that overt syphilis, progressive paralysis, and other manifestations of syphilis had a common aetiology. After 1906, it might have been too easy to dismiss unexplained symptoms as syphilitic: Other neuropsychiatric syndromes are described in *Grundriss* which were not otherwise recognized for many decades, when there could be no confusion with syphilis.

Reference to specific brain disorders includes *Parkinson's disease* and its festinating gait (L34 [p. 245]: 'This movement accelerates in a manner similar to propulsion in *Paralysis agitans*'). *Dyskinesias*—involuntary movements of mouth and tongue—are described (L19, p. 120) although Wernicke attributes them to vivid taste hallucinations in patients with general paralysis. *Landry's paralysis* (L27, p. 182) first described in 1859 by the French physician, Jean Baptiste Octave Landry de Thézillat [41], was known later as the *Guillain–Barré–Stohl syndrome*, after a publication in 1916 by Georges Guillain and Jean Alexande Barré. In modern definition it is an autoimmune condition of myelin sheaths, limited to peripheral nerves, often triggered by infection. In Wernicke's day, it was not separated from other polyneuropathies; and those due to thiamine deficiency could also affect the CNS. In L27 (p. 182), he refers to flaccid paralysis, absent tendon reflexes, and muscles sensitized to pressure. These symptoms are found in polyneuritis due to in thiamine deficiency. However, he writes: 'Oddly enough, I have never seen such severe cases of polyneuritis accompanied by polyneuritic psychosis'. The latter term, refers to CNS involvement; he hints at his suspicion of differences between the two syndromes.

Epileptic seizures are first mentioned occasionally in early lectures, and are dealt with in greater depth in L24 and L38. The full range of epileptic phenomena was not well documented in the 1890s. Hughlings Jackson's classification separated Petit-mal from Grand-mal, but included Vertigo [42, 43]. In L37 (p. 284) we read '… a specific muscle area such as the faciolingual region is affected, the onslaught then spreading further with familiar regularity'. This reminds one of Jackson's report of 1863, on the 'march of epilepsy', from which he inferred orderly representation of body parts in the brain; and the cortical region involved was known by 1875 [44]. Notably, Wernicke, who inferred this principle from other evidence, does not cite Jackson. He may have been unaware of his work, given that Jackson's most important papers on it were in journals which were probably inaccessible in Germany [45, 46]. The Asylum reports in which the later publication appeared became the journal *Brain*. In European centres, differentiation of epilepsy from hysteria was much-debated [16] and the word 'seizure' was used for both. Charcot was the first to attempt to distinguish the two, but differentiation was not easy in Wernicke's time. For instance, in L28, the so-called 'second state' could arise equally from hysterical or epileptic attacks. Wernicke's term 'hystero-epileptics' (L19, p. 122) presumably refers to what are now called 'pseudoseizures' or 'psychogenic convulsions'.

Wernicke mentions 'general weakness of memory' in L7 (p. 40; and in L8) where he describes early stages of a disorder akin to what came to be called Alzheimer's disease. In 1907, 2 years after Wernicke's death, Alois Alzheimer, of Kraepelin's institute in Munich, published the first description of the disorder, with details of neuropathology, after the patient he had studied for 5 years had died, and been subjected to autopsy. Clearly clinical aspects of Alzheimer's disease were known at the time of Wernicke's death; and the 'plaques' had also been described already by Marinesco [25], but not linked to dementia.

In L14 (p. 87) Wernicke refers to confabulation as '… the *positive* form of falsification of memory', described as 'incoherence in contents of consciousness', linked to "memory disturbance"'. A reference to Kraepelin is dated 1887, also the year of the doctoral thesis of S.S.Korsakoff in Moscow, defining what came to be called 'Korsakoff's psychosis'. This is related to chronic alcoholism and vitamin deficiency, prominent features of which are loss of memory for recent events and confabulation, with intact long-term memory. Since the vitamin deficiency caused both this and peripheral nerve problems, the syndrome was also called *Polyneuritic psychosis* in *Grundriss* (e.g. L26, p. 174). Regardless of whether Kraepelin or Korsakoff claims priority, Kraepelin's major contribution to the concept came later (1913), when it was identified as a feature of *paraphrenia* (see [47]).

Clinical Psychiatry: A phrase in L25 (p. 168); ('… if you follow the practical advice for clinical analysis …'), may imply that guidelines were taught in medical schools on ways to advance clinical knowledge. It is not clear whether this refers to psychiatry or more widely. It implies recognition that research and routine practice, for many practitioners were inseparable endeavours, unlike today. In any event, in Wernicke's day psychiatry was seen as an advancing frontier. With regard to then-current knowledge of clinical psychiatry, we start with general concepts, moving on to specific disease entities or prototype diagnoses.

Separation of positive from negative symptoms in psychiatry developed before Wernicke's day, being first proposed, in the context of childhood convulsions, by John Russell Reynolds in 1861 [48], and extended by Hughlings Jackson in 1881 to apply to neurological symptoms more generally. For Jackson, following the distinction was based on the hierarchical concept of brain organization, so that positive symptoms reflected release from inhibition coming from higher levels. In psychiatry, the same concept goes back to Meynert: (L33, p. 240): 'You can judge how far Meynert approximates the standpoint that I have always advocated in these demonstrations, from the fact that he always places in the foreground symptoms of functional deficit, that is the different grades of weakening of associations, and he considers symptoms of irritation to be a consequence of these.' These ideas appear as early as L2, where we read: 'absence of reactive movements is often just as characteristic and as valuable a symptom as their pathological modification'; and in L11 (p. 67) '… all changes in content of consciousness can then be likened to focal symptoms, and will behave just as do more familiar focal symptoms of brain diseases; but these naturally, will have a different clinical "weighting" depending on whether they correspond with the stimulus state or the paralysis state'; in L12 (p. 72) 'deficit symptoms' are contrasted with 'irritant symptoms'; in L14 positive and negative 'falsifications of memory' are separated (confabulation, vs. 'quasi-amnesia'). In L19 (p. 123) the idea is mentioned that the cerebral cortex can suppress subcortical activity, notably in the basal ganglia; and symptoms arise as release phenomena when such inhibition fails. The idea has been used often since then in accounts of symptomatology; yet we now know that, with minor exceptions, long-axons cortical neurones projecting to the basal ganglia are excitatory.

Another concept which Wernicke took from the past was that there are 'times of special vulnerability for development of various diseases of consciousness' (L5, p. 30). This derives from Kahlbaum, who proposed [49], in 1863 that certain psychiatric disorders tend to occur during transitional periods of life. The idea is developed in most detail in L38 where we read (p. 294) that 'times of normal physical change, such as puberty, menopause, and finally senescence, are particularly likely to predispose to onset of psychoses'.

The concept of 'degeneration' loomed large in social and psychiatric thought in late nineteenth century. The term (German: *Entartete*) was introduced by Griesinger, but its persistence had several origins; harmful effects of urbanization during the industrial revolution, concepts of social Darwinism and then biological evolution more generally, greater awareness of historical change of societies (as in Edward Gibbons' *Decline and Fall of the Roman Empire*), in psychiatry Benedict Morel's *Treatise on Degeneration,* and in forensic areas, Cesare Lombroso's writings on criminality in relation to anthropology. Valentin Mangan (1835–1916) developed the degeneration concept in a supposed evolutionary and genetic context, and published with Paul Sérieux, in 1892, *Le délire chronique a évolution systématique* ('Chronic delirium with systematic evolution'). The concept was losing currency by the outbreak of World War I, but can yet be seen as a precursor to both Kraepelin's *Dementia praecox* (for which by definition, full recovery was not possible), and later of eugenicist ideology adopted in Germany and elsewhere (with the word 'degenerate' [*entartete*] figuring prominently in propaganda of the Third Reich, especially in relation to art and music). Wernicke is scathing about the glib way in which the concept was sometimes used, as in L17 (p. 104) where we read of how other authors regarded 'chronic paranoia ... separate from all other mental illnesses, and the so-called degeneration, acknowledging the latter to have only one aetiology. He *does* sometimes use the term in a stricter sense, for instance in the context of alcoholism, or documented degeneration of nerve fibres. Only once does he use the word in a more prejudicial sense, when he hints that it occurs across generations in families, for instance, in L38 (p. 294): 'Appearance of degeneration, which can be followed in many families ...' He also refers to 'neurotic degeneration' (L30, p. 195; L31, p. 211), the exact meaning of which for him is unclear.

On genetics, clinicians routinely asked about family history. So, in L14 (p. 88) we read '... a strong family predisposition to mental illness was established in this middle-aged man'. Founding principles of genetics based on Gregor Mendel's work in the 1860s were not well known, and systematic study of the inheritance of mental disorders was some way in the future. Wernicke considered hereditary tendencies in most detail in L38 (p. 297 *seq.*). There is not so much as a hint of eugenicist notions, although such ideas had roots going back some years earlier, at least in Britain; and in Switzerland, Auguste Forel advocated such ideas [50]. On one occasion (L38, p. 297) he ventures on the difficult area where genetics and (social) environmental influences interact, and where the degeneration held sway (when he suggests that suicidal acts are attributed to effects of suggestion, even when they are familial traits). In L38 he also seems to give way to surrounding prejudices, when he makes passing comments on the social class of some patients with familial mental disorders.

Terms for classes of disorder, syndromes, and symptoms, used in Wernicke's day, are mentioned here. Use of Latin terms, with upper case initial letter for the first, was the style of Carl Linnaeus in his eighteenth century botanical taxonomy, and in the parallel taxonomy for diseases which he also developed in 1763 [51]. Named classes were then taken to be 'natural types', an implicit assumption adopted for diseases in the nineteenth century.

The old term '*melancholy*' appears first in L1, then in L17 (p. 81), and is discussed in detail in L30 as *Affective melancholia.* Two specific concepts come from Kahlbaum: *Hebephrenia,* was taken to be a form of adolescent insanity, mentioned several times in *Grundriss* (L14 [p. 87]; L17 [p. 107], and in detail in L39 and L40). The concept was elaborated by Ewald Hecker (1871) (assistant to Kahlbaum) as an offshoot from the then-new idea that adolescence could be conceptualized as a distinct developmental stage. The term rapidly gained acceptance, to be incorporated into Kraepelin's concept of *Dementia praecox* (following Heinrich Schüle [1880] and Arnold Pick

[1891]) [52, 53]. Today it survives as the 'disorganized' subtype of schizophrenia, or the 'disorganization' dimension of symptoms (although such sub-typing was abandoned in DSM-5). Kraam and Phillips [54], who review the concept, never mention confabulation, although this was widely seen as characteristic of hebephrenic schizophrenia. *Presbyophrenia* (L14; p. 87), a type of 'paraphrenia' (psychosis with onset during a period of transition in elderly people), a concept whose history is reviewed by Berrios [55], is long-abandoned, but is mentioned several times by Wernicke.

Paranoia is a very old concept, with a complex history [56, 57], complicated by popular misunderstandings. While broadly signifying 'delusional', variants focus on whether it is 'monodelusional' as believed today for 'delusional disorder' and advocated by Kraepelin [58]; and on the subject of delusions. Popular understanding today stresses persecutory content. It was divided by Theodor Ziehen ([17]; p. 210), assistant to Otto Binswanger at Jena, *Paranoia chronica simplex* being one of his four types, held to be a distinct disease. Wernicke disliked the term as referring to any disorder, but defined *paranoid states* as 'all those chronic mental disorders where we encounter falsification of content of consciousness' (L11, p. 65).

The term *neurasthenia* originated in New England [59], to become part of medical vocabulary (as 'nervous exhaustion'; L17, p. 106) in Wernicke's time, for instance in L37 (p. 280) when he mentions that tendon reflexes may be increased in neurasthenia. (This was reported by others, for instance by Dejerine and Gauckler [60]). The term is seldom used now in the West, but appears in some Western classification systems, and has greater currency in East Asian medicine.

Two terms appear in Wernicke's footnote (L1, p. 6), and later. *Verbigeration*—the monotonous, usually rhythmical, repetition of one or several words—and *Mutism:* 'By mutism we define the temporary speechlessness of the mentally ill.' These two were subsequently classed as catatonic symptoms, aspects of Kraepelin's *Dementia praecox*. However, Kretschmer, [61] argued that catatonic symptoms—or at least some of them—may be aspects of conversion hysteria. *Mutacismus* is also mentioned in L24 (p. 164), signifying voluntary muteness in mentally ill people, often selective according to circumstance, especially in catatonia.

In L23, under *Anxiety psychosis*, we are given a vivid description of what might also have been termed 'conversion hysteria' by Freud. Wernicke does not use this term, although the phenomenology is described clearly—severe hysterical anxiety leading to distinctive quasi-neurological symptoms (paralysis, sensory losses, etc.), whose detail fits no known neurological pattern. 'Blind thrashing behaviour' (L38, p. 164), seen in patients under extreme stress, is also discussed by Kretschmer [61] using the term 'instinctive motor flurry', which removes an animal from a danger zone only by chance. He hardly regarded it as defensive, but likened it to behaviour of a cornered animal, as did Wernicke. In addition, in L24 (p. 158 *seq.*), Wernicke recalls a case from the late 1870s, which—whatever else might have been present—included major components of delayed war neurosis ('shell-shock', as it came to be called in England), from the Franco-Prussian war. Images of bodily dismemberment probably derived from what he saw as a soldier (*névrose traumatique* and *hystérie traumatique,* according to Charcot). The framework in which Wernicke understood such syndromes would have been quite different from that of clinicians such as Freud (who had debated in 1886 in Vienna whether hysteria could occur in men.) History of the term 'conversion hysteria' since then has been complex. DSM-III abandoned 'hysteria' but kept 'conversion', which, in DSM 5, became 'Functional Neurological Symptom Disorder'. Three ideas may need to be defined (Conversion, Dissociation, Somatization), with but two terms usually recognized in diagnostic systems. DSM-III and DSM-IV separate dissociation from the others; ICD-10 splits somatization from dissociation/conversion.

VI. Wernicke's Underlying Philosophical Views

We come now to unique aspects of Wernicke's thought. In *Grundriss,* our eventual focus, of course, is on clinical issues for psychiatry, which have their own philosophical underpinnings; but underlying these are Wernicke's unique ideas on brain theory, and deeper than this his singular approach to methods and philosophy of science itself. To give a good account of his system of thought it is necessary to start with the latter topics first, and then work towards his special approach in psychiatry.

VI,(a). Wernicke's Adoption of the European Style of Natural Philosophy

Throughout *Grundriss,* we see a distinct contrast to pre-existing medical traditions. Wernicke's approach as a psychiatrist probably *was* unique, but as a scientist, it seems he drew lessons from outside medicine, from the most fundamental science, namely physics, or, to give it its original name, *natural philosophy.* Similarities in both content and method are to be found between much of Wernicke's thought and prevailing traditions of natural philosophy. Striking similarity is also evident, especially in L1–8, with the thought of Ernst Mach, placing Wernicke clearly within European traditions going back to Leibniz, rather than English ones tracing back to Newton. How the similarities with Mach were conveyed to Wernicke we do not know. In any case they support the view that if psychiatry is to be rational, it must be based on concepts as fundamental as those from which natural philosophy itself arose; and psychiatry then differs from most medical disciplines, whose basic concepts are 'givens', derived from elsewhere, requiring no original philosophical or metaphysical thought. (A *caveat* is needed here: Ernst Mach was avowedly *anti-metaphysical*; but this may have been in reaction to the emptiness of German idealist philosophy of the time, rather than a denial of centuries of metaphysical debate preceding and accompanying the birth of the natural sciences.)

At the *methodological* level, there are four striking features about Wernicke's thought. *First,* the author was a firm advocate of reasoning in science, as much in psychiatry as elsewhere. Systematically, he sought *reasons* for relationships between observations. This is typical of physics from its outset, where reasoning was usually mathematical; but it need not be mathematical, as in Wernicke's case. The contrast with biomedicine is that (with notable exceptions) relations between variables is established by statistical inference, which eventually becomes a proxy for causality.

Second, Wernicke is more willing than most biomedical scientists to base arguments on hypotheses about hidden variables, which, at the time, cannot be directly validated, and thus lack direct empirical proof. This is typical of physics, where many hypotheses or variables arose from their value in providing explanations, rather than from direct proof that the variables existed with properties ascribed to them. The archetype for the die-hard medical empiricism is the apostle St. Thomas—a physician—who could not believe in the Resurrection without feeling the holes in Christ's hands. In contrast, Wernicke writes often of 'internal connections' in the brain (information connections, not anatomical ones), which he could never observe directly, but inferred from their effects. So, in L11 (p. 66), we read of the 'indisputable connection', between active mental disturbance and chronic mental disorder in which the active process has subsided; and in L12 (p. 73) we read of 'internal relationship between hallucinations and autochthonous ideas.' In both cases, plausible inferences are made, as a physicist might argue without directly observing the process, or intervening variables. Likewise in L20 (p. 127), he writes: 'Gentlemen! You can see that just by getting to know all the internally connected symptoms puts the significance of the first left temporal convolution in the right light, as the site of 'phonemes', the most common—and you could almost say, the most important—of all the psychotic symptoms'. The same phrase is used in L29 (p. 198) for the relation between autochthonous ideas and phonemes; and in L30 (p. 208) for Affective melancholia and a variety of symptoms; and similarly elsewhere. Occasionally, the inference of hidden connections with explanatory power is applied to *individual* symptomatology, rather than a generic process, as in L38 (p. 283), where we read '... the entire clinical picture could be understood only as a circumscribed autopsychosis based on an overvalued idea': Reliance on unobserved internal processes is linked to his important concept of 'elementary symptoms' (see below), since links between such symptoms and secondary ones involve internal links.

A *third* related feature, is Wernicke's willingness to postulate ideal situations, far removed from any empirical demonstration as 'thought experiments', which aid clarity of thought. This way of thinking connects Wernicke directly to Mach. It was a concept gaining currency in the Germanic world at the time, as *Gedankenexperiment*, about which Mach wrote ('On thought experiments') in 1905 [62]. It is different from medical traditions where strict empiricism tends to rule, and is especially different from modern insistence that every statement be 'evidence-based'. As an example, in L2 he writes: 'If we do not expect a speaker to lead us astray, then we must recognize that in this case, in a normal person, answers will arise in a totally determined manner, to be predicted with approximate accuracy.' He acknowledges that 'total determination' is *not* reality, but uses the conjecture to advance an argument, just as a physicist postulates a 'frictionless surface'. In L5, to bring to life the idea that a person's body (and brain) are also part of the observable external world, he invites the reader to join in such a 'thought experiment', and in L6 to compare humans with molluscs. Other examples are evocative analogies.

The *Fourth,* and perhaps most fundamental similarity to the natural philosophy tradition is Wernicke's approach to validating concepts: When pioneers of the sixteenth and seventeenth century struggled to make rational the study of Nature, their struggle was, in part, to define concepts in a way which supported precise reasoning [63]. Definition and explanation are then interdependent. Proto-scientific pioneers in psychiatry, such as Pinel and Esquirol saw their role as being to describe what they saw, not to explain it. Gradually the emphasis shifted: For Kraepelin, classification (that is definition of concepts) had to come first, presumably on the basis of some sort of authority, and only then could explanation be attempted. Wernicke's approach was different from both. Rather than laying claim to personal authority, he states, early in L1: 'symptoms must be deduced from familiar features of the diseased organ'. By aiming to *deduce* symptoms from more basic knowledge (the only occasion on which the word *abzug* is used in *Grundriss*) he clearly sought explanations as understood in traditions of natural philosophy. There are of course many ways in which subjective experiences can be grouped as named symptoms. His statement appears to state that the groupings *he* recognized were those which could be deduced from actual or potential brain mechanisms, the neurosciences of his day, a procedure closer to that of physicists than of typical medical researchers. This makes him different from most psychiatrists, before or since, and possibly unique. Examples follow later; but as a general statement, he states (L11; p. 69) that 'only as an exception do you find an "objective" observer who experiences just the "foreignness" of emerging thoughts without attaching to them any far-fetched interpretation'. One may ask if, even in principle, description (and therefore classification) of experience can *ever* be wholly separated from interpretation, as Kraepelin wanted: All description uses pre-existing forms, analogies, or vocabulary.

We can now recognize what were the *founding* ***clinical*** *concepts* for Wernicke. The statement just quoted indicates that primary concepts for him were not any supposed disease entity (defined by a range of symptoms, accepted with little deeper analysis, as in Kraepelin's system), but symptoms themselves, as primary experiences, from which any disease entity is derived secondarily. However, with symptoms taken as the starting point, one should rely not on surface appearance, but on deeper understanding, to reveal commonalities, despite surface differences. Here we see interdependence of definition (or descriptive form) and explanation, allowing symptoms to be grouped together and named. We see striking parallels here with the thought of Ernst Mach. Mach's first university experience was teaching medical students (in which he excelled), and he was to make major contributions to analysis of sensory systems, especially the visual system. In important ways, he anticipated ideas which blossomed in the twentieth century as Gestalt psychology [64]. For Mach the foundation for natural philosophy could not be *derived* concepts—mass or force—but primary experience, that is *sensation*. His integration of physics with perceptual psychology is made clear in the title of his book first published in 1886, and extensively revised in 1905: 'The analysis of sensations and the relation of the physical to the psychical' [65]. His maxim was: 'The world consists of sensations, for the scientist and for the common man' ([3]; p. 126). He knew well that, when sensory systems register reality they impose their own biases and distortions of that reality, an insight stated centuries earlier by Francis Bacon, who wrote: 'It is a false assertion that the sense of man is the measure of things. On the contrary, all perceptions as well of the sense as of the mind are according to the measure of the individual and not according to the measure of the universe. And human understanding is like a false mirror, which, receiving rays irregularly, distorts and discolours the nature of things by mingling its own nature with it' [66]. Cohen ([3]; p. 131) comments that 'Mach's theory of science is a new and better version of Bacon's counsel of modesty, and warning against hubris.' It is in any case striking that Mach and Wernicke both based their science on primary experience rather than derived concepts.

Given that our sensory systems are akin to a distorting mirror, it follow that notions of absolute space, assumed in Newtonian physics, might be part of the distortion. Here again, we see striking kinship between Wernicke and Mach. In L5, when discussing the brain's representation of corporeality and the 'tone of a sensation', Wernicke bases our concept of space as having been acquired from association between adjacent points on a sensory surface, which are then captured within cortical connectivity. This principle is straightforward for the retina, more complex for cutaneous sensation, albeit similar in principle. The phrase 'local sign' is used already in L3. The phrase was not Wernicke's, but originated with Hermann Lotze in 1852 [67], and was later used by Hermann Helmholtz, Mach, and William James (who probably took it from Mach, whom he had visited in Prague). For Lotze and Helmholtz, local signs were learned associations, necessary to relate the position of each point of a sensory surface such as the retina, to a frame of reference such as the visual axis. However, the term was used in various ways, sometimes incorporating practical actions which helped define a position with respect to a frame of reference, and for Wernicke incorporating both 'emotional' quality of sensation at each sensitive point, and motor behaviour such as defensive movements associated with the 'emotion'. In discussing the spatial sense in the retina, with fixed orientation, arguments used are nevertheless reminiscent of those of Lotze, Helmholtz and Mach. There are many further similarities between Wernicke and Mach in their respective treatment of sensory systems, such as the role of motor systems in elaborating perception (L3, L6) ([65]; p. 127), terms such as 'sensation of movement' (L6) ([65]; p. 137), the importance for perception of constantly dealing with solid bodies (L4, L6, etc.) ([65]; p. 232), and even highly technical detail such as retinal after-images (L3) ([3]; p. 131).

Not only did Wernicke recognize distortion imposed by sensory systems on our perception of space, he also hints at distortion in perception of time. In L4, he suggests that two percepts are never experienced simultaneously: '... simultaneity of sensory perception is not possible, on account of the property designated as the "oneness" or perhaps as the "unity of consciousness". In truth, we always experience only one sensory percept at once; any second, apparently simultaneous percept happens either earlier or later. Association by simultaneity therefore appears to be but a special case of generic association through succession.' Simultaneity may be subjectively valid, yet, as Wernicke appears to accept, a unitary subjective percept arises objectively by association of more elementary components (although for elementary perception this is scarcely available to consciousness). These statements are not very precise indicators of Wernicke's thoughts, but later, in dealing with clinical matters he refers to definite distortions of sense of time in some of his patients. Thus, in L14 (p. 89), he describes how, normally '... memories are strung so close together that alien elements find no place between them. This temporal association must therefore be broken if the pseudo-experiences of confabulation are to be taken as true.' Again, in L18 (p. 219), he describes a patient who 'on one occasion … expressed his astonishment that the head warder had disappeared through one door of the hospital and simultaneously entered through another door. On another, food suddenly stood before him without any delay … Both events seemed supernatural and magical to him at the time. Now the patient gives us the explanation that he made errors of observation due to a lapses in attention.' Such distortions are no cause for surprise if our concepts of space and time arise from the associations of spatial or temporal data points, rather than the geometric absoluteness of space and time; and they match contemporary views: Subjective time is not a geometrically regular dimension. These ideas also appear to connect *Grundriss* with debates about distortion of space and time occurring in physics in the same era: Even before Einstein's special theory of relativity cast doubt that absolute simultaneity could ever exist, simultaneity was being discussed by Henri Poincaré and Hendrik Lorentz.

Beyond such parallels with physics, in one section, Wernicke questions the validity of the concept of causality, replacing it with something akin to a 'mathematical function' relating variables. Thus, in L4 (p. 23), he refers to 'causality', as an inbuilt error or bias in how we view the world. Admittedly he is not consistent, because in L5 (p. 30), now fully convinced of the validity of causality, he writes: 'Movement without *any* kind of cause, is inconceivable'. Nonetheless, we see echoed what David Hume had written in 1740 [68]: ''Tis not therefore reason which is the guide of life but custom. That alone determines the mind in all instances to suppose the future conformable to the past. However easy this step may seem, reason would never, to all eternity, be able to make it'. In a more recent precedent, when Fechner developed his strict psychophysical parallelism, he denied causation between mind and brain in either direction. In this, he followed a line taken two centuries earlier by another proponent of parallelism, Baruch Spinoza. A fundamental premise of Spinoza's was that entities with *nothing* in common, could not engage in causal interaction [69]. So, things which are extended in space might engage in *their* form of causal interaction, and things in the realm of thought (ideas) followed *their* own sequences; but since there is nothing in common between extension and thought, neither could there be causal interaction in either direction between 'body' and 'mind'. Instead, there was continual parallelism between the two, necessarily so, since the two were different aspects of a single entity.

Mach adapted this parallelism to physical 'causality' as a whole, and wrote: 'the old-fashioned idea of causality, is a little clumsy: A dose of cause is followed by a dose of effect. This represents a kind of primitive, pharmaceutical *Weltanschauung*, like in the doctrine of the four elements … connections in nature are rarely ever so simple that one can identify *one* cause and *one* effect. Consequently, I have tried for a long time to replace the concept of cause by the mathematical concept of the functional relation: dependency of the appearances from each other' [65, 70]. Such reasoning is likely to be a source which was to lead the physicist, Niels Bohr [71] to question the validity of *any* 'claim of causality'. In L4, Wernicke sometimes uses the word 'function' unmistakably in a mathematical sense, implying no causal relationships, merely a systematic description of events (albeit non-quantitative). For instance he writes (p. 23): 'Perhaps by now it is obvious that consciousness of the outside world has definite dependence on the outside world, or, we might say, is a function of it.' In the same lecture he writes: 'Always, when a certain sequence of events recurs without exception, we believe that a law is operating, and are particularly encouraged in this belief when we succeed in arbitrarily evoking the initial event, and then observe the subsequent one. Such an experiment has an irresistible persuasive power over us. However, clearly, this reveals no deeper connection between the two events—it proves merely the presence of that pathway which was claimed earlier in the same processes. Our need to infer causality, in short, is an inborn error or a bias of our brain.'

These ideas come in early sections of *Grundriss*. In clinical sections, Wernicke does not follow through on these ideas, and happily uses 'aetiology' as a synonym for biomedical cause. In L38 (p. 293), we read 'Every specialist is forced to some general notion: Very often we find some debilitating event being specified as a proximate cause'. In L26 (p. 174) he uses the phrase 'an unconditional cause-and-effect relationship'. It is possible that he was hinting here at a definition of 'cause' provided by John Stuart Mill a few years earlier [72]: 'the antecedent or combination of antecedents upon which an effect is invariably and unconditionally consequent'. 'Cause' itself is very hard, perhaps impossible, to define rigorously.

A view made clear in Mach's writings, probably shared by Fechner, possibly also by Wernicke, is that a scientist's task is to provide the most economical *description* of nature, not to *explain* it (if that implies 'finding its cause'; although 'explain' *could* encompass exact quantitative descriptions, and the reasoning leading to them). Here Mach's views probably coincided with those of Newton two centuries earlier, but definitely differ from ones prevailing in biomedicine, then and now.

Overall, there are numerous similarities between Fechner, Mach and Wernicke, on underlying methodology, the primacy of subjective experience, the conditional nature of reality conveyed by such experience, and the concept of causality. The similarities give strong support to the idea that it was Mach to whom Wernicke made his cryptic acknowledgement in the Foreword to the 1894 edition of *Grundriss;* and they connect this work with Einstein's approaching revolutionary ideas, where mass, length and time were all subject to distortion.

VI,(b). Wernicke on Mind/Brain Relationships

The debate about the relationship between mind and brain (otherwise expressed as that between mind and body, mind and matter, meaning versus mechanism, or subjective versus objective insights into reality) is central to Western philosophy, and can be traced back to Plato, even to Pythagoras. Wernicke's 'credo' announced in L1, that mental disorders are diseases of the brain, was adopted by most psychiatrists in Germany since Wilhelm Griesinger, this being central to debates between 'Psychikers' and 'Somatikers'. The Somatikers were clear about the materialism on which they based their views, although they often had sympathy for some views of the Psychikers, while rejecting less helpful notions, such as remaining ideas of demon possession and various types of quackery. Wernicke is caught between two opposed influences, the materialism of the 'Somatiker' ascendency in psychiatry, and the more metaphysical tendencies of Gustav Fechner and followers. It would be a mistake to take Wernicke's materialism as implying lack of subtlety or sensitivity to subjective realities (a charge often made later against behaviourists). We read, for instance in discussing cerebral representation of language (L2, p. 10): 'We need not assume that the entire process normally follows a set pattern, virtually in preformed pathways, so that the result is predictable.' Far from the determinism, which might be implied by reflex concepts of Wernicke's times, here he anticipates Chomsky on the creative aspects of language. Overall his stance became a curious mix, avoiding many implications of Fechner's strict psychophysical parallelism. Thus, for Wernicke, parallelism applies to some brain structures but not others, and not consistently. His ambivalence surfaces in L19 (p. 124) in terms of opinions of his former colleagues: He discusses the views of Meynert and Neumann that hallucinations might arise due to release from inhibition. The former, his earlier mentor, was clearly of the Somatiker persuasion, the latter, one of the few remaining Psychikers. The logic of their respective positions is similar—only the words differ—and while Wernicke suggests that Meynert's version might be strengthened by experiments on localized function, he prefers the impartiality of Neumann's views.

In more detail, in L2 (p. 11) we encounter the phrase 'the organ of consciousness, in other words, the organ of association'. The important point is that consciousness is defined by the act of association. This equation comes more easily in German than in English, since the German word for consciousness, *Bewusstsein*, contains the past participle of *wissen*, the verb 'to know', which knowledge, is, in some sense acquired by association. The phrase *sich bewusst sein*, could then be translated as 'to be aware of' or 'to be conscious of'. In L3 it becomes clear that Wernicke departs from classical 'two substance' dualism, suggesting instead the inseparable union of two different aspects of cerebral activity. However, this seems mainly limited to the cerebral cortex, when he writes (p. 17): 'Consciousness is a function of the central projection fields. If the assumption—that projection fields occupy the entire cortical mantle—is confirmed, then the corollary follows: Consciousness is a function of the cortical mantle.' His argument for the role of the cerebral cortex is based partly on comparison with animals, where both cortical structure and apparent perceptual capacity (as inferred from behaviour) differ from humans in corresponding ways. In L3 it is also implied that consciousness depends on neuronal *perikarya* in the cortex (the presumed site of association), not on axons or glial cells, when he writes (p. 16): '… when a memory … reaches a person's awareness via nerve pathways, it occurs specifically in nerve cell bodies.' Wernicke is thus far short of the fully fledged parallelism of Spinoza or Fechner, essentially more materialistic in tone.

Inconsistency in his proposed matching between mind and brain comes again in L6 (p. 33), where we read: 'The first spontaneous movements a child makes are apparently under control of organ sensations', in the newborn, with no continuity of retrievable memory with child or adult. Where he uses phrases such as 'sensations of movement' or 'representations of movement', the inference is that, even for simple reflexes in molluscs, sensory stimuli produce sensations. In L8 he writes (p. 49): 'Feelings of pleasure and pain in the spinal cord also seem to confer Affect to the organ of consciousness, except that here we cannot specify the grey matter as the sole bearer of the phenomenon'. He thus appears to be *guided* by Fechner's parallelism, although his views are not worked out so consistently as by Fechner. His parallelism is sometimes expansive, sometimes more restrictive.

Nonetheless, the influence of parallelism has a major impact on his whole approach to psychiatry. Wernicke, like Meynert, had no qualms about using subjective intuitions about how his own mind worked, in order to draw inferences about how the brain operated. Examples are his subtle, yet consistent distinction between 'feeling' (*Gefühl*), 'sensation' (*Sinnes*), and 'perception' (*Wahrnehmung*), and his grasp of Plato's point (see next) of the subjective difference between our perception of an object, and that of the *generality* or *idea* of the class of objects. Such intuitions are of course fallible, yet nonetheless a fruitful source of ideas for exploration.

VI,(c). Wernicke on Theory of Knowledge

Just as old as the debate about the relation between mind and body is Plato's theory of ideas, central to epistemology. In L4 (and note, L2), Wernicke considers the relation between representation of immediate perception of an object and that of the generalized concept of the object. He recognizes the distinction made by Plato 2000 years earlier. Subjectively, it arises from the everyday fact that we generalize from individual cases of an object to its generic form, which latter may have some vividness in our minds. The distinction was implicit, 50 years later, when Donald Hebb [73] formulated the 'neural assembly' concept. In Wernicke's original, letter-spacing of his preferred term is widened—k o n k r e t e n B e g r i f f e—('concrete concepts'), clearly his own special term. However, the conclusion implied by Wernicke, and made explicit by Hebb was very different from that of Plato: In contemporary thinking, we ascribe the origin of generalized concepts, as distinct from objects themselves not to the other-worldly realm of Plato's ideas, but to their manner of representation in the cerebral cortex, as captured by associative processes.

On other aspects of the theory of knowledge there are frequent indications of the influence of Immanuel Kant, and hints at that of John Locke.

The main debt to Kant is separation of 'form' from 'content' of experience. This appears first in L2 (p. 13): 'If the presenting symptom is an urge to talk, then by the same token this is a circumscribed *form* of hyperkinesia. If, on the other hand, his response is nonsensical speech, we could rightly regard this as a symptom of parakinesia. Here, however, one would need a more detailed account for each of these, because misunderstanding is to be expected. We will always be forced, on practical grounds, to distinguish two totally different aspects of speech: active movement as such, and the *content* of the spoken words.' (emphasis added). In psychiatry, this separation became central to writings of both Karl Jaspers and Kurt Schneider. In L3, Wernicke analyzes the difference between sensation and perception, perception involving coordination of many items of sensation, which conferred 'form' on them. This had been emphasized by Ernst Mach [64], and later was central to Gestalt psychology. The hint at John Locke comes in L4 (p. 22), when Wernicke distinguishes essential and non-essential features of a concept. Locke [74] had separated 'primary' from 'secondary' qualities (a split which, while not identical to Wernicke's, has some relation to it).

A different debt to Kant comes in L8 (p. 44), where he writes: 'Sensory perception that has never occurred previously ... remains not only misunderstood, but also very-imprecisely perceived'. This is supported by modern realization that, even for the most basic visual perception, we 'learn, by experience, how to see'. However, this sentence is followed by: '... complex thought processes usually take place along prescribed paths', and 'Overall, mental activity shows itself to depend on a long history of acquiring ideas, and arranging them in special ways'. This appears to be a close parallel (albeit a special case) to ideas presented in the opening of Kant's *Critique of Pure Reason*, [75] where it is argued that syllogistic logic, as previously conceived is always incomplete, strictly a *non sequitur*, because it relies on unstated, background notions ('synthetic *a priori*' statements, for Kant). Wernicke (but not Kant) implies that such knowledge is not *a priori*, but acquired.

In Wernicke's clinical lectures, notably when writing on delusions, he makes further assumptions on epistemology. In L9, the first clinical lecture, he explicitly identifies symptoms, which we call 'delusions', as '*falsification* of contents of consciousness'. This raises the unanswerable question, attributed in the Gospels to Pontius Pilate 'What is truth?', a question which is tautologous, since any answer has to be framed in terms of an assumption about the very matter at issue. Baruch Spinoza grasped the tautology well, when he wrote 'He who would distinguish the true from the false must have an adequate idea of what is true and false' [69].

The notion that delusions reflect *error* in thinking has a long history [76, 77]. Modern psychiatric thought usually identifies a delusion (as far as possible) by the *manner* in which a belief is held and expressed, and by how it was formed (if evidence on this is available). Wernicke, no doubt aware of difficult issues in epistemology raised by delusions, has prepared the ground well: In earlier lectures he emphasized how, based on current knowledge, the brain comes to represent individual stimuli, and their integral, reflecting the outside world in its entirety. In L4 (p. 22), he is quite explicit: 'We can also identify the sum of such concepts as *consciousness of the outside world*, for in these concepts we in fact possess a true picture of the outer world' (*ein getreues Bild der Außenwelt*).

The brain also acquires consciousness of the person's own body, and the updated sum, of all his/her life experiences so far. Altogether these three comprise, to a degree, an individual's concept of themselves as an integrated person. However, the brain's representation is not absolute, just an approximation, as Francis Bacon asserted. Given that the brain's representation is *potentially* fallible, it may become more seriously deceptive. Nevertheless, Wernicke's strong definition of truth and its separation from falsehood, based on understanding brain mechanisms implies that philosophical notions of truth depend on, and in a sense, 'bend the knee to' what is known, or inferred about brain processes. This reasoning also links with Mach's view, that our view of external reality is a distortion, although sensation is primary.

One specific aspect of distortion is introduced in L15 (p. 96), where Wernicke writes about 'overvalued ideas': 'In this lady there was no psychopathic basis from which the overvalued idea would have grown. However, you will not go far wrong if you take note of the "critical" age she had reached, combined with an excess of mental energy, and resulting improper lifestyle, as sufficient reason for occurrence of a sexually coloured, overvalued idea'. These sentences sum up his notions of 'overvalued ideas', and spell out with crystal clarity, a profound problem. Our evaluation of ideas, persons or events inevitably recruits basic functions of association, implemented by the cerebral cortex. Any mechanism designed to detect and register associations, must contain a 'set point' or 'threshold' above which the link becomes credible, and below which it is rejected as coincidental, and then forgotten. As in any statistical inference, conclusions are reached 'to degrees of probability', not as certainties. Thus, without any inference of psycho*pathology*, we are all prone to error. Depending on where the threshold is set—which varies from person to person—we may be more, or less error-prone. Overvaluation of ideas then reflects normal cerebral mechanisms in persons who are intrinsically error-prone, as are we all. For some of us, cultural traditions have given us an alternative faculty, that of deduction, which, when deployed systematically, can at least correct inconsistency, if not preventing error. L15 (also L14) deals with such corrective strategies. However, deduction is not a natural ability, but an artifice developed in some cultures. Even in the most sophisticated cultures, only a minority of the populace has sufficient ability and faith in the method for it to overrule their associationist instincts. Therein lies our problem!

VI,(d). Wernicke on Personhood, Unity of a Person, and 'Self-Consciousness'

The concept of personhood, the 'unity of a person', and—'mystery-of-all-mysteries'—'self-consciousness', are topics which arise as much in early lectures as in later clinical ones. Wernicke is not entirely consistent in his treatment of them. In L7 (also L12), following Meynert, the view is expressed that an individual's unchanging sense of 'corporeality' gives him his 'primary Ego', which also assimilates his knowledge of the outside world, and personal life story. However, by L14 (p. 86) he writes: 'Normally, in a complex brain mechanism, there should not exist the remotest corner that is in discord with all other parts, and which does not function under their influence': This view of normality is perhaps the dream of a philosopher, for whom rationality comes easily, who *does* try systematically to erase all inconsistency in his thought, and who (incorrectly) takes this as a universal norm. Such a philosopher may be over-influenced by Western religious thought which took rationality as the norm for human nature. However, deduction, and the quest to eliminate logical inconsistencies are *not* universal human endowments (whatever philosophers of earlier centuries had said): They are products of education, training honed by experience, and practice. The example given in L14, of a patient with a doctoral degree, is exactly the sort of person to have acquired this facility; but most unlettered people, however efficient and agile their minds, lack this facility, and operate on the basis of memory and inductive inference (which *are* universal cerebral processes) rather than by deduction. In L16, Wernicke, in effect, accepts this, when he compares recovery in two patients. In one, completely lacking insight when ill, and complaining about his illegal detention, recovered in an uneventful way; in another hypothetical but plausible patient, with extensive legal training, there is a persisting focus on legal injustice, with continued accretion of far-fetched explanatory delusions. However, subsequent *helpful* corrective explanations might also develop in those who have acquired a facility in reasoning.

The insight that the supposedly 'indivisible' Ego has a complex, ever-shifting structure, and can become overtly fragmented, is clear in some of Wernicke's lectures. In L12 (where he introduces the sejunction concept) he discusses patient Rother, and writes (p. 72): 'This individual consists simultaneously, as it were, of a number of different personalities', and that there is 'a disintegration of individuality'. Likewise in L28 (p. 193) he uses the phrase 'split personality' (*Spaltung der Persönlichkeit*). The composite nature of personhood is also found in writings of Ernst Mach who wrote that, although 'psychology and psycho-pathology teach us that the Ego is the bond which holds all my experience together, and the source of all my activity', it can 'grow and be enriched, can be impoverished and shrink, can become alien to itself, and can split up—in a word can change in important respects, in the course of its life' ([65]; p. 356). Quotations like this show that Mach—polymath that he was—could offer deep insights into psychiatry, from which Wernicke may have benefited. When we get to L28, and discussion of the 'second state' in some of his patients, the fragmentation of personality is explicit. A vivid personal account is given by a patient, of her experience of this state, its authenticity ensured by apparent lack of distortion by her awareness of any popularized concepts of 'multiple personality'. Wernicke clearly regarded the topic as very significant, because, after describing this case, he starts his comments with the words: 'To leave no doubt about the importance of this case ...' The so-called 'multiple personality' had occasionally been described in the previous century, in France especially by Charcot, who described a transient condition with disorder of consciousness: There was dissociation between automatic activities (which were coordinated, if sometimes outlandish or bizarre) and personality, to which these activities were foreign, or contrasted with education received. Pierre Janet described splitting of identity, in relation to psychic trauma. Wernicke's emphasis is different, with little stress on psychic trauma, and more on other ways in which such states might be precipitated, including epileptic seizures, and alcoholic binge drinking. Hysteria is mentioned in this context, and it is clear that Wernicke accepted it as a condition not limited to women. Some states of dissociation described by Wernicke fit the definition of 'fugue', a condition which, according to Ian Hacking [78] was, in part, a male equivalent of hysteria. The modern definition of fugue—a rare condition, usually related to psychic stress—has as exclusion criteria physical trauma, other medical conditions, and various psychiatric diagnoses. The case reported by Max Naef [79] (a doctoral thesis produced while working under Auguste Forel) which Wernicke describes in detail (L28, p. 190 *seq.*) would be excluded according to such criteria: This patient's problems probably combined consequences of hyperthermia-heat stroke and dengue fever, given the high air temperature in inland Australia, and railway carriages with no air conditioning in the 1890s (see [80]; on neuropsychiatric effects of hyperthermia).

In L7, the topic of '*self*-consciousness'—'riddle of all riddles' is Wernicke's phrase—is discussed, and Wernicke's scepticism about philosophy is interesting. He does not dismiss it out of hand, which would have been simplistic, given that the natural science tradition grew out of hard debates in past centuries on essentially philosophical issues; and Wernicke was clearly indebted to philosophers, especially Kant. However, he ends by pointing out that the seemingly 'indivisible unchanging ego' (implied by much of our language, culture and history), *is* actually a complex dynamic structure. This point can be made from many perspectives, suggesting that different parts, with different functions can 'cast their eye' over other parts, by looking back in time (Wernicke's point), or by looking around at the other parts of this complex entity. Such ideas were becoming accepted by clinicians, from work of Pierre Janet in Paris. By the time of the 1906 edition of *Grundriss*, more sophisticated views on this had been formulated across the Atlantic, by J. Royce and J.M.Baldwin (see ref [16]), whose work Wernicke is unlikely to have read. The line of thought was developed in the 1930s by George Herbert Mead [81] and a modern addition is found in a section of the doctoral thesis of Kate L. Ball [82]. The *non*-unified nature of the Ego was accepted by Mach, who writes of 'the instinctive, but untenable splitting up of the Ego into an object experienced and an active or observing subject—a problem which has tormented everybody long enough' ([65]; p. 332). Again: 'Whoever cannot get rid of the conception of the Ego as a reality which underlies everything, will also not be able to avoid drawing a fundamental distinction between my sensation and your sensation' ([65]; p. 356). Apart from anything else, this shows continuity between the thorough parallelism of Spinoza and Fechner, and the thought of Mach.

VI,(e). Wernicke on 'Will', and on Teleology

In L30 (p. 204), we read: 'For anyone to "will" a certain action presumes making a decision, unquestionably an action of pure thought … In content, this implies that two or more possibilities have been weighed against each other'. The German word for 'will'—*Das Wille*—resonates in German history. In combining '*Das Wille*' with 'pure thought' a link is made to earlier idealist philosophers such as G.F.W.Hegel (1770–1831) which belies the materialist tone with which *Grundriss* began. For Hegel, 'Will' is not 'free' until it is actualized, apparently unlimited by physical realities in the brain. Later, the monthly magazine of the Hitler Youth was to be entitled *Wille und Macht* ('Will and Power'). In discussion of freedom (or otherwise) of will by philosophers, the process of 'getting out of bed' is a widely used metaphor, as here (L30, p. 207). It appears in William James' (*The Will to Believe; and other essays in popular philosophy*, published in 1897 [83]), and may have started its life there. Wernicke side-steps the challenge to determinism-in-principle, based on overemphasizing '*Das Wille*', when he writes (L30, p. 207) '… of the error … that a person can control his thoughts and feelings, whereas actually the thoughts control the person'.

Possibly neither of these is right. Perhaps a person (or at least 'one side' of a person) *is* his or her thoughts. Descartes, after all, asserted 'I think therefore I am'. Referring back to the 'unity of personhood', Wernicke is not consistent in discussion of 'will'. He writes (L35, p. 267) 'To assume a unilateral condition of the will would be nonsense': Why nonsense, to assume that 'the will' resides in one hemisphere? Many clinical findings have shown that personhood is *not* indivisible. Here, rather than seeing personhood as the integral of many parts of consciousness, we fall back on older notions, perhaps related to an 'indivisible soul'. K.L.Ball, in her doctoral thesis [82] suggests that personhood is twofold, the right hemisphere characterized as 'the self experiencing, and acting *now*'; the left, as 'conceptualizing the self, the will, and controlling at least some thoughts'.

Hegel's concept of 'will' is pure teleology. In L8, Wernicke apologetically admits that his definition of Affect is also teleological. Teleological reasoning has a long history. The birth of the natural sciences depended (*inter alia*) on abandoning Aristotle's notion of 'final cause' (a cosmic form of teleology) in favour of 'antecedent cause'. For Freud teleological arguments were used widely, without restraint, this being a major criticism of his work. However, the behaviour of living things clearly often *does* work towards an end goal, and Ernst Mach himself argued that teleology was sometimes a valid account of nature, although not as Aristotle's 'final purpose', or with any *overall* purpose for living things. (Here he might be at odds with Richard Dawkins, and his concept of the 'selfish gene'). Today, no apology is needed for teleology, if a correct approach is adopted: Rigorous ways were devised to establish the teleological nature of behaviour, in work of ethologists such as Nikolaas Tinbergen and Konrad Lorenz, work that is highly relevant to psychiatry.

VII. Wernicke's Contribution to Neuroscience, Psychology and Overall Medical Knowledge

In the English-speaking world, Wernicke's name is linked with two ideas: cerebral localization of function, and—almost as strongly—a supposed 'associationist school' of thought. Less well known, yet fundamental to *Grundriss,* are his ideas on basic brain science. Here we deal with his additions to science and medical knowledge, and with important *gaps* in his understanding, which shaped some of his mistakes. His major contributions to thought about mental disorders come later.

VII,(a). Basic Neuroscience

At least in early lectures, Wernicke assumes that interactions between nerve cells were solely excitatory. In L8 (p. 43) he writes: 'We can demand no more from it [the brain] than the sequence of certain excitatory processes'. Later, he contradicts this, implying that inhibitory interactions might occur between cortical neurones. Sometimes this is ambiguous, when he mixes psychological and biological language. Thus, in L8 (p. 48), when introducing the topic of emotions he writes of 'a set of phenomena ... which very often have effects of slowing down [*hemmenden*] the course of mental activity, which are both decisive and disruptive, in equal measure.' In L19 (p. 123) he attributes the idea of 'mutual inhibition' to Meynert, whom he quotes in L33 (p. 236): 'The association intensity corresponds to the molecular tissue attraction as a source of strength. The mass of arching fibres, within which two sources of force, that of the idea of an "objective" and that of the initial idea, tend towards each other, as it were, in the act of thinking, always attaining vital force for elevation above the threshold of consciousness from two ideally centralized cortical areas, but the secondary association from only one of these areas: either that of the "objective" or that of the initial idea, according to whether for example the rhyme fits its word picture. The functional attraction is the weaker here, and is inhibited by the stronger'. In L35 (p. 235) he uses the curious phrase 'inhibitory thought' [*hemmende Gedanke*]. 'Inhibition' is mentioned again in L35 (p. 236) where we read: 'maintenance of certain abnormal positions may reveal only subjective sensations of changed balance between the motor impulse and its collateral and antagonistic activation of definite muscle areas, which cooperate in the normal position'. He adds (note): 'This representation is based on Duchenne's theory. The more recent works of Hering, Jr. have meanwhile proven that the assumption of an antagonistic muscle coordination is not tenable.' However, shortly after (L35, p. 269), he explicitly refers to inhibition *at a neuronal level* 'The same inhibition [*Hemmung*], which is responsible for immobility of the patient, transfers to such intercortical pathways, and then seems very well suited, just as in the speech area, to produce the paraphasia'.

Sherrington is acknowledged as the first to demonstrate neural inhibition clearly, inferred rather than proven, in the spinal cord. There were however a number of forerunners, such as the Edinburgh-based physiologists Charles and John Bell early in the nineteenth century, and others in Russia and Germany in the nineteenth century, cited by Sherrington in his Nobel Lecture of 1932. It is therefore interesting that the work of Hering in 1897, apparently denying the existence of inhibitory effects, and which Wernicke cites, has, as its co-author CS Sherrrington, who had travelled in Germany (where he met, and worked with Goltz [see biographic comments, below]). In *Reflex activity of the spinal cord* of 1933, Sherrington and colleagues [84] often used the phrase 'reciprocal innervation', and 'reciprocal inhibition' is used occasionally, stating (p. 67) 'There is as yet no experimental evidence for the existence of inhibition with neurones other than motoneurones'. *Direct* proof came in 1942, when spinal inhibition by the eponymously named Renshaw cell was discovered [85]. Overall Duchenne (and Meynert) were proved correct in this debate. Hering was proven incorrect, but may have influenced Wernicke.

Of great interest is that, as early as 1894, Wernicke had clear ideas for what is now called 'synaptic plasticity' as the physical basis of memory. This is mentioned in L3 (p. 16), where he writes: 'Pathways that are initially hard to access become more firmly trodden-in with each new training experience—you could say that they are "molded by experience"'. There are references to early German experiments (dated 1880 [Ward], and 1882 [Jarisch and Schiff]), showing the concept as a basis for memory to have been clear in his mind in 1894, and to be much older than its current reincarnation. (Other early references on synaptic plasticity are found to be in John [[86]; p. 198]). What is more, in discussing 'falsification of memory' (L14, p. 89), he shows awareness that there must be a complementary process: '... memory falsification requires a preceding break-up of associations.' Today, dissipation of associative memories is the subject of experimental study as 'long-term synaptic depression', a complement to 'long-term potentiation' which establishes them. Related to this, the temporal precision of association at a neuronal level, is mentioned in L3 (pp. 17, 18): 'I agree entirely with Sachs and Goldscheider, that only by assuming that functional links are acquired between *simultaneously excited* perceptual elements using existing connections can one explain the specific memory for respective forms of retinal images, defined by patterned stimulation of retinal points' (emphasis added). The modern slogan is 'cells which fire together, wire together'.

VII,(b). Wernicke and 'Associationism'

It is incorrect to regard 'Associationism' as a 'school of thought'. It is now fully accepted as a major bridge between neurobiology and psychology. Wernicke's view that the cerebral cortex was (above all other brain regions), *the* organ of association, is basically correct, as a three-word synopsis. In L33 (p. 236) the assumption behind this is stated in simplest form: 'If such functional differences of excitability are disregarded in the organ of association, the primordial condition of the childlike brain (Meynert's "genetic confusion"), in which any given association is possible, reappears to some extent, and may be retained for a while, because anatomically preformed combinations exist between any given two cortical areas'. Miller [87] developed a similar starting point as a basic substrate for forming associations, that all neurones are connected with all others in the organ of association—the 'omniconnecton principle'—although, of course, this does not—and cannot—occur in practice.

One can of course point out that other principles of organization need to be added. As mentioned above, for Wernicke, associations were not only spatial (between data represented simultaneously), but to a degree, temporal. However, he had no idea of the brain mechanisms by which temporal associations might be formed, nor the temporal limits within which they might apply. More fundamentally, associations in the cortex are potentially so ambiguous, that they need some sort of supervision or constraint to 'disambiguate' them. A recent theory [88] attempts to give an account of this process: By interplay between hippocampus and cerebral neo-cortex, the inherent ambiguity of associations in the latter structure could be resolved. It was also argued that such interplay sets up lasting configurations which represent *contexts* for cortical operations in specific situations, serving to disambiguate activity circulating in the 'organ of association'. These contexts, it was proposed, correspond to Kant's 'synthetic *a priori* notions', which Wernicke describes as the 'long history of acquiring ideas, and arranging them in special ways' (p. 44). There is one further major shortcoming in the view of the cortex as an 'organ of association': The motor region of the cortex, directly influencing lower motoneurones of brainstem and spinal cord, and the decision-making processes by which motor outflow is determined, do not fit the concept. Wernicke gets near to this in L35 (p. 267): 'From such arguments, it seems that in motility psychoses, consciousness of personality—in our sense, that "grand complex of ideas" which makes up the Ego—is to a certain degree detached from motor mechanisms of the body, over which "the Ego" has become used to exert control. As a witness, the "Ego" is confronted with motor processes, and also with the failure of this machine, and in turn, is initially affected by this'. By analysis at a psychological level, this appears to reach a conclusion which can now be put on a stronger footing: Operations of the motor system are not a natural component of the cortex, seen as the 'organ of association'. The motor cortex is anomalous, having a place in the parcellation of the cerebral cortex only because of other styles of processing imposed on it by the basal ganglia, and elsewhere.

Many implications of the concept of association are pursued in early lectures. Much of L3 is devoted to distinguishing perceptual images from memory images. In the tactile sense, he separates sensitivity—'ability to detect' a tactile stimulus—from what he terms *Tastvermögen*—using such stimuli for object recognition. In modern terms this is the distinction between sensation and perception, the former implying 'awareness' arising direct from sensory input, the latter implying added processes of interpretation or analysis of that input. We translate this as 'tactile perception'. Likewise, later in L3, he often uses the word *optische* and occasionally *visuell*. At one point he writes of 'visual impressions that attract our attention' using the word *Gesichtseindrücke*. In modern terms both this and *visuell* imply 'perception' as distinct from 'sensation'. Later (L20, p. 129) with a slightly different sense, he is at pains to separate perceptual images from 'thoughts' with no perceptual connotation (mental images devoid of perceptual imagery). The German word *Empfindungen* implies sensation itself rather than perception (*Wahrnehmung*) or remembered images of sensation, a subtle subjective distinction, discussed in relation to both visual and auditory sense. In translation we try to make the distinction as consistently as possible (for instance using 'visual' as opposed to 'visual perceptual', and avoiding the word *optische*).

Despite separating perception from memory images, Wernicke argues that similar associative processes apply at each level: He sees an exact parallel between formation of memory images in primary visual areas by linkage of 'perceptual elements', and those higher in the hierarchy which generalize from percepts to concepts. The arguments are another prescient forerunner of Hebb [73] in advancing the 'neural assembly' concept: Most representation is via networks of widely distributed, but connected nerve cells. In L3 and L4 his arguments amount to setting up a 'straw man', such that 'perception' and 'memory' are separate processes, represented in different groups of nerve cells; and he then proceeds to demolish the hypothesis, where he writes (p. 24): 'But as soon as you go beyond this initial physiological unit, the memory image, and envisage just the next higher level of visual images or even association between visual images and remembered images from another projection field, the difficulty of conceiving the process increases enormously.'

In L4 (p. 22) he refers to 'simple circuit operations'. He probably means what we now refer to as 'positive feedback': A 'suspicion' that 'something is the case' leads to a 'search backwards' for relevant evidence, and if it is found, it is fed forwards again, to strengthen the initial suspicion. In this way we arrive at sharp categorical judgments—'identifications' in Wernicke's terms—which go beyond objective assessment of the evidence. Wernicke is speaking of what we would now call 'pattern completion', a process which Braitenberg [89] calls 'ignition'—of representation of a whole, when only parts of are detected.

Wernicke's associationism is based on 'association based on signal continuity', a concept pursued by Pavlov and others in somewhat different contexts. Not long after Wernicke's death ideas emerged that there was another major type of association: North American psychologists developed the idea of association between an item of emitted behaviour and the subsequent *effect* of that behaviour. From this so-called *law of effect*, the concept of *reinforcement* was developed, along with associated lines of theory and experiment. This concept was mainly missing in Wernicke's thought, as far as it influenced behaviour.

VII,(c). Cerebral Localization of Function

The concept of cerebral localisation followed naturally from the ruling paradigm of general medicine, to relate symptoms to diseases in specific organs or body systems, defined by anatomy and pathology. This was inevitable when, with few objective markers of disease, symptoms were the prime source of evidence of disease processes in the living. The relation with general medicine is seen in L24, where Wernicke employs the localization concept to refer to *bodily* symptoms, bodily 'localization of function' being common clinical thinking at the time. Interestingly, throughout this lecture he refers to localization in the body of feelings of *anxiety*. Just as much as asking a patient 'where does it hurt?' he is at ease asking 'where does your anxiety come from?' This may seem strange today, but is logical, and has precedents from classical times, when the heart rather than the brain was held to be the seat of emotions. Similarly, a word root for 'schizophrenia' (and other terms in psychiatry) is that for the 'phrenic nerve' supplying the diaphragm. Curiously, yet logically, the word 'hypochondria' (literally, 'below the ribs') is occasionally applied to unusual states of happiness as well as to those of anxiety (p. 107; L29, p. 198).

The concept of cerebral localization arose in Wernicke's earliest work defining the brain region representing speech sounds, but had become more nuanced by the time *Grundriss* was written, although missing some points we accept today. Sometimes he presents localization as a hypothesis, without evidence, as in L1, when he suggests that semantic organization of speech uses brain regions different from those for phonetics. Sometimes he *infers* topographic mapping between connected regions, in absence of evidence, simply because it seems necessary. Sometimes his use of the concept is an analogy ('For purposes of this analysis, all changes in content of consciousness can then be likened to focal symptoms, and will behave just as do more familiar focal symptoms of brain diseases' [L11, p. 66]). Sometimes he refers to the concept in a quite metaphorical way. Sometimes he makes it clear that it is no more than a hope for the future that precise location can be found for symptoms he describes, as when he writes (L33, p. 236): 'the closed train of thought is a functional acquisition pointing towards a most minute localization in definite anatomical elements'. In stricter scientific vein, he concedes that much representation is diffuse, an insight closely connected to his ideas on modifiable connections between members of widely dispersed nerve cell networks. Nonetheless, in describing akinesia, hyperkinesia and parakinesia, which can occur independently in different muscle blocks (L35, p. 260), the inference that there *is* localized abnormality is strong, although the brain structure in which this exists (cortex, or perhaps basal ganglia) is unclear.

In early lectures (e.g. L2) the evidence he cites is clinical, either relating symptoms to identified lesions, or studies in animals using lesions and electrical stimulation. In L5 he cites experiments conducted by Munk, involving cortical lesions, with long-term follow-up, and study of behaviour, carried out mainly on dogs, with some on monkeys. The same principle assuredly applied in humans. Wernicke writes 'There can no longer be any doubt that each region represents the total sensibility and motility of the designated body part, the arm region, which thus constitutes the central projection field for sensibility and motility or, in other words, the entire nervous system of the arm.' This comment would not be held valid today: A 'second somatosensory area' was defined by Adrian in 1940 [90], spatially separate from the primary area, and now known to deal with aspects of somatic sensation different from those dealt with by the primary area. In L1 he refers to Broca's area as the 'motor speech pathway'. Modern neuroanatomists would avoid such a statement, knowing the relation to motor outflow to be less direct. In one respect, however, his localization is quite modern: In L36 (p. 274) he writes 'Affiliation of motility symptoms with changed body awareness is thus illustrated again': This view, iterated several times in this lecture, corresponds to a view which avoids separating functions of primary motor and somatosensory areas of cortex (for instance in the notion of 'active touch': [91]).

In L3, Wernicke discusses the difference between perceptual and memory images, and writes (p. 18): 'only those elements in the cortical projection area serving perception should correspond to points in the retina': He appears to assume one-to-one relations between neural elements in the retina and those in the visual cortex, a view which modern neuroanatomists would question. Likewise, in L6, there is reference to a conjecture that there be orderly connections between points on the cortical map of the retina and locations controlling activity of combinations of eye muscles, corresponding to these points; some empirical evidence for this is cited from Munk's experiments. However, empirical proof is lacking. This conjecture is intended to address a major problem for representation in the brain: How can object recognition generalize over different *sizes* of retinal image, different directions of viewing etc. We read (p. 18): 'An equilateral triangle or a cross can be recognized whether the triangle is standing on its base or its apex, or whether the cross is standing, lying, or standing at an angle. How could the same memory image be derived?' The explanation proposed seems far-fetched today. Moreover, given his more plausible account of *concept* formation in L4, which might also apply to percept generalization, it is unnecessary.

Diffuse representation is raised as early as L1, when the *supposed* Conceptualization Centre is mentioned. 'In truth, this supposed Conceptualization Centre is distributed to cortical sites far removed from one another'. In L2, any ambiguity is resolved, by asking whether this centre has a definite physical location, or is it more diffusely localized, perhaps 'localized' more exactly but more abstractly in a *logical* structure? In L7, when discussing the cerebral basis of personhood, he asks (p. 39): 'What spatial sense can we make of a personalized consciousness?' In answer, he refers to several types of disorder. Amongst those listed, it is unclear if they include what is now call 'mental illness', to which cerebral localization seldom applies, or to neurological conditions, where it often *does* apply. Overall, while, as a neurologist, Wernicke's name *is* rightly linked to the concept of cerebral localization of function, this concept is not central to *Grundriss.* At times he pulls away from localizationism in a fundamental way. Thus, in L36 (p. 274), he writes: 'There seems to be no compelling case for drawing an analogy between the differentiation amongst these cases [of akinetic motility psychosis'] and the quite circumscribed nature of direct focal symptoms in brain diseases'. Thus, he recognized that localizationist approaches, whatever their value in neurology, had limits as applied to realities of mental disorders.

At times cerebral localization is raised as a possible basis for future classification: '... I cannot emphasize strongly enough that the forthcoming principle of classification must be that of anatomical arrangement, giving a natural grouping and sequence of substantial changes' (L17, p. 104). Here he is flying his favourite kite, that correlations will one day be found between the site of brain pathology and symptoms exhibited by patients, not only in neurology (where this was well supported) but also in psychiatry. The relation between symptoms of progressive paralysis, for which neuropathological evidence was available, and other psychoses for which it was not, lent weight to localizationist views which he might have wanted to apply generally to psychoses (L37, p. 274). We now know that pathological changes in progressive paralysis/tertiary syphilis are greater than ever seen in endogenous psychoses, so the analogy may be false. Even so, in closing pages of L41 (p. 328), he rejects this hope: 'Do the few cases I have in mind allow us to conclude that *all* acute psychoses, as well as the less severe cases would reveal similar anatomical findings, were they to reach autopsy? . . In my opinion this question cannot be supported.'

VII,(d).'Psychic Reflexes'

The notion of 'psychic reflexes' was common talk at the time. Wernicke formalizes the concept, with distinctive italicized abbreviations: *sAZm,* signifying the various stages in the 'psychic reflex arc'. *s* and *m* are sensory and motor fields respectively, presumably in the cortex, while *A* and *Z*, are hypothetical staging posts where higher lever perceptual analysis and output planning are accomplished. This model is first described in L2 (p. 12), for instance in the following lines: 'Nervous excitation, which takes place along the pathway *sAZm* can be likened to a reflex process, and we can designate this pathway as a "psychic reflex arc". The movement activated from *m* then appears as the result—a discernible consequence—of this activation.' The model is used throughout *Grundriss,* for instance in L8 (p. 44), though expressed less clearly than in L2 '... [mental] activity triggered by the question as "registration"; and the result of mental activity included in the answer as "execution"'. An example is the symptom of negativism 'possibly having a significance similar to that of a "modified cortical reflex"' (L35, p. 266). Comparison with a monosynaptic 'stretch reflex' is hinted at, and the differential susceptibility he describes, to rapid as opposed to slow stretch, implies selectivity to 'phasic' as opposed to 'tonic' stretch, a distinction well-known for stretch reflexes. However, the two effects must have very different mechanisms.

Jackson's hierarchical concept of brain organization has already been mentioned. In L20, Wernicke deals with levels of coordinated motor behaviour, generated by the brain under different conditions. These were to be explored later by Kretschmer [61] in *Hysteria, Reflex and Instinct.* Curiously, in L20 (p. 131), he accounts for complex, but more-or-less automatic actions, as using a 'short-circuit' *within* cortical networks, as derived from the 'psychic reflex' concept. He uses the concept again in L24 (p. 157), to account for eruptions of 'senseless rage': 'These motor expressions bear the stamp of senseless rage, and would be correctly understood as a type of reflex response to violently increased organ sensations, and thus as hyperkinesia induced by psychosensory means, via a short-circuit'. An alternative view was possible, following Jackson's claim, that organization of motor responses shifts from cortex to subcortex. Something like this is suggested in L32 (p. 225): What appears to be 'body language' which is quite complex, is nonetheless instinctive, more-or-less automatic.

The psychic reflex perspective leads to other conclusions on voluntary actions, which are strange for modern readers. Wernicke writes (L35, p. 266): '... persisting contractions and those independent of passive movements are so invariably combined with states of unconsciousness or marked stupor, that one might be compelled to relate them to some form of volitional action. I confine myself to suggesting that there are sufficient clinical and experimental data to prove that central projection motor fields are the origin of tonic spasms and contractures': There is a disjunction here, in that evidence for involvement of primary motor cortex is taken as equivalent to voluntary action, even in patients who are unconscious or stuporous.

VII,(e). Wernicke on the Basal Ganglia

Wernicke has little to say about the basal ganglia. In L11 (p. 67) he does refer to a specific structure, the lentiform nucleus (*Linsenkern*); and in L19 (p. 123) to the idea (still current today) that the cerebral cortex has an inhibitory action on activity in the basal ganglia. He *was* aware in a general way, of issues raised today for understanding these structures. Thus, the fascinating lecture on melancholia (L30, p. 204 *seq.*), gives an incisive psychological account of decision-making, but referring to the cerebral cortex. This is incompatible with a view of the cortex as the 'organ of association', which can include neither 'decision making', nor competition between rival programs—implying inhibitory as well as excitatory processes. However, *mutatis mutandis,* it is a fine account of processes now thought to occur in the basal ganglia, where separate paths exist to initiate and to veto any possible action, the so-called 'direct' and 'indirect' pathways from striatum to motor thalamus and motor cortex; and within each of these—under most circumstances—for resolution of competition between rival courses of action [92]. In the process, Wernicke insists that at least one competitor should have access to motor outflow pathways. Today, that condition is not needed: Competition can occur entirely between intrapsychic ideas. He actually had evidence for this: Thus, in L29, where patients are discussed in whom the veto faculty is impaired, symptoms occur in one patient as unconstrained *motor outflow*, and in another as unconstrained *thoughts*.

Closely related to functions of the basal ganglia, Wernicke had little awareness of the reinforcement principle, either (as soon to be defined) in learning theory, or, following the Olds/Milner experiment of 1954 [93], at the biological level. He does *imply* a reinforcement process in L22 (p. 140), when he writes: 'we must attribute to Affective states the capacity to alter the normal value of ideas, in such a way that certain ideas are overvalued ...' This principle could clearly influence the representation of *ideas* and *perceptions*; its role in reinforcing behaviour is hard to find in *Grundriss.* In any case, with no explicit knowledge, he sought elsewhere for processes by which abnormal excessive (not epileptic) neural activation could occur. This was one aim of the 'sejunction theory' (see below).

VII,(f). Higher Levels of Functional Organization

At a higher level of organization, Wernicke makes an important distinction as early as L8, between *content* of consciousness (produced by permanent change) and *activity* of consciousness (its ever-fluctuating dynamics). This becomes a recurring theme throughout *Grundriss*. In terms of activity, he compares 'psychophysical motion' between sleep and waking (L8, p. 46), and seems aware that sleep is an active process (an issue resolved many years later). At times, he draws parallels, as many have done, between distortions of reality in dreaming, and in mental illnesses. In L9 (p. 55), he writes: 'Lack of insight into illness is, in effect, the same as an increase in the sum of a person's memories by a body of data not corresponding to reality, as we might gain from experiences in a dream. If we were to string these often highly adventurous dream experiences onto our store of memories, what incalculable consequences for our actions, or our judgment of people might it lead to!' More scientific issues about sleep are raised in L26, when discussing *Delirium tremens*, a severely abnormal state following withdrawal, after prolonged excess of alcohol consumption. We now know that similar states can be produced by withdrawal from other sedative/hypnotic drugs, such a benzodiazepines. He writes (p. 172): 'we are entitled to attribute another main symptom of *Delirium tremens*—total insomnia—to the stimulating effect of the dream-like hallucinations'. Today, insomnia is generally regarded as a sign of an impending or actual psychotic state (defined more narrowly than in Wernicke's day), rather than being precipitated *by* the hallucinations. Admittedly, hallucinations in other situations (effects of drugs, their withdrawal, or toxicity, brain injuries, general medical crises), which are often visual rather than auditory, *may* lead to, rather than follow insomnia.

An alternative view of *Delirium tremens* is possible, now we know of a specific 'pressure' for dreaming (rapid eye-movement) sleep: Insomnia could be a precursor to dream-like hallucinations, where the pressure for REM sleep and dreams is so great that it breaks through, even during apparent wakefulness. In this context, in L27 (p. 179), Wernicke refers to 'falsification of consciousness, and [the] belief in the lived reality of the dream experiences', and thus appears to imply this theory. It can now be based on solid evidence—the so-called REM dissociation [94]—for which there is some EEG evidence [95]. This idea is supported by a further similarity reported in L14 (p. 87) 'the total loss of memory during epileptic twilight states, alleged experience of *Delirium tremens*, or any other delirium from severe intoxication, hysteria, or lastly, during normal dreaming'. Amnesia for dreams is well known, and normal. There are however two differences between the state Wernicke describes and normal REM sleep, that in the latter, there is deep muscle relaxation, with no possibility of mental imagery influencing outward behaviour; and in the aftermath of delirium, after a period of sleep, imagery from the period of delirium *is* remembered for a while (L27, p. 179).

VIII. Wernicke's Distinctive Clinical Concepts in Psychiatry

VIII,(a). Is Clinical Science Even Possible in Psychiatry?

Wernicke was aware of this as a significant question. In the eighteenth century, when botanical classification was high on the scientific agenda, the acknowledged pioneer, Carl Linnaeus (1707–1778), was a Platonist (philosophically speaking), who believed in 'natural types'. A rival Frenchman, George Buffon (1707–1788) asserted, in contrast 'Nature knows only the individual'. Just the same issue arose as psychiatry invented itself. In L8 Wernicke writes: 'Despite all differences in social milieu, and the epoch in which we live, all individuals in full possession of their senses, have firmly laid down in their store of apperceptions, combinations of identical thoughts. In this regard therefore, we must guard against overestimating the diversity of individuals. This is definitely an advantage for psychiatry, making clinical observation possible'.

This basic step moves the researcher from what seems endless variety and uniqueness of persons, to their being somehow brought within a generic scheme. After this step, he implies, psychiatrists may be within reach of scientific study, even of diagnoses, rather than being limited to endless unfocused description in the style of the natural historian. Wernicke does this through a set of well-analyzed psychological processes, usually applicable as much to healthy as to disturbed individuals. Emil Kraepelin had the same basic objective, but approached it in a very different way.

VIII,(b). Role of Theory in Wernicke's Psychiatry

Theory plays a crucial role in *Grundriss,* especially in the first eight lectures. This is emphasized again in his closing sentence of L41: 'In conclusion, I want to draw your attention to one point, and that is that these, my last comments, should serve to remind you of the need for those theoretical considerations which occupied us in the first half of our clinical studies, but, for you, perhaps often quite difficult to understand.' At times he states explicitly that there are two roads to scientific truth—theory and empirical data; and that such truth is most secure when the two agree. In L28 (p. 188), commenting on the 'second state', he writes: 'Although I do not deny the theoretical interest in these most enigmatic states, this should not affect their factual status'. This distinction is most clear in comments on melancholia, a disorder defined by him most strongly in theoretical terms. So, in L35 (p. 261), we read: 'Affective melancholia presented us with an example where symptoms derived from a hypothetical scheme, and these alone, make up a clinical picture which, in reality, is met very often'; and yet shortly after, empirical demands prevail (L35, p. 262): 'sooner or later in their course, they give further signs, in that delusions of relatedness join in, this being entirely foreign to melancholia. Cessation of melancholia, which may last for a year or more, then usually gives way to a further, worsening stage of persecutory delirium, and soon of megalomania.' Again (L35, p. 260) we read: 'As we have seen above, it is in the nature of akinetic symptoms, that it is often totally impossible to decide how far they are intermingled with other identification disorders, and at other times this is possible only after the akinetic stage is over. So we must then take into account the possibility that the above clinical picture of akinetic motility psychosis, derived entirely empirically, is too broad, and still contains cases in which the motor symptom complex is merely grafted onto another syndrome, which is just as significant, and encompasses it': We see here his keen awareness of a methodological issue, that grouping of symptoms to form clinical entities is sometimes guided by theory, but, in its absence, by empirical associations; and we see his discipline in separating the two. Less explicitly, the same point is made in L34 (p. 256): 'Although this result is based on a statistical review of cases, it also confirms what we might already have expected'.

The balancing act between theory and empirical data was crucial to the birth of the natural sciences. The main difference from natural philosophy is that psychiatry is *much* more complex, and a would-be theoretician needs far more facts at their finger tips before venturing an explanation. This is hinted at in a comment on Kahlbaum (L34, p. 254) who '... has not escaped the fate of all authors who have laboured on monographs in a designated domain': He implies that his own more comprehensive approach, covering the whole field of mental disorders, as well as their basis in neuroscience allows him to suggest conceptualizations superior to those offered by those limited to single areas of psychological abnormality. This also underpins his profoundly holistic approach to the brain and his understanding of each patient as an individual.

In his final lecture, Wernicke gives us some clues to his methods in analyzing and distilling the wealth of clinical data at his disposal. 'My presentation is based on approximately 5,000 carefully kept medical records that have been prepared over the course of 15 years, under my direction and supervision' (L41, p. 325), one presumes between 1885 and 1900, his years at

Breslau. 'Unceasing study of these case histories, their monitoring by continuous observation, the comparison of similar cases with one another, in addition to special study of individual symptoms in these patients, required such an expenditure of time that it was impossible for me also to evaluate studies of other authors in the literature to the extent that would have been necessary for my purposes. The individual cases gave me the advantage that they were very fully examined for my purposes, especially since, through my photographs, which form an integral part of our medical records, I usually managed to call to mind the entire personality' (L41, p. 325). This paragraph, and the preceding one, gives us insight not only into his method, but also his into utter dedication to the task he had set himself.

VIII,(c). Relation Between Neurology and Psychiatry in Grundriss

Despite his opening assertion that mental disorders are brain disorders, Wernicke *does* understand (L1) that they are generally different, a different sort of brain disorder—*Geisteskrankheit* as opposed to *Hirnkrankheit*. He also sometimes makes a distinction between 'psychological' and 'organic' (i.e. neurological) drivers of abnormality, for instance of abnormal movements (L23, p. 148; L24, p. 154). Nonetheless, as a didactic method, he sometimes uses disorders from neurology as a spring-board from which to understand psychiatric conditions, when the two have similar symptoms. Examples include the case of transcortical aphasia in L1; 'hypermetamorphosis' introduced in L20 in a neurological context, to be developed in L22 in a psychiatric context; and mania after temporal lobe lesions, to lead into mania with no such lesion. (The only basis upon which he could have made this comparison is to have seen mania in a patient whose brain was subsequently examined *post-mortem*, referring to his own *Lehrbuch der Gehirn Krankheiten* [96]). Modern studies of secondary mania after brain injury *do* attribute it most often to damage in temporal basal polar regions [97]).

In drawing attention to Wernicke's strategy, we should however be aware that conditions which, to modern clinicians, are clearly neurological, fell easily within his area of practice. The first example (L1) is a patient with abnormality in semantic rather than phonetic organization of language. He draws an analogy between nonsensical speech and transcortical aphasia, a concept already defined. Other examples of 'crossover' are patients who turn continually in circles (L12, p. 74), ones with impaired speech but intact singing (L12, p. 75), or compulsive speech after a temporal lobe lesion (L20, p. 127). In L29 (p. 199) his description corresponds well to modern descriptions of obsessive-compulsive disorder (OCD, now a psychiatric disorder) or to the closely related Tourette's syndrome (now a disorder in neurology). Giles de la Tourette (1857–1904) described the latter syndrome in 1884, while working under Charcot. In these two syndromes, the balance between the ability to initiate and to veto actions is shifted to the former and away from the latter. Wernicke's comment about actions being 'softened by concomitant anxiety' is interesting, since OCD *is* often co-morbid with anxiety disorders, or occurs along with anxiety. The specific symptom of *Coprolalia* [from *kopros*=faeces] (L32, p. 232), with inability to suppress undesirable *speech* is discussed in an apparent case of Tourette's syndrome, as in L29 (p. 200).

Some disorders described by Wernicke straddle with ease the divide between today's neurology and psychiatry: In stroke patients we see the symptom of confabulation, or a patient (L39, p. 200), who 'believed the persecutor to be a man who lay beside her in bed and had taken possession of the paralyzed half of her body'. The commonality of processes of forming explanatory delusions between the latter case and many cases we now identify as mental disorders is striking. In L37 (p. 305) he states that '... bouts of cortical epilepsy tend to leave focal symptoms in their wake, including, quite remarkably even those of a sensory nature, such as sensory aphasia or hemiopia, and often also combined sensory symptoms right up to the level of asymbolia'. Presumably he implies that areas of association cortex as well as primary areas were affected. In L20 (p. 131) a recognizable symptom is given an accurate description—now called 'akathisia', a term introduced in 1902 by the Czech physician Ladislav Haskovec (1866–1904), working in Prague [98]. Wernicke does not use the term, and may not have known the latter's account. In L32 (p. 230) disturbing sensations are described by two patients, with either akathisia or what might now be called 'restless legs syndrome', and which were driving their unusual movements. The former is usually now seen as a side effect of therapy with neuroleptic medicines; the latter, mainly during sleep periods. The phenomenology is nevertheless similar. Overall, it is refreshing to see so many conditions described with so little awareness of today's frontier between neurology and psychiatry.

VIII,(d). Wernicke's Concept of Mental Illness/Disease

In L1 Wernicke's 'credo', that mental illnesses are brain diseases, was in part a continuation of an ancient debate, between those who viewed diseases as imbalances of factors intrinsic to each organism (a view fitting the doctrine of 'four humours'), and those who proposed that there were *essential* concepts of disease, to be classified in ways akin to botanical classification [99]. Essentialist notions grew, over the whole of medicine, as symptoms came to be correlated with pathology in specific organs or organ systems. This was the tradition Wernicke grew up with, and in L5 (p. 28), he refers to cases in neurology (presumably with lesions of known location) as 'cortical diseases'. Such ideas reached their peak in the late nineteenth century when infectious diseases were identified with specific microorganisms. Extension to mental disorders was (and still is) less convincing.

Wernicke's ambivalence on this large issue is discussed later in this essay. Here we limit comments to aspects which might have been 'lost in translation'. Psychiatry in the English-speaking world in the last century drew heavily on earlier German work. The English term 'disease', is the easiest translation of the German word *Krankheit,* which was Wernicke's usual word, used either narrowly or broadly. In English it might be extended to include effects of injury (although this is unusual). In L5 he *does* use the word to refer to brain injury, which is odd to English speakers. However, in English, there are several alternative words to chose from, with different shades of meaning ('disease', 'illness', 'ailment' 'disorder', 'sickness', 'condition', 'syndrome', etc.), with fewer alternatives in German. Some physicians separate 'disease' (a generic concept) from 'illness' (that is, how a generic disease has unique effects at an individual level). In German, *Krankheit* serves most purposes. In English, despite available alternatives, the restricted vocabulary of German has tended to prevail. Thus, one of the oldest anglophile psychiatry journals, founded in Wernicke's lifetime, followed German tradition by calling itself *Journal for Nervous and Mental Disease*.

Today, the debate is opening up again, part of a larger debate on use of medical models for mental disorders. Medical terms for mental disorders are now increasingly challenged by some of today's consumer activists. This is not new. One of Wernicke's critics, Karl Jaspers, based his criticism in part on exactly this—the use of medicalized 'disease' terms for mental disorders [100], this being the basis for his sharp line against Wernicke, as a purveyor of *Hirnmythologie* [101]. It is therefore indeed ironic that Wernicke never once uses the word *Psychopathologie* in *Grundriss*, while Jaspers is best known for his *magnum opus* entitled *Allgemeine Psychopathologie* [102]. (The original 1913 version of this work ran to only 332 pages; the English translation which is now read, comes from the 7th edition of 1959, with 748 pages.)

There are hints that Wernicke was aware of the alternative view, although he could not break free from medical terms. In L5 and later (L9), he uses the plural form, *Krankheiten*, when he has not yet mentioned any generic illness by name or given any diagnostic term. Sometimes he uses *Geistesstörungen*, rather than *Geisteskrankheiten* (in L9, apparently introduced to *Grundriss* in the 1900 revision of 1894 text [[52]; pp. 121]). In

L24 (p. 162) he applies the term to chronic mental disorders); and in L33 (p. 242) he uses the term *Zustandsbild,* literally, 'picture of an existing condition' He writes 'To demarcate such cases it would be well to remember the old differentiation between habitual forms and actual illnesses advocated especially by Kahlbaum. The state of exhaustion described above is evidently not to be regarded as an actual illness, but shows us asthenic confusion as a habitual form or, as recently termed, a *disorder* [*Zustandsbild*]'. Such details *might* indicate that Wernicke intended to convey the English concept of mental *illness* or *disturbance,* as distinct from disease. However, in L9 and L16, he uses *Geistesstörungen* to make another precise distinction (also made by Miller [[103]; p. 99]), between 'active psychosis' and 'psychotic symptoms persisting as a *hangover*, or *memory effect*' from past episodes.

It is worth summarizing the history of the word 'psychosis' here, and what it meant for Wernicke. According to Beer [52], Feuchtersleben was the first to use it in print, in 1847, but it may have been current for some time before that. He intended to stress *mental* concomitants of nervous disorders, in contrast to the word 'neurosis' which originally referred to objective signs of brain disorder. In any case, the word was not used to differentiate classes of mental disorder in Wernicke's day. At the time of the 1906 edition of *Grundriss,* Wernicke often used 'psychosis' as 'falsification of content of consciousness', with 'hallucinations' and 'delusions' as the main examples, a usage similar to today's prevailing meaning, but rather wider. (In today's parlance, 'psychosis' is often evidenced by *limited* forms of delusions and hallucinations. Thus, in today's terms, falsification of body perception in anorexia nervosa, or dissociation leading to falsification of personal identity are not classed as psychotic.) However, Wernicke also used 'psychosis' with a much wider range of meanings. Already in L1, he uses the phrase 'motility psychosis', and classes mutism and verbigeration as 'psychotic symptoms'. Some clarification is offered in the next paragraph where he explains that 'psychosis' refers to an active mental illness, to distinguish it from residual states after an active phase has subsided, for which he prefers 'chronic mental disturbance'. The term also spans anxiety psychosis (L22, p. 143) alcoholic psychosis (L38, p. 295) and hysterical psychosis (L39, p. 301). A section in L24 (p. 162) gives important clues about how, operationally, he used the terms 'psychosis' and 'neurosis', and, indeed what 'mental illness' was for him. It reads: 'For paralytic and hebephrenic somatopsychosis, severe organic loading is taken to be prognostically unfavourable when the limits of hypochondrial neurosis are exceeded and an undoubted mental illness is present'. 'Psychosis' becomes virtually synonymous with 'mental illness', requiring obvious distortion of a person's sense of reality (in any of the three domains of consciousness), while 'neurosis' is separate from both these terms. Overall, the best rendition of psychosis for Wernicke was probably 'a state leading at least transiently to loss of insight (loss of the sense of personal wholeness)'. However, he was probably still formulating the concept at the time of his death.

VIII,(e). Wernicke's Concept of Psychopathology

Wernicke *never* uses the word *Psychopathologie* in *Grundriss,* although the word had been in common use in the Germanic world for some decades. This is a fact of critical importance in deciding how far he accepted the medical notion of mental illness. The words *Pathologie* or *pathologische* are used frequently, but refer almost entirely to actual or potential findings in the brain, while a different word, *krankhafte*, is used to describe experiential or behavioural abnormality. Thus, in English, for the former ('pathology'), we translate here with words which are directly equivalent, and for the latter we use words such as 'abnormality', 'aberrant' or occasionally 'unhealthy'. His habitual usage might imply that, for him, experiential or behavioural features for which he used *krankhafte* might be *statistically* quite abnormal, but were not pathology *sensu stricto.* We identified just two exceptions, where *pathologie* (not *psychopathologie*) is linked to behavioural or experiential abnormality (see 'Psychopathology' in section XVI. 'Terminology'), and a third referring to 'sexual pathology' (p. 326). We also found two examples of tautology (such as *krankhafte Symptome*). The issue here is part of an older debate, on whether 'symptoms' of mental disorders are in continuity with normal experiences, or are qualitatively different in nature [104]. Clearly, in his sejunction theory, and in symptoms he thought to be derived from sejunction, he *did* have a clear concept of neuropathology underlying psychiatric symptoms; yet that theory could not withstand scrutiny (see below). For most other symptoms, our impression is that Wernicke mainly thought in terms of the 'continuity' alternative, although he never explicitly addresses the issue.

VIII,(f). Wernicke's Attitude to 'Symptoms'

Despite never using the term *Psychopathologie,* Wernicke often used the medical term *Symptome.* We have already seen how, like Mach, he based his reasoning on primary experiences. In L1–L8, this reasoning links neurobiology to psychology quite directly. In psychiatry reasoning from primary experiences meant that symptoms as reported by patients were the starting point. Like Jaspers, he tried to grasp the subjective experience of his patients, rather than relying only on objective manifestations. He rejected grouping by aetiology (by which he meant 'proximate cause'), because any one aetiology could lead to a wide variety of syndromes. He preferred grouping based on reasoning from more immediate data; and he suggested that analysis of each case may lead to conclusions at various levels of organization: as psychological formulations, as specified pathways or regions, and potentially as cellular or molecular pathology at such locations.

Much of his reasoning is about *psychological mechanisms* underlying symptoms. (Reasoning at other levels, if attempted, was usually hypothetical.) Thus links between symptoms and neurobiology were indirect; but they *did* exist, plausible if indirect. Most of his psychiatric practice appears to have been 'psychological medicine' in a strict sense. Sometimes the reasoning is exact and prescient. For instance, in L20 (p. 129) he discusses the idea that representation of some verbal thoughts—those 'which are mainly concrete, with a somewhat simplified thought content'—does not involve the left temporal lobe. This intriguing idea receives support from recent research on representation of language in Chinese script. In this case, the sequence from visual representation of symbols to that of their meaning can be direct, not (as in alphabetic script) mediated via initial acoustic coding [105].

Wernicke, defined and grouped symptoms in so far as he understood them on the basis of more basic scientific principles. In contrast, Jaspers took the basic categories of Kant as irreducible qualities [106, 107], but could not validate them in a fundamentally scientific way. His categories therefore had *no* link to any possible physical basis, and were thus independent of the common language of science. Wernicke like Jaspers, uses Kant's philosophy in emphasizing the distinction between content and form, yet drew on Mach's philosophy of science, to take primary experience as the key to the language of the natural sciences. In psychiatry, this meant that symptoms, albeit linked only indirectly to their physical substrate, were by no means independent of that substrate. Wernicke thus *did* succeed (in principle if not always in practice), in bringing the common language of science to bear on psychiatry. That was a huge achievement.

For Wernicke symptoms were by no means fixed entities, as they may be in general medicine. In L15, he argues that the class of symptom which emerges can depend on immediate events in a person's life: What starts as an overvalued idea, may subside, or be amplified to delusional proportions, depending on whether immediate events and the social environment are benign or malevolent. Likewise (L18; p. 114) the symptom-picture in a patient (not just its content, but the class of symptoms) depends on his pre-existing intellectual endowment (namely his capacity for 'well-ordered thinking'), whether it be intrinsic, or developed through education. In addition he recognized that the underlying driver of a symptom complex might show up as a variety of symptoms, depending on individual characteristics of each patient. Thus, in L13 (p. 81), we read: 'For a single form of illness (such as acute "anxiety psychosis"), which entails an essential mental content, one individual might portray that content itself, while another produces phonemes representing the same content'. Major symptoms such as hallucinations and delusions can occur in many conditions, and do not define any such condition in absence of other contextual detail; they are indications of significant mental disorder—no more—whose true nature must then be defined.

The primary aim of *Grundriss* was to teach about psychiatry and the abnormalities he called symptoms. There are just a few references to what is now called 'personality theory'. In L7 we read some of Wernicke's ideas about human individuality, the emphasis being on acquired rather than innate personality traits. This emphasis also features in the clinical lectures, sometimes in reference to habits of behaviour, but occasionally to personality as formed by habit. For instance, in L20 (p. 128), the term 'brain habits' is used, implying emphasis on *acquired* personality traits, rather than ones built into a person's brain processes *ab initio.* His comments on how basic processes appear as different symptoms according to each individual's traits suggests that he *was* aware of more fundamental differences. However, research studies on personality were not well developed at the time of writing.

VIII,(g). Wernicke's Concept of 'Elementary' Symptoms

In L13 (note) and L14 (p. 87) Wernicke introduces the term 'elementary symptom', (*Elementarsymptome*), an important concept in his attempt to bring reasoning to bear on psychiatry. It implied that, for each patient, a single symptom was usually fundamental, one from which all others were derived. The concept is not well presented in *Grundriss*, but is implicit throughout. Krahl and Schifferdecker [1] explore the idea, its origins, implications, and differences from ideas of other psychiatrists of the time, on the basis of Wernicke's extant conference presentations. His analysis of melancholia exemplifies the concept. According to this, disorder of mood is not primary; 'disorder of will' *is* primary. It is only a patient's awareness of how impaired he or she is that leads secondarily to lowered mood. Whether or not Wernicke's reasoning is robust, few other psychiatrists even made the attempt. It is however part and parcel of his essential holism: As each person constructs his sense of wholeness, all parts of the mind (approximately) might be in interaction with every other, continually changing their mutual relation in response to life events. It follows that a single abnormal experience can influence all aspects of psychology, thus producing many secondary symptoms. 'Symptoms' are thus not isolated, documented one-by-one, regardless of concurrent abnormal experiences, individual context, personal faculties, and life events. Wernicke appears to use the same concept for somatic symptoms, for instance when (L24, p. 156), he suggests that a variety of secondary symptoms can start with abnormal laryngeal sensation. A later psychiatrist, Eugen Bleuler, *was* influenced by Wernicke, and *did* distinguish primary from secondary symptoms of schizophrenia, apparently following Wernicke's lead.

A flaw in this approach is that abnormality at the neuropathological level (such as decreased myelination) might have impact on many pathways in the brain, giving rise to diverse psychological changes. The correlation between concurrent symptoms is then due to their common biological origin, not to interactions at the level of information. Moreover, at times Wernicke admits failure to derive all symptoms in a patient from a single 'elementary symptom'. Thus in L21 (p. 135) he writes: 'We will not be able to derive the fact of disorientation from experiences that you have just heard about, and they must be viewed as independent phenomena'; or in L28 (p. 149), in discussing a case of acute autopsychosis: 'Manifold abnormal sensations of which she complained belong here only in part; in other ways their importance is probably that of independent, hysterical concomitants'. In other lectures (e.g. L23, p. 149) he is at pains to point out that in the disorder he describes, symptoms occur 'in isolation', these being exceptions to his usual thesis.

The logic of interaction between symptoms is usually ignored in today's psychiatry in documents which operationalize detection of symptoms, as if they were independent entities. The concept of 'elementary symptoms' has much to recommend it in a field where scientific reasoning is rare. The history of the transition from Wernicke's style to today's, moves inexorably from Jasper's flexible approach to description [108]; to Schneider's first rank symptoms of schizophrenia, later codified, probably against the author's intention [109]; to the emphasis of Erwin Stengel, working for the World Health Organization in the 1950s, on standardized nomenclature [110]; and then to DSM III. This is largely the story of tension between gifted and imaginative clinicians who, above all, needed flexibility, and administrators requiring precision and replicability, whatever the validity of the concepts used.

Krahl and Schifferdecker [1] suggest reasons (other than his premature death) why Wernicke never developed the idea more fully. One such reason is that he preferred to focus on sejunction theory. However, in the opening paragraph of L15, sejunction and supposed 'elementary symptoms' are closely related, the former as a neuropathological process, generating the latter as primary symptoms. So, in showing how one elementary symptom leads to others, he refers to: 'the remaining content of consciousness, appearing, to a degree, to have disintegrated into fragments, a fact to which we gave the name "sejunction", in other words, detachment of individual components one from another. Such components initially form tight-knit structures, as complete experiences, but their sejunction is shown by the fact that memories which flatly contradict each other can co-exist. The sejunction hypothesis then led us to a closer understanding of certain symptoms of activation, first, of manifestations of disturbed conscious activity itself, and then of self-generated ideas and obsessions, then of hallucinations.'

Brief discussion is also needed on how Wernicke saw the relationship between positive and negative symptoms. He states '... more complex circumstances underlie pathological processes of *activation*, and in some way must be seen to depend on symptoms of deficit' (L14, p. 85). In other words, deficit ('negative') symptoms had more direct explanations than symptoms of activation ('positive' ones), which were usually secondary to the former. This assumption may have grown from the fact that, as a neurologist, he was mainly concerned with functional loss after discrete lesions. In his sejunction hypothesis, he sees positive symptoms as a bi-product of deficits. However, this rule is by no means absolute. In L33, in introducing 'confused mania' (p. 236), he is clear that the picture of positive symptoms 'as a symptom of stimulation—that is, one connected to flight of ideas and loquacity—is separated in principal from the corresponding state of deficit'. Moreover, in discussing states where hyperkinetic and akinetic phases are combined (L35), 'the hyperkinetic stage always comes first.' This issue was addressed by Miller [111], suggesting that, at least for schizophrenia, negative symptoms arise from activation underlying positive ones; repeated excess of nervous activity produces progressive cellular destruction (However, the author no longer accepts this inference). Many views are viable here.

VIII,(h). Affective Impact of Mental Illnesses

As part of Wernicke's thoroughly holistic approach, he gives considerable thought to the emotional impact of mental disorders. For this, he uses several terms—*Affekt*, *Gefühl* and *Emotionen* being the main ones—used carefully in different senses, and often using the word *Färbung* (coloration). A fourth word used occasionally is *Gemütsbewegungen* (literally 'movements of temper or disposition'). *Affekt* refers to an inner experiential reaction or state, learned about mainly from a patient's words. *Gefühl* is more of a 'visceral' feeling, an 'organ sensation', but not identified with any particular sensory modality, and closely linked to an automatic reflex reaction (often found in the compound noun *Organgefühl*); while *Emotionen* refers to objective manifestations of *Affekt*, a state with visible, non-verbal, autonomic or somatic signs of emotion, typical of hysteria (as becomes clear in L39). In L39 (p. 303) we also read an interesting line: 'Almost always in these cases, phrenic nerve insufficiency can be demonstrated as the basis for the fear'. This appears to refer to the theory of emotions proposed independently by William James [112] in 1884 and Carl Lange [113] in 1887: Emotions as experiential states originate as subjective responses to automatic autonomic and other stereotyped bodily reactions.

This is a difficult area for translation, where there may be more words in German than in English. In English 'emotion' is the term used in general speech, 'Affect' is a specialist term, although its use goes far back in history; and another word 'passion' is archaic, but with similar meaning. In our translation we use 'Affect' or 'Affective state' when Wernicke uses *Affekt* (retaining the upper case 'A', to avoid confusion with the English verb—'to affect'); and Emotion is used when he uses *Emotionen. Gefühl* is usually rendered as 'feeling'.

In L25 (p. 169) Wernicke suggests that in acute psychosis (*Acute hallucinosis*, in his terms) disturbed Affect recovers first, followed by hallucinations, while delusions persist longest. In addition, quite generally, he designates the Affective impact of mental disorders in acute mental illnesses, especially if they 'irrupt acutely' (p. 190), by the distinctive German word *Ratlosigkeit.* However, the impact is itself a product of another state, identified as *Desorientierung* (disorientation). Wernicke admits that he cannot define the latter properly, it being a matter for future work. It is presumably not in the realm of Affect or emotion itself, but possibly a precursor of these at a cognitive level. *Ratlosigkeit* appears to be the Affective state produced by awareness of conflict or incongruity between contents of the mind, produced by mental illness, as in L28, where we read (p. 190): 'It was only the newspaper article [reminding a patient of a former place of work] that awakened in him the Affective state of autopsychic disarray [*Ratlosigkeit*], and which caused him to seek medical help.'

In all psychoses, abnormal mental content appears in the context of the Affective state termed *Ratlosigkeit*, an insight probably based on Griesinger's concept of 'primordial delirium' (L18, p. 113). The word *Ratlosigkeit* requires some discussion. Its use predates Wernicke, for instance in writings of Kahlbaum [32], allied to the term 'confusion'. Wernicke knew it to be used sometimes by his patients to describe their state of mind; and he is also aware that it is distinctive to the German language (L21; p. 134). How should it be rendered in English? The usual translation has been 'perplexity', or 'helplessness'. Neither word is a correct rendition. It is different from 'disorientation', since, in L21 (p. 134), we read that sensory deception alone need not produce disorientation, but can lead to *Ratlosigkeit;* and in L27, a patient is described with*out Ratlosigkeit*, but with prominent allopsychic disorientation, (p. 181), contrasted with another in whom allopsychic disorientation *is* accompanied by *Ratlosigkeit* (p. 183). The difference appears to be that a person in a state of *Ratlosigkeit* knows that he/she is in this state; a disoriented person may lack such self-knowledge (presumably of an Affective state). The relation between disorientation and *Ratlosigkeit* is not entirely clear, but may depend on whether the disorientation is in the allo-, auto-, or somato-psychic domains: Intense emotional reactions to auto- or somato-psychic symptoms may exist, while allopsychic orientation is maintained.

Ratlosigkeit, is itself an abstract noun indicating loss of *Rat*—a German noun most often used as a 'counsel' or 'advisory body'—a group of people, such as a city or regional government, 'taking counsel', or 'providing advice'. Implicitly, then, *Ratlosigkeit,* suggests 'loss of the inner counsel' or 'deliberation amongst our various faculties', a meaning quite different from and more specific than either 'perplexity', or 'helplessness' (the latter implying 'loss of control'). There appears to be no equivalent word with the same sense in English. Most discussion of it in psychopathology appears to have occurred well after Wernicke's days, for instance in a monograph from 1939 by G.E. Störring (see unsigned review in *Journal of Nervous and Mental Disease,* in 1940 [114]). The two English words we feel get nearest to *Ratlosigkeit* are 'confound', usually as a verb, and 'disarray', as a noun. The former has shifted in meaning but its older meaning is captured in a line from the English national anthem 'confound their politics'; and in this older meaning sometimes meant 'to confuse, fail to distinguish, mix up'. While there is no satisfactory translation of this word, we choose 'disarray' to render *Ratlosigkeit.* This word captures the sense of lost coordination, sometimes of a social group, but not that of coordination of separate faculties. The usage should be read in conjunction with this explanatory paragraph. Occasionally we do use the word 'perplex' in a non-technical sense, and when we use 'helplessness', it is to translate a word other than *Ratlosigkeit.* Occasionally, our word 'disarray' is used to translate another German word (e.g. *Unordnung*: p. 86).

VIII,(i). Wernicke's Sejunction Theory

A central conjecture in Wernicke's account of mental disorder, apparently a process at the cellular level, is his *Sejunction Theory,* supposed to account for two striking observations. The first is the apparent illogical nature of utterances in many patients, blind to logical inconsistencies between different expressed beliefs. The second, as stated in the summary heading to L12 is 'to explain pathological excitatory symptoms'. Already in L2 he has given a breakdown of possible neuropathological bases for mental disorders: Three things could go wrong at a cellular level: Reduced, increased, or aberrant excitability. In this context, he refers to 'pathways' and to 'conduction' therein. His inclusion of causes other than frank lesions sounds modern, but gives no detail. The chief experiences which made him raise the topic of pathological excitation were probably symptoms of progressive paralysis, some of which he interpreted as abnormal excessive excitation at specific locations; his explanation of hallucinations in terms of the sejunction theory may have grown directly from such evidence. This theory also led him to view negative symptoms as primary, positive ones as secondary: 'I have represented sejunction as the fundamental process, and derived symptoms of irritation from this' (L33, p. 240). The German word for 'symptom of irritation', *Reizsymptome,* could also be translated as 'stimulation symptom'.

In no way does this theory stand the test of time, or could it ever have done so. It is a weakness, which in his day, fuelled the charge of 'neuromythology'. It is nevertheless instructive to examine the origins of the theory, the clinical facts which it purported to explain, and the facts he did *not* know, which had he known, might have held him back from this notion. In *Grundriss,* it is presented in L9 in connection with a patient named Rother (who is representative of many long-stay patients in his institution). There were also various accessory notions, to deal with other clinical facts. Here we deal with the core concept. Other detail, especially on the second aim of the theory, follows later in relation to specific symptoms.

Details of Rother, a gardener by trade, are as follows: Wernicke has known him since 1871, only one year after he graduated in medicine. He has been a stable, reliable member of the institution for many years, with little outward sign of abnormality, coherent in carrying out many daily tasks, interested in current affairs, capable of all normal courtesies, with a seemingly rational attitude to his being in the institution. However, when questioned, his answers are astonishing. Once we gain complete trust, in the chatting stage, he regales us unreservedly with his experiences. At first we are struck by the fact that he knows nothing about having overcome a mental illness; for his part he might have come into hospital only because of an acute febrile illness, and he actually considers it wrong—a mistake—that he has been held for so long, even though he admits that the doctors had always been kind to him. Then he tells of a conflict with one of his gardener's boys shortly before his admission to the institution. During the struggle he had been thrown down the stairs by this man, and had broken his neck.

I ask: "Who?"
"Well, me".
Question: "But aren't you alive and sitting here?"
"Well, yes, but the other one is probably still there."
Question: "What other one?"
"Well, Rother."
Question: "So, once you have been dead; is this possible?"
"Of course, everyone has a double."

He then recounts how he had experienced other quite different things that no-one would believe: he had once been a bull and, as such, had been tortured in a quite inhumane manner and then been slaughtered. He describes how they had drawn a ring through his nose and dragged him along. He had also been crucified once, together with two robbers.

Question: "Like Jesus Christ?"
"Yes, exactly like that."
Question: "Then you are probably Jesus Christ?"
"Yes, I am Jesus Christ."

In L12 (p. 72) where the term 'sejunction' is first introduced, Wernicke discusses Rother's state of mind. This section is more controversial than most of his writing in *Grundriss*; yet his insight, to our mind accurate, is that there *is* something important to be explained. In part, 'sejunction' is intended to account for supposedly abnormal co-existence of incompatible notions. Different interpretations of such distortions of personal identity are possible. Literally, Rother's words refer to the *Doppelgänger* (in English: 'alter ego'), a familiar concept through most of the nineteenth century. A second interpretation is a true multiple (as opposed to double) personality, a concept recognized after work of Pierre Janet in France, and today given the name Dissociative Identity Disorder in DSM-IV (still controversial). This may be revealed as multiple voices in conversation (three are referred to in L29, p. 198), a symptom now known to be more common in Dissociative Identity Disorder than in what is called schizophrenia. A third possibility is that an attempt is made to recreate for a person confined in an abnormal situation, a semblance of normality as a 'reconstructed persona'. A fourth, and most likely possibility, recently expounded by Ball [82] is that, in a chronic stage of schizophrenia, there is failure to unite two aspects of the 'self'—the 'self experiencing now', and the 'conceptualized objectivized self', normally represented (respectively) in right and left hemispheres. If the two are poorly integrated, a strong conceptualized self may see a weak 'self experiencing now' as an alter ego, sometimes referred to in the third person (see: L21, p. 135; L22, p. 143; L24, p. 159)—or here, using the patient's own surname. This is different from 'dissociative identity', where each identity, while to a degree separate, itself remains coherent.

Succinct statements of the core of the sejunction idea come in L14 ('the uncoupling of associations') and early in L15 '... "sejunction", in other words, detachment of individual components one from another': This phrase is reminiscent of that to be used by Eugen Bleuler in his 1911 work '*Dementia praecox or the group of schizophrenias*' [115] who wrote: 'In this malady the associations lose their continuity. Of the thousands of associative threads which guide our thinking, this disease seems to interrupt, quite haphazardly, sometimes such single threads, sometimes a whole group, and sometimes even large segments of them. In this way, thinking becomes illogical and often bizarre'. The similarity is no coincidence: Wernicke's *Grundriss,* and specifically the sejunction concept, *did* influence Bleuler [116]. 'Sejunction' (literally a *breaking* of associations, or a state of broken associations) is a better term than 'disjunction', or 'dissociation', both of which imply separation of internally coherent entities. There may also have been older origins to the concept, coming from Meynert, since Wernicke writes (L33, p. 241): 'I might assign such cases to the highest grade of weakened association [in confused mania] described by Meynert, which he compares to genetic confusion.' Meynert's concept was that in the childlike brain, associative connections are already very weak, which was probably linked to Kahlbaum's idea current in Meynert's day that adolescence was a time of vulnerability to psychosis. Implicitly, Wernicke believed the 'breaking' to have a clear basis, at a micro-anatomical level, rather than any gross lesion. As such, *sejunction* laid claim to be a fundamental and new neuropathological process underlying most major mental disorders. However, it lacked any supporting evidence at the neuronal level.

Part of the context for 'sejunction' is what Wernicke did *not* know, but which we know now. He had no idea, or did not use, the idea that active inhibition existed in the brain at neuronal levels, which, at psychological levels, could suppress one or more of a set of incompatible notions. Failure of inhibition *might* then give a better account of Rother's state. Even given his ignorance of neuronal inhibition, a major flaw in his reasoning is apparent: He confuses *statistical* incompatibility ('negative association') which could recruit inhibitory processes now understood, with *logical* incompatibility (whose physical basis would be quite different). Further gaps in Wernicke's knowledge which made possible the sejunction theory are mentioned below.

However, one might ask what *could* be the basis of the apparent loss of logical consistency in patient Rother? As pointed out in section VI,(c). "Wernicke, on Theory of Knowledge", the facility for deductive inference, and with it, awareness of logical inconsistencies and the need to eliminate them, is not a natural human endowment, but one in which some people excel, while others think in more natural ways, dependent on memory and association. Wernicke's assumption that personal identity is synonymous with *logical* consistency of information within an individual's mind is unrealistic, and would not separate normal persons from his patients. Regardless of this, to operate via deduction in the quest for consistency requires that 'ground rules' for a system of logic be in place, as a 'framework' for reasoning within which premises and conclusions can be 'located'. In terms of Immanuel Kant's *Critique of Pure Reason,* these are the 'synthetic *a priori* statements', needed (for instance) for numerical or spatial reasoning. In another work [88] a theory was developed to show how, by interplay between hippocampus and neo-cortex, the inherent ambiguity of associations in the latter structure could be resolved; and it was also argued that such interplay sets up lasting configurations representing *contexts* for operating in specific situations. In those humans who operate via deduction and logical consistency, such contexts encompass the operations needed for deduction, setting up hidden assumptions as the 'framework' needed for the system to operate. In those who do not operate in this way, likely to be those with little education such as patient Rother, contexts can still be established by interplay between neocortex and hippocampus, but serve other roles in the day-to-day lives of such people. In expressions of belief, inconsistencies may then exist, but since these are between relatively unremarkable notions, they attract little attention, although it may be hard to get such persons to grasp the incompatibility of co-existing beliefs. If however, such persons experience periods of active illness which introduce bizarre notions into their beliefs, there is again no way in which the incompatibility can be resolved; yet the bizarreness of their beliefs now makes it clear in social settings that they have been mentally ill. The more bizarre the beliefs acquired during periods of active illness, the more outlandish is the residue of strange beliefs outlasting the active phase; yet, with no ability in rational analysis, resolution of conflicts of beliefs is difficult, and may be impossible.

For Wernicke, primary abnormalities could be defined at either a biological, cellular level, or at a psychological level. Sejunction was supposed to be the primary biological abnormality. At the psychological level 'elementary' symptoms emerge, as in patient Rother. Some such symptoms are distorted perceptions (hallucinations); others are beliefs whose abnormality falls short of being delusional. With regard to beliefs, he introduced two terms, *autochthonous ideas* (L11, p. 68) and *overvalued ideas* (L15, p. 92), both linked to delusions.

VIII,(j). Hallucinations and Related Phenomena for Wernicke

For Wernicke, hallucinations are important symptoms, more primary than delusions (which are seen mainly as secondary attempts to explain), and, as such, a major class of 'elementary symptom'. This theme, which went back to Griesinger, may explain why, for Wernicke, a major subdivision of psychoses is 'hallucinosis' (with separate acute and chronic subtypes) a term which probably originated with him, and not widely used until after his death. He recognized the heterogeneity in both the clinical aspects of hallucinations, and their origin. His views on hallucinations appear in L13, L19, and L20. Although covering hallucinations in all modalities, as well as multimodal ones, he clearly states that '… for all hallucinations—with few exceptions—hallucinated speech sounds predominate' (L13; p. 80). Exceptions included psychoses of intoxication. On the 'incorrigibility' of hallucinations, he writes: 'The reality of a sensory deception is maintained against the testimony of all other senses and most fantastic attempts are made to explain it, leaving no room for doubt, or the possibility of their sense being deceptive' (L13, p. 80). Such an emphatic statement might not be made today, when many lay people know of the symptom, some of whom, when they themselves experience it, know immediately the experience to be deceptive, not a faithful reflection of external reality. In L21 (p. 134) in discussing patient K., Wernicke appears to accept this possibility.

Wernicke refers to the usual auditory hallucinations, which are verbal, as 'phonemes' (L13; p. 80), although he mentions non-verbal auditory hallucinations, (L19) which merge or transform into verbal ones. The word 'phoneme' came from Dufriche-Desgenettes in 1873. Use of the term for an abstract concept in linguistics started with Polish researchers, Jan Niecislaw Baudoiuin de Courtenay and Mokiloj Kruszewski, working at the University of Kazan in Russia between 1875 and 1895. Wernicke's use of the term has a different sense, indicating inner experiences of speech sounds, which might be projected as external voices (including dialogues [L13, p. 81]), or projected upon identified people in the vicinity (L13, p. 81), a manifestation with less favourable implications. He is strict in what he identities as hallucinated speech: 'In my opinion there is no reason to refer to hallucinations of the muscle sense, as Cramer (1889) does, in order to explain "hearing voices". The symptom of "thought echo" should be as restricted as possible, and understood in the sense that the patient recognizes these as their own thoughts, sounded out loud on certain occasions, such as, for example, when the patient is reading or writing. Cramer himself, and all his successors, left the symptom so broad, that it has lost its original value as an elementary symptom, and now still requires an explanation of its various routes of development' (L13, p. 80, note): Here he probably refers to a comment made in L6, that muscle sensation had previously been given undue emphasis for position sense.

Visual hallucinations are discussed in L19 (p. 120) '… patients themselves refer to them as "images", and … as shadows, or even as "ghosts", a term implying some form of explanatory delusion.' Whatever the perceptual component of a hallucination, the words with which it is described, such as 'poison', often imply explanation. Visual hallucinations, like auditory ones, capture the full focus of attention, but have a greater sense of unreality than phonemes, and are thus less compelling and 'incorrigible'. Tactile hallucinations, sometimes called 'delusions of infestation' today, leave open the idea that they originate from genuine disturbance of sensory input. A fine account is given (L19, p. 121) of multimodal ('combined') hallucinations, a topic rarely discussed today. These often combine senses with natural kinship (such as taste and smell). For such combinations, Wernicke uses the term 'dreamlike', etymologically similar to today's 'hypnogogic' but probably a separate experience. An issue of increasing relevance today, is whether these are re-enactments of past trauma.

Many suggestions are made on the origin of hallucinations. In L19, the possibility of abnormal sensory input is implied in both auditory and tactile sense. Somatization, a modern term, is not used, but the concept features prominently (L10, L24) especially in relation to intestinal sensation. Then (as today), patient complaints might be based on lay conceptualizations of the body, and current fads of the day. In L10 (p. 62) a patient is described for whom 'the suspicion we therefore had, that he was still suffering physical sensations, was confirmed when we examined him; for it revealed that the patient still felt an obstruction and constriction of the bowel immediately proximal to the anus, complained about extreme discomfort and all sorts of abnormal sensations during defaecation, albeit conveyed with a sense of hopelessness, and requested medical treatment for his actual suffering'. In L24 (p. 162) we hear of 'unbearable tickling sensation in the intestine'. L24 also contains descriptions of what might now be called 'Irritable Bowel Syndrome' a 'functional disorder' not otherwise recognized until the 1950s, and usually dealt with in gastroenterology. Prominence given to intestinal sensation (see also L5) may seem strange to a modern reader. However, the idea that 'autointoxication' from gut bacteria might cause mental disturbance was becoming popular at the time. It built on the germ theory of disease, starting with a paper in 1868 by Hermann Senator (1835–1911), professor in Berlin. It developed further, especially after Wernicke's time, in France, Germany and elsewhere [117]. Kraepelin regarded auto-intoxication as a possible cause of *Dementia praecox* [118]. In L24 (p. 161) we also read of 'the old theory of positional changes in the colon as the cause of mental illnesses', a belief whose origin we could not trace.

Another recently named syndrome *Persistent genital arousal disorder* (L24, p. 156) is also described. What is now called *delusion of infestation* is mentioned (L24, p. 163). Another possible case of exaggerated sensory input comes in L13 (p. 83): 'It often happened that the father pounded the table which drove him into the most powerful sexual arousal.' 'The very sight of his father was apparently associated with a morbid feeling that in this case was linked to morbid physical sensations about which he was uncomfortable. Such examples would probably have been called reflex hallucinations by Kahlbaum'. Wernicke likens it to what Kahlbaum called 'sensory delirium'. In either case it is an exaggerated sensation, rather than a quasi-perceptual image arising from (or distorted by) meaning constructed at higher levels (as are many of today's 'psychotic hallucinations'). Alternatively, it may be a case of what, in psychoanalytic theory, is called the 'electra complex', unusual only in its being directed from son to father. In any case, much of the description in L24 combines what might now be called somatization disorders, along with eating disorders, especially *anorexia nervosa,* which posed a threat to life, then as now (L24, p. 162).

In so far as some hallucinations arise from genuine amplification of sensory input to the cortex, with no change of stimulus parameters, they may signify an unrecognized, but general class of disorders, found in many, perhaps all sensory systems, dealt with sometimes in psychiatry as 'somatization', sometimes in various other specialties, as functional disorders in corresponding body systems. Their brain mechanisms may be the background for *some* types of hallucination—indeed, also for some delusions. Today, such sensory abnormalities are an active area of research, not yet assimilated into broad generalizations (see section IX,(d). "Wernicke's Approach to Classification of Mental Disorders" on theoretical validation of Wernicke's symptoms groups). With such advances nowhere in sight in Wernicke's day, it is no surprise that his concepts of hallucinations—and delusions—differ from today's.

Apart from unusually amplified sensory input to the cortex, Wernicke argues that sensory perceptions with no external stimuli, must originate in cortical regions for sensory perceptions; 'the difference from actual sensory perception is then limited, in that the origin of the stimulus in one case lies in the periphery, while for hallucinations it lies in central, transcortical sites, although the target location is the same in both situations' (p. 81). In part this statement may have arisen from his encounters with progressive paralysis patients in whom striking positive psychotic symptoms, as well as those of deficit were seen. On the exact means by which this occurs two quite different accounts are offered. The most plausible account comes towards the end of L19. Starting from early ideas of Müller, that there is genuine disturbance of sensory input or processing in sensory pathways, he excludes, step by step, each suggestion. As part of this, he rejects Meynert's view that hallucinations arise from over-activation of subcortical nuclei (L19; p. 123). This is based on the fact that hallucinations often convey complex meaningful images, along with the anatomical fact that, intrinsic to the cerebral cortex is a massive system of long and short association connections, while the thalamus and basal ganglia have no counterparts. Modern evidence supports the argument, in that principal neurons of the thalamus have no local axon collaterals, and the principal neurones of the striatum (caudate/putamen in humans), main nucleus of the basal ganglia, are inhibitory, not excitatory; so neither structure can support massive associative operations. In the end, he is forced to conclude that 'the essence of a hallucination [occurs when an] aberrant stimulus extends via the memory image to these carriers of the organ sensation; and a memory image becomes a visual image, and next, becomes a hallucination, as soon as it is makes contact with the associated organ sensation—by excitation of those perception cells.' This view can incorporate a comment made in L11 (p. 69) of 'thought becoming sound': the so-called 'audible thoughts', as a hypothesis for auditory verbal hallucinations, and (L12, p. 73) 'the finding that patients themselves do not know exactly whether they hear voices or only experience related thoughts, corresponds to a transitional state between autochthonous thoughts and hallucinations'.

This is Wernicke's most coherent account of hallucinations. However, at an earlier stage (L12) he offers other views, deriving from the theory of sejunction, which like the theory itself, is prone to diverse criticism. In L12 (p. 74) he writes 'hallucinations may occur even without an actual process being in place, merely by accumulation of nervous current at the point of sejunction'. Here the 'sejunction' concept, based on observations of haphazard disconnection of ideas, with scant awareness of their logical incompatibility, has shifted to a different class of events, namely subjective reports of hallucinations. The connection is not obvious until we read what follows (L12, p. 74) 'the perceived magnitude of the stimulus is amplified beyond the norm; consequently, excitation of sensory regions of the brain (*s*) may be expected to occur, even without an external stimulus, especially if the same process has occurred often, and therefore become habitual', and again (L13, p. 79) 'projection fields themselves, regardless of whether these fields are directly affected by a pathological stimulus, or are affected only indirectly as a result of a sejunction process and the *hypothetical backflow* of nervous current from complex associative structures' (emphasis added).

What is implied is that, when pathways for associative links are somehow broken, nervous activity in pathways lacking onward connection can build up, like a blocked stream, and propagate backwards ('hypothetical backflow') to irritate the site of origin, namely primary sensory areas. Pent-up nervous energy, so to speak, produces spurious retrograde activation of sensory regions. A specific example appears in L35 (p. 268): 'For primary auditory hallucinations, hearing is indeed to be regarded as a stimulation process that arouses not only acoustic patterns, but also related organ sensation; and, beyond the intensity of the original stimulus, it is only the presence of a well-worn pathway, which has always served for repetition, that explains irradiation into the motor speech area'. The latter can only be the well known pathway from Wernicke's to Broca's area, perhaps accounting for links between verbal hallucinations and uttered speech. A similar relation is implied in L34 (p. 251): 'Certain parakinetic symptoms, in hyperkinetic motility psychosis, about which we have already had a chance to learn, give us a better hope of their being traced back to processes of irritation'.

Another statement, of how sejunction could account jointly for broken associations and aberrant excesses of excitation appears in L26: 'We see in his allopsychic disorientation, a failure corresponding with paralysis; and we may assume that those complicated arrangements of mutually associated memory images which allow recognition of the immediate situation have become paralyzed or inexcitable. It is then perhaps not accidental that the irritant effect becomes so clear, in that analogous arrays of memory images, corresponding to whole situations and experiences, emerge spontaneously, and with abnormal clarity'. In these two sentences we see, in essence the twin processes of the sejunction concept—loss of habitual associations, and their replacement by spurious excesses. These words are in the context of *Delirium tremens*.

Three incorrect assumptions lie hidden here, all refuted by subsequent advances. *First,* at the anatomical level, it is assumed that primary sensory regions of cortex receive major inputs only from ascending sensory pathways, not from other cortical regions. This is incorrect: The overwhelming numerical majority of synapses on pyramidal neurones in primary sensory cortical regions are derived not from thalamic input but from other sources, mainly other cortical regions [119]. Thus, hallucinations *could* arise by abnormal predominance of 'top-down' control, which is usually overridden by sensory input. There are precedents for this: When sensory input is greatly reduced, the balance shifts, so that visual hallucinations may occur in sight-impaired people (Charles Bonnet syndrome), or when falling asleep. This is implied by Wernicke's account of hallucinations (L12, p. 76): '… combined hallucinations are not uncommon in all situations of reduced sensation.'

The *second,* incorrect assumption is that the 'hydraulic' metaphor which Wernicke uses is misapplied to transmission along nervous pathways. The mistake arises because he did not know that the all-or-none law applied to axonal conduction, making information transmission by axons largely independent of signal energetics. Without such knowledge, the two *could* be linked, so that the hydraulic metaphor might apply.

The *third* gap which sejunction attempted to fill, is Wernicke's lack of awareness of the concept of reinforcement. Much of L20 deals with a supposed pathological process by which points of excessive activation arise in the cerebral cortex, leading to abnormal added experience ('positive symptoms'). However, today, we might attribute such excess to overactive neural reinforcement, possibly arising directly in the striatum, and relayed from there to specific cortical foci. Overactive reinforcement is now a major hypothesis to explain psychotic symptoms.

Overall, Wernicke offers two incompatible accounts of hallucinations, one plausible and probably correct for at least some types of hallucination, the other based on the sejunction theory, which is quite implausible.

VIII,(k). Sejunction Used to Account for Phenomena Better Explained in Other Ways

In L12 the sejunction theory is used over-inclusively, to account for two clinical manifestations which we now know to have more plausible accounts. One of these (L12, p. 74) was a patient turning continually in circles: Apart from explanatory beliefs which a patient might construct, this is not psychosis, by modern concepts: Such a movement disorder is well known (and well-studied in animal models), arising in the basal ganglia from either asymmetrical damage or asymmetrical activation by drugs or internal processes. Description of the subjective impact of these motor symptoms is interesting and vivid, but the case put forward that these are examples of 'sejunction' is implausible. The second patient (L12, p. 75) is '… a female patient [who] began to sing, and you may still remember how clearly she spoke about the fact that she did this against her will, and did not feel like doing it … She typically showed a defective pattern of breathing … When singing however, she suddenly presented a normal respiratory pattern.' Wernicke writes: 'I believe that I have demonstrated conclusively that the explanation of this phenomenon is possible only based on the sejunction hypothesis'. This is unnecessary. The finding that motor disability disappears during singing is known elsewhere in neurology, perhaps related to unusual motor control, subject to unusual emotional influences.

VIII,(l). Delusions and Related Phenomena for Wernicke

There has long been unresolved debate over whether delusions arise by normal interpretation of experiences which are themselves abnormal, or as interpretations which are themselves abnormal (see Miller [120], while admitting that alternative views apply for some aberrant beliefs). For Wernicke delusions are 'falsification of contents of consciousness', and, with few exceptions, he advocates the first of these, mainly denying a role for abnormality of interpretation in forming delusions. This idea can be traced back to John Locke for whom delusions arise not from flaws in reasoning, but from faulty premises [77]. Thus in L11 (p. 67), he writes: 'Suffice it to say that we can trace back explanatory delusional ideas to every single one of the acute symptoms that we will encounter later'.

Later he clarifies this in one area: 'Patients differentiate quite well between their own thoughts, which, in the case of compulsive ideas compel them against their will, and "foreign" thoughts, in the case of *autochthonous ideas*' (emphasis added). The word 'autochthonous' appears to be Wernicke's special term, with no antecedents. Outside psychiatry, it refers to something arising locally (for instance in an indigenous society), rather than having wider currency, and introduced to a locality from outside. In psychiatry, an autochthonous idea is a strongly perceived notion, with no links to prior thought activity. It may be *perceived* as coming from an external, alien, perhaps malevolent source. This is confusing in relation to its wider meaning. It might be better rendered here as a 'self-generated idea' which preserves the wider meaning, but since it is a distinctive part of Wernicke's vocabulary, we retain 'autochthonous'. He writes (L11, p. 68) 'Patients notice the emergence of thoughts which they consider alien to themselves, not perceived as normal, that is, probably not created by the usual processes of association'. In L12 (note), we read that patients 'initially have no explanation' for autochthonous ideas. Usually however an explanation is immediately contrived, except occasionally (333) where he writes: 'Nevertheless, there are those like the patient who taught me only recently. In that particular case autochthonous ideas were the sole psychotic symptom, and they subsided again without being related to any explanatory delusions.' In L12 (p. 73) we read: 'We might also be tempted to seek a distinguishing feature related to sejunction, so that at one time—for compulsive thoughts—we might be dealing with an excitatory process whose continuity is preserved; and at another time—for autochthonous ideas—with an excitatory process, where it is partially lost'.

Wernicke assumes that the organ of consciousness is the organ of association, that association is based on excitatory processes, that it occurs in the full focus of consciousness, and is slow enough for us to know of its operation. Therefore, according to him, when a person is *not* aware how an idea sprang to mind, that is evidence of a primary abnormality, and perhaps a loss of excitatory processes. However, the premises in the argument can be questioned: Normally, we often do not know the precursors of ideas arising in our minds, although they are likely to be the result of continuous reverberation in our brains. Wernicke admits as much with the phrase 'unconscious mental activity', in L12 (p. 73). The phrase 'partially lost' again admits this as a possibility.

Closely related to autochthonous ideas is Wernicke's concept of 'overvalued ideas', a term similar to the then-popular phrase—*'idéé fixe* (which Wernicke uses occasionally [L15, p. 94; L41, p. 329]). This is developed in L15, where he writes that they '... are sharply distinguished from self-generated ideas in that they are evaluated within a patient's consciousness, and thus, by no means are to be viewed as alien intruders.' Overvalued ideas may remain as isolated symptoms, as in a case he describes in L15 (p. 93) of an elderly gentleman who, when outside the institution continually feels harassed by other people, especially a certain master carpenter '... everything always came back to the one master carpenter who, meanwhile, had served up the old story to other people, and notified the police of their observations of mental illness. Nowhere in the institution has anyone observed even a hint of a delusion or any other sign of mental illness in this patient'. An overvalued idea *may* lead to delusional elaboration, but since this is not a necessary feature, the two symptoms are separate, an overvalued idea being classed as an 'elementary symptom'; yet Wernicke admits that 'the mechanism of its formation remains unexplained' (p. 90).

Wernicke is clear that delusions themselves are acquired by a learning-like process, sometimes instantaneously, and can then persist as enduring beliefs. In L10, (p. 61) he documents cases where 'we have observed . .the time at which somatopsychic delusional ideas actually originate, and can thus provide evidence of their origin from abnormal physical sensations.' From this, the point he often makes in early clinical lectures, follows easily—that there is a difference between active illness, and beliefs that endure when the active phase is over ('stable conditions and diseases actually in the process of developing': L9, p. 34). Thus, delusions differ from hallucinations, which, while remembered, are immediate experiences. In L25 (p. 169) he makes this point for one patient, that 'recovery involves elimination of the hallucinations, despite tenacious retention of the system of delusions'. Recent research also shows that hallucinations are usually eliminated more quickly than delusions during antipsychotic drug therapy. Experiences which *could* be classed as abnormal, and from which, in Wernicke's, view, delusions arise, have been mentioned already—hallucinations (which may be projected into the external world as 'delusions of relatedness'; L11, p. 69; L13, p. 80) and autochthonous ideas (often projected on to a doctor; L11, p. 69). He also suggests that lack of insight may itself be a primary abnormality (L9, p. 56), often based on the fact of a patient's detention in hospital (L10, p. 64; L14, p. 88). This is seen as a primary effect of the sejunction process; but this is hard to accept: For a patient with no education about psychiatry, what needs to be explained is not so much *lack* of insight, which is to be expected, but that many patients *do* have, or *do gain* insight, even, to some degree, when acutely disturbed. Other origins are said to be other pre-existing symptoms, for instance when a persecutory delusion leads to delusions of grandiosity (L9, p. 56), or when past abnormal experiences are reinterpreted retrospectively (such as when knowledge that a person has had some sort of 'episode' leads to the belief that she has acquired a new style of thinking, or expertise in a new topic; L11, 68).

Beyond such origins of falsified beliefs, are other sources for delusions which need not be abnormal or pathological. Some involve changed sensory input (L10, p. 61, p. 63), especially in the sense of taste or smell (L11, p. 70), or for hearing, symptoms such as tinnitus (L19, p. 117). Wernicke attributes some falsifications to bodily changes, including ones due to physical abuse (L11, p. 67), which need have nothing to do with mental disorder. Likewise, manifest abnormality of motor function or behaviour (L12, p. 74), itself perhaps due to neurological rather than psychiatric disorders, or recovery of mobility (L12, p. 74) can be the origin for an explanatory delusion. Lastly, he mentions instances where awareness of sudden, loss of attention, not itself abnormal, becomes a source of delusional of explanation (L19, p. 114).

The classes of delusion for which the above experiences are a trigger, include delusions of reference, grandiosity, persecution or hypochondria. The first two of these are in the autopsychic domain, the third in the allopsychic domain, and the last in the somatopsychic domain. It follows that these four classes of delusion are not primary: They are subclasses of the two major types, *delusions of relatedness* or *explanatory delusions*. So, for instance in L17 (note, p. 107), on the subject of grandiosity, he writes: 'Here, I believe that I am in agreement with Snell, who also denies the primary occurrence of overestimation ideas essentially' [121]; and later in this lecture he discusses, but rejects Griesinger's idea that delusions of grandiosity or persecution might be primary symptoms.

Clarification of the terms we use in translation is needed here, especially with regard to 'delusion of reference'. Wernicke often uses the term *Beziehungswahn,* which we usually translate in a generic, abstract sense as 'delusion of relatedness'. However, that relatedness often involves a patient interpreting an event, an idea, a coincidence, or something else, as referring specifically to him- or her-self. For this we use the more specific, less abstract term 'delusion of reference', a term already current, after Neisser [122] drew attention to 'morbid self-reference' (*krankhafte Eigenbeziehung*). It became more precise in 1918 with the publication of Ernst Kretschmer's monograph *Der Sensitive Beziehungswahn* ('The sensitive delusion of reference'). The term is as in *Grundriss*, but Kretschmer allied it to a specially sensitive personality type. Wernicke makes a similar suggestion (L13, p. 170), referring to Raskolnikov, Dostoievsky's sensitive hero from *Crime and Punishment*: 'In a brutal habitual criminal, the state of mind of a Raskolnikov would be impossible'. In Wernicke's terms, such delusions have a strong autopsychic content. For delusions in the other two domains (allopsychic and somatopsychic) we retain the generic term 'delusion of relatedness'. There are other issues for translation. The German word *Wahn,* can mean either 'delusion' or 'an abnormal state in which delusions can occur' (i.e. 'madness'). We indicate which meaning is intended, whenever *Wahn* appears. Likewise the terms 'delusion' and 'delirium' can be confused (more in French than in German), and we have stuck close to Wernicke's words here.

Wernicke repeatedly stresses that the process of explanation of experience is usually not abnormal. So, 'explanatory delusions may have no independent significance' (L12, p. 77). This emphasis was common in the nineteenth century, when, for instance, delusions could be conceived as 'parasitic' on more primary symptoms such as hallucinations [77]. If more than one explanatory idea is conceived, a patient may be in honest doubt which of several to prefer. He supports his view with the comment (L16, p. 99) that 'individual circumstances can decide the outcome—another argument supporting our view that the formation of explanatory delusions cannot be based on an ongoing disease process.' 'Explanation' may also take the form of voices ('phonemes') or be built into ongoing experiences of voices (L13, p. 81). So, we read: 'The content of the phonemes consists overwhelmingly of "delusions of reference"' (L13, p. 82).

In delusion formation, abnormality of association itself, that is the very process by which experience is interpreted, is given less emphasis. Nonetheless, such abnormality is often implied. For instance, 'delusions only rarely stay limited to the initial delusional ideas (usually of persecution, see above) but often develop further in the most consistent manner, forever giving rise to new delusions' (L11, p. 67). Such 'spread' is not typical of 'normal' explanations by healthy people. In L10 (p. 61) we read that 'parables, similies, or analogies are … forced up to conscious levels, in distinctive ways for each patient, and are then used as a means of description', again seldom part of normal explanation. Wernicke writes (L10, p. 60) of experiences 'reconfigured … as is often the case, within just such a religious framework.' Why, one may ask, 'often the case'? An answer is provided, in that religious language, rich in parable, simile or metaphor, and necessarily symbolic in nature, offers the best scope for elaboration by hyperactive association; but he does not make this point. In L12 he states (p. 77) '… a pre-existing tendency to delusional interpretation is also supplied by abundant normal or near-normal material for processing and evaluation'. This admission shows that he felt a need to qualify his thesis, that delusions are quasi-rational explanations of abnormal experience, with hints that some personality traits favour delusions.

The phrase 'delusion of relatedness' itself almost implies hyperactive association, although Wernicke still attributes misinterpretation to faulty perception, in that raw sense impressions are given abnormal Affective overtones, often self-referential. In L18 (p. 115), where he is writing of acute rather than chronic disorders, he is more explicit: 'I presented this to you as an example of a somatopsychic delusion of relatedness; however, we cannot doubt that here too it was based on a process of aberrant elaboration of new associations. In our patient still other examples showed up in this connection, with somatopsychic delusions of relatedness forming via processes of *aberrant association.*' (emphasis added; the same phrase—*krankhafter Assoziation*—occurs in L19, p. 240). In addition, the concept of an overvalued idea, which Wernicke admitted he could not explain, is well accounted for as intrinsic hyperactivity of a kind of association—between matters of personal value, and surrounding events. Beyond this, the list of sources from which explanatory delusions arise, such as abnormal sensations (of taste/smell, or tinnitus), bodily change, or loss of attention, are normal experiences for us all, yet we do not use them to construct delusions. Events which occur from time to time for any of us—unusual motor performance or behaviour, knowledge of past mental abnormality (common after excess alcohol), the fact of detention (not limited to mentally ill people)—are not very abnormal (though perhaps strange for people experiencing them de novo), and are not normally given delusional interpretations. Thus, his emphasis seems unconvincing.

Despite what seem significant shortcomings in his exposition on delusions he makes shrewd comments about other influences on delusion formation. On whether delusions persist, we read, of a malcontent with a delusionally overvalued idea (note, L14): '… the repetition of the incapacitation decision was rejected by an expert because the malcontent's delusion was known to be incurable! But the result of this provocation itself, was that the patient was actually cured!' Later in this lecture a lady teacher's overvalued idea is related in part to her fastidious personality. Again, in L16 (p. 99) we read: 'If [a former patient] has to deal with foolish people who offer support for his misconceptions …he will delve just as injudiciously into newspaper reports about his fellow victims; he will again be excited by these and can hardly escape from delusions, which continue every day and week that passes after his discharge, unless he puts his allegations to the test, thinking this to be in his best interests, thus helping the inherently false focus of his attention to fade away'. Today, such factors are rarely discussed. In addition Wernicke offers some views on the different manifestations of delusions according to a person's habitual style of thinking. In L14 (p. 89), when discussing *post hoc* corrective adjustments to beliefs, he writes: 'Turning first to the subsequent correction, you will soon notice how closely the phenomenon is related to explanatory delusions… However, the subsequent correction possibly corresponds to a more refined psychological need, while explanatory delusions are driven by a coarser motive. Explanatory delusions take advantage of consciousness, usually quickly, through unconscious processes, and thus with much elemental power; subsequent corrections, on the other hand, take place slowly, as real, conscious thought processes leading to a conclusion after long brooding.' Likewise, he writes 'a prerequisite of such delusions by analogy is a facility for relatively well-ordered thinking' (L18, p. 113).

These determinants of the nature of delusions are in the immediate circumstances in which they form, the personality of the patient, or in their personal style of thinking. Today, there might be more awareness of how enduring traits, independent of anything driving a patient's psychosis might shape a person's 'cognitive flexibility' or 'rigidity', and therefore the ease with a they can change their beliefs. Rigidity would tend to make delusional beliefs persist longer. There may be a bias towards evidence which confirms rather than refutes beliefs, making recovery more protracted. 'Confirmation bias' is a topic of recent research, not least in relation to psychosis [123], but it is not yet clear how far it is an enduring trait, regardless of psychosis. Given that the balance between confirmation and refutation varies between people, and from time to time, Wernicke's sense that 'logic' is preserved in explanatory delusions should be qualified by examining that 'logic' (which is not a unitary skill).

VIII,(m). Other Symptoms of Psychosis According to Wernicke

Wernicke's concept of psychosis is broader than the one usually used today. Hence symptoms dealt with below may not be included in today's 'psychosis'. In L23, he describes and analyzes 'anxiety psychosis', an uncommon term today, yet clearly associated with delusions and hallucinations, which may be auto-, allo-, or somatopsychic in content. Anxiety itself, he states (L36, p. 491), 'can be regarded as a special somatopsychic form of disarray'. In L1 we are introduced to 'motility psychosis'—one of his special concepts, a topic expanded in later lectures. Many symptoms he describes started with Kalhbaum. After Wernicke such symptoms were commonly incorporated by both Kraepelin and Jaspers into the diffuse concept of 'catatonia' (Kahlbaum's term, meaning no more than 'movement'). He is thus 'delivering the goods' as announced in L2, following Meynert, that 'there is nothing else to find and observe than movements, and that the whole pathology of the mentally ill consists of nothing more than peculiarities of their motor behaviour.' Much later Karl Leonhard [124] adopted Wernicke's term, for psychoses which were neither manic bipolar nor schizophrenic.

Motility symptoms are described in greatest detail in L31–35. Symptoms, classed as 'hyperkinesia', 'akinesia' and 'parakinesia', are described. Hyperkinetic symptoms are partly features of mania (L31, L33); akinetic and parakinetic ones are described in L34 and L35. Hyperkinesia includes both motor and speech excesses (the latter termed *verbigeration*). Akinesia includes *immobility* which '…varies, as our cases show, according to its severity, in that sometimes it is so marked that it leads to cessation of almost all reactions, and causes a condition apparently similar to death' (L34, p. 249). Kretschmer, called this a 'death feint', likening it to responses in most mammalian species (widely studied, and referred to as 'animal hypnosis'). It could account for cases when people reach the morgue, and are found still to be alive. Another akinetic symptom is *rigidity*. Akinesia for speech is *mutism* (L34, p. 249; L1, note, and includes *reactive mutism* (L34, p. 253). In L35, (p. 267), we are given a specific example: '…failure to answer questions put by a physician'. In L35 (p. 264) we hear of 'the so-called *hypochondriacal palsies*', which 'provide evidence that elimination of will can be manifest in localized muscle areas… Of course they never amount to palsies of individual muscle and nerve areas, but of whole limbs, or at least of whole sections of limbs'. Hughlings Jackson's had suggested that the motor cortex, despite its orderly representation of body parts, did not represent individual muscles, but rather organized movements [125]. However, what is described appears to be different, a shut-down of a definite region of motor cortex (or a connected region of the striatum) giving regional impairment, rather than impairment of specific movements.

Parakinetic symptoms include *waxy flexibility* (*flexibilitas cerea*) described in detail, and what appears to be a milder form, sometimes called *mitgehen* ('going along with') in classic German psychopathology, a symptom '… in which any joint resistance is lacking' (L34, p. 252). *Negativism* (L34, p. 250) is motiveless resistance to any imposed passive movement. In L34 (p. 245) we read 'akinesia gradually remitted but stereotyped movements appeared'. *Stereotypy* is a term used by Kahlbaum, and by Kraepelin from the 1890s. Today it is widely used to identify behavioural pathologies in laboratory animals given stimulants and other agents.

Many of the movements described here—aimless, but identifiable as fragments of activity which in other circumstance might be purposeful—are common enough, though in less obvious form, amongst most people who never get the attention of a psychiatrist. We are thus reminded of the title of Freud's book from 1901 *The psychopathology of everyday life* [126]. However, if such manifestations—the 'symptoms' described by Freud—*are* everyday occurrences, present to a degree in any of us, this calls into question their being designated as psycho*pathology*. Rather, they might be taken to be normal manifestations of a motor system capable of acquiring complex behaviours for specific purposes, manifest even when those purposes are not engaged.

The clinical lectures in *Grundriss* deal with psychiatry rather than neurology, yet reveal a world-class pioneer neurologist at work. Today, it is often asked why such symptoms are seen so rarely in psychiatric practice. One might rather ask whether such symptoms *actually are* so rare. An alternative view might be that, as psychiatry split from neurology, symptoms which do exist, today as in Wernicke's day, are not now recognized for what they are. So, in L35 (p. 267), we read: 'When you encounter a new patient who responds to your questions with striking silence, and thus makes examination difficult, do not omit, gentlemen, to move his limbs and arrange them in certain positions'. This hints that symptoms are not found today, because physicians do not know what to look for. However this would not apply to profound akinesia lasting for weeks, described in L34, which could hardly be missed.

In L15 we read of the relationship between obsessions and two easily confused symptoms, overvalued ideas, and autochthonous (self-generated) ideas. Wernicke (L2, note) writes: 'Obsessions are only exceptionally an essential element of paranoid states, if you consider cases of inveterate habitual influence on actions by obsessional ideas bordering on mental disturbance, where they belong in my opinion. On the other hand I do not deny that between self-generated ideas, overvalued ideas, and obsessions, transitions exist, in which it is difficult to assign the symptom to its correct position. In general however, the three symptoms are easy to tell apart. When Friedmann [127], recently attributed obsessional ideas to the overvalued ideas in his perceptive work, and connected the latter to the principal element of delusions, he does me too much honour, and moves beyond the bedrock of clinical experience.' This explores the difference between paranoid states (with their complex, multifaceted, and at times fast-moving delusions), and what was once 'paranoia', now renamed 'delusional disorder', in which abnormal beliefs have a single theme, clung to with obsessive tenacity, with little wider influence on the rest of mental life, and unaccompanied by hallucinations. Today there are growing hints that some forms of delusional disorder may be similar to some types of obsessive compulsive disorder, yet the overlap is ill-defined, since both appear to be heterogeneous.

VIII,(n). Melancholia and Mania

Wernicke's brilliant analysis of melancholia (L30, p. 206), exemplifies his concept of an 'elementary symptom', from which all other symptoms flow. Melancholia is not primarily a mood disorder, but a deficit in 'will'. Thus the patient described at the start of L30 states that 'she could feel neither joy nor grief; her heart was turned to stone'. Any mood change (which he refers to as *deprimierte Stimmung*—'depressed mood') is secondary, as are fear of the future, feelings of inadequacy, self-accusatory or guilt-ridden ideas, world-weariness and suicidal thoughts. This is plausible: A person who regularly experiences periods of depression (in today's term), and learns that these have a predictable time course, and therefore that he or she will soon recover, may 'sit out the episode', undoubtedly impaired in decision-making, yet without desperate fall in mood. Conversely, as Wernicke acknowledges, lowered mood can be brought about in other ways (L28, p. 194), when he refers to a 'transient fit of melancholy mood, which could as well be really the impact of insights into [a different] illness.' The description is of what Wernicke calls 'Affective melancholia', a concept mainly separate from a more severe, but less well-defined concept, 'depressive melancholia' ('the *so-called* depressive melancholia': L34, p. 257), in which *outward signs* of changed mental state are present (patients stop talking, or doing anything). The modern word 'depression' does not capture this distinction.

The converse clinical picture, mania (L31) is excessive facilitation and acceleration of activity (implicitly in the cortex), and with it, excessive ease in making associations. Initially this gives rise to improved performance in many tasks, and secondarily, to elevated mood. As ideas crowd for attention, all are pushed to maximum levels, and there is a 'levelling of ideas' with excesses of association, which may lead at a later stage, to confusion and severe impairment. Wernicke makes interesting comments on the 'levelling of ideas' (L31, p. 218): 'We can understand this *levelling of ideas*, which is one of the most important symptoms of mania, when we take intrapsychic hyperfunction to be a *general* increase in excitability of intrapsychic paths. On the other hand, the normal overvaluation of ideas is to be explained by the physiological (functionally acquired) increase in excitability of *specific*, chosen paths'. On the basis of modern knowledge, the following inferences might be drawn: (a) Mania occurs due to generalized change in cortical neurones, making them more excitable; (b) Since mania is not permanent, but episodic or transient, such change is also transient—probably originating in neuronal biophysics, rather than permanent change at the level of neuronal structure; (c) This is different from enhanced excitability in specific pathways, brought about by cellular learning mechanisms.

The analysis of mania raises two interlocking issues: *First*, hitherto Wernicke has regarded loss—or breakage—of associations (mediated by sejunction) as different from hyperactivity of association (seen in mania). The first is the direct forerunner of the 'disorder of associations', regarded by Eugen Bleuler as a primary characteristic of the disorder for which he coined the term 'schizophrenia'. The metaphor of a 'knight's move' in thought (a modern phrase) has been used to describe that disorder. Interpreted literally, this is a move along unorthodox pathways, but still actually existing, if indirect, associative links. A commonly cited example is the link between 'lion' and 'stripes' (with 'tiger' as the hidden connecting link). However, the more the associative links become indirect, via hidden stages, the less likely is it that a clinician can detect them. Therefore to claim that a sudden shift of topic in a patient's discourse is 'incoherent' rather than a case of 'hyperactive association' is a subjective judgment on the part of a clinician, saying as much about his mental processes as about those of his patient. Cases where Wernicke makes the strongest statements about breakage of association are in early lectures, dealing with patients with very chronic disorders. This distinction might be made in error more often in such cases than in most acute cases considered later. One can thus argue that Wernicke's attempt to separate *breakage* of associations from their *hyperactivity* is flawed reasoning. In the disorder we now call schizophrenia, there *is* evidence of hyperactive associative processes, including an excess of indirect associations; but this is appears to be an enduring trait, not a transient state, as it is in mania. There may however be a more subtle distinction to be made here: Apart from enduring traits leading to excessive ease in association, in the transient psychotic phases of schizophrenia, delusions may arise because of hyperactive associations based on *strong motivational drives*. In contrast, flight of ideas in mania is not limited to ideas with strong motivational links; any recruitment of Affect-laden ideas, with consequent classic delusions, is then secondary.

A comment on motility disorders is made in (L35, p. 260), that 'more often ... the akinetic symptom is an expression of increased intensity'. In L35, Wernicke discusses the relations between mania and Affective melancholia, including topics such as 'cyclic psychosis', and the same idea is raised, as he hints, when he writes (L31, p. 220): 'A mild form of one illness generally tends to appear during convalescence from the others and signals its termination'. This has an equivalent in later paper by Court [128], advocating the view that mania and depression are not polar opposites. Rather there is a transition from normal, to depressed, to mixed and then to a manic state.

VIII,(o). Hebephrenia, Thought Disorder, and Forerunners of *Dementia Praecox*

'Hebephrenia' was a mental disorder defined by Kalhbaum and Hecker, typical of adolescence, characterized by 'thought disorder', that is disordered cognition, revealed as silly, foolish, meaningless talk. Today, thought disorder is evidenced by disordered content of speech. In L25 (p. 170) and L29 (p. 196) cases are mentioned in which any 'formal thought disorder' (*formale Denkstörung*) is absent, the first times in *Grundriss* this term is used. (It is to be distinguished from 'thought deficit'—*Gedächtnisdefekt*—which appears occasionally [e.g.: L27, p. 180]). The clearest account of thought disorder is in L40 (p. 325), in adolescents, although there it is called 'hebephrenic dementia' not 'thought disorder'. 'Hebephrenia' became part of Kraepelin's *Dementia praecox* (hebephrenic subtype), and survives now as 'disorganization' in the symptomatology of schizophrenia. *Dementia praecox*, defined in the 1896 edition of Kraepelin's textbook, had, by definition, a poor outlook, ending in dementia, however it started. The most direct reference to this is in L39

(p. 304): 'Thus the unfavourable prediction that Kräpelin makes for such cases, does not always apply to those during puberty'. This clearly refers to *Dementia praecox*; yet Wernicke never uses the term, and distances himself from its major implication, the inevitability of a poor long-term outcome.

Apart from this, there are statements in *Grundriss* where motility disorders present similarities to what became the catatonic subtype of *Dementia praecox*. Thus, in L32, (p. 228) Wernicke writes: 'After a few weeks in this hyperkinetic state, which was sometimes replaced by akinetic phases of apparent exhaustion, he became calm, but at the same time with rapid increase of feeble-mindedness, while his greatly reduced nutritional status gave way to a rapid increase in body weight. At present, you would scarcely recognize this ruddy, apparently profoundly demented patient, instantly refusing and unbiddable towards any demand to think. The contrast is provided by the evidently *un*intentional movements, reminiscent of the familiar jactation of unconscious states. Common to both is only the monotonous recurrence of the same form of movement'. Later in the same lecture, we read: (L32, p. 234): 'the special aetiology is thoroughly decisive for the prognosis, so that the paralytic form here leads to dementia, as it does in other paralytic psychoses. This is true in cases of hyperkinetic motility psychoses, which occur in the course of a real hebephrenia or other chronic, hebephrenic degenerative psychoses'. In L34 he writes that akinetic motility psychosis is most prevalent in young persons, especially girls; and in L39 (p. 303) he writes: 'Next most common might be motility psychoses of any kind, but particularly akinetic motility psychoses, which find their next occasion for occurrence at time of puberty'. He refers to 'the familiar tendency for akinetic motility psychosis to be transformed into dementia'. There are common points here between Wernicke's motility psychosis and *Dementia praecox*, yet what he describes does not match Kraepelin's concept. Likewise, in L31 (p. 219) a phrase occurs which we translate as 'early dementia' (*schon zeitig … Demenz:* literally 'early-onset dementia'). Despite the phrase being similar to Kraepelin's *Dementia praecox*, the intended meaning is quite different.

In L32 (p. 227 *seq.*) there is also a long verbatim transcript of speech pathology. Such examples were used deliberately in literary productions when surrealism took off after World War II, for instance in the incoherent 'speech' of Lucky, in Beckett's *Waiting for Godot* [129]. Such crossovers from psychiatry were intended to portray speech disorganization ('formal thought disorder') in schizophrenia.

VIII,(p). Dementia

Today, dementia is often seen as an end stage, with little to be done by way of either treatment or prevention, and, at least for Alzheimer's disease, defined partly by adverse, irreversible change in the brain. However, since Wernicke distances himself from Kraepelin's *Dementia praecox*, he has to define dementia independent of this. In L34 (p. 256), he maintains that dementia is not an irreversible end-stage; and he hints that at least some forms of dementia are a biproduct of severely disordered mental processing—mental *chaos*—as opposed to delusions which are *systematized* in some way. Likewise, much of L39 implies that psychoses occurring at transitional periods of life reflect in part the special stresses and confusion arising during those periods. If such suggestions are correct, some forms of dementia represent the unravelling of acquired schemata for understanding the world, the body, and the self, arising not so much from a biological disorder, but from disorder of the 'information economy' associated with extreme mental states. If so, the inevitability of transition to dementia would be less absolute, and possibilities for prevention, even reconstitution, would be more favourable. Sometimes combination of coinciding stressors (in L39 [p. 306], of menstrual difficulties and hebephrenic symptoms) is a prerequisite for transition to dementia. Pursuing this line of thought, L37 focuses on Progressive Paralysis, which, we note, commonly led to dementia. His criterion of lost insight, supposed to separate it from neurosyphilis (p. 286) raises an interesting question, given that most cases of progressive paralysis *were* forms of neurosyphilis. One might ask whether the loss of insight was a genuine consequence of underlying brain pathology, or rather of severe *psychological* reactions, including denial (=lack of insight) of awareness of a slowly progressing disorder, which was widely feared, publicly stigmatized—more even than other mental disorders—and ultimately fatal.

In L40 (p. 314) the more familiar side of dementia is prominent. In the nineteenth century, terms for different grades of intellectual deficiency varied, but usually three grades were recognized. The most severe was *idiocy*, and terms for other grades varied from one country to another. Generally the three grades were defined in terms of mental age (and, in the twentieth century, as I.Q.). The 'theoretical' basis was often in part racist (with more severe levels supposedly correspond to 'lesser races'), and also had some basis in Haeckel's recapitulation theory (which was also closely linked to his own racial ideas).

VIII,(q). Prognostic Indicators; Concepts of 'Cure', or 'Return to Health'

Wernicke often writes of the degree to which patients can recover from their illnesses, and we get various clues in *Grundriss* to the prognostic indicators he used. The word he usually uses is *Heilung*, which might be translated as either 'healing' or 'curing'. Occasionally he uses *Besserung* (strictly 'improvement'; e.g. L23, p. 151). Back-translation of the German word 'cure' includes both *Heilung*, and *Kur*, while that for 'heal' is limited to *Heilung*. We therefore prefer to translate *Heilung* as 'heal', 'restore to health,' or sometimes 'recover' as more accurate, terms that are less strongly medical, similar in implication to 'recovery', now widely favoured amongst community mental health groups. Occasionally (L11, p. 67) the word 'cure' is used, and then, in quotation marks, as if to signify that it is not a wholly valid concept.

Most of his prognostic indicators refer to psychological processes or factors, which are separate from any illness. In L15 (p. 94) we read '... when the extent of the disease is limited just to the first psychotic elements, it is possible for health to be restored through the gradual appearance of more powerful countervailing arguments'. Whereas today, various forms of psychotherapy or CBT might be sought to resolve conflicts of belief set up during periods of psychosis, Wernicke appears to consider that unaided processes of natural healing will occur, simply by a patient's awareness of contradictions existing amongst his or her beliefs. Later he writes: 'The clinical presentation of such cases has proved useful to me several times, as is the process of "internalization" itself, that is, a conscious ability to recognize mental illness'. The notion that, by use of a person's powers of introspection, self-knowledge can contribute to recovery, is a modern-sounding, and wise principle, but hard to support on the basis of strictly biomedical ideas of mental disorder as diagnosable diseases. Further hints of Wernicke's approach come in L16 (p. 98) for a patient who 'can hardly escape from delusions ... unless he puts his allegations to the test, thinking this to be in his best interests, thus helping the inherently false focus of his attention to fade away'. He acknowledges the role of social milieu in resurgence, progression or regression of symptoms: 'Gradually, and in favourable cases, patients themselves notice that return of awareness of their period of illness is unhelpful' (p. 99). Here he suggests what is now seen as good practice in 'early intervention' programs for psychotic disorders, that patients can be assisted to gain insight into warning signs of an incipient breakdown, which may help avert relapse. Sometimes Wernicke comments on the prognostic significance of different symptom profiles, for instance, for anxiety psychosis in L23, and for psychoses more generally in L40, where complete recovery can occur (he estimates) in about a third of cases. The word 'degeneration' (*Entartung*) when used, a concept already with a long history in the Germanic world, as in other countries, refers to the supposed irreversible nature of mental disorders, often related to alcohol abuse.

VIII,(r). Holism in Wernicke's Thought

When dealing with Wernicke's clinical style (section IV "Wernicke's Personal Style in Psychiatric Practice, Teaching, Writing, and in Scholarly Disputes"), the following sentence was quoted (L7): 'After a person has recovered from a mental illness, it is required that we ensure that he has achieved insight into the abnormality of the state he has experienced; for the sum must necessarily be inaccurate if it contains false elements'. We see here an impressive aspect of Wernicke's thought—his understanding of each individual striving to be a coherent whole. The individual's search for this sense of personal wholeness is found in other giants of psychiatry in early twentieth century (Jung, Kretschmer, and later Victor Frankl); but *nowhere* do we find it rooted so firmly in brain science as in Wernicke. We see the intrinsic holism at many levels. When referring to fundamental neural processes, he is never far from the concept of unified personhood: In L3, in discussing the relationship of perception to memory, we learn that, though the two words are separate, the respective functions are inseparable; and on 'remembered images' he writes of their 'solid *ownership*' (German: *Besitz*), implying that a person 'owns' them. Later, in L11 (p. 67) when commenting on normal large-scale patterns of association, he writes: 'We would then not be too bold were we to conclude that, in this sense, the set of "specific energies" of sensory elements may be transferred to the entire organ of association.' Even more remarkable, in L20 (p. 126) he mixes this physical metaphor, with another, that of 'resonance'. The first seems strange today, but the second is an astonishing forerunner of the modern idea (still debated), that the 'binding problem' of unifying percepts and concepts across dispersed cortical regions is solved by resonance of electrographic activity shared across regions [130].

He is at home with the idea that cognitive and Affective processes are in continual interaction as parts of the unified whole. We read (L8, p. 49): 'It will not surprise you that the content of apperceptions in mental activity also exerts influence on accompanying Affect'; and in introducing clinical topics in L9 (p. 54), he writes: 'We can define acute mental illnesses as the process of altering the content of consciousness, which we see taking place in a defined time period. Such changes are often linked with Affects and emotions, just as they are under conditions of healthy mental life.' The latter idea is expanded greatly in L22, where Affective states are taken to be the driving force behind illusions, hallucinations and other symptoms.

In the clinical lectures, he incorporates into his account of symptoms a person's entire trove of life experiences, their employment, training, and acquired habits of thought (if not so much their intrinsic personality traits). He has little to say on a topic thought important today, the impact of psychic trauma as a cause of (or at least an influence on) mental disorders: Nevertheless, in L37 (p. 281) we read: 'Whoever finds himself forced to work beyond his individual strength, under tight time pressure, taking on responsibilities beyond his capacity, must struggle with excitement, grief, and sorrow, that can easily cause damage in purely intellectual work. Undoubtedly all-pervading careerism encourages such damage. From this, and similarly from the increased prevalence of syphilitic infection, we can explain the significant predominance of the male sex, particularly amongst educated classes'. Surprisingly, this is in the lecture on Progressive Paralysis. He alludes to a common myth (which one of the authors has met in a Chinese context), that psychosis occurs 'because a person thinks too much'. We see here a habit of inference emerging in other situations, when the true cause of an ailment is not clearly defined: All manner of supposed social factors are seen as 'causes', or contributory ones. A modern example is gastric ulcers, once attributed to 'stress', now known to be due to a bacterium which flourishes in acid environments. How far this applies to mental disorders as understood today is unsure.

All this is underpinned by an account in L7 of how each person constructs their own sense of personhood, by assimilating the three components of their trove of memories—the enduring sense of their own bodies, experiences of the external world, and their personal life story—into a remarkably unified whole (for most people). Wernicke had no access to insights we now have, such as one made by Geschwind [131] that in sub-primate animals, where prefrontal areas are small, multimodal convergence in areas occurs mainly in limbic areas, notably the hippocampus; while in humans, it occurs extensively in the neocortex itself. Geschwind suggests that this might be a prerequisite for appearance of language; but it also allows each of us to construct a sense of personal wholeness, however far this falls short of any ideal. In his grasp of the intrinsic holism of a human person, Wernicke, in our view, is ahead of where many practitioners in mainstream psychiatry are today, dominated by categorical diagnoses in which a patient's search for inner unity has no place; and where the profession rarely teaches trainees how, as doctors, they could foster the rebuilding of the sense of wholeness in their patients. Other traditions however (such as that of Carl Gustav Jung) do retain this emphasis, but are not mainstream.

These issues are related to one discussed later, namely whether medical concepts of disease, defined as disorders in specific organs or body systems are adequate as an analogy for mental disorders. In one sense Wernicke's holism implies that personhood arises because of close interaction of *all* system (or at least of their cerebral representation), which is perhaps a less medical conceptualization. However, in another sense, he might be saying that the 'system' which is disordered in conditions he describes, namely the brain *as a whole*, is precisely the system representing, as far as possible, that personhood, unified to whatever degree is possible. In that sense, he succeeds magnificently, and this can then be seen to fit within medical paradigms, albeit ones which are significantly stretched.

Admittedly, our fulsome praise has to be qualified, because Wernicke apparently entertained the idea that human beings are entirely 'rational' in their mental operations, this being not just an ideal, but the expected norm. Departure from this norm is then, by definition, a form of pathology, or mental disorder. This point became central in the critique of psychiatry by Michel Foucault [132]. Another possible criticism of Wernicke's approach (for which today's psychiatry is a better target), is for specialists to over-pathologize experiences (especially hallucinations and delusions) which are part of normal human experience. One might mention the transition by imperceptible steps from normal overvalued ideas to frank delusions; or that in many cultures 'hearing voices' is accepted as normal, even as a 'gift'.

VIII,(s). Wernicke's Links to the Emerging Dynamic Tradition in Psychiatry

At the time when Wernicke practised in Breslau, major changes were occurring in European centres in the emerging profession of psychiatry. Three strands of mental health care were in interaction—care and administration in institutions; teaching, research, and practice by academic neurologists; and the gradual, uneasy incorporation into orthodox medicine of what had been folk medicine for centuries, but became the dynamic tradition in psychiatry. The last of these is analyzed in detail by Henri Ellenberger [16]. The point is that they *were* in fruitful interaction at the time, and leading physicians crossed from one to the other, apparently with no overwhelming sense of 'cognitive dissonance' (although both Freud and Jung had periods of crisis—referred to as 'creative illness'). In addition there were many interactions between this emerging discipline and experimental psychology of the day. Key figures included Charcot, Freud, Janet, and later Jung, Kretschmer and many others. Meynert can also claim to have crossed some frontiers. Many clinicians of the time, from respectable academic positions, had experimented with hypnosis, either themselves being hypnotized, or by administering it as physicians; and Wernicke refers to it occasionally (e.g. L14, p. 90). Hypnosis was a 'bridgehead' by which dynamic psychiatry spread within orthodox practice.

Wernicke himself was, it appears, also one of those intrepid 'frontiersmen'. Over many years, he had sporadic contacts with Freud, whose first independent work, an 1891 monograph on aphasias, was partly a response to Wernicke's work. Freud had seven of Wernicke's works in his library, and in 1896 Wernicke referred a patient to Freud.

In 1898 Freud's first truly psychoanalytical study (of the Signorelli parapraxis) appeared in *Monatsschrift für Psychiatrie und Neurologie*, edited by Wernicke and Ziehen [133]. Wernicke cites Charcot several times, whose work in Paris started the acceptance of dynamic psychiatry. In any case, he indicates at the start of *Grundriss* his awareness of alternative models for mental disorder: a footnote (L1, p. 4) to his statement that 'mental disorders are disorders of the brain' declares: 'A difference of opinion prevails only over how far they [that is mental illnesses] are of a functional nature or are determined by palpable changes.' This probably refers to the debate at the time, about psychogenic syndromes studied by pioneers of dynamic psychiatry, such as Charcot, Janet and Freud, where symptom patterns unknown in neurology occurred—later to be called 'conversion symptoms'.

Apart from these links, much of Wernicke's engagement with the emerging dynamic tradition is captured by his use of key terms or concepts, usually ones featured in Freud's works. Perhaps the most telling words are *unconscious* and *subconscious*. In L2 he writes that ultimately all symptoms boil down to *movements* of one sort or another, a view concordant with the materialism of the Somatiker school. However, he then 'exclude[s] ... intentional movements of which other people are aware before they reach the consciousness of the patient him- or her-self'. In this, he hints at advances in France and Vienna, where unconscious or subconscious processes (which control seemingly deliberate behaviour) were recognized. He acknowledges that symptoms arising in the autonomic nervous system may be relevant, although never in *Grundriss*, do they have the importance implied by dynamic psychiatrists of his day. On the hinterland between conscious and unconscious (L5; note) we read: 'We will be confronted again and again with the contrasts between functioning and latent consciousness; they correspond apparently to different states of one and the same anatomical substrate. However, precisely for that reason, we have not the slightest inclination to examine it more closely, for the time being.' This shows his awareness of contemporary discussion on subconscious processing. In L8 (p. 47), he writes of 'intense pain, such as violent toothache, [which] immediately signals to our subconscious to redirect attention to our senses'. This is the first time Wernicke uses the word 'subconscious' (German: *Ohnmacht*). In a later lecture (L24, p. 162) he writes 'When the functioning of organs which usually goes unnoticed, reaches perception...', phraseology which clearly indicates his awareness of varying levels of consciousness. In L34 (p. 251) he writes '... balance evidently cannot be maintained based on a particular level of mental ability, the only possibility remaining is unconscious compensation, in other words, adjustment acting exclusively within consciousness of corporeality'. The contradiction between the two last phrases implies that Wernicke accepted that that component of 'contents of consciousness' which was most familiar to each patient—consciousness of corporeality—had, by its familiarity, sunk below usual levels for conscious awareness.

In Freud's writings, the *Ego* (German: *das Ich*) is a term of great importance. As a noun, it had currency in German philosophy long before Freud used it (around 1920) in his structural model of the human psyche. For instance, it appeared in writings of Max Stirner (1806–1856) and of Theodor Meynert—mentor to both Freud and Wernicke—who used the term 'primary Ego' in his treatise *Psychiatry*: *Diseases of the Forebrain* [134]. For Wernicke, like Meynert, but unlike Freud in the 1920s, the concept was rooted in what was known about sensory and motor systems. It is hard to find in Freud's extensive writings a precise definition of what he meant by the term 'Ego', and it was probably used in more than one sense. Freud only occasionally cites Wernicke, although in *New Introduction to Psychoanalysis* [135], he acknowledges a point which Wernicke stressed, that the Ego (unlike Freud's *Id* and *Superego*) *was* at the interface with the external world. Wernicke's usage contrasts with religious or metaphysical ideas of an entity defining a person's essence (his/her 'soul' in Western tradition) often taken to be immortal. As the 'essence' of personal identity, this entity may be held to be indivisible, but reasons put forward for quasi-indivisibility of personal identity by Wernicke are quite different, in no way suggesting immortality.

The phrase 'symptom complex' is usually thought to be intrinsic to psychoanalytic thought, but its history is interesting. The noun 'complex' goes back to the seventeenth century. Wernicke's 1874 paper on aphasia was actually entitled *Der aphasische Symptomencomplex; Eine psychologische studie aufanatomische basis*. In *Grundriss*, the phrase 'symptom complex' occurs a number of times (pp. 17, 132, 150, 162), and on p. 72 we have a reference to the 'Ego complex': 'The fact that, in the brain, different ideas and idea-complexes are not merely juxtaposed, but are normally combined into larger groups, and finally into unity of the ego, can, in the final analysis, be due only to associative processes.'

Neurosis is a term much used by Freud. It originated in the eighteenth century with the Scottish physician, William Cullen, meaning an objective disturbance in the brain. By the time of Freud and Wernicke its meaning had shifted completely [52]. As the 'Somatikers' gained ascendency, 'psychosis' took over from the earlier word, while 'neurosis' became accepted as a term for disorders arising from emotional conflict; and 'psychosis' by Wernicke's day was also becoming split into 'organic' and 'functional' types, the respective home ground for neurology and psychiatry.

Wernicke, no doubt aware of these shifts, sometimes 'flags' the areas of contention. In L29, in dealing with the relation between obsessions and autochthonous ideas, he writes (p. 199): 'In no other area is it more difficult to separate psychosis from neurosis: Thus, to identify both the degenerative aetiology as well as the elementary symptoms as lying within the range of mental normality, it might be fitting to speak solely of *obsessional neurosis*.' Mainly he uses 'neurosis' in the new sense, but sometimes in the older way. His first use of the term (L8, p. 47), refers to '... neuroses (following head injuries, railway accidents and the like)' has hints of both meanings. In the late nineteenth century, with expansion of the rail network, railway accidents had become common (see also L27, p. 182), and an issue for public debate (depicted in closing sections of Tolstoy's *Anna Karenina*—published in serial form between 1873 and 1878). Related to this was the question of how far disability was genuinely injury-related, or exaggerated by conscious or subconscious processes to obtain insurance payouts, or other secondary benefits. (In the now-unified Germany, national health insurance had been introduced under Bismarck in 1883.) This debate lay behind one of Freud's early public presentations (in 1886) ([16]. Ellenberger, 1970, p. 438). The term 'railway neurosis' could thus be used in a Freudian sense. Such a usage is found in L11 (p. 68), when discussing a patient with somatopsychic delusions. Wernicke writes '... with such a round-about description of the change in content of his consciousness, he is seen by many doctors as a hypochondriac, that is, suffering from neurosis'. The term 'neurosis' is sometimes used with hints of the older sense of William Cullen. So, in L37 (p. 284) we read of 'epileptic neurosis', a curious juxtaposition which would not be written today, reflecting the undefined border between hysterical and epileptic seizures; and in L41 (p. 329) we read of '... neurosis in a subcortical vascular centre'.

Conversion symptoms are closely linked to severe anxiety. In L23 (p. 150) Wernicke introduces the term 'anxiety neurosis', and asks how 'anxiety psychosis' (perhaps equivalent to conversion hysteria) differed from 'anxiety neurosis': 'In no other area of mental illness are there so many points of contact with the functional disorders of the nervous system.' 'Functional disorder' implies a disorder with no clear structural basis [136]. Wernicke uses the term only a few times, and not very consistently. In L16 (p. 99) he writes '... for such cases one must concede the possibility that these symptoms persist to some extent as a purely functional disorder'. In L32, (p. 231) it is applied to abnormal movements of chorea, a claim hardly made today.

Both 'anxiety' and 'neurosis' are terms with interesting histories, long predating Wernicke. Their combined use became prominent in 1894, at a time when the concept of 'neurasthenia' was introduced from North America. Freud stated that 'anxiety neurosis' should include: 'general irritability, anxious expectation, anxiety attacks, and [somatic] equivalents such as cardiovascular and respiratory symptoms, sweating, tremor, shuddering, ravenous hunger, diarrhoea, vertigo, congestion, paraesthesia, awakening in fright, obsessional symptoms, agoraphobia, and nausea' [137]. Wernicke's use of the phrase suggests that it already had wide currency, if only in informal use. Most specifically, he occasionally refers to symptoms (notably psychogenic amnesia) which other clinicians were calling *conversion hysteria*. In L14 (p. 90) when referring to lapses of memory, he writes that 'the close relationship between the content of these memory lapses and the overvalued idea points to the fact that the associative link is not entirely missing, but is heavily biased towards and limited to the overvalued idea, without which insight the apparently conscious act could not be explained. So this probably represents a narrowing of consciousness, as it is known otherwise only from states of high Affect ... However, we cannot exploit this moment, because it remains unexplained why only certain types of mental patient show this symptom'. The idea of loss of memory at times of high Affect is similar to 'hysterical amnesia' which Freud attributed to repression; 'narrowing of consciousness' (also L39, p. 301) at such times was a theme of Janet, in his exploration of automatism ([16]; p. 224). Amnesia described by these writers was often more extensive than in cases referred to by Wernicke, whose explanation is quite different. In L25 (p. 306), Wernicke *does* use the term 'defensive reaction', but it is not clear that this referred to 'psychological defence' as understood in the emerging dynamic tradition. Today, such amnesia might be attributed mainly to high selectivity of 'selective attention', a concept not well formulated in Wernicke's day. Nowadays its selectivity is known to vary between people as a trait, and (as a state variable), from time to time in one person. Wernicke hints that he understands both. Another hint at evidence from which others developed the concept of repression comes in L16 (p. 99). Wernicke refers to '... patients who are "right back into" their life, and who are independent enough to earn their own bread; yet they are very reluctant to talk about their periods of illness, even setting up major barriers to clinical probing'. Likewise, in (L16, p. 99) we read: 'Gradually, and in favourable cases, patients themselves notice that return of awareness of their period illness is unhelpful'. Reticence about talking of periods of past illness may have bases other than fear of reactivating psychosis (as implied here). It might reflect fear of something that utterly defies a patient's comprehension, for which they have no language or frame of reference, leading to avoidance of anything linked to the experience, and possibly to genuine amnesia. These two may be the same, since retrieval of memory depends on activating the context or 'framework' in which a memory was embedded.

IX. Wernicke's Approach to Classification of Mental Disorders

IX,(a). Historical Introduction

No system for classifying anything can be rational, until the purpose is specified. Wernicke accepted prevailing traditions and concepts, yet appears to struggle to break free from them. Alternative approaches of Linnaeus and Buffon in the eighteenth century have been mentioned, and Wernicke tried to reconcile competing claims for mental disorders. From time to time it is clear that he, like Linnaeus, sought a 'natural order' in what he saw in the clinic (and debates about the word 'nature' were critical in the seventeenth century in emergence of the *natural* sciences—not least in writings of Robert Boyle). We read (p. 4): 'However, since in Nature combinations of symptoms are far more diverse and complex, it has been necessary to construct an artificial framework, sometimes more widely, and sometimes more narrowly, accomplished by different observers in very different ways'; and again 'Symptoms must be deduced from familiar features of the diseased organ, in order to treat the illness—in our case from features of the brain.

Only in this way do we have the prospect of obtaining a classification and overview of symptoms which is both natural (i.e. based on the nature of things) and, at the same time, exhaustive.' In L21 (p. 133) we read 'Disorientation disorders included in our schema represent only the *route* by which nature brings about such disorientation; but every psychiatric patient is in some way disoriented'.

Despite his quest for 'natural types', he can also focus on the uniqueness of each patient; and in L20, stands back from any system he might impose, with the following words (p. 131): 'We should always remember, simply, that any schema, ours included, has value merely of a means of teaching and understanding, and becomes superfluous as soon as a better, simpler, or more correct grouping of the facts is found. Rest assured, gentlemen, nobody is more aware of this than I, and that respect for the facts when searching for a way to represent mental illness as seen in the clinic is my primary consideration.' Clearly, in his own field, he was aware of counterarguments, such as a contemporary Buffon might have urged.

The 20-year period after 1890 in Germany was critical for emergence of what we now take for granted, that mental disorders are defined as categories; yet Wernicke was unhappy with the growing trend. He preferred to take as his starting point symptoms and the processes by which they arise, rather than supposed disease entities. There are several steps between his position and the notion of mental disorders as categorical 'diseases': In his frequent use of the word *Krankheit* he probably implied no more than a 'process' (such as sejunction); and occasionally he uses *Geistesstörungen* as a 'catch-all' term, rather than *Krankheit* ('disturbance' rather than 'illness' or 'disease'). As early as L11, he writes (p. 66): '… let us face the question of nomenclature. According to current labels, all those patients would be examples of "chronic insanity" or "paranoia" … We can avoid this misunderstanding if we talk of *paranoid states*, which include all those chronic mental disorders where we encounter falsification of content of consciousness, while conscious activity remains well preserved.' In L17, he is sharply critical of Ziehen (and others) for implying that there are definite 'diseaseconditions' (*Krankheitszustand*). The next step, that there are categorically separate 'diseases' probably had little currency in 1894, but the 1896 edition of Kraepelin's textbook promoted this notion, and took hold increasingly, so that, by the time of Wernicke's death it may have prevailed. Gradual emergence of the disease concept for psychotic disorders is discussed by Beer [52].

Another issue for classification, which hardly applies today, comes in L9. Wernicke contrasts 'internal' and 'external' origins of mental disorders, and the phrase 'external cause' is used in L23 (p. 146), referring to an event in a patient's life. This followed Kraepelin's early (1881) classification, separating endogenous from exogenous origins to mental disorder. The latter included infectious causes: At the time, there were several links between infectious disease and mental disorder. Quarantine measures for patients with dangerous infections were in places not unlike those for compulsory detention in psychiatric institutions. Early attempts to define concepts of medical ethics applied in both fields. At a time when unlettered people understood little of their own bodies, symptoms of infectious disorders could be incorporated into psychotic delusions (L10; p. 61); and of course, syphilis, whose late stages include psychiatric syndromes, fitted Kraepelin's scheme, especially after the spirochete had been discovered (although today, when syphilis is rare, the dichotomy is less relevant). A bacterial toxin was seen as a potential cause of mental disorders.

IX,(b). Purposes of Taxonomy

Wernicke was aware that different systems of classification are needed for different purposes. In L10 he refers to the issue of how to separate 'curable' from 'incurable' cases, this being an *administrator's* classification. In L11 (p. 66) he sketches his classification of psychoses, using *scientific-clinical* principles—somatopsychic, allopsychic, and autopsychic classes of psychosis.

Clearly he saw the two purposes as separate, adding (p. 66): '… you could emphasize the importance of that group of patients in whom the disease process had apparently run its course, and the patients have recovered, without their having gained any insight into their illness'; and continues: 'The necessity of the latter distinction can, however, lead us to introduce other, somewhat-simplified terms into the field.' This second, simpler, more pragmatic classification serves the interests of institutional administrators in identifying patients who recovered or were improved sufficiently to be discharged, and those needing continued institutional care. A similar purpose for classification, dealt with in L40, is to define severity. In L40 (p. 314), in discussing mental deficiency, he writes: 'Separating these three [types] one from another is of course quite artificial, and in many borderline cases cannot be achieved; but otherwise, it is easily applied in practice': Here he accepts both the pragmatic need for, and the limitations of categorical classification of persons. However, generally, he separates the two purposes.

In Kraepelin's system, emerging at the same time, classification (at least to separate *Dementia praecox* from *manic depressive illness*) was based *jointly* on patterns of symptom, and long-term evolution of each case, especially on whether a patient recovered sufficient to be discharged. The distinction between an administrator's and a scientist/clinician's purposes was thus not so clear: The administrator's classes became part of a supposed scientific classification. Granted, classification based on long-term outcome *does* have a scientific side, and in L17 Wernicke *does* explore how acute syndromes progress to chronic ones. Merging of classification systems, which *should* be kept separate, because they serve different purposes still prevails. Systems such as DSM-III, DSM-IV and DSM 5, purportedly serving clinical purposes, are widely used in USA and elsewhere for decisions on finance, insurance, and medico-legal or forensic matters. Likewise, ICD, though now widely used for clinical purposes, started life as an administrator's document for collected mortality statistics.

IX,(c). Broad Versus Narrow Criteria

Wernicke's critique of then-current categories was not a rejection of categorization of mental disorders in principle, and he *did* have his own distinctive categories: Most of his criticism was targeted at over-inclusive definitions. We see this as early as L11 (p. 65): '… if we wanted to *comprehend* it in this way—that paranoia was a well-characterized clinical form of illness then the floodgates of greatest confusion of concepts would be opened, for the cases show very great differences one from another.' In L38 (p. 294) we also read: 'Nevertheless, if, by way of example you speak, hear, or read of "exhaustion psychoses" as a specific clinical entity, this is the same misunderstanding to which I have already repeatedly drawn attention. Even more can one say, with some justification, that in the sense just discussed, by far the majority of acute psychoses are "exhaustion psychoses"'. More broadly, he writes (L17, pp. 101, 102): 'The "general impression" sometimes relied on even by better-known representatives of our profession, when they fail to elicit definite psychotic symptoms, is no better than everyday parlance and must elicit the deepest suspicion, when used as the basis of diagnosis of a paranoid state'. Today, in much the same way, the 'cause of psychosis' is often attributed to 'trauma', without either trauma or psychosis being defined precisely enough to specify the nature of the relationship, except most vaguely as 'proximate cause'. The positive side of this, Wernicke's preference for *narrow* definitions (which also applied to symptoms, such as verbal hallucinations) appears several times, for instance in L34 (p. 254): 'Only where [motility symptoms] constitute the clinical picture, solely or in greater part … are we justified in accepting a special *illness* whose essential symptoms are motor in content. I would particularly emphasize that "catatonic"—or, in our sense, specific motor—symptoms, tend to appear in the majority of chronic progressive psychoses at some phase of the illness. We are thereby warned to confine our clinical picture of akinetic motility psychosis within the narrowest possible limits.' Again in L35 (p. 261), he cautions himself: 'So we must then take into account the possibility that the above clinical picture of akinetic motility psychosis, derived entirely empirically, is too broad'. The same criterion could be said to apply to another of his more specific entities—Affective melancholia. Here we get an important clue to one of his criteria to determine when, if ever, he could think of specific illness or disease entities: They should be defined as narrowly as possible in terms of symptoms, thus avoiding the conundrum of today's nosologist—that entities overlap so much that spurious co-morbidity, is not just an exception, but the norm.

Occasionally, however, when seeking to define and name ill-defined concepts, he recommends broader concepts as in L28 (p. 192), where he refers to 'the concept of the second state, which is unambiguous in itself—yet currently always too narrowly defined'.

IX,(d). Psychiatric Taxonomy in Practice: Issues of Co-morbidity, Illness Trajectory, and Severity

Concepts identified in a scientific taxonomy of disease need not be identical to those recognized in official systems of diagnosis, although the two should be closely related. Whatever his critique of categories current at the time, Wernicke *did* often make use of specific diagnoses. Sometimes he refers to established diagnosis (*Delirium tremens*, Progressive paralysis), which today would hardly be seen as *psychiatric* diagnoses. In L23, in relation to 'anxiety psychosis' we read (p. 148): 'In *diagnostic* terms, the assumption is that the illness will often develop further, forming no more than the initial stage of a more complex disease picture'. Here he refers to one of his *own* concepts unambiguously as a diagnosis; but often his special terms, although presented as if they are diagnoses, seem to be highly specific to one or a few cases, and say more about analysis of those cases than of disease entities (e.g. 'acute expansive autopsychosis mediated by autochthonous ideas'; p. 199).

Wernicke *did* recognize that any disorder might include a variety of symptoms, and that any symptom could occur in various disorders. Today, especially in DSM, it is habitual to list collections of symptoms which jointly define each condition. Inevitably, many patients fit diagnostic criteria for a number of disorders, which is almost certainly mainly an artefact of how diagnoses are defined. In an attempt to avoid such high prevalence of co-morbidity, systems such as DSM often impose by *fiat* exclusion as well as inclusion criteria in their definitions; but this has been criticized. '… by defining some diagnoses in terms of exclusion as well as inclusion criteria, arbitrary separation is enforced between disorders which are actually closely related, and a possibly arbitrary hierarchy between disorders is generated' [138]. However, Wernicke's approach, where, in each patient, one symptom is usually fundamental, the others secondary, related to the first by psychological reasoning, is a stronger way to avoid spurious co-morbidity arising from facile categorization.

Separation of acute from chronic disease goes back to the first and second centuries CE, in writings (whose originals are lost) of Soranus of Ephesus [139, 140]. By the nineteenth century, the distinction was accepted as important in medical descriptive writing. In psychiatry, the issue was of widespread interest, and central to Kraepelin's systematization. Coming from a medical background, with all that goes along with concepts of disease, Wernicke naturally wanted to make a similar separation; and as early as L14 (p. 86) he writes: 'We set out initially to study alterations in the content of consciousness. We identified acute and chronic mental illnesses according to the processes by which they arose'. This habit came partly from Meynert, since in L37 (p. 284) he writes, on progressive paralysis: 'Whenever actual psychoses appear during the course, the illness always shows an acute character, at least temporarily, and Meynert explicitly classed it with the acute psychoses'. In L17 and L18, the subject matter of *Grundriss* shifts from chronic to acute conditions, and Wernicke discusses ways to differentiate the two (L18; p. 111), partly on the basis of duration (up to a few weeks still being acute) but mainly on the basis of the processes: Chronic mental disorder reflects changed *content* of consciousness; acute disorder reflects changed *activity* of conscious processes (p. 111). Later (L40, p. 310), he refers to finer distinctions: 'We must subdivide the acute psychoses according to their time course into per-acute, acute, and subacute psychoses. This distinction is of practical importance; however, we would only apply it when we are dealing with a clinical picture of acute coloration which has developed slowly over time, to distinguish it from chronic psychosis'. Clearly he *does* think there are distinctions to be made, which are practically important; yet he seems to struggle to separate acute from chronic syndromes, and in the end finds clinical realities scarcely permit this. Thus, in L17 (p. 105) we read 'Each newly emerging symptom of mental disorder may have an acute character. Most chronic mental illnesses can even be characterized by their acute episodes, with new symptoms which may occur at any period along their course. I have intentionally avoided describing these states wherever possible, because they belong with acute psychoses; but this was not wholly successful for separating such episodes from new-emerging individual symptoms, because even there, just as everywhere else in nature, imperceptible transitions take place'. Likewise in L40 (p. 310) he writes: 'We … differentiate chronic and acute psychoses. However, closer examination of these differences of the course over time soon showed that acute clinical pictures are occasionally to be found as in chronic cases, somewhere along their time-line'.

In L40 (and several times earlier) Wernicke writes of the practical need to chart the severity of each illness across its course. In L34 (p. 255) he concludes that 'range' of symptoms is not independent of severity, and therefore the former is not a secure criterion for classification. In L40 he again considers separate dimensions of 'range' and 'intensity' of symptoms, but finds considerable difficulties in their use in practice: 'We must not hide from the difficulties in the way of such an undertaking' (L40, p. 111). A striking feature of cases presented in *Grundriss* is nevertheless his ability to recognize patterns in the longitudinal course of individual illnesses. In this respect, his descriptions may be better than can be made today, partly because, with better treatment, long-term evolution of severe illnesses is seldom seen, and partly because organization of mental health services today make longitudinal follow-up by a single clinician more difficult.

IX,(e). Wernicke's Prototype Classificatory System

Descriptive schemes, based on a researcher's intuitions may claim to be theoretically neutral, but there are often implicit theoretical assumptions, even if unintended or well-hidden. In L2, as mentioned, Wernicke gives his classification of all possible symptoms in a three-by-three table, with columns identified as 'Psychosensory', 'Psychomotor', and 'Intrapsychic', the rows as 'loss of', 'excessive', or 'aberrant' excitability. Given the lack of reasoning underlying the scheme, and that it encompasses all conceivable possibilities, it probably has few hidden assumptions. It probably *is* strictly descriptive.

Beyond this, in L1 to L8, a more significant system for description is advanced, derived cogently from basic brain science. Contents of consciousness fall into one of three domains: allo-, somato-, and auto-psychic. This provides a three-way classification of phenomena he sees in his patients. This is not the whole of Wernicke's scheme for classifying symptoms. Motility symptoms and disorders are a special feature in his thinking, although he often suggests that they are linked closely with somatopsychic phenomena; and Affective reactions to other psychopathology, differing according to the nature of the latter are incorporated into his descriptions throughout. In early clinical lectures, the three fundamental terms are used to describe various types of 'falsification of consciousness'—allopsychic, somatopsychic, and autopsychic (L9). Between L24 and L29 there are clinical presentations of acute *disorders* dominated by each symptom domain—somatopsychic in L24, allopsychic in L25 to L27, and autopsychic in L28 and L29.

Somatopsychosis	Allopsychosis	Autopsychosis	Motility psychosis
Anxiety psychosis	Acute hallucinosis	Acute autopsychosis ('second state')	Hyperkinetic motility psychosis
Hypochondriasis	Delirium tremens	Hysterical absences	Akinetic motility psychosis
(Eating disorders)	Polyneuritic psychosis	Acute expansive autopsychosis mediated by autochthonous ideas	Combined hyperkinetic and akinetic disorders
		Obsessions	
		Affective melancholia	
		Mania	
		Confused mania	
Compound and mixed psychoses			
Progressive paralysis			
Hebephrenia			
Dementia			

The emphasis is nevertheless on symptoms (rather than diagnoses), some of which, with modern names, can be assigned to Wernicke's categories: Delusions of persecution are allopsychic. Misperceived body image (in *Anorexia nervosa*) is somatopsychic. Delusions of reference, and usually overvalued ideas, are autopsychic. Only later does he use the three-way split to define disorders themselves, subdivisions of the all-encompassing term 'psychosis': somatopsych*osis*, allopsych*osis*, autopsych*osis*, and motility psych*osis*. Specific diagnoses then fall under each of the latter terms. Some of these are Wernicke's own concepts, usually based on a deeper level of abstraction than most diagnoses with we are familiar today, a few which we recognize and to which can assign modern terms. In the Table above are some of the diagnoses (mainly for acute disorders) appearing in *Grundriss*.

Given the care with which he derives the system, there are bound to be theoretical implications. For instance, Wernicke implies that there is some symmetry in the three (or four) components of consciousness. Thus, in one area after another—falsification of contents of consciousness, explanatory delusions, delusions of relatedness, disarray and disorientation, other Affective reactions, overvalued ideas—he uses the same three-way split to organize his descriptions. Despite the clarity of reasoning behind this, one can ask three questions:

1. Is the implied symmetry scientifically valid?
2. Is the classification clinically useful?
3. Are the three symptom groups statistically independent?

The first question is theoretical, to be answered on the basis of brain theory. The other two are empirical matters, some of which were clearly beyond the methodology of his time. Empirical evaluation of this three-way split may be the most important way forward from what Wernicke wrote in *Grundriss*, but it is a complex task. However, he *does* provide a language, which condenses many details he heard from his patients into generic concepts. He uses that language, in part to describe *individual* cases, often in very interesting ways, for instance:

L11 (p. 66): According to this classification the first patient presented, the gardener Rother, would be classified as an example of a total chronic psychosis; Frau Reisewitz, a chronic auto-allopsychotic; the patient Tscheike, a chronic auto-somatopsychotic; the Biega, case, a pure somatopsychotic; Frau Schmidt, a combined chronic allo-somatopsychotic; and Frau Reising, a chronic allopsychotic.

L33 (p. 239): Previous attacks of the illness, especially the first, which appeared along with menstruation, were pure manias. Actual disorientation in the allopsychic area never occurred; in the autopsychic area it had characteristics of grandiose delusion, understandable in the context of mania—this having religious coloration, corresponding with the patient's personality; and in the somatic domain, disorientation consisted essentially of abnormal sensations, perhaps linked with menstruation, and an explanatory delusion for the pseudospontaneous movements, particularly of her trunk.

(p. 274): … somatopsychic disorientation may be limited to delusions of pregnancy, autopsychic disorientation to accompanying ideas of having sinned, and allopsychic disorientation restricted only to certain time periods and certain relationships, so that the prevailing situation can still be recognized correctly.

Such comments are some way distant from generalizations with which science usually deals; but there are also many *general* statements, ones with which research *can* deal. However, the sophisticated logic pervading *Grundriss* is necessarily a complex pattern. Moreover, because the 41 lectures were delivered as clinical presentations, the merits of his language for describing symptoms is not at once apparent: generalizations are scattered through the lectures in a seemingly uncoordinated way. To clarify these dispersed statements, and to illustrate their potential—were his system better known and understood—a few of the clearest (and most oft-repeated) generalizations in each area of symptomatology are given below. The analysis avoids conditions whose specific cause we now know, especially alcoholism and syphilis. The intention is then to focus, as far as possible, on what we now recognize as endogenous mental disorders. These paragraphs might point to future work; but, of course, if this line is to be followed, the first step would be to devise authenticated instruments, as mandated by modern standards, for rating his three categories—allo-, somato-, and auto-psychic aspects of his several clinical variables.

Using his language, Wernicke's many generalizations have no accompanying detail to document their veracity, as needed today; but it would be unwise to ignore statements from an observer and analytic thinker as shrewd as Wernicke, even if rigorous proof is lacking. Most of the roughly 5,000 careful clinical records from Breslau have not survived, except for the around 150 published as *Krankenvorstellungen aus der psychiatrischen Klinik in Breslau*. However, from his short period in Halle records have survived, and Frank Pillmann, who has access to them, has attempted to evaluate Wernicke's system on the basis of 889 cases so documented [18]. He seeks to validate Wernicke's special diagnoses as mutually exclusive categories, as might be expected today. However, the core of Wernicke's system was not diagnoses, but symptoms. Pillmann is therefore judging Wernicke based on today's assumptions, which Wernicke may not have shared, rather than starting from a *tabula rasa*, as, in a sense, he himself did, with no automatic assumption that there *must* be categorical diagnoses. In the paragraphs below, we discuss the three questions just raised:

1. *Theoretical validity*. Several objections can be raised against the implied symmetry of the three domains of psychopathology. *First*, memories involved in building our notion of personal identity are of a different type from those giving us a sense of bodily integrity, and, quantitatively if not qualitatively, from those which represent the outside world. The difference can now be based on that between 'episodic memory'—a trove of memories of unique events occurring throughout our life—and 'semantic' memory—usually acquired by repetition of events, a distinction not yet formulated in Wernicke's day. Episodic memory is more important in constructing a person's sense of identity than in representing his body, and possibly also in representing' the outside world. It is now thought to involve interaction of neocortex with the hippocampus [88], in ways which apply less to the other contents of

consciousness. *Second*, the account of *Delirium tremens* (L26) emphasizes dramatic allopsychic disorientation, while autopsychic orientation is remarkably preserved. The probable explanation, (section VII,(f). 'Higher Levels of Functional Organization'), is that the syndrome described is what is now called 'REM dissociation' (a breakthrough of dreaming, after prolonged insomnia, within a state more akin to wakefulness). This is such an abnormal state that any suggestion of symmetry with contents acquired in other ways can be dismissed. *Third*, 'autopsychosis' as described in L28 does not match psychosis in other domains (if cases of epilepsy, alcoholism or other obvious assaults are excluded): Regardless of the area in which content is described, there is nothing fitting usual definitions of either hallucinations or delusions; and these *should* occur in Wernicke's scheme, since, in L30 (p. 204), the point is added that 'such a disorder of identification [is] assumed to occur in psychosensory areas'. In any case, the 'alternative personhoods' described in L28 are relatively coherent, not dominated by any such symptoms. *Fourth*, if motility psychosis is taken as a fourth component, we should be reminded that brain mechanisms underlying movement differ vastly from most of those of the cerebral cortex seen just as an 'organ of association'. Despite presence of a motor cortical region, the important role of the basal ganglia and cerebellum (amongst other structures) make symmetry with other contents of consciousness most unlikely. The difference between motility functions and the other domains is implicitly recognized when Wernicke refers to 'independent development of akinetic and parakinetic mobility symptoms, separate from normal mechanisms of association' (L12, p. 74).

Given this, several positive things can be said about Wernicke's broadened concept of psychosis. Many cases discussed in L23 and L24 appear to arise from disordered sensory processing. Modern research shows that sensory thresholds and sensitivities across several modalities often correlate (e.g. [141–143]) findings most easily accounted for by some generic feature of the cortex as a whole. If so, it is at least plausible to incorporate Wernicke's somatopsychic disorders into the broader scheme, where other symptoms also arise in the cortex. The point he makes in later lectures, about affinity between somatopsychic and motility phenomena has support from modern neuroscience, in which primary areas for somatic sensation and motor function are increasingly seen to be functionally interdependent. At the same time, it makes scientific sense to separate somato-psychic functions (depending on somato- and proprio-ceptive inputs, whose patterned inputs stay fairly stable over long periods of time) from allo-psychic ones (depending on ever-changing inputs from distance senses), the corresponding cortical areas being some way distant from each other. The conceptual separation of auto- and allo-psychosis was crucial in his differential diagnosis of *Delirium tremens* (L26). Lastly, his distinctive 'anxiety psychosis' and 'hypochondriacal psychosis' concepts *do* have features in common with today's concept of psychosis—especially delusions and hallucinations—although the content is quite different.

2. *Predictive validity in the clinic*. Is Wernicke's system for describing symptoms useful in predicting early signs, development, course, and eventual outcome of different conditions, and possibly in predicting the relative effectiveness of different treatments? One of the broadest generalizations based on his system is about the sequence in which symptoms appear and disappear during acute syndromes: Autopsychic phenomena appear first, and, during recovery, disappear last. Thus, when discussing a young patient with a fluctuating state of consciousness he writes (L18, p. 116): 'We can discern, amongst the internal stimuli mixed together in the centre of his radiant mind, abnormal sensations, self-generated ideas, and simple disorientating phonemes. Disorientation occurs predominantly in the autopsychic area, followed by the allopsychic area.' Many examples of this principle are reported in the context of

anxiety states. In L23 (p. 146), for a patient with anxiety psychosis, we read: 'These autopsychic ideas of anxiety existed on their own in the initial period of illness, and only shortly before his admission were they joined by those of fantastic threats, and at the same time, there was an increase in the patient's restlessness which became so noticeable that it was inevitable that he be transferred to an institution'. In L23 (p. 147) he offers a view that 'Such anxiety regularly leads to emergence of various ideas, which therefore deserve to be called 'anxiety ideas'. They show grades of intensity such that the autopsychic ideas of anxiety correspond to lower intensity, the allopsychic and somatopsychic ones to more severe anxiety'. Then, as a generalization, he writes (p. 147): 'When the disease starts, and as it subsides only autopsychic ideas of anxiety are usually present. In some cases anxiety persists, accompanied just by such ideas; far more often the ideas are "dressed up" as phonemes. At the height of the anxiety state, hallucinations can also appear temporarily in other modalities, and in some of the most acute cases, as in the example of anxiety in a case of epilepsy described above, can occur simultaneously in all senses, as combined hallucinations.' On p. 253 we read: 'it seems to be intrinsic to such cases of agitated melancholia that autopsychic ideas of anxiety outweigh by far any others in their content, even though allopsychic ideas may never be totally absent.' Later, (L40, p. 311) he notes that 'most anxiety psychoses are examples of such a remitting course, in which anxiety, and the autopsychic disorientation based upon it, usually exist in a persistent fashion, but are increased in attacks that lead to allopsychic disarray, and corresponding ideas of allopsychic anxiety in the guise of phonemes.' He also extends the generalization to exacerbations in chronic illness (p. 199): 'We have concerned ourselves earlier with more sophisticated ideas; but if we consider just the time course to be the decisive factor, we often have to attribute new stages of these to acute autopsychoses, occurring during a chronic course of illness.'

Suggestions that autopsychic symptoms appear first and disappear last, compared to symptoms in the other domains makes theoretical sense. For Wernicke, autopsychic symptoms appear to have been more difficult and complex than allo- or somato-psychic ones, since they are discussed from L26 onwards, after first discussing the latter two. In L33 (p. 240) he offers this rationale: 'The situation may arise that the firmest associative links exist in the domain of consciousness of the body, the next firmest in consciousness of the environment, and the loosest—and likewise the last to be acquired, with the greatest individual differences—in consciousness of personhood. Correspondingly, a similar measure of severity of illness, or, according to Meynert's concept, of general weakness of association, was always manifested first in the autopsychic region, and second and third in allopsychic and somatopsychic domains.' Today, much stronger reasoning lends support to this rationale: As already mentioned, the sense of personhood each of us constructs depends on a trove of unique memories of individual events, while our sense of corporeality and of the outside world, are usually acquired by a degree of repetition of events. Retrieving the former, acquired by episodic memory depends largely on reinstating the neural context which prevailed when they were acquired. At the level of brain function, the contexts for each memory depend on interaction between neocortex and hippocampus, more so than do the other types of memory. These are the most sophisticated brain mechanisms we have, the most vulnerable to failure, and likewise the last to be reinstated.

Some of Wernicke's generalizations are about *grading* the intensity of a mental disorder. The intensity of Affective reaction, according to Wernicke, is important in determining overall severity of an illness. So, we read (p. 161) '... the autopsychic area shows itself always to be involved, to varying degrees, corresponding with the Affective state induced by anxiety or somatopsychic disarray.' In L40 (p. 310) we read: '... most acute psychoses, especially all subacute ones, initially show a worsening course. An example of this is given by acute hallucinosis ... The clinical picture, apparently rises rapidly to full disease intensity according to its Affective coloration ...' Again (p. 312): 'There are essential variations in the degree of orientation here, and these depend in a distinctive way on the intensity of Affect. The name we give—autopsychic anxiety ideas (we might also call them "misfortune ideas", undermining ideas of happiness)—shows their derivation from an Affective state.' However, the relation to intensity of the Affective response may vary across the course of an illness: In contrast to the above statements, he writes (p. 281): 'The most severe hypochondriac presentations show themselves with hardly any Affective component, such as having no head, no heart, no lungs, no stomach, or being completely hollow, "only a tube", as one educated patient put it so starkly ... However, for weeks in an earlier acute stage of his illness, the same patient had presented the picture of most severe somatopsychic disarray, admittedly not as agitation, but only as almost total inaccessibility and helplessness, while only occasionally were there isolated expressions and actions pointing to total loss of bodily orientation.'

There are also many straightforward generalizations about course of illness, prevalence at various ages, and prognostic signs of favourable and unfavourable outcomes, which need not be repeated here. In addition, there is nothing to predict which specific treatments might be appropriate, and effective in different disorders, since there *were* no specific treatments in his day. Nonetheless, questions are raised for today: If it is true that there is some kinship between symptoms arising in different domains, because of their origin in different areas of the one structure—the cerebral cortex—some treatments now used in one class of disorders may be usefully applied in others. The cases in point are kinship between somatopsychic and allopsychic domains, and between somatopsychic and motility disorders. Whether psychosis (as defined by Wernicke) in different domains respond to today's antipsychotic medicine in similar ways is an empirical question, which, at present, cannot be given a definite answer. However, single case studies have reported remarkable benefits for body dysmorphic disorder by treatment with antipsychotic medicines [144–146], a disorder which, as defined, may include delusions. Understandably, there have been no controlled studies, given the vast conceptual divide between the disorder in question and those for which antipsychotic medicines are usually prescribed.

3. *Statistical independence of the three domains of psychopathology*. To assess properly the statistical relation between symptoms in Wernicke's three domains, the first requirement would be to have authenticated instruments for assessing each; and then, after collecting suitable data sets, deployment of methods such as factor analysis. This *might* be possible with the data to which Pillman [18] had access. As a beginning, we can search among Wernicke's general statements looking particularly for ones about association or dissociation across the different domains.

With regard to statements about *associations*, the most abundant are *between auto- and allopsychic domains*:

L10 (p. 62): She had no abnormalities of sensation, nor did her general condition reveal any disturbances. Nevertheless, more extensive examination showed other severe changes, noted as defects, which encroached principally into allopsychic and autopsychic areas.

L23 (p. 147): Often, only autopsychic ideas are present, at a moderate level; or there may even be a combination of autopsychic and allopsychic ideas of anxiety, with added phonemes only at times when anxiety intensifies.

L23 (p. 147): Common contents of autopsychic ideas of anxiety and matching phonemes express concern for family members, for the financial situation, challenges to personal honour, and there may be micromania, self-recrimination, with corresponding abusive phonemes. The content of allopsychic ideas of anxiety is usually a threat to life or of ignominious disciplinary actions, abuse, etc.

L25 (p. 166): The main symptoms we know about are phonemes, whose content, corresponding with his anxious state, is partly of a threatening nature, and partly expresses his reduced personal status (that is, part allopsychic part autopsychic notions of anxiety).

L25 (p. 170): A specific characteristic of acute hallucinosis seems to be the occurrence of phonemes on a grand scale, their content being autopsychic and allopsychic delusions of reference.

L29 (p. 201): In addition, everything that people in the neighborhood say or do is assessed as if those people know the patient's thoughts; and so it reaches the point, symptomatically, of generalized autopsychic delusions of reference, with corresponding reinterpretation of the outside world. Allopsychic orientation will then also be impaired.

L33 (p. 242): Cases of weakened association, with autopsychic and allopsychic deficit symptoms but no motor excitatory symptoms (therefore: 'asthenic autoallopsychoses') which I have often seen in very acutely ill young girls.

L36 (p. 278): Residual sequelae involved severe confusion with autopsychic and allopsychic disorientation corresponding to previous hallucinations and a moderately irritatable mood.

Those for association of auto- and somatopsychic symptoms include:

L10 (p. 61): We will talk later about the processes by which such falsifications of consciousness—partly somatopsychic, partly autopsychic—actually arise.

L24 (p. 154): However, the dolour and autopsychic focus of her anxiety remained, as did the somatopsychic perception of anxiety about having small bowel movements.

L 24 (p. 158): When the noise was bad, restlessness in her heart and anxiety also occurred. Also present were severe unhappiness, hopelessness, autopsychic ideas of anxiety with a self-accusatory content—which at the same time she rejected—insomnia, fear of silence at night when the noise increased, and thoughts of suicide.

L28 (p. 188): From our point of view the case is also very clear, because it presents a typical example of autopsychic disarray and disorientation. The addition of somatopsychic disarray and disorientation should not distract us from this view, but will, on the contrary, strengthen it.

Associations between allo- and somato-psychic domains are few, including:

L10 (p. 63): The patient was apparently suffering a slowly developing paranoia, the basis for which could be found mainly in a series of morbid sensations and tactile hallucinations. The patient notices changes in her body but, in contrast to the previous patient, attributes these to outside influences; and thus she reaches allopsychic—in addition to somatopsychic—falsification of consciousness.

L36 (p. 272): Moreover, there exists an internal connection between somatopsychic symptoms, and (in this case), allopsychic symptoms, due partly to simple explanatory delusions, and in part to the elementary symptom of somatopsychic delusions of reference, which, at the time, we categorized as newly formed associations.

L39 (p. 306): Moreover there are some—mainly severe—clinical pictures of psychoses related to the puerperium, especially when, apart from the puerperium, other harmful circumstances are present, such as excessive lactation, febrile illness, or painful mastitis, that have reduced the levels of energy. In such circumstances the most severe hypochondriacal psychoses may occur, with allopsychic disorientation.

Associations of motility symptoms with other domains include:

L39 (p. 303): Almost always in these cases, phrenic nerve insufficiency can be demonstrated as the basis for the fear. Twilight states lasting several days sometimes occur in young people in connection with major emotions, with total allopsychic disorientation almost to the point of asymbolia, blended with episodes of parakinetic symptoms.

L39 (p. 306): Of the mixed forms, a special introduction is needed to manic allopsychosis and manic hyperkinetic allopsychosis.

L39 (p. 307): To all these delirious states, apart from familiar symptoms of hallucinations (in particular the dreamlike hallucinations), occasional ideas of anxiety, and a restlessness more-or-less reminiscent of jactation, an allopsychic disorientation appears always to be distinctive, at least temporarily.

Statements on *dissociation* between domains are also interesting. *Ones where allo-psychic experience is normal, while symptoms abound in other domains include*:

L10 (p. 60): You will observe the contrast between this case with such pronounced allopsychic falsification of consciousness and another patient, in whom consciousness of the outside world is in no way involved over the entire course of the illness right up to the present time, while the main alterations are in awareness of physicality, and, in due course, of personhood as well. We can take it as an example of residual, mainly somatopsychic falsification of consciousness.

L23 (p. 149): … in acute hallucinosis, a characteristic paranoid stage develops very early, which is not the case for simple anxiety psychosis. In the latter condition, allopsychic orientation remains intact, unlike the anxiety-laden state found in *Delirium tremens*.

L25 (p. 170): The rapid, comprehensive, and indeed allopsychic falsification of content, and the emergence of a manner of being persecuted physically, and usually soon directed against specific persons of groups of persons, is highly characteristic acute hallucinosis; while in acute anxiety psychosis, except for certain less common cases with chronic progression, this is absent.

L25 (p. 170): … the predominant features of acute hallucinosis, the preserved allopsychic orientation, and the absence of any formal thought disorder, can persist for weeks, until an increase in defensive emotions and the occurrence of new symptoms mark the progression of the illness.

L30 (p. 210): Affective melancholia totally lacks ideas of allopsychic anxiety so typical of most cases of anxiety psychosis.

L33 (p. 239): Recovery in this case was accomplished, in that the last attacks acquired a form more of pure mania, while the first attack, even more than the second just described, bore an overwhelming stamp of hyperkinetic motility psychosis. Allopsychic orientation in this case was completely intact.

L33 (p. 239): Previous attacks of the illness, especially the first, which appeared along with menstruation, were pure manias. Actual disorientation in the allopsychic area never occurred; in the autopsychic area it had characteristics of grandiose delirium, understandable in the context of mania.

L33 (p. 240): Preceding attacks had a form more akin to hyperkinetic motility psychoses, while the following sixth attack and last attack was purely manic followed by permanent restitution, once a stage of exhaustion had passed. This patient always remained perfectly orientated in the allopsychic domain.

L35 (p. 261): At other times the fantastic menacing delusional state occurring within well-retained allopsychic orientation is to be seen in the same paranoic stage, combined only with hypochondriacal sensations mainly intestinal in nature.

L36 (p. 274): Nonetheless, I want to emphasize explicitly that a definite combination, specifically that with hypochondriacal symptoms, makes up an almost normal picture; again this indicates that motility psychoses should be included with the broader concept of somatopsychoses. On the other hand, in many cases, the fact that complete allopsychic orientation is retained, has been established with reasonable certainty.

In other situations allopsychic symptoms alone predominate (often as exceptions to the idea that autopsychic symptoms are the first to appear and the last to disappear):

L33 (p. 240): Confused mania, in the sense we give to the name, does not by any means embrace all cases of the so-called periodic mania. Quite often, attacks of periodic mania do indeed correspond to the clinical picture outlined, yet allopsychic disorientation is also present, manifested as ignorance—or mistaking the place—of the situation and persons, often even of objects ... We will therefore proceed correctly, if we regard such cases not as confused mania, but as *periodic manic allopsychosis*—and they are often also totally sensory psychoses.

L33 (p. 242): In one case of this kind, the principal characteristics of the state of exhaustion were found as previously described, namely a certain defect in spontaneity; failure of ideation in more complex demands; attentiveness retained just through excitement; but very poor memory retention and simultaneous allopsychic disorientation, accompanied by symptoms of motor and sensory irritation of moderate nature.

A few statements mention dissociation between different abnormalities in the same domain:

L27 (p. 181): Nevertheless, the existing [memory] deficit will explain the fact that no trace of disarray was present, in obvious contrast to the severe allopsychic disorientation.

L36 (p. 275): The combination of allopsychotic symptoms with mania is important practically, and deserves special mention. The clinical picture of *choleric mania*, found quite often as an independent illness, consists essentially of a combination of mania with ideas of anxiety and corresponding phonemes, but without any necessary allopsychic disorientation. Usually however, allopsychic delusions of relatedness and hypermetamorphosis are present.

Normal autopsychic experience with symptoms appearing in other domains is mentioned occasionally:

L26 (p. 230): Results of the clinical examination so far can be summarized, that we are dealing with a patient who, in contrast to near-completely preserved autopsychic orientation—up to the last 2 days—presents severe allopsychic disorientation.

L26 (p. 176): the contrast between well-preserved autopsychic orientation and severe allopsychic disorientation which provides a decisive criterion. No other illness that I know provides such a striking contrast.

Normality of somatopsychic experience while symptoms appear elsewhere is seldom mentioned.

L36 (p. 274): I want to emphasize explicitly that a definite combination, specifically that with hypochondriacal symptoms, makes up an almost normal picture; again this indicates that motility psychoses should be included with the broader concept of somatopsychoses ... In one such case, there was complete somatopsychic orientation, but complicated by fantastic micromania, and in general by a picture of Affective melancholia.

Occasionally, Wernicke's three-way split allows him to make differential diagnoses:

L25 (p. 170): The illness [acute hallucinosis] is easily differentiated from *Delirium tremens* because of the point of difference from the former—the fundamental symptom of allopsychic disorientation in its strict sense.

L25 (p. 170): The differential diagnosis [of *Delirium tremens*] from acute anxiety psychosis can easily lead to confusion, because of the main point in common between the two, which we should acknowledge: the abusive and fantastically threatening character of phonemes, and that they arise out of ideas of anxiety of an autopsychic and allopsychic nature is undoubtedly common to both. But with anxiety psychoses, ideas of autopsychic anxiety namely those of belittlement, quite often predominate, these being grouped not so often into phonemes, as here.

To the best of our knowledge, no one has ever developed Wernicke's language for symptoms along the lines of modern research. Admittedly, his language has theoretical flaws, yet they are no worse than those of instruments in use today. It is nevertheless an interesting language, and if untried, seems useful at least as a descriptive scheme. The above section, where some associations and dissociations appear frequently, others rarely, suggests that there is structure yet to be discovered, with important developments yet to come, were this to be attempted. A case in point is that the association of allo- and somato-psychic abnormalities is relatively rarely reported. The three (or four) broad domains for symptoms may correspond well to large regions of cerebral cortex, which are some way distant from each other; and if so, these broad concepts seem well suited for modern studies with functional imaging, seeking excesses or deficits in cerebral activity in large cortical regions corresponding to the predominant symptom domains.

X. Wernicke's Struggle to Adapt Medical Concepts to Clinical Reality

The 20 years from 1885 during which Wernicke practiced psychiatry were of critical importance for the emerging discipline in continental Europe. This is partly because interactions often occurred between the three components of psychiatry, which came together to form the modern profession, arguably more fruitful than in later years. In addition, it was during this period that the idea took root that mental disorders could be subdivided (as elsewhere in medicine) as named categories. Wernicke's medical training, and the assumption that mental disorders *were* diseases like those being defined elsewhere in medicine inevitably led him to apply medical concepts to what he saw in his clinics. However, there are signs that he struggled in this attempt. We have already seen his scorn for many categories of mental disorder gaining currency in his day, although he did not deny that valid categories might be revealed by later research, and he defined a few such himself. His psychological reasoning, guided by general principles and acute awareness of cerebral functioning, is often highly individualized based on immediate or distant events in each patient's life, and on individual habits of thought acquired during education or employment. This personalized approach might have been more familiar in the newly emerging dynamic psychiatry, rather than within medical paradigms, and does not easily fit into diagnostic concepts, applied in a generic manner. His three-way split of symptom domains was of value to him in *describing* what he saw, but by no means were they separate disease entities, or even separate pathological processes, with separate causes, courses, and treatments.

In the preceding section, we saw how Wernicke struggled to adapt the traditional distinction between chronic and acute disorders to realities in his clinic. Likewise, in L11, he has difficulty separating illnesses which have 'run their course' from those that are still active. The fact that these decisions proved largely beyond him may indicate that his model of mental disorders based on medical precedents required major amendment to match clinical realities. In particular, if his essentially holistic view of human nature, including each person's never-ending quest to integrate past with present experience, is correct, it might make sharp separation between acute and chronic illnesses impossible in principle, except by administrative *fiat*. This appears to be the conclusion to which he is forced in L17.

Wernicke's struggle is similarly evident in his attempts to define prognosis. In L16 (p. 150) he writes of '… cases where active illness is fully extinguished …' Clearly he uses medical terminology, with implications about 'prognosis'. To speak of 'fully extinguished cases' appears to imply a physical disease process with its natural course, rather than a rift in a person's sense of 'wholeness', which might be healed during that person's later journey through life. In any case, the prognostic indicators to which he *does* refer are of a quite different nature: the natural healing a patient might derive from his awareness of inherent contradictions in belief, the impact of malign social environments which provoke return of symptoms, dangers of undue rumination for resurgence of symptoms, and the difference between unlettered people and educated rationalists in coming to terms with past episodes of illness. Again we see unresolved tension between medical training and clinical experience.

An aspect of mental disorders on which we have more appreciation today, and which casts doubt on medical conceptualization of such disorders, is that these disorders are by no means purely negative in their impact, but an inseparable amalgam of negative and positive features, although the latter are given little weight by doctors trained to detect psycho*pathology*. This does not easily fit medical concepts of disease. Wernicke shows some awareness of the principle.

He is aware that in some acute conditions, patients may have sharper attentional focus than normal. A patient 'on one occasion … expressed his astonishment that the head warder had disappeared through one door of the hospital and simultaneously entered through another door. On another, food suddenly stood before him without any delay, a process that reminded him of the fairy tale "wishing table"' (L18: p. 114): Both events indicate a break in temporal continuity, due to total lapses of attention to the outside world. (See section XV. 'Allusions Requiring Clarification' for clarification of 'wishing table'). He comments (L18, p. 116): 'The state of distraction is reminiscent of delirium, and appears to be associated with a dream-like clouding of consciousness. We can conceive of no sharper contrast than the attentive, razor-sharp consciousness, which follows immediately afterwards'. However, from brain theory, or psychological theory, we realize that these two states, apparently dramatically different, are closely related: If attention has an excessively sharp focus, it can focus either on internal information, or on the external world, in either case excluding anything else. Since both are represented in the cerebral cortex, a state of sharpened attention to one may apply to the other. Wernicke also suggests that in acutely disordered states, patients may have a better-than-normal sense of sound localization (L5, p. 29). In L19 (p. 118) he elaborates thus: 'Usually the direction from which voices appear to come can be precisely specified; and patients often develop, in this regard, quite striking ability to localize, found only in cases of illness. The source of the voices is indicated not only by the direction, but even by the very precise location and distance from the ear.' What is missing in *Grundriss* is an awareness of how enduring personality traits combine an inextricable mix of both impairment (even severe disability), and, in other faculties, major strengths, which may amount to outstanding talent. That is also missing in much of today's psychiatry, although it is now a possible development, with our greater awareness of the intrinsic diversity of personality types.

A major sign of Wernicke's struggle to apply medical concepts is his rejection of aetiology as a basis for classification. Admittedly, he knew little of *fundamental* causes, and usually replaced this with 'proximate causes', substituting correlation for causation. Even so, he firmly rejects aetiology, defying principles established elsewhere in medicine (notably for infectious diseases). So, in L39 (p. 307) he writes of '… the maxim that, so often, I sought to instil, that aetiological consideration offers a benefit only if we separate it sharply from clinical definition of the various psychoses, making no claims to artificial construction, or certain clinical forms defined exclusively by aetiology'. Similar statements occur throughout *Grundriss*. Clinical pictures of diverse kinds arise from any one aetiology; the two are in no specific relation to each other. What, one might then ask, *could* determine which clinical picture emerges in each patient? For Wernicke, we have some hints: Stage of life, accumulation of past experiences of mental disorder, education, employment, sophistication of baseline mental processes, and other life experiences in the recent or remote past—mainly social factors not medical ones. A modern writer might add baseline personality.

Perhaps the most fundamental source of tension evident in *Grundriss*, perhaps intrinsic to psychiatry as a whole, is between *mechanism and meaning*, or alternatively between *physical disorder and informational discord*. Wernicke 'cut his teeth' as a neurologist on clinico-anatomical correlations; as a psychiatrist, he naturally sought neuronal pathology as a basis for mental disorders he studied. The sejunction theory was supposed to provide this basis. While quite hypothetical, it showed him striving to fit mental disorder into medical concepts; yet, even in his day, it failed. In L14 (p. 74), in an account of retrospective delusional explanations, he writes that 'modified contents of consciousness must be reconciled, according to our prevailing notions of causality, with old, as yet unchanged domains'; and yet he clarifies this as occurring 'according to strict standards of logic'. However, causality and logic are not the same! In L20 (p. 125) he confronts the ambiguous status of mental disorders as diseases akin to those of general medicine. Pathologies along these lines, he argues, like cortical lesions in neurology, should be random ('subject to chance'). We find this echoed later in Bleuler's words on schizophrenia: 'This disease seems to interrupt, quite haphazardly, sometimes such single threads, sometimes a whole group, and sometimes even large segments of them'. In contrast, Wernicke suggests that hallucinations are *not* random, *not* haphazard; not so much a deranged *mechanism*, but rather a disturbance in processing *meaning*.

Overall, throughout *Grundriss*, he gives little direct evidence of a *neuro*pathological basis for any mental disorder, apart from disorders now clearly part of neurology. Perhaps there is *no* such qualitative pathology, at a cellular level, such as would be understood by a competent neuropathologist. Abnormalities at this level which *are* now evident, are more likely to be subtle quantitative departures from the norm in cellular make-up, which do not amount to pathology; and these can then combine to produce unstable vicious circles in large-scale functioning of the brain. 'Pathology' (if that is the right word), is then at the level of whole-person functioning, especially in social functioning, which is beyond a person's normal capacity for reintegration. The implicit definition of Wernicke's term *Geisteskrankheit*, thus becomes 'loss of sense of personal wholeness'—a non-medical concept, which does not fit within system-based ideas of disease. The fundamental question posed is then: Can medical paradigms assimilate disorders whose essence is the brain's handling of information, and therefore in its apprehension of meaning? There is another huge imponderable: Had he lived longer, would he ever have resolved the tension? … and if so, how would he have done it?

At this point, it is appropriate to mention differences between the clinical style of Wernicke, and that of his contemporary, Emil Kraepelin, who outlived him, and whose influence continues to this day. Most of the points summarized here have already been mentioned in other contexts, and are brought together here to show the sharp contrast between the two researchers. Both wanted to adopt standards and methods of general medicine, to give psychiatry the status they thought it deserved. In L8, Wernicke asks: Is clinical science in psychiatry even possible? The answers of the two were quite different, and hinged around their respective approach to classification. For Kraepelin, classification had to come before explanation. Wherever possible, it should be based on pathology or aetiology. However, Kraepelin accepted by the mid-1890s that for key concepts this was no more possible than in Wernicke's system. He therefore focused on symptom clusters and long-term outcome; but the ways in which complexities of symptoms were to be assimilated could not be strictly rational, but, based on 'long experience', ultimately reliant on personal authority—especially his own. Kraepelin was under the influence (as was Wernicke) of the neo-Kantian revival, led by Hermann Cohen (1848–1918), dating back to the 1870s. Kraepelin took basic categories of Kant—especially 'cognition' and 'emotion' as separate and irreducible faculties [106]—as the basis for distinct disease types; but Wernicke gets closer to the core of Kant's philosophy, in emphasizing the distinction between content and form (as did Jaspers), but also took primary experience as the key to the language of the natural sciences. In psychiatry, this meant symptoms, albeit used *indirectly* via their sensory and motor representation in the brain, and supported by reasoning from neuroscience. In contrast, Kraepelin's disorders of cognition and affect (respectively *Dementia praecox*, with its supposed characteristic of 'thought disorder', and Manic-Depressive psychosis), were rooted *directly* in Kant's philosophy and his psychological categories, with *no* link to their physical basis, and thus separated from the common language of science. Kraepelin—at least in separating *Dementia praecox* from manic depressive psychosis, and with long term outcome as a criterion—fused clinico-scientific and administrative requirements giving supposed scientific disease categories, while Wernicke acknowledging that the two required different, co-existing systems of classification, criticized over-use of terms such as degeneration, and never uses the *Dementia praecox* concept.

The categorical typology of Kraepelin, and especially the implied gloomy prognosis of *Dementia praecox* undermined any attempt to see mental disorders as dysfunctions at the level of personal wholeness, and any implications this might have for a clinician trying to rebuild that sense in his patients. Wernicke's system of thought was altogether more holistic, and more optimistic, not only in his approach to classification, but also in his ability to make explanations at an individual level. We see this in his neuroscience-based concept of personal wholeness, where the three components of memory are brought together to form a single larger entity. We also see it in his accepting that emotional and cognitive aspects of experience are parts of this same whole, always interacting, whether in health or in disorder. His holism is also seen in his search, wherever possible for ways by which different symptoms interact, one symptom often taken as 'elementary', the root of all others, a style not found in Kraepelin. For him, *Dementia praecox* was a disorder primarily of cognition, manic depressive psychosis one of mood; his work on *Dementia praecox*, seldom mentions abnormal emotions.

In terms of overall style, Wernicke is impressive in that he attempts to bring scientific reasoning—albeit of an unusual style—to bear on psychiatry. He believed that neurology and psychiatry were different parts of a single discipline, or at least natural partners, unlike Kraepelin, who want psychiatry to be an independent discipline. By his faith in reasoning—and in other ways—Wernicke tried to distance himself from any personal authority he might have had; nor did he easily accept the authority of others. Kraepelin, by contrast, both accepted authority (such as psychological categories of Kant), and expected that he himself should wield such authority. Wernicke, of course did have power conferred on him by virtue of his position, but appears to have been aware of his need constantly to earn it, in daily interactions with many people. It is perhaps no coincidence that, in this period, when militarism was growing in Germany, involving many psychiatrists, Kraepelin was actively involved in military research [5], while Wernicke, who certainly knew about military matters, 'stood somewhat apart from the main stream and military roads of science', according to Theodor Ziehen's obituary. The debate continues to this day, enlivened now by vocal contributions from service users. The definitive answer still escapes us.

XI. Wernicke's Reasoning

XI,(a). Style of Reasoning

Already in his first lecture we sense the great care with which Wernicke constructs his arguments: His word *Begriffszentrum*, translated as 'Conceptualization Centre', is qualified as 'supposed' (*supponierten*), suggesting that he is setting up a hypothesis for later modification; and this is how it unfolds in L2. Sometimes he sets up a 'straw man', with the intention, later, of showing it up for what it is. In L3, in relation to visual after-images, he sets up a hypothesis, in order to present counter-arguments, and so gain better understanding, almost a classic *reductio ad absurdum* argument. In addition, he often uses a style common in natural philosophy (and important for Ernst Mach), of putting forward a scenario, which is not realistic, just to clarify an argument. Overall, the more we have worked on his German text, in our attempt to get the most accurate rendition in English, the more are we impressed by his attempts to use terms in his very complex system of thought in a consistent way, which does not blur his essential concepts. His reasoning is often subtle, but, especially in later lectures, complex, and at times hard to follow. For example, in L36 (p. 271), he writes of the relationship between three concepts of melancholia—hypochondriacal, depressive and Affective. We view this as a contrast between hypochondriacal and depressive melancholia, while Affective melancholia, referred to in passing, provides further explanation—but it is hard to be certain.

In the *first eight lectures*, Wernicke's reasoning is mainly 'psychobiological', that is 'cross-level reasoning' as found elsewhere in the natural sciences. Specifically, he establishes rational links between, on the one hand, facts from neuroanatomy (the abundant long and short cortico-cortical connections) and from putative physiological principles (modifiability of these connections), and on the other hand psychological facts of memory, that memories of quite different types and acquired at different times are assimilated to provide a somewhat integrated sense of personhood. In the *clinical lectures*, a more special and distinctive form of reasoning becomes prominent, by which symptoms are related to each other (usually from 'elementary' to secondary symptoms), to events in a person's life, to habits of thought acquired during education or training and employment, or to immediate social circumstances in which a person might find himself, such as after discharge. The relationships are not mere correlations; nor are they 'causal' in the sense that they employ known causal principles from elsewhere in science; nor are they strictly logical relations in the usual deductive sense. The relation between elementary symptoms and explanatory delusions is formally the *reverse* of normal deduction, a word which Wernicke uses seldom (the exception in L1 being: 'Symptoms must be *deduced*'). Thus the premise for an argument (e.g. the fact of an explanatory delusional belief) *follows* rather than precedes (in the patient's mind) the thing to be explained—an experience which is primarily abnormal. So (L10, p. 60) '... everything is identified in a reconfigured manner to match certain prevailing notions'. A preformed conclusion suggests 'how the evidence is to seen'. This style is of course common in everyday life, sometimes adopted deliberately when expedient, for instance when a person needs to defend themselves against charges of wrong-doing. For those with little experience in reasoning, and no alternative model of inference, it is quite instinctive. Provision of an explanation for a new experience is initially then an exercise in imagination, only later checked deductively for consistency. As such it is similar to a creative scientist seeking an explanation, a process far more complex than syllogistic deduction. This, of course, is the *patient's* style. Wernicke's reconstruction of this style *is* genuine scientific reasoning, albeit of a form unusual in science.

The way Wernicke formulates patients' thought process includes some fascinating elaborations. Mainly he sees the process of delusion formation as near-normal in terms of rationality, but, with sejunction, that rationality, that awareness of the existence of inconsistencies, and the imperative that such inconsistencies should be eradicated, all fail. He is keenly aware of the anomaly in many patients, when 'The very fact that this patient is unaware of contradictions between his various misconceptions, suggests that the combination of all higher associations into a single unit, the ego, has ceased' (L12; p. 72). However, he also suggests that use of explanatory delusions in a 'corrective' sense is important in retrospective review of psychotic beliefs, especially in educated in people with habits of logical thought. So, in L14, we read: 'The more that discernment can be regained or has been retained during chronic psychoses, the more mental activity takes place according to strict standards of logic, and the more imperative it is to restore some semblance of order in structures brought into disarray by illness'. Again, when discussing mania: 'As long as this "circumspect collectedness" is not lost, secondary associations may be noticed to an intensified degree, and yet the main association is retained. This possibility exists particularly in highly trained minds' (L31, p. 216). These are good examples where life experience, work experience, or education provides skills which counteract 'mental illness'. However, sometimes, a facility in reasoning *hinders* resolution of conflicts of belief acquired during psychosis, as in the case suggested in L16, of a patient with a highly trained legal mind, who applies his training to provide ever-more elaborate accretions to his sense of injustice about involuntary detention. A rational habit which benefits one person can be devastating in another.

Some would argue that the highly individualized style of Wernicke's reasoning reduces its scientific status; but it is hard to uphold such objections in the face of Wernicke's skilled arguments, where a patient's education, professional activity, and social milieu after discharge are built into his understanding of how delusional material arises, declines, or is subject to progressive increment or decrement.

Wernicke occasionally uses the word 'experiment', but usually as Mach's 'thought experiment', or as experiments conducted in animals by researchers in other fields. In L20 (p. 129) he describes what he actually did, to establish hypermetamorphosis: 'by bringing favourite sensory stimuli into the vicinity of the patient: for example, pulling out a watch, a handkerchief, the stock market report, or noting how objects are casually played with, to give a sense of sight …' In L13 (p. 81) he writes 'In this example, in one case only ideas full of anxiety, or "anxiety ideas", as I call them, in the other, frightening and threatening phonemes, that is the same ideas, but put into words. We can assess such experience …' He appears to refer to tests which may have been carried out on his patients, possibly word association tests. Such tests were first used by Francis Galton, and, developed further by Wilhelm Wundt, with reaction time as the dependent measure. Theodor Ziehen was the first to explore the method thoroughly in 1898 [147], and it was from him that C.G. Jung learned the method to use on his patients at the Burghölzli Mental Asylum in early years of the twentieth century [148]. It is thus plausible to suggest that Wernicke also used the method in some form. In any case the idea of innocuous experiments to test hypotheses about motives or cognitive strategies used by individuals was elaborated further in later years by ethologists and child psychologists such as Jean Piaget, and Nikolaas Tinbergen.

Wernicke cites exact quantitative data only once (L37, p. 288 *seq.*), Meynert's rather than his own, on brain weights in various patient groups. He claims that the data for progressive paralysis show greater proportionate loss in frontal compared to other regions. The values presented hardly prove this in males, where the percentage losses in frontal, temporal, and occipital lobes are 16 %, 14 %, and 11 %, respectively; and in females do so only in so far as the temporal lobe in paralytics loses 5 % of the weight of the comparison group, compared to 20 % and 15 % losses in frontal and occipital lobes. Variance is not reported, this being before the days of statistical analysis.

XI,(b). Reasoning by Analogy

It has been pointed out already that, when trying to understand a new field, reasoning by analogy, despite its shortcomings, is often the only way forwards. Exactly the same style is found, most eloquently, three centuries earlier, and for exactly the same reason, in Francis Bacon's *Novum Organum* [66] a founding text for the natural sciences as a whole. For Wernicke, the 'conceptual gap', which forced him to adopt this strategy, was his ignorance of basic processes, especially the physical basis of nervous signals.

Many examples of analogies have already been given, some predating Wernicke, such as those from Meynert. He refers to Meynert's image of an 'enclosed pipe system', and in L4 (p. 23) and L8 (p. 46) extends this to a 'wave of psychophysical motion', citing Fechner, but referring to his earlier work on aphasia, in which a succession of associations is described as 'a wave motion in an enclosed pipe system'. Sometimes analogies are drawn from his earlier works, as when (LI) he draws the analogy between nonsensical speech in psychiatric patients, and transcortical aphasia, a concept already defined; and when in (L4) he points out the similarity in forming perceptions from sensation, as for concepts from percepts. Sometimes analogies come by broadening the meaning of accepted terms, as when he clarifies the notion of the Conceptualization Centre (L2): He refers to inputs to it, using the word *versinnlich*, usually translated as 'sensual', although the situation is strictly neither sensual, nor sensory. He implies that a person's *understanding* (of a question just posed) becomes a quasi-'sensory' input to subsequent stages of processing, where formulation of the answer occurs.

The boldest and most far-reaching analogies are usually based on recent advances in other areas of science, a recurring feature in *Grundriss*. The first example is in L1, when, to clarify the indirectness of relay between cortical regions, he refers, to telegraphy. Presumably he referred to cables and Morse code, not radio-telegraphy—'wireless'—since it was only in 1894 that Nicola Tesla first demonstrated the 'wireless' principle, and the first commercial system of radio transmission, patented by Guglielmo Marconi, was not in use until 1906. Electrical metaphors ('resistance' in L19 and L30; 'short-circuit' in L20, p. 131) occur periodically. In L4 and L8, and often thereafter, he refers to a physicist's graphical display on rectangular coordinates, to depict interaction of two interdependent psychological variables. In L4 these are 'strength' (or 'intensity') and 'extent' (or 'circumference'). In L8, they are the 'level' and 'extension' of consciousness, the former also expressed as intensity of excitation or activation by a stimulus. The word 'extent' is often replaced in our translation by 'range'.

The most prevalent physical analogy is the concept of energy (*Kraft*). Originally this term was akin to 'life force', a metaphor often used by scientists or philosophers (J.F.Herbart, Fechner, Helmholtz) in nineteenth century German psychology, and by Sigmund Freud in psychiatry. The scientific concept of energy emerged slowly from this, and in mid-nineteenth century, various forms of physical energy were unified in the field of thermodynamics. The first use of *Kraft* in *Grundriss* is in L2, where the word identifies potentialities latent in any stored memory (and again in L8). In L30 (p. 206) we read of 'necessary expenditure of energy'. 'Potential energy' is specific term, coined in the nineteenth century by the Scottish physicist William Rankine. Its use in L8, draws a conscious analogy with the physicist's concept, where Wernicke refers (p. 46) to there being 'only a certain store of "life force" available in the brain for psychophysical movement'; and in L32 (p. 223) his words (our translation) are: 'all her energy has been quite used up'. These phrases hint at a conservation law for (psychic) energy, as did Freud's hydraulic metaphor. Conservation of energy is a concept with a long history, but had been formulated concisely within living memory by Helmholtz. It is no coincidence that Ernst Mach had also published in 1872 a book entitled *History and Roots of the Principle of Conservation of Energy* [149] (strictly 'conservation of work': *Erhaltung der Arbeit*). Modern concepts of fixed limits to 'processing resources' for attention have similar implications.

Sometimes Wernicke takes physical analogies too far: In L11 (p. 66) the term 'specific energies', like 'potential energy', is adopted from thermodynamics, but its meaning—'specific' in so far as it is linked with specific patterns of information—is quite different from its use in physics ('energy per unit mass' or 'energy density'). In developing the sejunction hypothesis in L12, he mixes several analogies, in part mechanical, hydraulic and electrical, including reference to 'resistance' (L20, p. 126). He invokes localization of function far beyond any empirical evidence; and uses the concept of energy less precisely than as the robust physical variable we now know. In phrases such as 'build up of nervous energy' he seems to draw on the concept of conservation of energy. He may also have drawn on the fact that novel events force themselves on us with unusual vigour if suppressed (as he argues in L8, p. 46, when describing how a miller is awakened from sleep when machinery in his mill *stops* its steady grind). Inevitably, inferences are made about underlying physical processes, which lacked any empirical support.

Sometimes analogies lead to serious errors, and, from today's perspective it is easy to see mistakes from undue reliance on analogies. Memories are not 'stores of energy'; discharge of nervous activity along associative links does not 'drain away' anything; failure of such discharge does not lead to 'build up' of energy (the supposed 'irritant' for symptoms such as hallucinations). Often he draws analogies between neurology and psychiatry, which turn out to be false. So, in L11 (p. 67) he writes: 'We can fairly equate residual alteration in content as a localized process, with changes in content when psychoses progress slowly', implying that changed content of consciousness (like focal brain injury) is irreversible, an error based on his choice of analogy. In his analogy between progressive paralysis and other psychoses (L37, p. 280), we now know that the pathological change in the former is greater than ever documented in endogenous psychoses. Sometimes, in use of analogy, close juxtaposition of error and visionary foresight is startling. In L20 (p. 126) the 'specific energy' metaphor is used to point to the intrinsic holism of the entire associative machine, a metaphor which may seem strange to us today; but then he mixes this with the metaphor of 'resonance'. Use of this analogy is astonishing because it was 30 years before any reliable method of recording the EEG was available.

Errors in inference by analogy are not flaws in reasoning: They are expected in this style of inference, to be recognized and, in due course, corrected. However, conclusions based on analogies should never be given credence greater than at the time of their origin. The concept of 'mental illness', as analogous to illnesses of general medicine is a case in point. Is it an appropriate? Is it given greater credence than it deserves? Does it survive just on the basis of habitual use? These questions need to be posed.

Throughout *Grundriss*, we see Wernicke searching for simplicity and symmetry, but sometimes, in hindsight it is simplistic. As already argued, the implied symmetry of the three-way split of contents of consciousness, is inexact. He also implies symmetry between melancholia and mania, opposite sides of the same coin, namely excessive ease or impairment in exercising 'will'. However, the underlying mechanisms, even as analyzed by Wernicke, are not opposites of one another, and modern research would show this more clearly; so, there is no true symmetry.

XI,(c). Flaws in Wernicke's Reasoning

Hindsight, it is said, is a wonderful thing. With the benefit of 120 years' hindsight, it is easy to find flaws in Wernicke's reasoning. The same can be said of those intrepid pioneers, the first who had the temerity to venture into *terra incognita*, by attempting to bring Reason to bear on Nature. Johannes Kepler, for instance, was one such pioneer, and, despite great achievements, could resort to 'mystical numerology', supposing there to be simple whole-number ratios between distances of different planets from the sun. Here he followed the precedent of Pythagoras, who found that simple whole-number ratios of lengths of vibrating strings produced harmonious musical intervals; and he was followed by John Dalton, whose successful hunch along similar lines was critical in the reasoning supporting his atomic hypothesis; yet in this Kepler was incorrect. The following comments are therefore offered, with full awareness that, with Wernicke, we deal with another intrepid pioneer. Some flaws we identify are small details, others more profound and far reaching, and some quite subtle.

Unidentified assumptions; *inconsistency in using assumptions*: In L4, Wernicke discusses the number of concepts we might have in our heads, and writes 'The number of words gives us a clue to the number of concepts': Of course there is a flaw: Any word (perhaps more so in English than German) has a variety of uses: Many words are ambiguous until the context is specified. The claim that Shakespeare used an unmatched variety of different words is commonly made, but has been questioned. Studies using modern methods do not find Shakespeare's vocabulary exceptional, compared to many other eminent writers. In developing the sejunction theory, an assumption is implied which is inconsistent with one made later in *Grundriss*. Thus, in L13, 'sejunction' is seen to involve build-up and 'back-propagation' of energy along forwardly projecting pathways from primary sensory areas to higher areas, as if there are no direct pathways in the opposite direction; but as early as L6 (and in L19; p. 124), it is clear that concepts (especially that of 'corporeality') are elaborated through associative interconnections with 'perception cells', implying (as we now know) that primary sensory areas receive inputs from higher cortical areas, distant in forward-projecting connectional terms from primary sensory areas. The inconsistency reveals the struggle in Wernicke's mind to explain hallucinations, and the incompleteness of his system. Another inconsistency is his assumption about inhibitory interactions in the 'organ of association' (implicitly the cerebral cortex). In L8 he states his belief that there are only excitatory interactions between neurones, but very soon, and in later lectures implies inhibitory interaction (see section VII,(a). 'Wernicke's Contribution to Neuroscience, Psychology and Overall Medical Knowledge', *Basic neuroscience*).

Confusion of neuronal with psychological language: Wernicke often jumps too easily between biological (neuronal) statements and psychological ones, as if they were the same. Philosophers might call this a 'category error': It is also another way in which analogies lead to errors. An example is where he writes (L14, p. 85) that '... breakdown of nervous structure, a change occurring at a definite location, leads to signs of deficit, with no possibility of recovery ...It seems that dissolution of associations in some circumstances is equivalent to destruction of certain psychological units': This paragraph has obvious ambiguity, over whether deficits referred to are primarily in physical (nervous) structure or in psychological (information) structure. Nevertheless, in his comparison of the views of Meynert and Neumann on hallucinations (p. 123) and the way he uses the word 'pathology' (never 'psychopathology') he shows a keen awareness of this very issue.

Overinclusiveness: Sometimes Wernicke's arguments are based on *supposed* areas with specified functions, *supposed* pathways, or *supposed* lesions, without anatomical or pathological proof. This style is common in today's clinical neuroscience, and is criticized by purists. In truth, it is hard to avoid, but best taken as 'hypotheses to be explored' not as known facts or conclusions based on secure deduction. Imaginative construction of explanatory hypothesis is part of Wernicke's style, as it is in the natural philosophy tradition. The concept of 'motility', an abstract noun related to 'movement', is also extended in ways some might call overinclusive (such as the pressure to speak), although his rationale is made clear in suitable places.

Failure to Separate Deductive from Inductive Inference: This has been referred to several times already, along with the idea that what Wernicke claims to be missing in some of his patients is a faculty which—in truth—most people never had. The supposed lost ability is closely related to one of the classical 'laws of thought'—the Principle of Non-contradiction—going back as far as Aristotle, and formalized in Russell and Whitehead's *Principia Mathematica*, published 4 years after the 1906 edition of *Grundriss.* Wernicke—logician that he was—may have regarded this principle as more of a universal human norm than it actually is.

XII. Treatments and Medical Technology of the Day

Specific treatments for any disorder were very limited in Wernicke's day; rational chemotherapy of any disorder was some way in the future. For mental disorders the best that could be offered was often little more than high quality nursing care, and restoring proper nutrition. There is no indication that Wernicke adopted treatments which were innovative, beyond high quality in this area, and his personal attention. Some supposedly specific treatments were hang-overs from days when medicine had no pretentions to a scientific basis. The few available medicines aimed to alleviate immediate symptoms and ensure good sleep rather than address fundamental issues. The history of medicines in psychiatry in this period is reviewed by Healy [150].

Of the few medicines used in mental hospitals, several were herbal. Most often mentioned in *Grundriss* is opium, used in various contexts, without prescription, and not mainly for pain relief. It appears to have been widely used in late nineteenth century Germany for disorders of mood, anxiety, or the two combined [150, 151], and in L23 (p. 149) its use in anxiety psychosis is mentioned. Such treatment may not have been complication-free: Thus, in L25 (p. 305) we read 'A strict bed regime must then be imposed, to ensure adequate sleep and nutrition, and to combat occasional fits of anxiety induced by opium'. Again, in L35 (p. 262), in a case of 'severe loss of intrapsychic function along with hypochondriacal symptoms', we read: 'At times of remission, or with a favourable response to a medication such as opium, you may hear from patients that they feel too ill to think, or speak or to do anything.' In L32 (p. 234) we read: 'Use of narcotics in hyperkinetic motility psychoses is generally contraindicated'. Modern support for this statement is that, in Tourette's syndrome, opioid agonists, far from alleviating symptoms, may exacerbate them [152] and opiate antagonists may be effective treatment [153]. For 'restless legs syndrome', a condition to which some patients in L32 may correspond, they may be effective treatment [154].

Another product originally extracted from plants (now manufactured synthetically) was camphor. Its medicinal use was mainly by external application to the skin, but it was used in small doses orally to strengthen the heart, during heart failure (L26, p. 173). Hyoscine (scopolamine), an alkaloid extracted from henbane, and a muscarinic antagonist, was used from mid-nineteenth century, with both sedative and euphoriant properties. It is mentioned in L23 (p. 149) for treating anxiety psychosis (in combination with opium), and recommended doses are given. In L32 (pp. 223, 225) it is recommended for treating hyperkinetic disorders, and as a sedative in patients with such disorders. It is not mentioned as treatment for melancholia (nor is *any* medication recommended for this condition). This is noteworthy, since one of today's hypotheses for depression is based on overactivity of muscarininc cholinergic systems, and anticholinergics are effective in some cases of depression.

Amongst synthetic products, *bromide*, introduced in the 1860s, was used as a sedative and sleeping draught (L28, p. 192) [155]. Bromide overdose has toxic effects, but there is no mention of this in *Grundriss*. However, in L34 (p. 246) we read: 'Stress and many sleeping drugs were given as the cause of the illness'. Then as now, hazards of regular use of sleeping pills seem to have been well known. *Amyl hydrate* is a product mentioned in L20 (p. 134), as having an 'immediate calming effect' in relation to psychosis with epilepsy. This may have been amyl alcohol, which, although a natural product of fermentation, was being produced industrially at the time, and was used as a sedative and anaesthetic between 1880 and 1950. Amyl hydrate also has properties as a vasodilator. *Paraldehyde* was first synthesized in 1829 by Wildenbusch and introduced into medical practice in 1882, by Vincenzo Cervello, as a central depressant. It was found to be anticonvulsant as well as sedative, and is administered in various ways. It is mentioned in L25 (p. 167); and in L26 (p. 176) recommendations on dose as a hypnotic are given which correspond well to modern recommendations, according to Medsafe, New Zealand [156]. In L25 (p. 166) there is mention of *Phenacetin*, first synthesized in the USA, and chemically related to paracetamol (its metabolite). It was introduced clinically in 1887, as a non-opioid analgesic, and fever-reducing drug, but was banned by the FDA in the USA in 1983, because of evidence of serious side effects. *Trional*, mentioned in L29 (p. 197) was first prepared in 1888, and introduced clinically in the same year, as a sedative and hypnotic. The chemist behind this was Eugen Baumann (1846–1896), and the specialist in internal medicine, Alfred Kast (1856–1903), worked at Breslau from 1892. It is now known to have neuronal inhibitory actions, related to GABA. There is no mention of any overall drug treatment for psychoses as understood either by Wernicke or in today's concept, but a combination of opium and hyoscine was probably used widely, since we also read in L23 (p. 150): 'Incidentally, treatment of anxiety psychoses gives outcomes just the same as those for psychoses generally'.

Treatment of syphilis is mentioned in L37 (p. 287). For centuries this had made use of mercury, applied externally to lesions. From 1843 potassium iodide by mouth was introduced, combined with mercury. That Wernicke recommended it for paralytic psychoses, which he differentiated from cerebral syphilis, indicates the unresolved relationship between the two disorders in his thinking. No other treatment was available until salvarsan was introduced in 1910, which also was relatively ineffective.

Other biological or physical treatments are mentioned. Magnetic cures, mentioned in L29 (p. 199) had a long history, and a century earlier in Europe had been popularized by Anton Mesmer (1734–1815). They were still recommended in some medical textbooks in Wernicke's day for mental disorders, convulsions, insomnia, migraine, fatigue or arthritis [157]. In L10 (p. 60) we hear of '"vaporization" of chloroform and the "electrical treatment"': Chloroform and various means of electrical stimulation were used in asylums in many countries in the late nineteenth century. Electrical stimulation in neurology clinics is also mentioned in L27 (p. 182), it being used widely in both Europe and Britain in the second half of the nineteenth century [158]. Use of leeches to initiate menstruation went back long before Wernicke's day, but was still apparently in use (L32, p. 234).

Medical technology was very basic. 'Infusion' is mentioned in L24 (p. 155), but it is not clear what is meant. Intravenous injection was a difficult procedure at the time, being favoured just for some medicines, and into the first decade of the twentieth century, at which time it was still a surgical procedure. In L32, (p. 223) we read of 'injection of hyoscine and morphine' as a sleeping draught for a hyperkinetic patient who would not stop singing. This was a subcutaneous injection (L23, p. 150; L32, p. 235), which was easier [159]. In L26 (p. 174) *Papilla nervi optici* is mentioned, no doubt visualized by ophthalmoscopy. The ophthalmoscope was invented in 1851 by von Helmholtz (although some say primacy goes to Charles Babbage, 4 years earlier). Its design underwent improvement after Wernicke's death.

There is little on any psychological approach to treatment in *Grundriss*, and nothing comparable to any form of psychotherapy. However, in L30, there is detailed guidance, on the sort of nursing care most conductive to recovery from Affective melancholia, along lines which follow easily from the concept of this disorder Wernicke describes. Likewise in L32 (p. 233; also L20, p. 130) he writes 'If sources of hypermetamorphosis are removed by seclusion of patients, such motor impulses subside quite predictably': Today, in good mental health facilities, the corresponding strategy is to use rooms specially designed to limit all kinds of sensory stimulation. Wernicke also gives his views on indications and contraindications for using seclusion (L41, p. 324).

XIII. Update on Scientific Issues Raised

In preceding sections there has already been discussion of some scientific issues raised by Wernicke, in the light of modern research findings. Here we summarize modern views on further issues raised in *Grundriss*.

Neuroanatomy: The number of nerve cells in the cortex (L4, p. 22) was 'about a *milliarde*, by Meynert's count' (about one billion). Modern estimates put the figure much higher—19 and 23 billion (mean figures for female and male respectively, with large individual variation: [160]).

Neuropathology is mentioned occasionally in *Grundriss*. The neuropathology of progressive paralysis is mentioned in several places, and Wernicke makes very bold conjectures in L7, where he suggests that there is pathology in an outer lamina of the cerebral cortex. In L41 (p. 326) we read: 'As Lissauer has shown, this loss of fibres [in progressive paralysis] has now been proved to be a systematic loss, corresponding to secondary degeneration; and Lissauer also succeeded in demonstrating the source of this secondary generation in the destruction of entire cell layers, in certain cases'. A later examination of neuropathology in cases of progressive paralysis [161], discusses the original findings and subsequent ones, concluding that the pathology can be attributed to a variety of factors, not directly related to the spirochete.

Defined neurological disorders: 'Visual agnosia' (first mentioned in L3, p. 16) was originally defined by Lissauer. Wernicke mentions it in cases of polyneuritic psychosis (Wernicke-Korsakoff syndrome) (L38, p. 295). Modern evidence shows that visual problems can occur in thiamine deficiency, albeit rarely (e.g. [162]), and that this is also associated with widespread cortical damage [163].

In L30 (p. 208) Wernicke comments on the high prevalence of seizures in cases of melancholia. This is echoed in today's research literature [164–169] the likelihood being that there are causal components in common between the two disorders rather than seizures being either cause or consequence of melancholia or depression. There may be atypical features to depression when the two occur together. The relationship is hard to define precisely because 'seizures' may be non-epileptic, and when they *are* epileptic, it is at present unclear which, of many types of epilepsy collected under the single term, is involved.

Wernicke's comment (L29, p. 200) that compulsive acts are more common at time of menstruation has modern support: Both motor compulsions ('tics') and obsessive thoughts are known to increase in the premenstrual period in some patients with OCD or Tourette's syndrome [170, 171].

Symptomatology: Although Wernicke knew little of the principle of psychological reinforcement, he makes an interesting point in this context (L8, p. 49) that 'all more complex processes of association—"mental processes" as we called them—are accompanied by a moderate degree of Affect', and again 'mental activity is usually associated with a slight degree of Affect.' He writes: 'Whatever is conducive to consciousness of personhood—the Ego—evokes a pleasant state of mind; whatever is harmful to it, evokes an unpleasant state of mind.' This *might* be questioned, since unpleasant emotion—such as 'shame'—may involve intense consciousness of personhood. Nonetheless, the notion conveyed, especially in the first quotation, is that the very act of association is itself subjectively attractive, perhaps because 'things start to make sense'. This idea has a long history, from St Augustine's 'Eros of the Mind', through Alfred North Whitehead's [172] first stage of learning ('Romantic emotion is essentially the excitement consequent on the transition from the bare facts to the first realizations of the import of their unexplored relationships').

In terms of symptoms, Wernicke also writes the following on mania (L31, p. 216): '… everything seems just as easy for a person who is manic as it is hard for one who is melancholic'. An assumption here is that free association is rewarding (reinforcing); but the implication is that overactive reward is a *consequence*, not the *cause* of flight of ideas, a point of relevance to today's dopamine hypothesis of schizophrenia (or 'of psychosis'). I also have used the idea, in that to construct an explanation is itself a reinforcement ([103]; p. 86). If, in addition, reinforcement itself can encourage some type of association, a positive feedback loop is closed, so that mania would then progressively accelerate. In L31 (p. 216) Wernicke also writes '… such manifestations of grandiosity usually remain within limits not far removed from what is possible, or which are manifest only conditionally, as opinions and expectations, or which are expressed ironically, as though the patient were joking, and indulging in "make-believe"'. That is, the full veracity of belief is not recruited, suggesting its origin is *not* overactive reinforcement. Pierre Janet, about the same time, thought that much psychotic thought was akin to 'play acting' ([16]; p. 218). On the other hand, some delusions appear to be backed by the full force of belief. There is an important issue here, with implications for diagnosis as well as treatment. Possibly the first mechanism is a general lowering of neuronal activation threshold, so increasing the ease with which threshold is reached, this being a dynamic shift, spread across the whole of the cortex, but without new learning. That for the second style of delusion formation may be dopaminergic excess, acting in the basal ganglia to shape beliefs in a more fundamental way.

In L30 (p. 208) Wernicke takes failure of imagery, or of imagination, as equivalent to a wider failure of association, possibly a subjective manifestation of the very process of sejunction. However, imagery and association are not identical. Modern literature, based on 'semantic priming' methods fail to find any abnormality in the process of association in major depressive disorder [173–175]. A non-tachistoscopic method ('spreading activation') suggests that students scoring high on a depression scale have *freer* access to a wider range of associated words than controls [176]. However, with regard to reduced imagery in depressed patients, Wernicke is supported by two modern studies [177, 178]. Curiously, in modern literature, it is in schizophrenia as diagnosed, where increased association is found, at least with the semantic priming method, along with reduced cognitive inhibition documented in various ways [103] both of which would lead to excesses of association. In euthymic bipolar disorder, there are few studies, but one shows no abnormality in the semantic priming task [179] and another shows *reduced* priming [180], while yet another [181] investigating cognitive inhibition produced evidence of reduction which was rather equivocal. In mania itself there are no such studies, presumably because of the practical difficulties of the experiment.

Defined mental disorders: In L34 (p. 256) Wernicke comments on the prevalence of motility psychosis as a function of age and gender: The comparison with Kraepelin's *Dementia praecox* has to be made, and clearly, the young age of onset is a point of similarity; but from what we now know about schizophrenia—the concept derived from *Dementia praecox*—it tends to occur more commonly in young *males* than females of similar age, in contrast to Wernicke's statement.

Modern research has rarely compared heritability of melancholia or depressive disorders between adolescent and adult illness, but when it has [182, 183] results confirm Wernicke's statement (L30, p. 213) that the childhood variety is more strongly heritable. Modern evidence also supports Wernicke's view that bipolar disorder has a stronger genetic basis than unipolar depression (L31, p. 219); and that obsessive disorders, or at least some of their forms of it, are also strongly inherited, (L29, p. 201; L38, p. 297) in common with Tourette's syndrome [184]. Wernicke also makes a more general comment (L38, p. 294): 'I want to make just one point here, that I still do not find sufficiently emphasized: that a strong hereditary predisposition may be present without its ever leading to acute or a chronic psychosis'. This fact is firmly supported today: Risk of psychotic disorders in those with familial loading for psychosis, although elevated compared to the general population, is still quite small. Following through from this, eugenic measures such as were soon to be deployed were unlikely to reduce the prevalence of such weakly heritable disorders.

In L38 (p. 296) Wernicke refers to psychoses in users of cocaine and morphine. In modern literature, paranoid psychosis induced by cocaine is well-known, but almost completely unknown for morphine; and there is no evidence of any enhancement of the psychotogenic effect when morphine is added to cocaine. Clearly, what he saw was cocaine-induced paranoid psychosis.

XIV. Historical Context

XIV,(a). Identified Researchers or Clinicians

These profiles include most of the researchers cited by Wernicke, but for some (usually doctoral theses) details were unobtainable. To this list can be added profiles of some of Wernicke's own students (included in section IV: Wernicke's Personal Style etc).

Alois Alzheimer (1864–1915), a Bavarian psychiatrist and neuropathologist, and colleague of Emil Kraepelin. In 1906, a patient he had been studying died and her brain was subjected to analysis using the Nissl's silver staining method. This was the first documented case of what became known as Alzheimer's disease. Alzheimer was appointed professor at the University of Breslau in 1912, but died 3 years later, probably as a result of rheumatic heart disease (L41, p. 328).

Oskar Berger (1844–1885), studied at Breslau, Berlin, and Vienna, a student of Griesinger, a neuropathologist, and an expert on electrotherapy (L29, p. 200).

Jules Gabriel François Baillarger (1809–1890), a French neurologist and psychiatrist, student of Esquirol, the first to describe the layered structure of the cerebral cortex, and as a psychiatrist, continued Esquirol's analysis of hallucinations (L31, p. 220).

Otto Ludwig Binswanger (1852–1929), a Swiss psychiatrist and neurologist. After studies at Heidelberg, Strasburg, and Zurich, he worked at a psychiatric clinic in Göttingen, and in 1880 worked under Karl Westphal in at Charité Hospital Berlin (at which time Wernicke was also working in Berlin). From 1882 to 1919 he held a chair in psychology at the University of Jena. His publications include studies of epilepsy (on which he wrote a textbook), neurasthenia and hysteria, and included research on neuropathology (L37, p. 291).

Paul Broca (1824–1880), a French physician, surgeon, and anatomist, the first, in 1861, to describe a relationship of a specific psychic function and a specific cortical region ('Broca's area' in the left frontal lobe). As a neuroanatomist he contributed to defining what is now known as the 'limbic lobe' (L37, p. 291).

Jean Martin Charcot (1825–1893), a French pioneering neurologist and neuropathologist, student of Duchenne, and founder of the neurology clinic at *Hôpital de la Salpêtrière*, in Paris. Apart from defining many neurological syndromes, he was one of the first academic physicians to take seriously the phenomenon of hypnotism, leading to the incorporation of dynamic psychiatry into mainstream medicine (L7, p. 40; L22, p. 142; L35, pp. 264, 265).

Julius F Cohnheim (1838–1884), a pathologist, first to show that accumulation of pus was due to migration of white blood cells. He worked at Breslau from 1872 to 1878, later at Leipzig, and would have been known to Wernicke (L7, p. 41; L36, p. 273).

August Cramer (1860–1912), published, in 1889, the first description of proprioceptive and kinesthetic hallucinations (L11, p. 69; L13, p. 83; L28, p. 201; L34, p. 251; L41, p. 326).

Duchenne de Boulogne—often referred to as 'Duchenne'—Guillaume-Benjamin Amand Duchenne (de Boulogne) (1806–1875), a pioneer and, arguably, the founder of neurology in post-revolutionary France (L5, p. 28; L6, p. 33).

Hermann Emminghaus (1845–1904), a German psychiatrist, studied at Göttingen and Jena, and worked later at Würzburg, before taking up in 1886 the chair in psychiatry at the University of Dorpat (then 'East Prussia'; now Tartu, in Estonia), in which position he was to be succeeded by Emil Kraepelin. He is best known for his writings on psychopathology (L1, p. 4; L28, p. 185; L40, p. 314; L41, p. 326).

Jean-Étienne Esquirol (1772–1840), a pioneer of psychiatry in France, a pupil of and successor to Philippe Pinel, at *Hôpital de la Salpêtrière*, in Paris (L19, p. 117).

Sigismund Exner (1846–1926), an Austrian physiologist, best known for work on comparative psychology, and on perceptual psychology (especially of colour), and structure of the visual cortex (L37, p. 289).

Jean Pierre Falret (1794–1870), a French psychiatrist, a disciple of Pinel and Esquirol, is best known for the concept of *folie circulaire*. A strict philosophical dualist, he believed that mental illness rose from an abnormal interaction between body and soul. He was also the first to suggest a principle adopted by Kraepelin, that the course of an illness was useful in delineating psychiatric entities: 'for… the idea of a natural course of illness that can be foreseen presupposes the existence of a natural kind of disease' [185] (L31, p. 220).

Gustav Fechner (1801–1887), a philosopher, physicist, pioneer of experimental psychology, and with a great influence, which spread far beyond psychology. Educated in what is now western Poland, he studied medicine in Dresden and Leipzig (where he spent most of his life). At an early stage in his career he held a professorship in physics, but resigned this after he developed an eye disorder. His scientific contributions are many and varied, but he is perhaps best known for formulating what is now called the 'Weber-Fechner law', based on 'just noticeable differences' which allows subjective sensation to be studied quantitatively. In philosophical terms he espoused a rigorous version of psychophysical parallelism (L8, p. 46).

Auguste Forel (1848–1931), a Swiss neuroanatomist and psychiatrist, acknowledged by Cajal as one of the contributors to the neurone theory. As professor of psychiatry, he ran the Burghölzli asylum (established in 1870) for 20 years. His writings include works on sexology, and on the biology of ants. Attention has also recently been drawn to the fact that eugenic ideas pervaded much of his work [50], but he had abandoned such ideas, and, in 1920, became a member of the Bahá'í Faith (which originated in mid-nineteenth century in Persia) (L28, p. 190 *seq.*).

Carl Samuel Freund (1862–1932), a German psychiatrist and neurologist, born in Breslau, and studied medicine there and in Zürich, and later with Westphal in Berlin and Charcot in Paris. Later, In Breslau, he became chair of the *Psychiatrische-neurologische Vereinigung.* Married the sister of Fitz Haber, Nobel laureate in Chemistry (L7, p. 40).

Gustav Fritsch (1838–1927), a neuroanatomist and physiologist, who studied natural science and medicine at Berlin, Breslau, and Heidelberg. With Edouard Hitzig (see below) he is best known for pioneering use of electrical stimulation of the exposed cortex of unanaesthetized dogs, which helped establish the principle of cerebral localization of function. The publication on this in 1870 also included ablation of the same cortical regions, as mentioned in L40 (p. 320).

Sigbert Josef Maria Ganser (1853–1931), a German psychiatrist, and a neuroanatomist who assisted Bernhard von Gudden in Munich. He is best known for work on a hysterical disorder (Ganser syndrome, now seen as a dissociative disorder, originally described in prisoners—sometimes called 'prison psychosis') (L39, p. 301).

Friedrick Goltz (1834–1902). In the experiment referred to in L34, reported in 1869, Goltz took two frogs, decapitated one and blinded the other to prevent any voluntary motions that might arise from visual sense. He placed both animals in a vessel of water and gradually raised the temperature. Both frogs kept quiet until the temperature rose to 25 °C; at this point the frog whose brain was uninjured showed signs of discomfort; and as heat increased, tried to escape, and died at 42 ° C. During this entire time the other frog sat perfectly still, and gave *no* evidences of distress or pain, and did not die until temperature reached 50 °C. The experiment was purported to prove that the brain itself was needed for conscious sensation, a conclusion which, needless to say, aroused much subsequent debate (L34, p. 250).

William Richard Gowers (1845–1915), a British neurologist, the most outstanding of his time. He is the only British physician mentioned in *Grundriss*, for his method of measuring blood haemoglobin (L27, p. 181).

Wilhelm Griesinger (1817–1868), born in Stuttgart, studied medicine at Zürich. Later he was professor of medicine in Tübingen, helped in planning the Burghölzli Mental Asylum in Zürich. He was a reformer for asylums of the day, believed in integration of former patients back into society, supported the 'Somatiker' viewpoint and opposed the 'Psychiker' school of thought (L1, p. 4; L8, p. 83; L17, pp. 103, 105 *seq.*; L18, p. 113; L28, p. 185; L30, p. 204; L38, p. 294; L41, p. 326).

Friederich Wilhelm Hagen (1814–1888), a German pioneer of psychopathology, who, amongst other achievements, developed the concept of 'delusional mood'. On hallucinations, in 1897s, Edmund Parish [186] wrote of Hagen's ideas, as follows: 'If an energetic ideational stimulus could arouse a corresponding activity in the sensory centres, hallucinations, and especially voluntary hallucinations, would be much more frequent phenomena of sane life than they are. In order to escape these difficulties, Hagen refers to 'subcortical sensory centres' as the seat of hallucination [187, 188]. Tamburini [189] writes: 'according to Hagen all peripheral stimuli arriving at the sensory centres are immediately diverted to two destinations: the ideational centres (where they will generate images in consciousness) and back to the periphery (by the principle of external projection). Stimuli generated in the brain sites themselves would suffer the same fate, thereby giving rise to apparent perceptions' (L19, p. 123).

Ewald Hecker (1843–1909), a German psychiatrist, a student and collaborator of Kahlbaum. Together they challenged the idea of a 'unitary psychosis', and constructed their own system for classifying mental disorders (L38, p. 303; L41, p. 320).

Hermann Ludwig Ferdinand von Helmholtz (1821–1894): Born at Potsdam, near Berlin, he initially trained in physiology (and might have become a medical student). Later he held various academic posts—at Königsberg, Bonn, Heidelberg, and then professor of physiology at the University of Berlin. His scientific contributions included both physical sciences (mechanics, conservation of energy, acoustics, electromagnetism) and physiology and neuroscience (sensory physiology, nerve conduction, ophthalmic optics) (L1, p. 6).

Heinrich Ewald Hering (1866–1948), best known for defining respiratory reflexes controlling inspiration and expiration (L35, note).

Johann Otto Leonhard Heubner (1843–1926), a pioneer of paediatrics (and director of the children's clinic at the Charité Hospital in Berlin). He was also an expert on infectious disease, and one of the first to use the newly prepared diphtheria antitoxin in his practise. Co-author of Handbook of Acute Infections (1874). Referred to, in context of 'luetic infections' in L37 (p. 262).

Hirth, CGLO. Biographical details not located. A paper of his is cited (L20, p. 126) on older concept of 'epigenesis' (see section 'Terminology').

Edouard Hitzig (1839–1907), a neurologist and psychiatrist, studied medicine at Würzburg and Berlin. He is well known for experiments at

Berlin with Gustav Fritsch (above) and later became director of the Burghölzli asylum in Zürich, and later became professor at Halle until he retired in 1903 (L40, p. 320).

Adolf Jarisch (1850–1902), an Austrian dermatologist, and a specialist in syphilis, cited in L3 (p. 16) as an early researcher into modifiability of spinal reflexes as a result of repetitive stimulation.

Friedrich Jolly (1844–1904), a neurologist and psychiatrist from Heidelberg. His work includes studies of hypochondria, and pioneering electrophysiology on myasthenia gravis. He is cited in *Grundriss* as approving the naming of 'Korsakoff's psychosis' (L38, p. 296).

Karl Ludwig Kahlbaum (1828–1899), obtained training at Berlin University, and worked first at an asylum near Königsburg, then as a lecturer in that city, before buying a private asylum, of which he became director, at Görlitz, a German city close to borders with present-day Poland and Czech Republic. He never had an academic position, but was a noted pioneer in psychiatry, challenging the idea of 'unitary psychosis', introducing a focus on the long-term course of illness into psychiatry, with suggestions that different forms of mental disorder occurred at different transitional periods of life. With Ewald Hecker he defined motor ('catatonic') symptoms [190] (L1, 4; L13, p. 83; L19, pp. 118, 119, 122, 124; L22, p. 141; L24, pp. 162, 163; L28, p. 194; L31, p. 220; L34, pp. 253, 254; L37, p. 280; L39, p. 303; L40, p. 320).

Jacobus Ludovicus Conradus Schroeder van der Kolk (1707–1862): a Dutch psychiatric reformer, and a defender of vitalism against encroaching materialism in Germanic and French thought (L19; pp. 123, 24).

Sergei Sergeevich Korsakoff (1854–1900), a pioneering Russian neuropsychiatrist, student of Meynert, later based at the Preobrazhenski mental hospital in Moscow, and founder of journal which still bears his name. His work encompassed psychiatry, neuropathology, forensic medicine, and alcoholism. He is best known for the syndrome of memory loss seen in chronic alcoholism (L38, p. 296).

Emil Kraepelin (1856–1926) studied medicine at Leipzig (and neuropathology under Paul Flechsig, and experimental psychology under Wilhelm Wundt), and also at Würzburg. In 1883 he published the first edition of his textbook on psychiatry. In 1886, he was appointed to the chair of psychiatry at the University of Dorpat (Tartu, present-day Estonia), and was later head of psychiatry in Heidelberg, and then Munich. His concept of *Dementia praecox* was first formulated in the 1896 edition of his textbook, on the basis of his clinical studies; and this and related concepts formed the basis for a system of classification which is still the mainstay of the profession in many countries. After the First World War, he founded a German Institute for Psychiatric Research. Later he advocated social Darwinist policies and eugenics (L14, p. 87; L30, p. 234 L34, p. 256; L39, p. 304).

Richard Krafft-Ebing (1840–1902) was an Austro-German psychiatrist, best known for his work on sexual pathology, and his work on this entitled *Psychopathia Sexualis* (L32, p. 234; L41, p. 275).

Jean Baptiste Octave Landry de Thézillat (1826–1865), a French physician and researcher, who, in 1859, discovered the paralytic disorder now known as Guillain–Barré syndrome (L27, p. 182).

Henri Le Grand du Saulle (1830–1886). His book, from 1875, entitled *La folie du doute (avec délire du toucher)* (Madness of doubt, with fear of contact by external objects) is cited by Wernicke (L29, p. 200).

Heinrich Lissauer (1861–1891), a neurologist and neuropathologist at the psychiatric institute in Breslau. Despite his early death, his name is associated with several important advances, being the first to describe visual agnosia, as well as studies on pathology of Progressive paralysis, and a tract in the spinal cord being named after him. Cleary Wernicke thought very highly of him (L20, p. 128; L37, pp. 284–286, 289–291; L41, p. 326).

Jules Bernard Luys (1828–1887), a French neuroanatomist, and a neuropsychiatrist, who led the way in defining connections of the basal ganglia, the first to describe the subthalamic nucleus (sometimes still called '*corpus Luysii*'), and the first to produce a photographic brain atlas. From the late 1880s, he was fascinated by hypnotism and hysteria, using extravagant experiments, and sometimes public demonstrations. His enthusiasm made him the most widely caricatured of those exploring such topics [191] (L19; p. 123).

Valentin Magnan (1835–1916) studied medicine in Lyon and Paris, and became an influential psychiatrist. He focused on the concept of 'degeneration' and also on the adverse effects of alcohol and street drugs. His system of classification, which was influential in France, but was superseded by Kraepelin's system, held that mental disorders were of just two types, which were quite separate, one based on hereditary degeneracy, the other defined by presence of delusions. 'Magnan's sign' refers to parasthesias, which can arise in cocaine addict (L17, note; L38, p. 297).

Adolf Meyer (1866–1950), with a medical degree from the University of Zürich, studied subsequently with Auguste Forel and Constantin von Monakow. In 1892, he found that he could not secure a university position, emigrated to the USA to become the first chief psychiatrist at Johns Hopkins Hospital. Subsequently he was to challenge the idea that mental disorders were natural types of disease, replacing the concept with that of 'reaction types'. The paper cited on p. 291 (L37) was published 2 years before he emigrated.

Ludwig Meyer (1827–1900), obtained a medical degree from the University of Berlin, and from 1866 to his death was professor of psychiatry at the University of Göttingen. He studied inflammatory changes in the brain in Progressive paralysis, and, in 1867, with Wilhelm Griesinger, founded *Archiv für Psychiatrie und Nervenkrankheiten* (L31, p. 221).

Theodor Hermann Meynert (1833–1892), polymath and pioneer in neuroanatomy and neuropsychiatry, amongst whose students are included Carl Wernicke, Sigmund Freud, Auguste Forel, Sergei Korsakoff, and Julius Wagner Jauregg. He gave the first detailed description of the laminar architecture of the cerebral cortex, and various brain structures are named after him (notable the *nucleus basalis of Meynert*). He was also a well-published poet. In L36 (p. 336), reference is made to 'Meynert's celebrated optic thalamus case'. It is not clear what this case was. However, Meynert and his doctoral student at the time, Auguste Forel, are credited with defining in 1872 the anatomy of the optic thalamus (L1, p. 4; L2, p. 11; L4, pp. 22, 23; L5, pp. 26, 27, 29, 30; L6, p. 34; L17, p. 106; L19, pp. 123–124; L21, p. 135; L26, p.172; L30, pp. 210, 211, 213; L33, pp. 236, 237, 240; L34, pp. 243–252, 253; L36, pp. 275, 277; L37, pp. 284, 285, 288, 290, 292; L40, pp. 314, 315, 318, 319, L41, p. 326).

Constantin Von Monakow (1853–1930), a Russian neuropathologist from the region north of Moscow, spent much of his life in Switzerland, as a student in, and then at the Burghölzli Mental Asylum under Edouard Hitzig, subsequently becoming leader of the Brain Anatomy Institute in Zürich. He made many contributions to neuroanatomy, and in conceptual terms recognized that the different localized mental faculties needed to be integrated, as were thalamus and cerebral cortex. In 1925, with Georg Koskinas, he published the most detailed cytoarchitectonic map of the human cerebral cortex (L37, p. 290).

Johannes Peter Müller (1801–1858), a German physiologist from Koblenz. In neuroscience he is noted for formulating the 'law of specific energies', from which Wundt could later derive the 'law of isolated conduction' (L1, p. 4; L19, p. 124).

Hermann Munk (1839–1912), a Professor of Physiology at the University of Berlin, from 1876 (L5, p. 26; L6, p. 36).

Clemens Neisser (1861–1942), a German psychiatrist, working in north Germany (today, Poland). His 'morbid self-reference' ([112]. Neisser, 1891) is mentioned as origin to delusions of reference (L13, p. 82; L37 p. 208; L38, pp. 285, 298).

Heinrich Wilhelm Neumann (1814–1884), of Breslau, one of the last German 'Psychiker' psychiatrists, and therefore potentially an opponent of Griesinger. He was director of the Breslau Psychiatric Institute, with Wernicke as an assistant, until his death, when Wernicke took over. In a footnote (L20, p. 130) Wernicke acknowledges him to be discoverer of the symptom of hypermetamorphosis. Despite his having an opposed philosophy for mental disorder, Wernicke does not hesitate to cite, and commend his work. (L1, p. 4; L19, p. 124; L20, p. 130; L22, p. 141).

Franz Nissl (1860–1919), a neurohistologist and pathologist, studied medicine at the University of Munich, with Bernard Gudden as one of his professors. He is best remembered for the 'Nissl' stain for cytoplasmic granules within neuronal cell bodies. Later he became a collaborator with Alois Alzheimer, and joined Kraepelin first at Heidelberg, and later, as full-time professor, in Munich (L37, p. 290; L41, p. 326).

Edouard Friedrich Wilhelm Pflüger (1829–1910), born at Hanau (near Frankfurt am Main), studied medicine at Marburg and Berlin, later to become professor of physiology at the University of Bonn. He contributed research in diverse areas of physiology, and, in 1868, founded the journal *Archiv für die gesammte Physiologie des Menschen und der Thiere* (now: Pflügers Archiv: European Journal of Physiology) (L5, p. 27).

Arnold Pick (1851–1924), a Czech neurologist and psychiatrist, trained under Karl Westphal in Berlin, and later headed the Prague institute for neuropathology. He was one of those to use the term *Dementia praecox* before Kraepelin adopted the term (L19, p. 126).

Wilhelm Sander (1838–1922), a German psychiatrist and neurologist (L17; p. 107).

Schütz H, Little details could be found about this pathologist, but, his 1891 paper cited in L37 came from the laboratory of Paul Flechsig in Leipzig. He held the position of 'Privatdozent' and 'erster Assistent der Klinik'.

Ludwig Snell (1817–1892), a psychiatrist and asylum director, who refuted the concept of 'unitary psychosis', and is cited in *Grundriss* for the concept of monomania (L17, pp. 105, 106), and (L17, note), for the view that grandiosity is not a primary symptom.

Herbert Spencer (1820–1903), a wide-ranging philosopher, and a social commentator, who was writing about social evolution some years before the publication of Darwin's *Origin of Species,* and it was he, not Darwin, who coined the phrase 'survival of the fittest'. His work 'Principles of Psychology' was published in 1855 (L7, p. 39).

Josef Starlinger (1862–1943), an Austrian physician and psychiatrist, studied medicine in Vienna, worked under Meynert and then under Julius Wagner-Jauregg. Little details could be found about him, but he was clearly abreast of developments in neurohistology, in using the osmium-based method of Vittorio Marchi for staining degenerating myelinated fibres, with potassium bi-chromate added to prevent normal myelinated fibres being stained. (L41, p. 326).

Franz Tuczek (1852–1925) studied medicine in Berlin with Westphal and in Munich with von Gudden, and then ran a psychiatric facility in Marburg. His research work was mainly in neuropathology, in relation to various conditions (ergot poisoning, progressive paralysis pellagra, alcoholism) (L37, pp. 289–291).

Rodolf Virchow (1821–1902), a pioneer in the discipline of pathology at a time when the doctrine of the humours still had influence. He studied under Johannes Peter Müller in Berlin, and later worked at the Charité Hospital there. Later he became the foundation professor of Pathological Anatomy at Würzburg, and later returned to a chair in Berlin University. Apart from his prodigious scientific work he was politically very active, including support for the revolution of 1848, a strong advocate for public health measures, and a strong opponent of Darwin's theory of evolution (and of his own student Ernst Haeckel). He declined the ennobling title 'von Virchow' (L37, p. 289).

Carl von Voit (1831–1908), a German physiologist and dietician regarded by many as the 'father of dietetics' (L34, p. 258).

James Ward (1843–1925), a British philosopher and psychologist. From Kingston upon Hull, he originally trained as a congregational minister, but won a scholarship to Germany, where he worked under Hermann Lotze (section 'Wernicke's Underlying Philosophical Views', *Wernicke's Adoption of the European Style of Natural Philosophy.*) On return to Britain he entered Cambridge University, with a scholarship to Trinity College, and published a paper entitled 'An interpretation of Fechner's Law'. His two papers on physiology in 1879 and 1880 were in German language journals, and one is cited in *Grundriss* (L3, p. 16). It is the only work by a British scientist he cites.

Karl Weigert (1845–1904), a pathologist and neurohistologist, who developed important methods for selective staining for myelin, and for glial cells. He had worked at Breslau, and held a chair in pathological anatomy at Frankfurt am Main at the time of the first edition of *Grundriss*) (L16, L41, etc.) (L37, p. 289; L41, p. 328).

Carl Friedrich Otto Westphal (1833–1890), a neurologist and psychiatrist from Berlin, under whom Wernicke worked in the late 1870s. He coined the term 'agoraphobia', and also showed the relationship between *Tabes dorsalis,* and Progressive paralysis. In L37 (p. 283) he is cited as supporting Wernicke's view—that paralysis almost always allows one to detect early signs of dementia (L29, p. 200; L36, p. 283).

H. Zacher. Few details could be found about this pathologist, cited in L37 (pp. 291, 292). Clearly he studied neuropathology of progressive paralysis and also published on syringomyelia (Fuestner and Zacher, 1883. *Arch f Psychiatrie* band. XIV).

Theodor Ziehen (1862–1950), studied medicine at Würzburg and Berlin, after which he worked under Kahlbaum at Görlitz, and then as assistant to Binswanger at Jena (where one of his patients was Friedrich Nietzsche). After a brief period at Halle he became an expert on mental disorders of childhood, and from 1917 was a professor of philosophy, again at Halle. He retired in 1930 (L3, p. 18; L4, p. 23; L33, p. 236; L36, p. 276).

XIV,(b). Other Medical or Scientific Topics

L27 (p. 182): 'Gastroenterostomosis': This operation for cancer in the lower part of the stomach, or pylorus, was very advanced for its day, and involved reconnecting the rest of the stomach to the jejunum. It was first accomplished by Theodor Bilroth (1829–1894) in 1881, at which time he held a professorship in Vienna. Bilroth was a pioneer of surgery and a gifted amateur musician and friend of Johannes Brahms.

L27 (p. 181): Blood haemoglobin measurement is mentioned '... haemoglobin content (Gowers) of only 55 %'. The crystalline form of the red pigment in erythrocytes had been seen as early as 1848, and Hoppe-Seyler identified the constituent, now called haemoglobin in 1868. He devised a method of measuring haemoglobin content, subsequently improved in various ways. The method of W.R. Gowers (1845–1915), who was primarily a neurologist, is referred to by Wernicke [192].

L28 (p. 186): The description of railway journeys of the time ('... the journey home in a railway compartment was particularly terrible; she felt that she had to leap out of the compartment') seems to be a case of what had recently been called 'claustrophobia', first documented in the 1870s in France, when dense urban dwelling was common.

L35 (p. 267): We read of '... "reactive mutism"; and the fact that it emerges when confronting a physician, is immediately understood, if I remind you of the distinction favoured by a temperamental colleague, between a "super-" and a "sub-consciousness"': This is unlikely to have been Sigmund Freud, but may have been Albert Schäffle, a Schwäbian sociologist, political theorist and journalist with roots in German idealist thought. His four-volume work *Bau und Leben des sozialen Körpers,* appeared in its second edition in 1896 [193].

L36 (p. 277): The idea that sexual abstinence was a cause of psychopathology was made popular by Freud, but had older roots. Freud for instance cited Schoppenhauer in this context, and the idea can even be traced back to Galen, who had suggested that hysteria in women was the result of sexual abstinence.

XV. Allusions Requiring Clarification

These allusions are usually made by Wernicke's patients, but are occasionally ones by Wernicke himself:

L9 (p. 57): 'Gottfried von Bouillon': A medieval Frankish knight, leader of the first crusade from the year 1096, and in the successful siege of Jerusalem in 1099. By the nineteenth century, he was a somewhat mythical figure, but several accounts of the crusades in the second half of that century would have made him a plausible theme for delusions.

L10 (p. 59) 'Dalldorf': presumably refers to one of the asylums in Berlin.

L10 (p. 60) 'Duchess of Arco': probably refers to 'Duchess of *Arcos,* member of a long-established line in the Spanish nobility. 'Kaiser Friedrich': who, in 1888, succeeded Kaiser William (King of Prussia, and German Emperor), but who died from throat cancer after only 99 days.

L10 (p. 60) '... the patient, having now survived the examination period, to play the role of a priest or prophetess': The imagery is reminiscent of the plot in Mozart's *Zauberflöte.*

L10 (p. 61) '... at the time that she felt that a prehistoric man, or a bloodthirsty man, or a lancelet ... had entered her body': This and the following description draws heavily on writings of Ernst Haeckel (1834–1919) a biologist and popular science writer, who introduced a version of Darwinism to German readers. 'Primitive man' (*Urmensch*) and *lancelet* (a species important in early arguments about evolution, also called *amphioxus*), figured prominently in his writings. From the late 1860s Haekel promoted the idea that 'ontogeny recapitulates phylogeny', illustrated with drawings of dubious scientific authenticity. By the time of Wernicke's *Grundriss* these ideas were well-enough known to be distorted in imagery in psychotic illness, and here, appear to make use of the illustrations in Haeckel's books. Later: 'She mentions the book *Häckel Urmensch oder Lanzettfisch*, but believes that *Häckel* means something like binding, or belonging together' (derivation obscure). Sometimes Wernicke himself hints at Haeckel's concepts, but it is unclear whether he refers to phylogeny or ontogeny, as in L8 (p. 49), where he writes: 'we see a protective or defensive device that the brain may have acquired during its development'. In L37 (p. 280) he writes '... we again need to hold onto our view that the progressive paralysis represents no more than an aetiological recapitulation of psychoses, which otherwise differ widely from each other': The phraseology here again hints at Haeckel's maxim.

L10 (p. 61) 'Since that time she had doubled everything—double nerves, double heart beat, even a double brain.': Concepts of a 'double brain' circulated widely in popular versions of neuroscience in the late nineteenth century [194], and in this case may have drawn on recent findings—including Wernicke's own—about cerebral asymmetry and language.

L10 (p. 61) 'According to her, a person has 27 senses': The reference is curious. The phrase '27 senses' is associated, especially in Norway, with the name Kurt Schwitters, a German artist, one of the Dadaist movement, and refugee during WWII. Born in 1887, he can hardly have been the inspiration for this patient's imagery, but there may have been an earlier source for their use of the phrase.

L11 (p. 68) 'Duke of Sagan': Old title, in French aristocracy, linked to the name Talleyrand, French diplomat from the Napoleonic area.

L11 (p. 70) Patients' explanation of auditory hallucinations in terms of telephone transmission: The telephone, and (just as important) the telephone exchange, predated Wernicke's 1894 edition of *Grundriss* by 15–20 years. 'Telephone' also referred to in L25 (p. 166).

L12 (p. 74): '... movement makes an increasing contribution to the entire personality, as levels of schooling increase': This comment may reflect the special emphasis in German schools on physical education, strongly present in most of the nineteenth century. Increased bodily awareness to which it led may have been one of the influences which led first Meynert, and then Wernicke to emphasize continuity of body awareness as the first source of personhood (the 'Ego').

L13 (p. 82) Raskolnikov: Principle character in Fyodor Dostoievsky's '*Crime and Punishment'*, first published in 1866 (also p. 193).

L14 (p. 87) '... their perceptions show every nuance of referential delusions, which an outstanding psychiatrist has described succinctly with the words "*tua res agitur*"': 'It is a matter that concerns you', a quotation deriving from Horace Book I, epistle 18, line 84: '… you too are in danger when you neighbour's house is on fire'.

L14 (p. 88) 'Götz': A contraction of 'Gottfried'. The person referred to (Götz von Berlichingen, 'of the Iron Hand') was a stormy nobleman from what is now southern Germany, involved in many battles and feuds in the sixteenth century. This left him with an iron prosthesis, after losing an arm. A play based on his life by Goethe had appeared in 1799. The offending defiant phrase and gesture, which Wernicke is too polite to specify, is found in Wikipedia: 'He can lick my arse', with the universal accompanying gesture of a bared backside.

L15 (pp. note) Animosity between Wernicke and Hitzig: 'These prejudices are related to what I claim to be the often misunderstood partiality of the disease in such cases. In what sense I conceive this partiality will become more readily apparent from the presentation given here, so that I shall probably refrain from a detailed refutation of the attack directed against me by Hitzig (1895)'.

L17 (p. 106) 'animal delirium': a literal translation, 'delirium of being an animal' (a.k.a. lycanthropy).

L18 (p. 113) 'Wotan', 'Ahlbrecht the Bear': There is a mixture of images here. 'Wotan' is from ancient Norse/Germanic mythology, incorporated by Richard Wagner into *Die Walküre*, the second part of his four-part cycle *Der Ring des Nibelung,* first performed in 1870. 'Ahlbrecht the Bear', otherwise known as Albert I (c 1100–1170) was the first Margrave of Brandenburg, from which 'The Bear' became a symbol for the city of Berlin. However, the allusion here may again be to Wagner's *Ring cycle*, since the first part of the cycle (*Das Rheingold*) includes a character with the name Alberich. As Wernicke notes, the patient appeared to believe in 'transmigration of souls', a common belief in the Germanic world in the nineteenth century, partly resulting from recent scholarship on eastern religions. Wagner's operas, not least his *Ring cycle* make continual reference to this belief [195].

L18 (p. 114) 'Head warder': Presumably this was a warder at the hospital, not a character from post-revolutionary France.

L18 (p. 114) Reference to a 'wishing table': This is based on a fairy tale of Brothers Grimm: 'The Wishing-Table, the Gold-Ass, and the Cudgel in the Sack'. For English text see Taylor [196]. The key section reads—'… a little table … made of common wood … had one good property; if anyone set it out, and said, "Little table, spread thyself," the good little table was at once covered with a clean little cloth, and a plate was there, and a knife and fork beside it, and dishes with boiled meats and roasted meats, as many as there was room for, and a great glass of red wine shone so that it made the heart glad. The young journeyman thought, "With this thou hast enough for thy whole life:"'.

L18 (p. 115) 'He was both a Christian and a Jew, and had a previous existence; and he refuted my doubt by pointing to the third article of Faith, that relates to the resurrection from the dead': This statement presumably relates to one of the Christian creeds, used in church services, and often written as three paragraphs, in the third of which comes the statement about resurrection from the dead.

L19 (p. 121) '… the spirits which he also heard wanted to conduct various procedures on him on purpose, for the spectators, even the dream images that he described': The patient's imagery is reminiscent of a clinical demonstration.

L19 (p. 124) '… the vestiges of aural mobility, which humans still possess': Vestigial organs—those similar to functioning organs in other species, but themselves lacking any obvious function—have been recognized since antiquity. They became objects of scientific study in the later part of the eighteenth century, and after Darwin's *Origin of Species* were widely seen to indicate a species' ancestry. Wernicke is well aware of this, an idea which was also prominent in writings of Ernst Haeckel.

L21 (p. 135) 'Diaconate institution': An institution for training deacons, a position in Christian churches which can be traced back to the Gospels, whose role is care of and ministry to the poor.

L22 (p. 140) 'Pleasure garden': A concept going back to antiquity, but which flourished in most European cities from the eighteenth century. Pleasures gardens (or their modern equivalent, 'Theme parks' or 'Entertainment parks') could provide various forms of entertainment, but, in cities with overcrowded homes, were also always places for romantic encounters.

L22 (p. 146): 'He would receive 50 lashes, counted-out'. We have interpolated the word 'lashes' as we understand his context.

L25 (p. 166) 'Several times the criminal bell had rung, as if he were now going to his death': In some jurisdictions in Europe, in the not too-distant past, bells were rung at the time of an execution.

L25 (p. 167) 'Last prayer': Presumably refers to Catholic ritual, this being (present-day) Poland, now a Catholic country. In Wernicke's day Catholic faith, while not adhered to by the majority, was adhered to by a large minority (~35 % of the populace).

L25 (p. 169) 'Lawyer of the right, lawyer of the left' (*Rechtsanwalt, Linksanwalt*, etc.): This satirical song is based around word-play, and double meanings, in German, as in English of the words 'Rechts' and 'Links' ('right' and 'left'). *Rechtsanwalt* means an attorney, whose concerns is with legal rights; *Linksanwalt,* is a term used in jest, a deceiver, a shyster, one who twists the law.

L25 (p. 169) 'Into the well, and under the water with him; he should be pumped full and cut open; then into the puddle with him; put him to death': In medieval Europe, as in Scotland, drowning was a more common means of capital punishment than hanging, surviving there until the seventeenth, even the eighteenth century. Dismemberment after execution (including dissection in an anatomy school), was also possible as an extreme measure, for instance in cases of attempted regicide in eighteenth century France, supposedly to prevent 'resurrection of the body.'

L25 (p. 169) 'Sewn into a cow-hide': Two possible interpretations are offered Rudolph IV, a Hapsburg ruler died in Milan in 1365; his body was carried back to Vienna, sewn into a cowhide, to preserve the body. 'According to the directions of the medieval Passion plays from Donaueschingen and Freiburg, the young priest who played the role of Judas first had to be sewn into a cowhide. Underneath, onto his chest, were to be placed the intestines of a sheep together with a live blackbird, or even a live black squirrel, symbolizing the damned (i.e. black) soul. During the act of hanging, which was performed rather realistically, the cowhide had to burst from the priest's chest downwards in order to let out the blackbird or squirrel and to show the intestines' [197].

L25 (p. 169) 'Wenceslas is coming': King Wenceslas, a Bohemian monarch, who died in the tenth century (but who is remembered in a popular English Christmas Carol), was a potent symbolic figure in central Europe, commemorated in Wenceslas Square, in central Prague.

L26 (p. 172): '... He knows the key dates of the last war; knows about Bismarck, Moltke, and the three Kaisers, his participation in the election': The German empire had full adult male suffrage since the election in 1871. The reference here is probably to the election in 1887.

L26 (p. 172): 'Krupp's cannon': The Krupp family, long-established as industrialists in the Ruhr district of Germany, started manufacturing cannons from 1840, under Alfred Krupp. By the late 1880s this amounted to about 50 % of Krupp's total output.

L26 (p. 173) '... the walls closing together or threatening to collapse': Does this image refer to events in Edgar Allen Poe's story, 'The Pit and the Pendulum', published in 1843, based loosely on torture during the Spanish Inquisition? (Poe himself had a lurid life-style, in which personal experience of *Delirium tremens* may have inspired some of his writing).

L26 (p. 173) 'When alcohol abuse deserves to be punished, it is bestowed in abundance, which leads to delirium': Does this refer to the maritime legend (echoes of which are found in RL Stevenson's *Treasure Island*), of Blackbeard, a notorious English pirate, who abandoned 15 crew members on Dead Chest Island for a month, leaving each with no more than a bottle of rum, and a sword?

L27 (p. 183): 'Choleric', indicating a fiery temperament, excitable, extrovert, and egocentric (or, in terms of body fluid, influenced by 'yellow bile'). It is interesting to see a term derived from the doctrine of the four humours appearing in *Grundriss.*

L28 (p. 189): '… delusion of being President of France and of his being appointed to Warsaw by the Tsar first': Warsaw at this time was under Russian suzerainty.

L28 (p. 191): 'if you want to validate the popular expression 'drunkard', note simply that, through external circumstances, the opportunity to drink alcohol and seek out like-minded company, is repeated each quarter year for certain social classes': This may refer to the fact that, following a decree in July 1888, Kaiser Wilhelm had decreed a succession of public holidays throughout the year across the German empire [198].

L29 (p. 195): *Staatsexamen*: A university qualification, required for teaching. At this time, the bias in this state examination favoured the nobility, but varied between *länder* and according to the year; and, until some years later, it excluded females.

L29 (p. 196): 'special providence': Shakespeare uses the phrase ('there is special providence in the fall of a sparrow'; Hamlet, Act V, scene 2). It reflects Protestant rather than Catholic theology, in that divine intervention was achieved not so much by dramatic miracles as objective public events, but by subtle workings of natural laws. In any case, this reference reflects very well the details of Wernicke's approach as a clinician, exploring details of this patient's delusions, and how well he was attuned to the culture and popular imagery of his times.

L29 (p. 196): 'He could only regard his time here as probation imposed upon him': The imagery is perhaps of purgatory, although this concept is rejected in most Protestant traditions.

L29 (p. 196) '30,000 Marks': A huge sum of money. With Germany since 1876 using the Gold standard, 1 kg pure gold exchanged for, at most, a few thousand Marks.

L29 (p. 196): 'Niederwald monument': Located at Rüdesheim, in the Rhine Gorge, commemorated the founding of the German Empire, after the Franco-Prussian war, in September 1871.

L29 (p. 196): 'Julian tower': Probably referring to a Romanesque church tower, of ancient origin, at Sankt Julian, not far south of Rüdesheim.

L29 (p. 197): '… go into the Oder': Colloquial term for a suicide attempt by drowning, probably a common method in northern Europe at the time. Peter Tchaikovsky made such an attempt in 1877 in St. Petersburg.

L29 (p. 198): 'two witnesses': Mentioned in the New Testament Book of Revelation [Chapter 11]. The role of the two witnesses is to decry the reign of the Antichrist-Beast.

L29 (p. 198) '… handed over to anatomy': In many medical schools of the time, bodies for dissection were those remaining unclaimed, who died in asylums.

L29 (p. 200): 'Panel doctor': Presumably a physician charged with official duties authorized by government.

L29 (p. 201): 'Journeyman': Tradesman's qualification from an apprenticeship, not yet qualified as a 'master' able to employ others. Journeymen were often travelling tradesmen. This system of qualifications still exists in parts of Europe.

L30 (p. 204): 'How did you find *me*, Professor?' We felt this lady may have been a bit seductive, hence our added intalicization of 'me'.

L30 (p. 203): 'even were war to be declared'. This lecture was presumably prepared in the late 1890s, at which time across Europe there were already forebodings of a major war to come.

L32 (p. 225): 'enforced exaggeration in the expressive movements of a minuet': The minuet was really a dance (or rather an important social occasion) of the seventeenth and eighteenth century, which was transformed into the Waltz by the nineteenth century. However, the title 'Waltz-minuet' was well known in central Europe in the nineteenth century.

L32 (p. 226): 'Occupational deliria': Elaborate pantomimes, as if continuing a usual occupation in the hospital bed, possibly depicted as a caricature in Charlie Chaplin's portrayal of assembly line employment in his '*Modern Times*'.

L32 (p. 232): 'Dr. Sch': This refers to 'the patient' with a PhD, not a medical doctor. In any case this patient seems to attribute his disruptive motor symptoms easily to divine intervention.

L32 (p. 233): 'sight of … a slate … brings patients … to write on the slate.' presumably the 'slate' used in schools, in preference to paper, for handwriting.

L33 (p. 240): 'Chansonette': Roughly a 'cabaret singer'. 'Cabaret' emerged in France from around 1881, and did not appear in Germany until the turn of the century, to reach its definitive German form during the years of the Weimar republic.

L34 (p. 244) '… she crosses her legs in a totally inappropriate manner': Presumably a breach of lady-like etiquette.

L34 (p. 247): 'Prince Bismarck came and gave him a malicious look': This patient, encountered during Wernicke's Berlin period, was seen at a time when Bismarck was politically powerful. (He was removed from power in 1890 by Kaiser Wilhelm I).

L34 (p. 249): 'Sleeping uhlan': A military metaphor. The Polish word 'Uhlan' ('Ulan' in German) refers to Polish light cavalry, armed with lances. The metaphor is thus similar to that of a fierce animal 'lying doggo'.

L37 (p. 284): 'For a year and a day': This curious phrase (*über Jahr und Tag*), has its origin in customary legal settings, both in England and in Europe, for instance wherein a person who dies more than 'a year and a day' after some assault, can no longer be deemed to be a murder victim; or where a couple must be married 'for a year and a day' before a spouse can claim a share of inheritable property. In medieval Europe, a runaway serf became free after 'a year and a day'. On the continent of Europe, laws codified as legal statutes had greater significance than precedents in the English common law tradition, especially after the French revolution. Nonetheless, in Europe, legal statutes *were* influenced by customary law, and the use of this phrase by Wernicke derives from this fact. This is why his use of this phrase is interesting. Today, in English as in German—it means 'for an indefinite period into the future'.

L37 (p. 288): 'medullary strips of the gyri and the common underlying white matter' *Die Markleisten der Windungen und das gemeinschaftliche Marklager zeigen sich ebenfalls beträchtlich verschmärlert.* We infer that this refers to white matter between the walls of a gyrus, and that lying deep to the gyrus.

L38 (p. 294): 'The acquired predisposition to mental illness is based usually on adverse influences that are also expressed as organic changes in the brain. These include *Hydrocephalus internus* [W], even if this has reached the stage of recovery, as we often see; but we also see it even where no conspicuous alteration of the head has been left behind': Head-shape is referred to here: A bulbous skull, then being seen as a consequence of *Hydrocephalus*, presumably the only way this condition might be identified in vivo at the time.

L40 (p. 314): '… if you challenge an elderly physician, lawyer, or mathematician with a test of word form in ancient Greek': This presumably refers to the classical education in ancient Greek, which educated people are likely to have received at an early age in Wernicke's time.

L40 (p. 316): 'Karlchen Mießnick': Pseudonym for Friedrich Wilhelm Ernst Dohm (born, Breslau, 1819; died Berlin, 1883), a translator, actor and editor (of, *inter alia*, a satirical magazine *Kladderadatsch*).

L40 (p. 316) 'Berliner Wespen': 'Berlin Wasps', a satirical magazine, founded in 1868 by Julius Stettenheim (of Hamburg) known as 'Wippchen', which, amongst other campaigns, fought against growing anti-Semitism.

XVI. Terminology

'*Abusus spirituosorum*' (L25, p. 168): Alcohol abuse went under a variety of names, such as Marcel's *Folie des ivrognes*; Kraepelin's *akuter halluzinatorischer Alkoholwahnsinn*, etc.

'Abulia' (L35, p. 267): The 1906 German medical dictionary defines 'Abulie' as 'want of will-power'.

'Acousma': This term, used in L19 (p. 207), is scarcely known today, referring to simple acoustic experiences, illusory non-verbal auditory sensations.

'Activation' (e.g. 'Nervous activation of muscle' [L6, p. 32]): *Muskelinnervation*). We do not translate 'innervation' directly because, in English, it refers to structure not function.

'Aegophony' (egophony) (L37, p. 280): Changed vocal quality, with lower frequencies filtered out, resulting in high-pitched bleating or nasal timbre.

'Affect': see section VIII,(h). 'Wernicke's Distinctive Clinical Concepts in Psychiatry' (*Affective impact of mental illness*).

'Alcoholic psychosis': 'most acute form of alcoholic psychosis' (L26, p. 174) a.k.a: 'drunkenness'.

'Amentia' (L33, p. 235), a term originally used by William Cullen (1777) to mean 'mental retardation'. For Meynert in his 1890 clinical lectures, the meaning had shifted—a sudden-onset state of confusion, as a disorder of thinking—contrasted with 'dementia', which for him was 'deterioration of personality' [199]. Symptoms of Meynert's (p. 240) 'amentia' ranged from excitement to stupor, occasionally ending in deterioration.

'Anxiety' (*Angst*) (L23, p. 145): We almost always render the German word as 'anxiety', only occasionally as 'fear', since 'anxiety' is more familiar in psychiatry, and fear implies 'fear *of something*', which is often not the case for anxiety states.

'Apperception' (first used in L2, p. 9: *Vorstellung*). The German word has many shades of meaning. 'Perception' is one rendition in English, but, as becomes clear by L8 (p. 43), the English word 'perception' usually refers to *sensory* perception, while here, a higher-level process is meant. When used in this sense, the English word 'apperception' will be used, whose definitions (OED) is: 'perception with recognition or identification by association with previous ideas'.

'Apoplexy': 'Stroke' is the common English term, Up to the end of the nineteenth century, 'apoplexy' referred to any sudden death with sudden loss of consciousness, today given the term 'stroke'. Literally it refers to bleeding of internal organs. 'Apoplect*iform*' implies *as if* leading to sudden death, usually describing what is now called 'stroke'. (See also L28, p. 186; L37, p. 284).

'Arsenic green' (L38, p. 296): This is probably the same as 'Paris green', a highly toxic compound of arsenic (copper acetate triarsenite), used in Paris as a rat poison (in sewers). From about 1900 it was used in America and elsewhere in agriculture, as an insecticide.

'Ascending' (*aszendierend*'): Although Wernicke frequently uses the metaphorical German word, we replace it by 'worsening', except when the German word is used in another sense.

'Asymbolia' (*Asymbolie*; also to be translated as *asemia* or *asemasia*) (L27, p. 183), a severe form of aphasia, in which there is inability to understand (and for the latter terms, perhaps also to use) symbols in communication. (See also L20, p. 128; L38, p. 295).

'Atonicity' (L34, p. 253): Pathological lack of muscle tone.

'Atrophy' (*Atrophie*) First appears on L38, p. 295 *Atrophie der Optici*; then L38, p. 288 *Atrophie des Großhirnmantels*; pp. 288, 289; L40, p. 317 *Optikusatrophie*. It invariably refers to biological change.

'Autochthonous': We usually retain Wernicke's word, although 'self-generated' may be less ambiguous. (Section VIII,(i). 'Wernicke's Distinctive Clinical Concepts in Psychiatry', *Delusions and Related Phenomena for Wernicke*).

'Brain-softening' (*Encephalomalacia*) (L11, p. 67) was an accepted medical term in the late nineteenth century, deriving from autopsy examinations of the brain, and later entered popular vocabulary. It referred to localized change in the brain, due to haemorrhage or inflammation. Three varieties, distinguished by colour, represented different stages of morbid processes, known respectively as red, yellow, and white softening. In Wernicke's day such changes were commonly seen post-mortem in aged people and in those dying from syphilis, as well as in cases of stroke.

'Cause': We take this to be a debated concept, and avoid using it except in special circumstances. It meaning is different from 'aetiology' which we translate directly from the German.

'Channeling' (*Bahnung*), first used in L22 (p. 139). The root word (*Bahn*) is common (*Bahnhof, Eisenbahn*, etc.). Dictionary translation of *Bahnung* includes 'canalization' or 'channeling', terms originating in engineering at a time when major rivers in Europe were being made navigable. We use 'channeling' as a more familiar word than 'canalization'. The meaning of *Bahnung* is captured in Wernicke's phrases such as 'frequent repetition' and 'deliberate practice', suggesting 'a pathway created by frequent use', 'stamping in' or 'blazing' of a trail. In psychology it means an ever-narrowing focus of attention and of motives for behaviour—as a result of mental disturbance, education, or other life events. This term 'canalization' appears to have originated with Pierre Janet as early as 1889. It is unlikely that it originated with Wernicke, to be adopted later by Janet, because Janet had little ability to read German [200]. The term *Bahnung* was also known in France and translated as *frayage*, (*'facilitation associative par répétition'*). Freud used it in *Entwurf einer Psychologie* [201], also named *Erinnerungsspur* ('memory trace'). 'Canalization' was used later by Gardner Murphy [202], acknowledging Janet as the source. Its use in psychology has diversified since Murphy's monograph. *Bahnung* has been used metaphorically in science in various other contexts, including genetics (after Waddington). In physiology it was first used by Sigismund Exner [203] and was explained through an electrotechnical analogy. The coincidence of dates of Exner's Wernicke's and Freud's publications using the term suggests that it captured a widely recognized concept for German-speakers [204].

'Blasé' (*Blasiertheit*) (L30, p. 207): This does not have quite the meaning of the French 'blasé' ('indifferent to normal sources of interest because they are familiar'; or 'indifferent as a result of excessive earlier indulgence'). Wernicke implies 'indifferent due to repeated failure to find enjoyment in usual source of interest.'

'Catalepsy', 'cataleptic attack' (L28, p. 191): This is the first mention of the term 'cataleptic' or 'catalepsy'. It is an old term, whose meaning has varied, and has included a variety of different conditions or states. According to Berrios [190], in its complete form, it is a state of overall motor paralysis, sometimes with normal muscle tone, or increased tone, sensory disconnection without anaesthesia or analgesia, passive posturing, and total amnesia for the period of its presence. In early nineteenth century it was classed amongst the 'neuroses' in the original sense of William Cullen (along with paralysis, tetanus, and epilepsy). It was important to Kahlbaum, is referred to by Wernicke in L34 (p. 253), and is mentioned by Ernst Kretschmer [61], for whom it was very similar to the instinctive 'death feint' known in most mammalian species. Curiously it is not reported today in humans, although it is a term widely used in animal studies of psychopharmacology (e.g. 'neuroleptic-induced catalepsy' in laboratory animals), which is probably different from the condition described by Wernicke, even when one restricts the comparison to motor signs.

'Chorea minor' (L32, p. 231): Sydenham's chorea, occurring after streptococcal injection affecting the brain.

'Column disease' ('L37 (p. 274): *Strangerkrankung. Strang* is a somewhat outdated German word for (spinal) column; *Erkrankung* is a more general, less specific word than *Krankheit,* referring to the start of a disease process.

'Complex': see section VIII,(s). 'Wernicke's Distinctive Clinical Concepts in Psychiatry' (*Wernicke's Links to the Emerging Dynamic Tradition in Psychiatry.*)

'Conform' 'The requirement for intellectual material to "conform"' (L40, p. 313): The sense here is of discourse to 'conform' to what is accepted (for instance to church doctrine).

'Confusion' (*Verwirrtheit*): We take this to indicate a state when conflict between mental contents becomes overwhelming. Likewise 'bewilderment'.

'Consolidating': '*um so fester*' (L4, p. 22). 'Consolidation'—of memory—is accepted terminology for memory researchers today, introduced by Muller and Pilzecker [205] but Wernicke does not use *Konsolidierung.*

'Crests of the gyri' (L37, p. 288): *Windungskuppen* site where localized pathology develops after brain injury.

'Crime against morality' (L25, p. 168): Presumably a sexual crime.

'Cure' see section III. 'The Medical Scene at Breslau in Wernicke's Day; Typical Psychiatric Practice', on criteria for discharge; and section VIII,(q). 'Wernicke's Distinctive Clinical Concepts in Psychiatry' (*Prognostic Indicators; Concepts of 'Cure', or 'Return to Health'*).

'Curve': This idea is used to characterize the plot of illness extent or intensity over time. This word captures Wernicke's meaning more exactly than 'plot' or 'graph'.

'Daimonion' (L29, p. 196): Roughly 'a daemon'; and, according to Merriam-Webster dictionary: 'an inward mentor conceived as partaking of the nature of a demon or inspired by one'. The legendary Socrates also experienced an inner voice giving advice (now perhaps called 'command hallucinations').

'Deduce' (*Abzug*): Used only once in *Grundriss* (L1, p. 4).

'Deficit': We prefer this to 'Defect' to render the German *Defekt.*

'Degeneration' (*Entartete,* or *Degeneration*). See section V. 'Contemporary Knowledge in Neuroscience; Contemporary Practice in General Medicine and Psychiatry in Wernicke's Day', paragraph on 'degeneration'.

'Delirium' (*Delirien*) is almost always separate from 'Delusion' (*Wahn*), but p. 211, where Wernicke cites Meynert is an exception. The German text often uses *deliriant,* but we avoid this term in our translation.

'Delusion' (*Wahn*): The German word can refer either to a delusion or to a state where delusions can occur. We have attempted to indicate which meaning is intended.

'Delusion of belittlement' (*Kleinheitswahn*) (L29, p. 200), a term with a slightly different sense from 'micromania' (see below).

'Delusion of persecution': *Verfolgungswahn.*

'Delusion of relatedness', 'delusion of reference' see section VIII,(l). 'Wernicke's Distinctive Clinical Concepts in Psychiatry' (*Delusions and Related Phenomena for Wernicke*).

'Depression'/'Depressed': see 'Melancholia'.

'Descending' (*Descendierend*). See above under 'Ascending'.

'Disarray': see section VIII,(h). 'Wernicke's Distinctive Clinical Concepts in Psychiatry' (*Affective impact of mental illnesses*).

'Disorientation': see section VIII,(h). 'Wernicke's Distinctive Clinical Concepts in Psychiatry' (*Affective impact of mental illnesses*).

'Drive': Wernicke's usual word is *Antrieb,* usually implying a degree of voluntariness, but sometimes, a response driven by a sensory stimulus, sometimes a behavioural urge, occasionally 'voluntary effort'. The word *Zwang* is used only once

'Dyspneic' (L39, p. 307): Short of breath.

'Eburnisation' (L37, p. 289): Degenerative process of bone occurring at sites of articular cartilage erosion commonly found in patients with osteoarthritis.

'Elementary symptom': see section VIII, (g). 'Wernicke's Distinctive Clinical Concepts in Psychiatry' (*Wernicke's Concept of 'Elementary' symptoms*)

'Emotions' (L8, p. 48): see section VIII,(h). 'Wernicke's Distinctive Clinical Concepts in Psychiatry' (*Affective Impact of Mental Illness*).

'Emotional incontinence' (L40, p. 320): It is not clear where this term originated in the English-speaking world. For many years it appears to have been little used, but recently, a number of papers on stroke patients in East Asia have used the term.

'Endowment': *Besitzstand.*

'Energy': Usually Wernicke's word is *Kraft,* but the word *Energie* occurs sometimes, especially when used for a specifically physical metaphor (p. 43: *pontentiellen Energien;* p. 66: *specifische Energie*; p. 73: 'drained away,' 'balancing up', 'build up': *Energie strom*; p. 80: 'damming up of nerve energy;' p. 81: *nerven Energie*; p. 86: 'perpetual motion'; p. 89: 'energy accumulated etc'; p. 126: 'specific energy'; BUT p. 183: 'verbal utterance, and their *energy*' (*enkraften*). p. 218: 'unrestrained energy'). (See section XI,(b). 'Wernicke's Reasoning', *Reasoning by analogy*).

'Envenomation' (L26, p. 176): This word implies some toxin of exogenous origin; but the exact meaning is unclear.

'*Ependymitis granulosus*' (L37, p. 25): Inflammation of the ventricular lining, with accumulation of granular tissue.

'Epigenetic': Use of this term (L20, p. 125) is confusing to a modern reader. Today the noun form 'epigenetics', introduced by Waddington in 1942, refers to the fact that the genome does not unfold in a manner determined solely by its own nature, but is subject to numerous influences during development, including, indirectly, ones from the outer environment [206]. However, in adjectival form ('epigenetic'), the term is much older, rooted in a theory of 'epigenesis', that the germ is brought into existence (by successive accretions), and not merely developed, in the process of reproduction [207].

'Experiment': see section XI,(a). 'Style of Reasoning'.

'Extent': This word is used to characterize the extent of an illness. We use this word, except when the German refers to a collection of specific symptoms, when we use the word 'range'.

'Faradisation' (*Faradisation*) (e.g. 'Faradic excitability of a nerve', L3, p. 16): This was a common term at the time, although 'electricity', 'electrisation', were also in common use. The sense of terms such as 'electricity' or 'electric' has shifted over the centuries, and was not precise in Wernicke's day. Strictly, 'faradisation' meant 'alternating current', which, by Wernicke's time, had superseded direct current in clinical situations.

'Fear': see 'Anxiety' above.

'Feeling tone': see 'Organ sensation'.

'Feudal estate' (L27, p. 180): The German word is *Herrschaft*, indicating the fiefdom of a feudal lord of earlier days.

'*Fibrae propriae*' (Meynert) (L37, p. 290): The coherent band of white matter lying immediately deep to the cortical grey matter.

'Fixed idea'(*fixen Ideen*) (L41, p. 329), obviously a direct translation from the French *idée fixe.*

'*Flexibilitas cerea*' (L34, p. 250): This is a latinized version of the term 'waxy flexibility' which Wernicke also used; but he appears to use the two terms as though they have slightly different meanings.

'Forgery': 'Forgery of consciousness' (L40, p. 313): Whereas 'falsification' of contents of consciousness' (*Fälschung des Bewußtseinsinhaltes*) need be no more than a one-off error, 'forgery of consciousness' (*Bewußtseinsfälschung*) is a more systematic, comprehensive and finalized version of such error.

'f.S. artery' (L11, p. 67): Presumably the artery supplying the superior longitudinal fasciculus (major hemispheric white matter tract).

'Ganglion cell' (*Ganglienzellen*), first used in L3 (p. 16): This was Wernicke's word for a cell body, or perikaryon of a neurone, However, the term is used in various ways, often in L3 referring to a specific neuronal type in the retina, and elsewhere just to indicate 'a central neurone'. In the latter context, he usually referred to long-axon (projection) neurones, although Cajal had already distinguished these from the 'local circuit neurones' (in the cerebral cortex).

'Gastric catarrh' (L26, p. 173); now 'Gastritis'.

'Genetic confusion' (L33, p. 236): see section VII,(b). 'Wernicke's Contribution to Neuroscience, Psychology and Overall Medical Knowledge' (*Wernicke and 'Associationism'*).

'Globus pharynges' (L22, p. 143): This term can be traced back to Hippocrates, and refers to persistent, but benign sensations originating in the pharynx or larynx, otherwise known as 'globus sensation', just 'globus', or in older terminology 'globus hystericus'—in common parlance 'a lump in one's throat'. As with many psychosomatic disorders there has been debate about whether it has a physical origin in the throat or related structures, or a psychological one [208]. Here Wernicke appears to use the term to refer to normal anatomical structures from where such sensations sometimes arise, rather than to the symptoms themselves. (See also L30, p. 208).

'Grandiosity' (*Grössenwahn*), first used in L8 (p. 200). We avoid 'megalomania' (which has too many connotations in English vernacular), and 'delusions of grandeur' (which are described later); and we wish to avoid confusion with true 'mania' for which Wernicke has a precise conceptualization.

'Granular cell' (L41, p. 326): This is somewhat dated terminology, referring to some layers of the cerebral cortex as 'granule cell layers' or 'granular layers'. Their main neuronal type is not sharply different from those in other layers, being pyramidal cells (*Ganglienzellen* in Wernicke's terminology); but they are smaller and more densely packed than in the layers (notably layer V) containing larger pyramidal cells, hence the term 'granular'. Lissauer defined cell loss in laminae II and III, which were referred to as 'granular layers'. It is not clear what 'laborious' method was used by Lissauer to trace the degenerating connecting of these cells. The Marchi method is based on detection of degenerating myelin, and Lissauer may have used an earlier version of this method.

'Hallucination': The usual German word is *Halluzination.* An alternative word is *Sinnestäuschungen* (sensory deception, sometimes including delusions as well as hallucinations). Visual hallucinations are referred to as *Halluzination*, but tactile ones as *Sinnestäuschungen*. '"Hallucinations of common sensation", which we will deal with in more detail later.' (L19, p. 121) We are not sure of the exact meaning of this phrase.

'Helplessness': see 'Disarray'.

'*Homo tardus*' (L31, p. 216): This may have been one of Wernicke's own terms. It is of interest, because the latinate binomial nomenclature, devised by Carl Linnaeus for both botanical classification and for classification of diseases, appears here to be used here to designate a personality type, rather than a disorder.

'*Hydrops ventriculorum*' (L38, p. 296): Literally, ventricular oedema.

'Hypermetamorphosis' '(L20, p. 125): This term originated with Heinrich Neumann, Wernicke's predecessor at Breslau [209], but also has a meaning in entomology. Today the term is not used, but perhaps should be reintroduced. It has similarities to syndromes seen after definite cortical lesions [210], including instinctive 'grasp reactions', tactile 'avoidance reactions' or 'instinctive visual fixation'. The term was to be used later by Klüver and Bucy [211] in descriptions of a syndrome produced in macaque monkeys after bilateral temporal lobectomy. However, their use referred to an 'excessive tendency to take notice of and to attend and react to every *visual* stimulus'. Wernicke gives no indication that the syndrome he describes in psychiatric patients is related to any cortical lesion, and excess of attentional fixation can occur in *any* sensory modality, but differing from one patient to another. It appears to correspond to various perceptual sensitivities (such as sensitivity to noise, or to visual movement), and can be seen as aspects of selective attention specific to one (or more) sensory modalities.

'Idiocy' (L37, p. 292); *Blödsinn.*

'*Impotentia coeundi*' (L24 (p. 160): erectile dysfunction.

'Inhibition': see section VII,(a). 'Wernicke's Contribution to Neuroscience, Psychology and Overall Medical Knowledge' (*Basic neuroscience*).

'Insane', 'Insanity': In current English usage these are legal rather than medical terms, although the two were not separated in Wernicke's day. We therefore avoid them unless they were already historic, were a patient's own words, or were referring to words of another clinician.

'Insolation' (L41, p. 328): Exposure to solar radiation, equivalent to 'sunstroke', which may be relevant to the case of the fugitive from Australia to Switzerland (see also L28).

'Jactation' (L20, p. 131): As used medically, this term (also 'jactitation') indicates abnormal, restless tossing or throwing about of the body.

'Lateral column symptoms' (L39, p. 301): Presumably differential loss of pain and temperature sense, while discriminative sensation remains intact.

'Lunatics' (*Irrenwesen*—first used in L1, p. 4; likewise: 'Mad-doctor': *Irrenärzte;* 'Lunatic asylum': *Irrenhaus,* L32, p. 229, literally 'madhouse'). These terms are the contemporary English equivalents, according to Lang [212]. The term 'lunatic' was removed from British law in the 1930 Mental Treatment Act, but not from US Federal law, until 6th December 2012. We often use *alienist* interchangeably for *Irrenärzte,* although Wernicke does not use the equivalent German term. German words for madness do not refer to the moon. The German word *Laune,* has a lunar origin, but is more benign than 'Lunatic' (indicating 'mood', 'whim' or 'caprice').

'Manic aphasia' (L20, p. 127): A term coined earlier by Wernicke, from which he now appears to be distancing himself.

'Manifestation': The word *Ereignis* consistently refers to 'outward signs' of mental disorder, while *Erscheinung,* sometimes refers to inner experience, and is better rendered as 'phenomenon'.

'Marasmus' (L24, p. 159): Signs of severe malnutrition.

'Megalomania' (L14, p. 95), a term that originated as the French *megalomanie*, used by Hecker [213] including the phrase 'exalted megalomanic lying', and first appearing in English in 1890. Wernicke used the term occasionally, but to refer to other physicians' usage, not his own. In German, it could be straight from French, or it could become '*der Grössenwahn*'. However, the latter term refers to *delusions* of grandiosity, or to a state where such delusions can occur.

'*Menstruatio nimia*' (L32, p. 225): excessive menstrual bleeding. (Also L38, p. 294).

'Mental illness': Despite his assertion at the start of L1 (following Griesinger) that mental illnesses are brain diseases, Wernicke uses separate words, respectively *Geisteskrankheiten* versus *Gehirnkrankheiten*, and, from time to time points out differences between psychiatry and neurology. His word for mental illness—*Geisteskrankheiten*—clearly shows that he identified the problems he encountered in his patients as a form of illness, for which medical terms were appropriate. '*Geisteskrankheiten*' or '*Geistesstoerungen*': Usually the first of these is used by Wernicke. Cases where the second is used include the following (with our rendition)—p. 54: 'mental disturbance'; p. 65 'all chronic mental disorders'; p. 66 'be advisable to reserve the term 'chronic mental disorder' just for residual cases'; p. 71: 'residual chronic mental disturbance'; p. 72 'equally for chronic and acute mental disorders'; p. 101 'right to declare a person mentally ill'; p. 102 'paranoid states are mental disorders', 'all chronic mental disorders' p. 105 'each newly emerging symptom of mental disorder' (and yet, on the same page we have 'most chronic mental illnesses' [*Geisteskrankheit*]; p. 158 'or senile mental disorder'; p. 161 'accessible to the lay man'; p. 162 'chronic mental disorder'; p. 180: 'We obtained a report of the exact time of onset of her acute mental disorder which was very inaccurate', (but on the same page, *Geisteskrankheit* is used, referring to onset of menstrual bleeding); p. 220 'circular mental disorder'; p. 275 'either chronic mental disorder or dementia'; p. 309: 'chronic mental disorder remains'; p. 313 'residual mental disorder'. In summary, *Geistesstoerungen* is usually used when referring to mental disorders generically, or in a less specialized way.

'Maceration' (L37, p. 288): strictly, 'softening by soaking', but used in a variety of situations. In pathology, refers to tissue degeneration after death (for instance in a still-borne infant).

'Medulla oblongata': *Oblongata.*

'Medullary degeneration': *Markdegeneration.*

'Medullary pyramid': *Markkagel.*

'Melancholia'/'melancholy': This is almost always the equivalent word in German. We use Wernicke's 'melancholia' in most cases except when it is in adjectival form, or when it refers to the history of the concept, when we use 'melancholy'. Only occasionally do we use *depressed* (p. 219), when the German word is *deprimiert.*

'Meteorism' (L34, p. 247): Gaseous distension of stomach or intestines.

'Metritis' (L24, p. 157): otherwise known as 'Pelvic inflammatory disease', an inflammation on the uterine wall, as opposed to 'endometritis', an inflammation of the functional lining of the uterus.

'Micromania' (L23, p. 147): A modern dictionary definition is 'excessive or unbridled enthusiasm for self-deprecation', or 'delusions of littleness or belittlement', ('low self-esteem' perhaps in modern terms; an autopsychic delusion in Wernicke's terms). 'Micromania' in this sense is the opposite of megalomania, and Wernicke term is usually *Kleinheitswahn*. We almost always use 'belittlement' rather than 'micromania', except when citing Meynert. Pierre Janet [214] gave 'micromania' a quite different meaning, when he writes as follows: 'Micromania deserves attention: It is evident that many of these patients grant more importance to that which is small than that which is big, Chu…, a woman of 36 years, anxiously searches for the "small crumbs of grease, crumbs of dirt" but does not take care of "big dirtinesses." Bow… is afraid of "small noises," not of the "big ones". A canon blow does not do anything to me, but I want to kill the people that chew, who pick their teeth, who cough… Mr. Stadelmann of Würzburg relates a nice observation of a man of 30 years, bothered since puberty by the preoccupation of what various insignificant objects will become in the future, a fly that flies, a lifeless match, the ash of the cigar, the spots of candle fallen to earth, etc. Mr. Farez also relates obsessions and disgust for very small objects, match tips, candle stains. It is needless to emphasize the importance that patients attach to the "little bugs." Into this preoccupation with what is small enters, of course, the mania of attention and precision.' [214]. This alternative meaning does not refer to the patient's self, but to how he/she experiences the outside world (allopsychic in Wernicke's terms); and since there are differences between right and left hemispheres in perception of large versus small images (at least in the visual sense), Janet may be referring to an abnormality of cerebral asymmetry.

'*Milliarde*' (L4, p. 22): one thousand million, according to terminology of the period, 'one billion', in today's terminology.

'Molecular' (L8, p. 43): This is implicitly contrasted with the term 'molar', as in chemistry, and as sometimes in psychology. This contrasts 'low-level details' of individual elements, and 'high-level properties' emerging collectively from many such elements. Wernicke, in effect, acknowledges that 'cross-level' explanations are the cornerstone of the most important scientific explanations.

'Molimina alvi': (L30, p. 208). Archaic term for premenstrual diarrhoea.

'Molimina uterina' (L30, p. 208): Archaic term for premenstrual uterine symptoms.

'Motility psychosis': Significantly, this is a disorder for which Wernicke appears to have had a special affinity, since he starts *Grundriss* by mentioning this disorder (L1, p. 6) and also finishes the series (L41, p. 329).

'Motor impulse' (L6), and 'Impulse' (used extensively in L31 and L32) to indicate a driver of motor activity. 'Impulsive' is also used a number of times in L32. It is not clear whether he was using 'impulse' as a deliberate analogy drawn from physical science (as he did with other terms, such as 'energy').

'Mytacism' (L27, p. 180). Excessive use of the letter 'm', or an equivalent sound.

'Negativity' (L34, p. 243): *Negativismus*.

'Nerve' (*Nerven*) (e.g. L3, p. 16) leaves it unclear whether it refers to a nucleus, a pathway, or to peripheral versus central nervous system.

'Nervous' (L29, p. 196): Apart from its use in neurology and neuroscience, this word has a vernacular meaning in English. The German word *nervös* is probably more stigmatizing than is 'nervous' in English, approximate synonyms being 'edgy', 'irritable' and 'agitated'.

'Neurosis': see section VIII,(s). 'Wernicke's Distinctive Clinical Concepts in Psychiatry' (*Wernicke's links to the emerging dynamic tradition in Psychiatry*).

'Nucleus' (L19, p. 123) has had a variety of meanings in science. In biology, its first use for the intracellular organ in each cell dates from 1831 (Online etymological dictionary). The use of the term in neuroanatomy for a collection of nerve cells, or discrete block of grey matter can be traced back as far as 1828, and was used in the 1875 edition of *Encyclopedia Britannica* (OED). After that time it had become standard terminology. Wernicke occasionally uses the German equivalent—*Kern*—as in *Linsenkern* (Lentiform nucleus: L11, p. 67), but in another instance (L19, p. 123), as the *sogenannten Kerne* ('the so-called nucleus'—possibly what is now called the dorsal column nuclei).

'Nurses'/'Warders': Wernicke never uses 'Schwesterin' only 'Warter' and 'Warterin' except on p. 180 (*Krankenschwester*: 'the attendant nurse' as a delusion). We therefore use warder' rather than 'nurse'.

'Organ sensation'. In L5 (p. 25) our translation reads 'Feeling tone of sensations': (*Gefühlston der Emfindungen*). Wernicke contrasts the 'tone' of sensation, with its 'sensory content'. (See also: L30, p. 207: 'tone of feeling' vs. 'quality of sensations'). The former might be clarified as 'emotional tone'. However, *Gefühlston*, is used in a sense different from both *Emotionen*, and *Affekt* (section VIII,(h). 'Wernicke's Distinctive Clinical Concepts in Psychiatry' [*Affective Impact of Mental Illnesses*]). He refers here to aspects of a stimulus associated with some inner 'drive' or motive for action. The term then becomes synonymous with 'organ sensation' (again in L6 and later), usually in the original as *Organempfindung*, or *Organgefühl*. The unifying theme appears to be that 'organ sensations' are ones whose primary role is related to near-automatic reflex or behavioural responses, rather than to detailed conscious awareness. This is not the same as 'emotional tone' where the emphasis is on sensory quality which may be linked to behaviour, but not to behaviour which may be disassociated from any necessary sensory quality. Organ sensations, with their implication for automatic reflexive behaviour, *may* be linked with perception at entry to the cortex, but not with memory images elaborated from these perceptions in higher cortical regions. The term translated here as 'organ sensation' has a complex history in nineteenth century German scientific thought. They can be traced back to Johannes Müller's *Elements of Physiology* [215], and, for him, had a relation to an unresolved issue about vitalism [216]. They were also linked to sensations arising in definite organs (which included sense organs such as the skin, eyes or inner ear), and these were sensations which, he thought, had a definite emotional 'colouration'. We resist the temptation to translate the term as 'organic sensation': Wernicke does sometimes use the adjective *organisch,* which has a different meaning. We can see the difference in the following terms we translate: 'the "organ of consciousness"', or the 'organ of association', in contrast with 'organic brain disease' or 'organic (versus functional) psychosis'. There is also a relation to a conceptual distinction published 2 years after *Grundriss,* by Rivers and Head [217], who separated 'protopathic sensation' (poorly localized, conveying sensations of heat, cold and pain), from 'epicritic sensation' (permitting better spatial localization of touch, pressure, etc.). These two were also separated by their different rates of recovery ('protopathic' sooner than 'epicritic') after experimental severing of peripheral nerves in the hand (the experimental subject in this case being Henry Head himself). Wernicke's use of the term 'organ sensation' is broader in scope than 'protopathic sensation', and does not appear to imply vagueness of spatial localization, and, unlike the latter term, includes sensory input from muscles and joints ('proprioception' in English terms), and that controlling eye movements.

'*Papilla optica*' (L26. p. 174): optic nerve papilla, the slight swelling, where nerve axons originating in the retina head towards the optic nerve, and the brain.

'Parametrium' (L24, p. 157): The fibrous layer between the bladder anteriorly, and the supravaginal cervix, posteriorly.

'Paranoia': generically, for Wernicke this meant a state where there is falsification of contents of consciousness (*not* 'persecution delusion'—which is a vernacular meaning today). Wernicke preferred 'paranoid state'.

'Pathological'/'Pathology' (*pathologische/ krankhafte; Pathologie*): Wernicke limits this almost entirely to abnormal findings at a biological level, rather than at an experiential, psychological or social level. For abnormality at the later levels he is almost completely consistent in using *Krankhafte*.

'*Pavor nocturnus*' (L39, p. 301): night terrors.

'Peak of illness': The German word *Krankheitshöhe* can mean either 'level' or 'peak' of illness.

'Perception' (*Wahrnehmung*). See above for separation from 'Apperception'.

'Perplexity': see 'Disarray'

'Personality'/'Personhood': see *Synopsis, L7,* for use of terms. See section VI,(d). 'Wernicke's Underlying Philosophical Views' (*Wernicke on Personhood, Unity of a Person, and 'Self-consciousness'*)

'Perytyphlitis' (L39, p. 307): Inflammation of the connective tissue about the caecum and appendix: in other words 'appendicitis'.

'Phenazismen' (L19, p. 117) archaic, exact meaning unclear

'Phrenic nerve insufficiency': (L12, p. 75; L30, p. 211). This phrase—probably Wernicke's own—does not refer to actual pathology in the phrenic nerve, but to a style of breathing, dominated by costal rather than diaphragmatic musculature, likely to be a symptom of hysteria rather than a disorder of the peripheral nervous system.

'Physiological' (e.g. L13, p. 82): '... *physiological* delusions of reference...' This word is contrasted with 'pathological', indicating, 'within the normal physiological range', or 'relatively normal, in the prevailing context' (also L15, p. 33). However, the word is sometimes used in a more general sense (e.g. L39; p. 307).

'Politzer method' (L24, p. 158): A manoeuvre devised by Adam Politzer in Vienna in 1863, using increased air pressure in the nasopharynx during the act of swallowing in order to reopen blocked Eustachian tubes, and to equalize pressures in the sinuses.

'Polyneuritic psychosis' (L27, p. 179): a.k.a. 'Korsakoff syndrome'.

'Psychiatry/Psychiatrie/Psychiater' (L34, p. 253). These terms came into used after term Johanne Christien Reil in 1808 coined the term *Psychiatrie*; and they were introduced in France, from 1846. They are rarely used in *Grundriss* (Title of book; pp. 253, 326).

'Psychopathology': Wernicke *never* uses the word *psychopathologie* (although, on a single instance, on p. 96, he uses 'psychopathische'—a meaning separate from the English word 'psychopath'). This is an important point in contrasting Wernicke's ideas with those of Jaspers. The only possible exceptions are on p. 67, where 'pathological principles' (*pathologischen Prinzipes*) are seen to underlie explanatory delusions; and on p. 111, where we read: 'To show how symptoms of mental illness are derived from this schema, and to put their occurrence and importance in various mental illnesses in their proper perspective, would be a separate and independent teaching exercise; yet any such attempt might take us too far from our real task, which is to become familiar with specific cases of illness. I shall therefore restrict myself just to the most important problems of identification from a theoretical point of view: I shall discuss these separately, in some detail, as ones which are quite essential for understanding the general *pathology* of mental illnesses. These are mainly symptoms falling in the domain of hallucinations or which have internal links with such symptoms.' (emphasis added)

'Psychophysical': A significant word, invented by Fechner. (See pp. 46, 68, 73, 80).

'Psychophysiology' In L13 (p. 80) we read: 'When introducing psychophysiology, I commented ...' This is the only time he uses this word in his main text, but he appears to refer back to the general heading for L1–8, where the word appears only at the start of his 'Contents' list.

'Psychosis': see section VIII,(d). 'Wernicke's Distinctive Clinical Concepts in Psychiatry' (*Wernicke's Concept of Mental Illness/Disease.*)

'Puerperium' (L32, p. 224), more commonly called the 'post-partum period' of ~6 weeks.

'Registration' (first used in L2, p. 13): In accord with the *sAZm* sequence, Wernicke refers to the result of the stage *s* to *A* as *Ausgangsvorstellung* (literally 'output presentation', but sometimes rendered as 'initial perception'). Here and subsequently (e.g. L8, L2, L29) we use the term 'registration'.

'Resistance' (L34, p. 244): German: *Widerstand*

'Seizure' In Wernicke's day this was not limited to epileptic seizures, an ambiguity recognized in Lang's medical dictionary of [213].

'Silly': *Dumm.*

'Spiritual *acquis*' ('endowment') (L39, p. 301; L40, p. 314): *geistigen Besitzstand.*

'Stimulation'/'Stimuli': The usual German word is 'Reiz'.

'Strength' (of a concept: *Festigkeit*) first used in L4 (p. 22) implying 'security' or 'robustness'.

'Substantial': *ehebliche* or *wesentlich.*

'Substantive': *enhaltlich.*

'Symptom' (*Symptome*): In English the word 'symptom' is sometimes restricted to what a patient complains about, while 'sign' is something a doctor observes for him- or her-self. This usage is not very consistent, but is a significant distinction. Wernicke does not make this distinction for the word *Symptome* (first used, L1, p. 4, see for example, L37, p. 280, where the word includes objective evidence from neurological examination, and subjective evidence—a patient's complaints.); so 'grandiosity,' for Wernicke, is a *Symptome,* although observed by him, rather than being a patient's complaint. Since the distinction is not made consistently in English, we translate it as 'symptom'.

'Tangible' (L41, p. 328), presumably a change at the level of gross, rather than microscopic anatomy.

'Tenesmus' (L24, p. 155): A feeling of constantly needing to pass stools, or void urine, despite empty rectum or bladder.

'Thought disorder': *Denkstoerung.*

'Transitivism' (L21, p. 137): Wernicke introduced the term, to describe patients who show no sign of psychological malaise, but whose entire way of thinking and feeling led him to abandon any assumption of similarity in trains of thought, behaviour and conduct, which he otherwise would apply. The word became part of psychoanalytic vocabulary, discussed especially by child psychologists such as Charlotte Bühler (1893–1974) and Jacques Lacan (1901–1981). For such writers, the concept is closely linked to development of a sense of personal identity, and for Bühler, was revealed by the fact that very young children often do not distinguish sharply between their own experiences and those of others. Transitivism as defined by Bühler is relatively normal, the abnormality coming when it is lost. Thus, for Wernicke the meaning of the term appears to be almost the opposite of that given it by later writers. However, the later writers distinguish 'true' from 'morbid' transitivism, which may reconcile these divergent views.

'Transitory psychosis' (p. 240): the so-called 'twilight states'.

'Trichinae' (L24, p. 159): Small parasitic nematode worm.

'Trophic' (p. 273) anatomical change due mainly to nutritional deficiency.

'Tuberculosis'/'Phthisis': usually German is'*Lungenschwindsucht*'.

'The urge to be active' (L31, p. 217): The German word *Tätigkeitsdrang* has no exact English equivalent. 'Impulsiveness' has a different meaning. The word 'impulse', or more often 'impulsive' has a long history of use to refer to a more specific psychological urge. 'Impulse' was adapted in Newtonian mechanics to have a more specific quantitative meaning (integral of force over time). (See also 'Motor impulse').

'Vicarious melancholia' (L30, p. 215), an attack of recurrent mania is replaced by one of Affective melancholia (see also L33, p. 239).

'Visual': In L6 Wernicke often uses *optische*, which, in English coveys more of a physics- than a brain-based notion. We render *optische* as either 'visual' or 'visual perception/perceptual'.

'Visual agnosia' (*Seelenblindheit*), literally 'blindness in the mind', usually translated as 'visual agnosia' (first used in L3, p. 16), but sometimes as 'psychic blindness'. 'Visual agnosia' means literally 'failure of visual knowledge'. In the context of a person born blind 'visual agnosia' is not exact.

Wernicke's Latin and Greek expression (excluding medical terms):

L3, p. 19 *Cum grano salis* ('with a grain of salt')
L7, p. 39: *κατ' εζοχην* ('to a prominent degree')
L13, p. 79: *Causa efficiens* ('efficient cause' [after Aristotle])
L13, p. 82: *sit venia verbo* ('forgive the word')
L14, p. 87: *tua res agitur* ('It is a matter that concerns you')

L18, p. 112: *a priori* ('from the outset')
L18, p. 114: *Pater familias* ('father of the family')
L34, p. 258: *prognosis quo/ad vitam* ('Prognosis and life expectancy')

XVII. References

1. Krahl A, Schifferdecker M, Beveridge A. Carl Wernicke and the concept of 'elementary symptom'. Hist Psychiatry. 1998;9(36):503–8.
2. Bartsch AJ, Neumärker KJ, Franzek E, Beckmann H. Karl Kleist, 1879-1960. Am J Psychiatry. 2000;157(5):703.
3. Cohen RS, Seeger RJ, editors. Ernst Mach, physicist and philosopher. Dordrecht: D Reidel; 1970.
4. Ziehen T, Wernicke C. Monatsschr Psychiatr Neurol. 1906;18:I–IV.
5. Lengwiler M. Psychiatry beyond the asylum: the origins of German military psychiatry before World War I. Hist Psychiatry. 2003;14:41–62.
6. Sherlock EB. Lunacy practice in Germany. Lancet. 1905;166(4291):1565–8.
7. Dock LL. The rise of the German free sisters. In: Dock LL, Nutting MA editors. A history of nursing, from the earliest times to the present day with special reference to the work of the past thirty years. New York: GP Putnam's Sons; 1912.
8. European Charter of Patients' Rights. 2002. http://ec.europa.eu/health/ph overview/co operation/mobility/docs/health services co108 en.pdf
9. NHS Patients' Rights. 2013. http://www.nhs.uk/choiceintheNHS/Rightsandpledges/NHSConstitution/Documents/2013/handbook-to-the-nhs-constitution.pdf
10. Centers for Medicare & Medicaid Services (CMS), HHS; Final Rule. Medicare and Medicaid Programs: Changes to the Hospital and Critical Access Hospital Conditions of Participation to Ensure Visitation Rights for All Patients. Federal Register. 2010;75:70831–44.
11. Storch E. Psychologische Untersuchungen über die Funktionen der Hirnrinde, zugleich eine Vorstudie zur Lehre von der Afasie [dissertation]. Breslau: Universität Breslau; 1901.
12. Berrios GE, Beer D. The notion of unitary psychosis: a conceptual history. Hist Psychiatry. 1994;5(17): 13–36.
13. Mann L. Klinische und anatomische Beiträge zur Lehre von der spinalen hemiplegia. Dtsch Z Nervenheilkd. 1896;10:1–66.
14. Miller R. Approaches to learning spatial relationships in gross anatomy: perspective from wider principles of learning. Clin Anat. 2000;13:439–43.
15. Levelt WJM. A history of psycholinguistics: the pre-Chomskyan era. Oxford: Oxford University Press; 2012. p. 383.
16. Ellenberger HF. Discovery of the unconscious: the history and evolution of dynamic psychiatry. New York: Basic Books; 1970.
17. Ziehen T. Psychiatrie für Ärzte und Studierende. Berlin: F Wreden; 1894.
18. Pillman F. Carl Wernicke (1848-1905). J Neurol. 2003;250:1390–1.
19. Seitelberger F. Theodor Meynert (1833-1892) pioneer and visionary of brain research. J Hist Neurosci. 1997;6:264–74.
20. Whitrow M. Theodor Meynert (1833-1892): his life and poetry. Hist Psychiatry. 1996;7:615–28.
21. Dalzell TG. Freud and the Viennese psychiatrists. In: Dalzell T, editor Freud's Schreber between psychiatry and psychoanalysis. On subjective disposition to psychosis. London: Karnac Books; 2011. p. 149–98.
22. Meynert T. Psychiatry; a clinical treatise on diseases of the fore-brain based upon a study of its structure, functions, and nutrition. Part I. New York and London: GP Putnam's Sons; 1885/1968. p. 247.
23. von Kölliker RA. Neurologische Bemerkungen. Z wissen Zool. 1849;1:153–63.
24. Weigert C. Beiträge zur Kenntnis der menschlichen Neuroglia. Frankfurt am Main: M Diesterweg; 1895.
25. Buda O, Arsene D, Ceausu M, Dermengiu DE, Curca GC. Georges Marinesco and the early research in neuropathology. Neurology. 2009;72(1):88–91.
26. Wundt WM. Grundzüge der physiologischen Psychologie. Leipzig: Engelmann; 1874.
27. Pareti G. The 'all-or-none' law in skeletal muscle and nerve fibres. Arch Ital Biol. 2007;145(1):39–54.
28. May CA. Description and function of the ciliary nerves - some historical remarks on choroidal innervation. Exp Eye Res. 1997;65(1):1–5.
29. Parent A. The history of the basal ganglia: the contribution of Karl Friedrich Burdach. Neurosci Med. 2012;3:374–9.
30. Haas L. Theodor Meynert (1833-92). J Neurol Neurosurg Psychiatry. 1999;66(3):330.
31. Clarke PGH. pers. com. 19.08.2013.
32. Kahlbaum KL. The clinico-diagnostic perspective in psychopathology (transl. Berrios GE), Die klinische-diagnostische Gesichtspunkte der Psychopathologie. Sammlung klinischer Vorträge 1878;126:1127–46. Hist Psychiatry. 2007;18(2): 231–3.
33. Bräunig P, Krüger S. Karl Ludwig Kahlbaum (1828-1899) - a protagonist in modern psychiatry. Psychiatr Prax. 2000;27(3):112–8.
34. Yaprak M. The axon reflex. Neuroanatomy. 2008;7:17–9.
35. Spencer H. The principles of psychology. London: Longman, Brown, Green and Longman; 1855.
36. Rainy H. On the action of diphtheria toxin on the spinal stichochrome cells. J Pathol Bacteriol. 1900;6(4):435–58.
37. Mickle WJ. General paralysis of the insane. London: HK Lewis; 1886.

38. Nitrini R. The history of tabes dorsalis and the impact of observational studies in neurology. Arch Neurol. 2000;57(4):605–6.
39. Argyll Robertson DMCL. Four cases of spinal miosis: with remarks on the action of light on the pupil. Edinburg Med J. 1869;15:487–93.
40. Folsom CF. The early diagnosis of progressive paralysis of the insane. Boston Med Surg J. 1881;104: 558–60.
41. Pfeiffer JAF. A case of Landry's paralysis with especial reference to the anatomical changes. Brain. 1913;35:293–305.
42. Gowers WR. On the borderland of epilepsy: vertigo. Br Med J. 1906;2(2377):128–31.
43. Lopez Piñero JM. The work of John Hughlings Jackson: Part 2. Hist Psychiatry. 2010;21:224–36.
44. Eadie MJ. Cortical epileptogenesis - Hughlings Jackson and his predecessors. Epilepsia. 2007;48(11):2010–5.
45. Jackson JH. A study of convulsions. Trans St Andrews Med Grad Assoc. 1870;3:162–204.
46. Jackson JH. On temporary mental disorders after epileptic paroxysms. West Riding Lunatic Asylum Medical Reports. 1875;5:105–129.
47. McKenna PJ, Lorente-Rovira E, Berrios GE. Confabulation as a psychiatric symptom. In: Kirstein W, editor. Confabulation: views from neuroscience, psychiatry, psychology and philosophy. Oxford: Oxford University Press; 2009.
48. Pearce JMS. Positive and negative cerebral symptoms: the roles of Russell Reynolds and Hughlings Jackson. J Neurol Neurosurg Psychiatry. 2004;75(8):1148.
49. Kahlbaum KL. Die Gruppirung der psychischen Krankheiten und die Einteilung der Seelenstörungen. Danzig: AW Kafeman; 1863.
50. Kuechenhoff B. The psychiatrist Auguste Forel and his attitude to eugenics. Hist Psychiatry. 2008;19:215–23.
51. Egdahl A. Linnaeus' 'Genera Morborum' and some of his other medical works. Med Library Hist J. 1907;5(3):185–93.
52. Beer MD. Psychosis: from mental disorder to disease concept. Hist Psychiatry. 1995;6:177–200.
53. Noll R. Dementia praecox, 1886: a new turning point? Hist Psychiatry. 2012;23:255–6.
54. Kraam A, Phillips P. Hebephrenia: a conceptual history. Hist Psychiatry. 2012;23(4):387–403.
55. Berrios GE. Presbyophrenia: the rise and fall of a concept. Psychol Med. 1986;16:267–75.
56. Schifferdecker A, Peters UH. The origin of the concept of paranoia. Psychiatr Clin North Am. 1995;18:231–49.
57. Dowbiggin I. Delusional diagnosis? The history of paranoia as a disease concept in the modern era. Hist Psychiatry. 2000;11:37–69.
58. Munro A. Delusional disorder: paranoia and related illness. Cambridge: Cambridge University Press; 1999.
59. Beard GM. Neurasthenia, or nervous exhaustion. Boston Med Surg J. 1869;80:217–21.
60. Dejerine JJ, Gauckler E. Les manifestations fonctionelles des psychonévroses et leur traitement par la psychothérapie. Paris: Masson; 1905.
61. Kretschmer E. Hysteria, reflex and instinct. New York: Philosophical Library; 1923/1960.
62. Mach E. On thought experiments. In: Erkenntnis und Irrtum. Leipzig: JA Barth; 1905.
63. Miller R. Validating concepts of mental disorder: precedents from the history of science. Biol Cybern. 2014;108(5):689–99.
64. Blüh O. Ernst Mach: his life as a teacher and thinker. In: Cohen RS, Seeger RJ, editors. Ernst Mach – physicist and philosopher. Dordrecht: D Reidel; 1970.
65. Mach E. The analysis of sensations and the relation of the physical to the psychical. 1886/1905: (transl. Williams CM, Waterlow S (editor)); New York: Dover; 1959.
66. Bacon F. Novum Organum, 1620 (repr. Fowler T (editor)). Oxford: Clarendon Press; 1888
67. Lotze H. Medizinische Psychologie oder Physiologie der Seele. Leipzig: Weidmann; 1852.
68. Hume D. An abstract of a treatise on human nature. Keynes JM, Sraffa P, editors. Hamden, CT: Archon Books; An abstract of treatise in human nature. 1740/1965.
69. Spinoza B. Ethics. 1677: (transl. Curley EM), The collected writings of spinoza, vol. 1. Princeton: Princeton University Press; 1985.
70. Heidelberger M. Functional relations and causality in Fechner and Mach. Philos Psychol. 2010;23(2):163–72.
71. Bohr N. The quantum postulate and the recent development of atomic theory. Nature. 1928;121:580–90.
72. Mill JS. A system of logic. London: Longman, Green; 1879.
73. Hebb DO. The organization of behavior: a neuropsychological theory. New York: Wiley; 1949.
74. Locke J. An essay concerning human understanding. London: Penguin Books; 1689/2004.
75. Kant I. Critique of pure reason (transl. Meiklejohn JMD). London: JM Dent & Sons Ltd; 1781/1934.
76. Mojtabai R. Delusion as error: the history of a metaphor. Hist Psychiatry. 2000;11:3–14.
77. Berrios GE. Delusions as 'wrong beliefs': a conceptual history. Br J Psychiatry. 1991;159 suppl 14:6–13.
78. Hacking I. Les Aliénés voyageurs: how fugue became a medical entity. Hist Psychiatry. 1996;7:425–49.
79. Naef M. Ein Fall von temporärer totaler teilweiser retrograder Amnesie [dissertation]. Universität Zürich; 1898.
80. Megarbane B, Resiere D, Shabafrouz K, Dutholt G, Delahaye A, Delerme S, Baud F. Descriptive study of patients admitted to an intensive care unit during the heat wave of August 2003 in France. Presse Med. 2003;32:1690–8.
81. Mead GH. Mind, self and society from the perspective of a social behaviorist. Chicago: University of Chicago Press; 1934.
82. Ball KL. Non-psychotic traits of schizophrenia as abnormalities of cerebral asymmetry: development

of a potential early screening instrument [dissertation]. Dunedin NZ: University of Otago; 2011.
83. James W. The will to believe; and other essays in popular philosophy. New York: Longmans, Green & Co.; 1897.
84. Creed RS, Denny-Brown DE, Eccles JC, Liddell EGT, Sherrington CS. Reflex activity of the spinal cord. Oxford: Clarendon Press; 1932.
85. Grant G. The 1932 and 1944 Nobel Prizes in physiology or medicine: rewards for ground-breaking studies in neurophysiology. J Hist Neurosci. 2006;15(4):341–57.
86. John ER. Mechanisms of memory. New York: Academic Press; 1968.
87. Miller R. Meaning and purpose in the intact brain. Oxford: Oxford University Press; 1981.
88. Miller R. Cortico-hippocampal interplay and the representation of contexts in the brain. Heidelberg: Springer; 1991.
89. Braitenberg V. Cell assemblies in the cerebral cortex. In: Heim R, Palm G, editors. Lecture notes on biomathematics, vol. 21. Heidelberg: Springer; 1978. p. 171–88.
90. Adrian ED. Double representation of the feet in the sensory cortex of the cat. J Physiol. 1940;98:16–8.
91. Gordon G. Active touch. The mechanism of recognition of objects by manipulation: a multi-disciplinary approach, 1977. Oxford: Pergamon Press; 1978.
92. Miller R. A theory of the basal ganglia and their disorders. Boca Raton (FL): CRC Press; 2008.
93. Olds J, Milner PM. Positive reinforcement produced by electrical stimulation of septal and other areas of rat brain. J Comp Physiol Psychol. 1954;47: 419–27.
94. Manni R. Rapid eye movement sleep, non-rapid eye movement sleep, dreams, and hallucinations. Curr Psychiatry Rep. 2005;7(3):196–2000.
95. Plazzi G, Montagna P, Meletti S, Lugaresi E. Polysomnographic study of sleeplessness and oneirisms in the alcohol withdrawal syndrome. Sleep Med. 2002;3:279–82.
96. Wernicke C. Lehrbuch der Gehirnkrankheiten, für Ärzte und Studierende. Kassel: Th. Fischer; 1881.
97. Jorge RE, Robinson RG, Starkstein SE, Arndt SV, Forrester AW, Geisler FH. Secondary mania following traumatic brain injury. Am J Psychiatry. 1993;150:916–21.
98. Mohr P, Volavka J. Ladislav Haskovec and akathisia: 100th anniversary. Br J Psychiatry. 2002;181:537.
99. Khushf G. Why bioethics needs the philosophy of medicine: some implications of reflection on concepts of health and disease. Theor Med. 1997;18(1–2):145–63.
100. Maj M. Mental disorders as "brain diseases" and Jaspers' legacy. World Psychiatry. 2013;12(1):1–3.
101. Thome J. Centenary of Karl Jaspers's general psychopathology: implications for molecular psychiatry. J Mol Psychiatry. 2014;2(1):3.
102. Jaspers K. General psychopathology. Baltimore: The Johns Hopkins University Press; 1997.
103. Miller R. A neurodynamic theory of schizophrenia and related disorders. Morrisville (NC): Lulu Enterprises; 2008.
104. Berrios GE. Descriptive psychopathology: conceptual and historical aspects. Psychol Med. 1984;14(2): 303–14.
105. Chen HC, Flores d'Arcais GB, Cheung SL. Orthographic and phonological activation in recognizing Chinese characters. Psychol Res. 1995;58:144–53.
106. Kihlstrom JF. To honor Kraepelin. From symptoms to pathology in the diagnosis of mental illness. In: Beutler LE, Malik ML, editors. Rethinking the DSM: a psychological perspective, Decade of behaviour. Washington, DC: Am Psychol Assoc; 2002. p. 279–303.
107. Berrios GE. Jaspers and the first edition of Allgemeine Psychopathologie. Br J Psychiatry. 2013;202:433.
108. Mullen PE. A modest proposal for another phenomenological approach to psychopathology. Schizophr Bull. 2007;33(1):113–21.
109. Hoenig J. Schneider's first rank symptoms and the tabulators. Compr Psychiatry. 1984;25(1):77–87.
110. Widiger TA, Crego C. Diagnosis and classification. In: Weiner I, Stricker G, Widiger TA, editors. Wiley handbook of clinical psychology. New York: Wiley; 2013. p. 3–18.
111. Miller R. Schizophrenia as a progressive disorder: relations to EEG, CT, neuropathological and other evidence. Prog Neurobiol. 1989;33:17–44.
112. James W. What is an emotion? In: James W, editor. Collected essays and reviews. 1884/1969. New York: Russell and Russell; 1969. p. 244–80.
113. Lange C. The emotions. In: Dunlap K, editor. Psychology classics. Baltimore: Williams & Wilkins; 1922. p. 33–90.
114. Störring GE. Wesen und Bedeutung des Symptoms der Ratlosigkeit bei psychischen Erkrankungen. Leipzig: Thieme; 1939. Review J Nerv Ment Dis. 1940;92:798.
115. Bleuler E. Dementia praecox: or the group of schizophrenias (transl. Zinkin J) 1911/1950. New York: International University Press; 1950.
116. Moskowitz A, Helm G. Eugen Bleuler's Dementia Praecox or the Group of Schizophrenias (1911): a centenary appreciation and reconsideration. Schizophr Bull. 2011;37(3):471–9.
117. Bested AC, Logan AC, Selhub EM. Intestinal microbiota, probiotics and mental health: from Metchnikoff to modern advances: Part I – autointoxication revisited. Gut Pathog. 2013;5:5.
118. Noll R. Kraepelin's 'lost biological psychiatry'? Autointoxication, organo-therapy, and surgery for dementia praecox. Hist Psychiatry. 2007;18: 301–20.
119. Peters A, Payne BR. Numerical relationships between geniculo-cortical afferents and pyramidal cell modules in cat primary sensory cortex. Cereb Cortex. 1993;3:69–78.

120. Miller R. Striatal dopamine in reward and attention: a system for understanding the symptomatology of acute schizophrenia and mania. Int Rev Neurobiol. 1993;35:161–268.
121. Snell L. Die Ueberschätzungsideen der Paranoia. Allg Z Psychiat. 1890;46:447–60.
122. Neisser C. Dissertation on paranoia from the clinical point of view. 1892. In: Alvarez JM, Hill F, editors. Classics paranoia. Spain: DOR Editions Ltd; 1997. p. 85–112.
123. Balzan R, Delfabbro P, Galletly C, Woodward T. Confirmation bias across the psychosis continuum: the contribution of hypersalient evidence-hypothesis matches. Br J Clin Psychol. 2013;52(1):53–69.
124. Leonhard K. Cycloid psychoses - endogenous psychoses which are neither schizophrenic nor manic depressive. Br J Psychiatry. 1961;107:633–48.
125. Phillips CG. Cortical localization and 'sensorimotor processes' at the 'middle level' in primates. Proc R Soc Med. 1973;66:987–1002.
126. Freud S. The psychopathology of everyday life 1901/1914 (transl. Brill AA). London: T Fisher Unwin; 1914.
127. Friedmann M. Über den Wahn, eine klinisch-physiologische Unterstellung, nebst einer Darstellung der normalen Intelligenzvorgänge. Wiesbaden: JF Bergmann; 1894.
128. Court JH. Manic-depressive psychosis: an alternative conceptual model. Br J Psychiatry. 1968;114: 1523–30.
129. Keatinge B. Beckett and language pathology. J Mod Lit. 2007;31(4):86–101.
130. Doesburg SM, Kitajo K, Ward LM. Increased gamma-band synchrony precedes switching of conscious perceptual objects in binocular rivalry. Neuroreport. 2005;16:1139–42.
131. Geschwind N. Disconnexion syndromes in animals and man. Part I. Brain. 1965;88(2):237–94.
132. Foucault M. Folie de déraison: Histoire de la folie à l'âge classique. Paris: Union Générale d'Éditions; 1961.
133. Molnar M. pers. com. 1.04.2014.
134. Meynert T. Psychiatry: a clinical treatise on diseases of the fore-brain based upon a study of its structure, functions, and nutrition (transl. Sachs B). New York: GB Putnam's Sons; 1885.
135. Freud S. New introduction to psychoanalysis. 1920/1973. Harmondsworth: Penguin Books; 1973.
136. Beer MD. The dichotomies: psychosis/neurosis and functional/organic: a historical perspective. Hist Psychiatry. 1996;7:231–55.
137. Freud S. The justification for detaching from neurasthenia a particular syndrome: the anxiety neurosis. 1894/1953, Collected papers, Vol 1. London: The Hogarth Press; p. 76–106.
138. Slade T, Andrews G. Exclusion criteria in the diagnostic classifications of DSM-IV and ICD-10: revisiting the co-occurrence of psychiatric symptoms. Psychol Med. 2002;32(7):1203–11.
139. Drabkin IE. Caelius Aurelianus: on acute diseases and on chronic diseases. Chicago: University of Chicago Press; 1950.
140. Dysert A. Capturing medical tradition: Caelius Aurelianus' on acute diseases. Hirundo. 2006–2007;5:161–73.
141. Haier RJ. Pain sensitivity, evoked potentials and the dexamethasone suppression test in depressed patients. Psychiatry Res. 1983;10(3):201–6.
142. Öhrström E, Rylander R, Björkman M. Noise annoyance with regard to neurophysiological sensitivity, subjective noise sensitivity and personality variables. Psychol Med. 1988;18:605–13.
143. Whitehead WE, Holtkotter B, Enck P, Hoelzl R, Holmes KD, Anthony J, Shabsin HS, Schuster MM. Tolerance for rectosigmoid distention in irritable bowel syndrome. Gastroenterology. 1990;98: 1187–92.
144. Nakaaki S, Murata Y, Furukawa TA. Efficacy of olanzapine augmentation of paroxetine therapy in patients with severe body dysmorphic disorder. Psychiatry Clin Neurosci. 2008;62(3):370.
145. Uzun Ö, Özdemir B. Aripiprazole as an augmentation agent in treatment-resistant body dysmorphic disorder. Clin Drug Investig. 2010;30(10):707–10.
146. Loréa N, Van Wijnendaele R. Body dysmorphic disorder and psychosis. Case reports and discussion. Encéphale. 2012;38(1):37–41.
147. Ziehen T. Die Ideenassoziation des Kindes. Samml Abh Geb pädagog. Psychol Physiol. 1898;1:1–66.
148. Kohs SC. The association method in its relation to the complex and complex indicators. Am J Psychol. 1914;25:544–94.
149. Mach E. Die Geschichte und die Wurzel des Satzes von der Erhaltung der Arbeit. Prague: JG Calve; 1872.
150. Healy D. Some continuities and discontinuities in the pharmacotherapy of nervous conditions before and after chlorpromazine and imipramine. Hist Psychiatry. 2000;11:393–412.
151. Weber MM, Emrich HM. Current and historical concepts of opiate treatment in psychiatric disorders. Int Clin Psychopharmacol. 1988;3(3):255–66.
152. Sandyk R. Naloxone withdrawal exacerbates Tourette's syndrome. J Clin Psychopharmacol. 1986;6(1):58–9.
153. Sandyk R. The effects of naloxone in Tourette's syndrome. Ann Neurol. 1985;18(3):367–8.
154. Hening WA, Walters AS, Kavey N, Gidro-Frank S, Cote L, Fahn S. Dyskinesias while awake and periodic movements in sleep in restless legs syndrome: treatment with opioids. Neurology. 1986;36:1363–6.
155. Eadie MJ. Sir Charles Locock and potassium bromide. J R Coll Physicians Edinb. 2012;42(3):274–9.
156. Medsafe New Zealand. Data Sheet. Paraldehyde injection solution 100 %. 2009. http://www.medsafe.govt.nz/profs/datasheet/p/Paraldehydeinj.pdf
157. Philpott WH, Kalita DK, Goldberg B. A brief history of magnet therapy. 1996. http://www.innerself.com/Health/history magnets.htm

158. Steinberg H. Electrotherapeutic disputes: the 'Frankfurt Council' of 1891. Brain. 2011;134: 1229–43.
159. Exchange Supplies. The history of injecting and the development of the syringe. 2014. http://www.exchangesupplies.org/article history of injecting and development of the syringe.php
160. Pakkenberg B, Gundersen HJG. Neocortical neuron number in humans: effect of sex and age. J Comp Neurol. 1997;384(2):312–20.
161. Malamud N. Lissauer's dementia paralytica: a study of its pathogenesis. Arch NeurPsych. 1937;38(1):27–42.
162. Hung SC, Hung SH, Tarng DC, Yang WC, Chen TW, Huang TP. Thiamine deficiency and unexplained encephalopathy in hemodialysis and peritoneal dialysis patients. Am J Kidney Dis. 2001;38(5): 941–7.
163. Jacobson RR, Lishman WA. Cortical and diencephalic lesions in Korsakoff's syndrome: a clinical and CT scan study. Psychol Med. 1990;20(1): 63–75.
164. Forsgren L, Nyström L. An incident case-referent study of epileptic seizures in adults. Epilepsy Res. 1990;6(1):66–81.
165. Hesdorffer DC, Hauser WA, Annegers JF, Cascino G. Major depression is a risk factor for seizures in older adults. Ann Neurol. 2000;47(2):246–9.
166. Hesdorffer DC, Ludvigsson P, Hauser WA, Olafsson E. Depression is a risk factor for epilepsy in children. Epilepsia. 1998;39 suppl 6:222A.
167. Kanner AM. Depression in epilepsy: prevalence, clinical semiology, pathogenic mechanisms, and treatment. Biol Psychiatry. 2003;54(3):388–98.
168. Kanner AM, Schachter SC, Barry JJ, Hersdorffer DC, Mula M, Trimble M, Hermann B, Ettinger AE, Dunn D, Caplan R, Ryvlin P, Gilliam F, LaFrance Jr WC. Depression and epilepsy, pain and psychogenic non-epileptic seizures: clinical and therapeutic perspectives. Epilepsy Behav. 2012;24(2):169–81.
169. Cramer JA, Blum D, Reed M, Fanning K, Epilepsy Impact Project Group. The influence of comorbid depression on seizure severity. Epilepsia. 2003;44(12):1578–84.
170. Schwabe MJ, Konkol RJ. Menstrual cycle-related fluctuations of tics in Tourette syndrome. Pediatr Neurol. 1992;8(1):43–6.
171. Moreira L, Bins H, Toressan R, Ferro C, Hartmann T, Petribú K, Juruena MF, Rosaro MCD, Ferrão YA. An exploratory dimensional approach to premenstrual manifestation of obsessive compulsive disorder symptoms: a multicentre study. J Psychosom Res. 2013;74(4):313–9.
172. Whitehead AN. The aims of education, and other essays. 2nd ed. New York: MacMillan Company; 1929.
173. Georgieff N, Dominey PF, Michel F, Marie-Cardine M, Dalery J. Semantic priming in major depressive state. Psychiatry Res. 1998;78(1-2):29–44.
174. Besche-Richard C, Passerieux C, Hardy-Baylé C. Lexical decision tasks in depressive patients: semantic priming before and after clinical improvement. Eur Psychiatry. 2002;17(2):69–74.
175. Dannlowski U, Kersting A, Arolt V, Lalee-Mentzel J, Donges US, Suslow T. Unimpaired automatic processing of verbal information in the course of clinical depression. Depress Anxiety. 2006;23(6):325–30.
176. Foster PS, Yung RC, Branch KK, Stringer K, Ferguson BJ, Sullivan W, Drago V. Increased spreading activation in depression. Brain Cogn. 2011;77(2): 265–70.
177. Hart RP, Kwentus JA, Hamer RM, Taylor JR. Selective reminding procedure in depression and dementia. Psychol Aging. 1987;2(2):111–5.
178. Morina N, Deeprose C, Pusowski C, Schmid M, Holmes EA. Prospective mental imagery in patients with major depressive disorder or anxiety disorders. J Anxiety Disord. 2011;25(8):1032–7.
179. Kwapil TR, Hegley DC, Chapman LJ, Chapman JP. Facilitation of word recognition by semantic priming in schizophrenia. J Abnorm Psychol. 1990;99(3):215–21.
180. Andreou C, Bozikas VP, Ramnalis A, Giannakou M, Fokas K. Semantic priming in remitted patients with bipolar disorder. J Behav Ther Exp Psychiatry. 2013;44(1):48–52.
181. Besnier N, Richard F, Zendjidjian X, Kaladjian A, Mazzola-Pomietto P, Adida M, Azorin JM. Stroop and emotional Stroop interference in unaffected relatives of patients with schizophrenic and bipolar disorders: distinct markers of vulnerability. World J Biol Psychiatry. 2009;10(4 Pt 3):809–18.
182. Weissman MM, Wickramaratne P, Merikangas KR, Leckman JF, Prusoff BA, Caruso KA, Kidd KK, Gammon GD. Onset of major depression in early adulthood: increased familial loading and specificity. Arch Gen Psychiatry. 1984;41(2):1136–43.
183. Todd RD, Botteron KN. Etiology and genetic of early-onset mood disorders. Child Adolesc Psychiatr Clin N Am. 2002;11(3):499–518.
184. Pauls DL. The genetics of obsessive compulsive disorder and Gilles de la Tourette's syndrome. Psychiatr Clin North Am. 1992;15(4):759–66.
185. Beaumont PJV. Phenomenology and the history of psychiatry. Aust NZ J Psychiatry. 1992;26:532–45.
186. Parish E. Hallucinations and illusions: a study of the fallacies of perception. London: Walter Scott Publishers; 1897.
187. Hagen FW. Die Sinnestäuschungen in Bezug auf Psychologie, Heilkunde und Rechtspflege. Leipzig: Otto Wigand; 1837.
188. Hagen FW. Zur Theorie der Hallucinationen. Allg Z f Psych. 1868;25:1–113.
189. Tamburini A. A theory of hallucinations. Hist Psychiatry. 1990;1:151–6.
190. Berrios GE. The history of mental symptoms: descriptive psychopathology since the nineteenth century. Cambridge: Cambridge University Press; 1996.
191. Parent A, Parent M, Leroux-Hugon V. Jules Bernard Luys: a singular figure of 19th century neurology. Can J Neurol Sci. 2002;29(3):282–8.

192. Rolleston H. The history of haematology. Proc R Soc Med. 1934;27(9):1161–78.
193. Schäffle A. Bau und Leben des sozialen Körpers. Tübingen: Laupp; 1896.
194. Stiles A. Robert Louis Stevenson's Jekyll and Hyde, and the double brain, 1500-1900. Stud Engl Lit. 2006;46(4):879–900.
195. App U. Richard Wagner and Buddhism. Rorschach/Kyoto: UniversityMedia; 2011.
196. Taylor M. 'The Wishing-table, the Gold-ass, and the Cudgel in the Sack' by The Brothers Grimm. 1884. http://classiclit.about.com/library/bl-etexts/grimm/bl-grimm-wishingtable.htm
197. Frojmovic E. Imagining the self, imagining the other: visual representation and Jewish-Christian dynamics in the Middle Ages and early modern period. Leiden: Brill; 2002.
198. Sösemann B. Hollow-sounding jubilees: forms and effects of public self-display in Wilhelmine Germany. In: Mombauer A, Deist W, editors. The Kaiser. New Research on Wilhelm II's Role in Imperial Germany. Cambridge: Cambridge University Press; 2003. p. 37–62.
199. Shorter E. A historical dictionary of psychiatry. New York: Oxford University Press; 2005.
200. Moscovitz A. pers comm. 23.05.2014
201. Freud S. Entwurf einer psychologie. 1895. In: Bonaparte M, Freud A, Kris E, editors. Aus den Anfängen der ischer, Frankfurt AM, 1950/1975. p.297–384 Psychoanalyse 1887–1902.
202. Murphy G. Personality, a biosocial approach to origin and structure. New York: Harper and Row; 1947.
203. Exner S. Entwurf zu einer physiologischen Erklärung der psychischen Erscheinungen. Leipzig: F Deuticke; 1894.
204. Heim G. pers comm. 26. 05. 2014.
205. Muller GE, Pilzecker A. Experimentelle Beiträge zur Lehre vom Gedächtnis. Zeitschr Psych. 1900;1:1–300.
206. Holliday R. Epigenetics: a historical overview. Epigenetics. 2006;1(2):76–80.
207. Haig D. The (dual) origin of epigenetics. Cold Spring Harb Symp Quant Biol. 2004;69:67–70.
208. Moser G, Vacariu-Granser GV, Schneider C, Abatzi TA, Pokieser P, Stacher-Janotta G, Gaupmann G, Weber U, Wenzel T, Roden M, Stacher G. High incidence of esophageal motor disorders in consecutive patients with globus sensation. Gastroenterology. 1991;101:1512–21.
209. Danek A. 'Hypermetamorphosis'. Heinrich Neumann's (1814-1884) legacy. Nervenarzt. 2007;78(3):342–6.
210. Denny-Brown D. Cerebral control of movement. Liverpool: Liverpool University Press; 1966.
211. Klüver H, Bucy PC. An analysis of certain effects of bilateral temporal lobectomy in the rhesus monkey with special reference to 'psychic blindess'. J Psychol. 1938;5:33–54.
212. Lang H. A German-English dictionary of terms used in medicine and the allied sciences. Philadelphia: P Blakistons's Son & Co; 1907.
213. Hecker E. Zur klinischen Diagnostik und Prognostik der psychischen Krankheiten. Allg Z Psychiatrie. 1877;33:602–20.
214. Janet PMF. Major symptoms of hysteria. New York: Macmillan; 1906. p. 329–32.
215. Müller JP. Handbuch der Physiologie des Menschen für Vorlesungen. Coblenz: J Hölscher; 1833.
216. Finger S, Wade NJ. The neuroscience of Helmholtz and the theories of Johannes Müller: Part 1: nerve cell structure, vitalism and the nerve impulse. J Hist Neurosci. 2002;11:136–55.
217. Rivers WHR, Head H. A human experiment in nerve division. Brain. 1908;31:323–45.

Index

R. Miller, K.J. Dennison (eds.), *An Outline of Psychiatry in Clinical Lectures*,
DOI 10.1007/978-3-319-18051-9

B

I

R

T

U

V

W

GPSR Compliance
The European Union's (EU) General Product Safety Regulation (GPSR) is a set of rules that requires consumer products to be safe and our obligations to ensure this.

If you have any concerns about our products, you can contact us on

ProductSafety@springernature.com

In case Publisher is established outside the EU, the EU authorized representative is:

Springer Nature Customer Service Center GmbH
Europaplatz 3
69115 Heidelberg, Germany

www.ingramcontent.com/pod-product-compliance
Lightning Source LLC
Chambersburg PA
CBHW061151240926
51846CB00006B/985
* 9 7 8 3 3 1 9 3 4 8 4 0 7 *